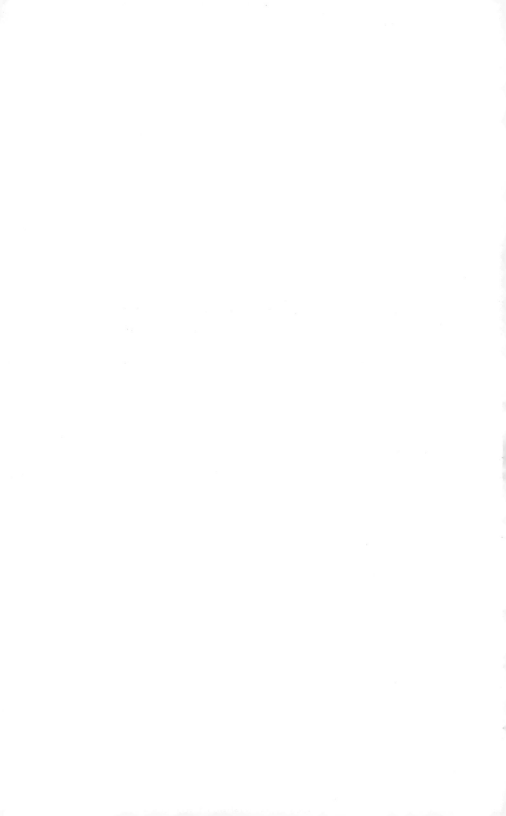

Benders' Dictionary of Nutrition and Food Technology

Benders' Dictionary of Nutrition and Food Technology

Seventh Edition

David A Bender
BSc, PhD, RNutr

Senior Lecturer
Department of Biochemistry and Molecular Biology
University College London

and

Arnold E Bender
DSc (hc), PhD, HonMAPHA, HonFRSH, FIFST

Emeritus Professor of Nutrition
University of London

(CRC)

CRC Press
Boca Raton Boston New York Washington, DC

WOODHEAD PUBLISHING LIMITED
Cambridge England

Published by Woodhead Publishing Limited, Abington Hall, Abington
Cambridge CB1 6AH, England

Published in North and South America by CRC Press LLC,
2000 Corporate Blvd, NW
Boca Raton FL 33431, USA

First published 1960
Second edition 1965
Third edition 1968
Fourth edition Newnes-Butterworth 1975
Fifth edition Butterworth Scientific 1982
Reprinted 1984
Sixth edition 1990
Reprinted 1998 Woodhead Publishing Ltd
Seventh edition 1999, Woodhead Publishing Ltd and CRC Press LLC
© 1999, Woodhead Publishing Ltd
The authors have asserted their moral rights.

British Library Cataloguing in Publication Data
A catalogue record for this book is available from the British Library.

Library of Congress Cataloging in Publication Data
A catalog record for this book is available from the Library of Congress.

Woodhead Publishing ISBN 1 85573 475 3
CRC Press ISBN 0-8493-0018-5
CRC Press order number: WP0018

Cover design by The ColourStudio
Typeset by Best-set Typesetter Ltd, Hong Kong
Printed by T J International, Cornwall, England

Contents

Preface

The study of food and nutrition covers a wide range of disciplines, from agriculture and horticulture, through the chemistry, physics and technology of food processing and manufacture (including domestic food preparation), the physiology and biochemistry of nutrition and metabolism, molecular biology, genetics and bio-technology, via social sciences and the law, anthropology and epidemiology to clinical medicine, disease prevention and health promotion. This means that anyone interested in food and nutrition will be reading articles written from a variety of disciplines and hearing lectures by specialists in a variety of fields. We will all come across unfamiliar terms, or terms that are familiar, but used in a new context, as the jargon of a different discipline.

At the same time, new terms are introduced as our knowledge increases, and as new techniques are introduced, old terms become obsolete, dropping out of current textbooks, so that the reader of earlier literature may be at a loss.

All of this provides the *raison d'être* of this Dictionary, the first edition of which was published 40 years ago, with definitions of 2000 terms. Over the years it has grown so that in this edition it includes more than 5000 entries.

At the front of the first and following editions, there was the following note:

Should this book become sufficiently familiar through usage to earn the title 'Bender's Dictionary', it would probably be more correct to call it 'Benders' Dictionary', in view of the valuable assistance of D., D.A. and B.G., guided, if not driven, by A.E.

The publisher suggested that the seventh edition should indeed be called 'Bender's Dictionary of Nutrition and Food Technology'. I was proud that my father invited me to join him as a full co-author, so that it could be called Benders' Dictionary. Sadly he died in February 1999, before the typescript was completed. I hope that I have done justice to his memory and to the book that was the first of many that he wrote.

David A Bender
April 1999

A note on food composition

This book contains nutrient composition data for 287 foods. This is Crown copyright material from *The Composition of Foods, Fifth Edition* and its supplements which has been reproduced with the permission of the Controller of Her Majesty's Stationery Office.

In addition to the nutrient content per 100 g, we have calculated nutrient yields per serving, and shown the information as a note that a specified serving is a source, good source or rich source of various nutrients. A rich source means that the serving provides more than 30%, a good source 20–30%, and a source 10–20% of the recommended daily amount of that nutrient (based on the EU nutrition labelling figures shown in Table 2).

Any specified food will differ in composition from one variety to another, and from sample to sample of the same variety, depending on the conditions under which the animal was raised or the plant grown, so that the values quoted here should not be considered to be accurate to better than about ±10%, at best; the variation in micronutrient content may be even greater.

List of Figures

A

abalone   A SHELLFISH (mollusc), *Haliotus splendens, H. rufescens, H. cracherodii*, also sometimes called ormer, or sea ear. Found especially in waters around Australia, and also California and Japan, the Channel Islands and France.

abscisic acid   Plant hormone with growth inhibitory action; the dormancy-inducing hormone, responsible for shedding of leaves by deciduous trees. In herbaceous plants can lead to dwarf or compact plants with normal or enhanced fruit production. Used horticulturally to inhibit growth, and as a defoliant.

absinthe   A herb LIQUEUR flavoured with wormwood (*Artemisia absinthium*); it is toxic and banned in many countries.
See also VERMOUTH.

absolute alcohol   Pure ethyl ALCOHOL.

absorption spectrometry   Analytical technique based on absorbance of light of a specific wavelength by a solute.

acarbose   The name of a group of complex CARBOHYDRATES (oligosaccharides) which inhibit the enzymes of STARCH and DISACCHARIDE digestion; used experimentally to reduce the digestion of starch and so slow the rate of absorption of carbohydrates. Has been marketed for use in association with weight-reducing diet regimes as a 'starch blocker', but there is no evidence of efficacy.

acaricides   Pesticides used to kill mites and ticks (Acaridae) which cause animal diseases and the spoilage of flour and other foods in storage.

accelase   A mixture of enzymes which HYDROLYSE PROTEINS, including an EXOPEPTIDASE from the bacterium *Streptococcus lactis*, which is one of the starter organisms in dairy processing. The mixed enzymes are used to shorten the maturation time of cheeses and intensify the flavour of processed cheese.

accelerated freeze drying   See FREEZE DRYING.

Acceptable Daily Intake (ADI)   The amount of a food ADDITIVE that could be taken daily for an entire life-span without appreciable risk. Determined by measuring the highest dose of the substance that has no effect on experimental animals, then dividing by a safety factor of 100. Substances that are not given an

1

ADI are regarded as having no adverse effect at any level of intake.

See also NO EFFECT LEVEL.

accoub Edible thistle (*Goundelia tournefortii*) growing in Mediterranean countries and Middle East. The flower buds when cooked have a flavour resembling that of ASPARAGUS or globe ARTICHOKE; the shoots can be eaten in the same way as ASPARAGUS and the roots as SALSIFY.

accuracy Of an assay; the closeness of the result to the 'true' result.

See also PRECISION.

ACE Angiotensin converting enzyme (EC 3.4.15.1), a peptidase in the blood vessels of the lungs which converts angiotensin I to active angiotensin II. Many of the drugs for treatment of HYPERTENSION are ACE inhibitors.

acerola See CHERRY, WEST INDIAN.

acesulphame (acesulfame) Methyl-oxathiazinone dioxide, a non-nutritive or intense (artificial) SWEETENER. The potassium salt, acesulphame-K, is some 200 times as sweet as SUCROSE. It is not metabolised, and is excreted unchanged.

acetic acid (ethanoic acid) One of the simplest organic acids, CH_3COOH. It is the acid of VINEGAR and is formed, together with LACTIC ACID, in pickled (fermented) foods. It is added to foods and sauces as a preservative.

Acetobacter Genus of bacteria (family Bacteriaceae) which oxidise ethyl alcohol to ACETIC ACID (secondary fermentation). *Acetobacter pasteurianus* (also known as *Mycoderma aceti*, *Bacterium aceti* or *B. pasteuranum*) is used in the manufacture of VINEGAR.

acetoglycerides One or two of the long chain fatty acids esterified to glycerol in a TRIACYLGLYCEROL is replaced by ACETIC ACID. There are three types: diacetomonoglycerides (e.g. diacetomono-stearin); monoacetodiglycerides (e.g. monoacetodistearin); monoacetomonoglycerides (e.g. monoacetomonostearin) in which one hydroxyl group of the glycerol is free. Also known as partial glyceride esters.

They are non-greasy and have lower melting points than the corresponding triacylglycerol and are used in shortenings and spreads, as films for coating foods and as plasticisers for hard fats.

acetohexamide Oral HYPOGLYCAEMIC AGENT used to treat non-insulin-dependent DIABETES mellitus.

acetoin Acetyl methyl carbinol, a precursor of DIACETYL, which is one of the constituents of the flavour of butter. Acetoin and DIACETYL are produced by bacteria during the ripening of BUTTER.

acetomenaphthone Synthetic compound with VITAMIN K activity; vitamin K_3, also known as menaquinone-0.

acetone One of the KETONE bodies formed in the body in FASTING. Also used as a solvent, e.g. in varnishes and lacquer. Chemically dimethyl ketone or propan-2-one $(CH_3.C{=}O.CH_3)$.

acetylcholine The acetyl ester of CHOLINE, produced as a neuro-transmitter at cholinergic nerve endings in the brain and at neuromuscular junctions.

ACH index Arm, chest, hip index. A method of assessing a person's nutritional status by measuring the arm circumference, chest diameter and hip width.

See also ANTHROPOMETRY.

achalasia Disturbance of the normal muscular function of the OESOPHAGUS, delaying the passage of food and sometimes causing regurgitation and severe chest pain.

achene Botanical term for small, dry one-seeded fruit which does not open to liberate the seed, e.g. nuts.

achlorhydria Failure of secretion of GASTRIC ACID and INTRINSIC FACTOR, which are secreted by the gastric parietal (oxyntic) cells. Commonly associated with atrophy of the gastric mucosa with advancing age.

See also ANAEMIA, PERNICIOUS.

acholia Absence or deficiency of BILE SECRETION.

achote See ANNATTO.

achrodextrin DEXTRINS formed during enzymic hydrolysis of STARCH which give no colour (achromos) when tested with iodine.

achromotricia Loss of the pigment of hair. One of the signs of PANTOTHENIC ACID deficiency in animals, but there is no evidence that pantothenic acid affects loss of hair colour in human beings.

achylia Absence of a secretion, e.g. achylia gastrica is absence of gastric secretion.

acid–base balance Body fluids are maintained just on the alkaline side of neutrality, pH 7.35–7.45, by buffers in the blood and tissues. Buffers include proteins, phosphates and carbon dioxide/bicarbonate, and are termed the alkaline reserve.

Acidic products of metabolism are excreted in the urine combined with bases such as sodium and potassium which are thus lost to the body. The acid–base balance is maintained by replacing them from the diet.

acid drops Boiled sweets with sharp flavour from tartaric acid (originally acidulated drops); known as sourballs in USA.

acid foods, basic foods These terms refer to the residue of the METABOLISM of foods. The MINERALS SODIUM, POTASSIUM, MAGNESIUM and CALCIUM are base-forming, while phosphorus, SULPHUR and chlorine are acid-forming. Which of these predominates in foods determines whether the residue is acidic or basic (alkaline); meat, cheese, eggs and cereals leave an acidic residue, while milk, vegetables and some fruits leave a basic residue. Fats and sugars have no mineral content and so leave a neutral residue. Although fruits have an acid taste caused by organic acids and their salts, the acids are completely oxidised and the sodium and potassium salts yield an alkaline residue.

acidity regulators See BUFFERS.

acid number, acid value (of a fat) A measure of RANCIDITY due to hydrolysis (see HYDROLYSE), releasing free FATTY ACIDS from the TRIACYLGLYCEROL of the fat; serves as an index of the efficiency of refining since the fatty acids are removed during refining and increase with deterioration during storage. Defined as milligrams of potassium hydroxide required to neutralise the free fatty acids in 1 g of fat.

acidophilus milk Heat-treated milk inoculated with 1–2% *Lactobacillus acidophilus* or *Bifidobacterium bifidum* (*Lactobacillus bifidus*) which ferment milk slowly at 39°C and form lactic and acetic acids, with small amounts of propionic and butyric acids, with final pH 3.9–4.4%; more than 10^6 live bacterial cells/mL. Claimed to enhance the growth of beneficial bacteria in the intestine.

Sweet acidophilus milk is made with a heavy inoculation of starter added to cold pasteurised milk to preserve the bacteria in the product.

See also PROBIOTICS.

acidosis An increase in the acidity of BLOOD PLASMA to below the normal range of pH 7.35–7.45, resulting from a loss of the buffering capacity of the plasma, alteration in the excretion of carbon dioxide, excessive loss of base from the body or metabolic overproduction of acids.

See also ACID–BASE BALANCE.

acids, fruit ORGANIC ACIDS such as citric, malic, tartaric, etc which give the sharp or sour flavour to fruits; often added to processed foods for taste.

ackee (akee) Fruit of Caribbean tree *Blighia sapida*. Toxic when unripe because of the presence of hypoglycin (α-amino-β-methylene-cyclopropanyl-propionic acid) which can reduce blood sugar levels and cause 'vomiting sickness', coma and death.

acorn sugar Quercitol, pentahydroxycyclohexane, extracted from acorns (fruit of *Quercus* spp).

ACP Acid calcium phosphate, see PHOSPHATE.

acraldehyde See ACROLEIN.

acrodermatitis enteropathica Severe functional ZINC deficiency, leading to dermatitis, due to failure to secrete an endogenous zinc binding ligand in pancreatic juice, and hence failure to absorb zinc. The zinc binding ligand has not been unequivocally identified, but may be the TRYPTOPHAN metabolite picolinic acid.

acrodynia Dermatitis seen in VITAMIN B₆ deficient animals; no evidence for a similar dermatitis in human deficiency.

acrolein (acraldehyde) An ALDEHYDE formed when GLYCEROL is heated to a high temperature. It is responsible for the acrid odour and lachrymatory (tear-causing) vapour produced when fats are overheated. Chemically $CH_2=CH.CHO$.

Acronize Trade name for the ANTIBIOTIC CHLORTETRACYCLINE; 'acronized' is used to describe products that have been treated with chlortetracycline, as, for example, 'acronized ice'.

ACTH See ADRENOCORTICOTROPHIC HORMONE.

actin One of the contractile PROTEINS of MUSCLE.

active oxygen method A method of measuring the stability of fats and oils to oxidative damage by bubbling air through the heated material and following the formation of peroxides. Also known as the Swift stability test.

actomyosin See MUSCLE.

acute phase proteins A variety of serum proteins synthesised in increased (or sometimes decreased) amounts in response to trauma and infection, so confounding their use as indices of nutritional status.

Adam's fig See PLANTAIN.

Addisonian pernicious anaemia See ANAEMIA, PERNICIOUS.

Addison's disease Degeneration or destruction of the cortex of the adrenal glands, leading to loss of GLUCOCORTICOID and MINERALOCORTICOID adrenal hormones, and resulting in low blood pressure, anaemia, muscular weakness, sodium loss and a low METABOLIC RATE. Treatment is by administration of synthetic adrenocortical hormones.

adenine A NUCLEOTIDE, one of the PURINE bases of the NUCLEIC ACIDS (DNA and RNA). The compound formed between adenine and RIBOSE is the nucleoside adenosine, and can form four phosphorylated derivatives important in metabolism: adenosine monophosphate (AMP, also known as adenylic acid); adenosine diphosphate (ADP); adenosine triphosphate (ATP) and cyclic adenosine monophosphate (cAMP).

See also ATP; ENERGY METABOLISM.

adenosine See ADENINE.

adermin Obsolete name for VITAMIN B₆.

ADH Antidiuretic hormone, see VASOPRESSIN.

ADI See ACCEPTABLE DAILY INTAKE.

adipectomy Surgical removal of subcutaneous fat.

adipocyte   A fat-containing cell in ADIPOSE TISSUE.

adipose tissue   Body fat, the cells that synthesise and store FAT, releasing it for METABOLISM in FASTING. Also known as white adipose tissue, to distinguish it from the metabolically more active BROWN ADIPOSE TISSUE, which is involved in heat production to maintain body temperature. Much of the body fat reserve is subcutaneous; in addition there is adipose tissue around the organs, which serves to protect them from physical damage.

In lean people, between 20–25% of body weight is adipose tissue, increasing with age; the proportion is greater in people who are OVERWEIGHT or OBESE. Adipose tissue contains 82–88% fat, 2–2.6% protein and 10–14% water. The energy yield of adipose tissue is 34–38 MJ (8000–9000 kcal)/kg or 15.1–16.8 MJ (3600–4000 kcal)/lb.

adiposis   Presence of an abnormally large accumulation of fat in the body, also known as liposis. Adiposis dolorosa is painful fatty swellings associated with nervous system defects.

See also OBESITY.

adipsia   Absence of thirst.

adirondack bread   American baked product made from ground MAIZE, butter, wheat flour, eggs and sugar.

adlay   The seeds of a wild grass (Job's tears, *Coix lachryma-jobi*) botanically related to MAIZE, growing wild in parts of Africa and Asia and eaten especially in the SE Pacific region.

ADP   Adenosine diphosphate, see ADENINE; ATP.

adrenal glands   Also called the suprarenal glands, small ENDOCRINE GLANDS situated just above the kidneys. The inner medulla secretes the HORMONES ADRENALINE and NORADRENALINE, while the outer cortex secretes STEROID hormones known as corticosteroids, including cortisol and ALDOSTERONE.

adrenaline (epinephrine)   A hormone secreted by the medulla of the ADRENAL GLAND, especially in times of stress or in response to fright or shock. Its main actions are to increase blood pressure and to mobilise tissue reserves of GLUCOSE (leading to an increase in the blood glucose concentration) and fat, in preparation for flight or fighting.

adrenocorticotrophic hormone (ACTH)   A HORMONE secreted by the anterior part of the PITUITARY GLAND which stimulates the ADRENAL GLAND to secrete CORTICOSTEROIDS.

aduki beans   See BEAN, ADZUKI.

adulteration   The addition of substances to foods, etc, in order to increase the bulk and reduce the cost, with the intent to defraud the purchaser. Common adulterants were starch in spices, water in milk and beer, etc. The British Food and Drugs Act (1860) was the first legislation to prevent such practices.

adverse reactions to foods (1) Food aversion, unpleasant reactions caused by emotional responses to certain foods rather than to the foods themselves, which are unlikely to occur in blind testing when the foods are disguised.

(2) Food ALLERGY, physiological reactions to specific foods or ingredients due to an immunological response. ANTIBODIES to the ALLERGEN are formed as a result of previous exposure or sensitisation, and cause a variety of symptoms when the food is eaten, including gastrointestinal disturbances, skin rashes, asthma, and, in severe cases, anaphylactic shock, which may be fatal.

(3) Food intolerance, physiological reactions to specific foods or ingredients which are not due to immunological responses, but may result from the irritant action of spices, pharmacological actions of naturally occurring compounds or an inability to metabolise a component of the food as a result of an enzyme defect.

See also AMINO ACID DISORDERS; DISACCHARIDE INTOLERANCE; GENETIC DISEASES.

adzuki bean See BEANS, ADZUKI.

aerobic (1) Aerobic microorganisms (aerobes) are those that require oxygen for growth; obligate aerobes cannot survive in the absence of oxygen. The opposite are anaerobic organisms, which do not require oxygen for growth; obligate anaerobes cannot survive in the presence of oxygen.

(2) Aerobic exercise is a sustained level of exercise without excessive breathlessness; the main metabolic pathways are aerobic GLYCOLYSIS and citric acid cycle, and β-oxidation of fatty acids, as opposed to maximum exertion, when muscle can metabolise anaerobically, producing LACTIC ACID, which is metabolised later, creating a need for increased respiration after the exercise has ceased (so-called oxygen debt).

See also ANAEROBIC THRESHOLD.

Aeromonas **spp** Food poisoning microorganisms that produce ENDOTOXINS after adhering to epithelial cells in the gut. Infective dose 10^6–10^8 organisms, onset 6–48h, duration 24–48h; TX 3.1.1.1.

aerophagy Swallowing of air.

aerosol cream Cream STERILISED and packaged in aerosol canisters with a propellant gas to expel it from the container, giving conveniently available WHIPPED CREAM. GELLING AGENTS and STABILISERS may also be added.

aerosporin See POLYMIXINS.

aesculin (esculin) A glucoside of dihydroxycoumarin found in the leaves and bark of the horse chestnut tree (*Aesculus hippocastanum*) which has an effect on CAPILLARY FRAGILITY.

AFD Accelerated freeze drying, see FREEZE DRYING.

aflatoxins Group of carcinogenic MYCOTOXINS formed by *Aspergillus flavus, A. parasiticus* and *A. nominus* growing on nuts, cereals, dried fruit and cheese, especially when stored under damp warm conditions. Fungal spoilage of foods with *A. flavus* is a common problem in many tropical areas, and aflatoxin is believed to be a cause of liver cancer in parts of Africa. Aflatoxins can be secreted in milk, so there is strict control of the level in cattle feed.

agalactia Failure of the mother to secrete enough milk to feed a suckling infant.

agar Dried extracts from various seaweeds, including *Gelidium* and *Gracilaria* spp. It is a partially soluble NON-STARCH POLYSAC-CHARIDE, composed of GALACTOSE units, which swells with water to form a GEL, and is used in soups, jellies, ice-cream and meat products. Also used as the basis of bacteriological culture media, as an adhesive, for sizing silk and as a stabiliser for emulsions. Also called agar-agar, macassar gum, vegetable gelatine. Blood agar is a microbiological culture medium containing 5–10% horse blood.

ageing (1) As wines age, they develop bouquet and a smooth mellow flavour, associated with slow oxidation and the formation of ESTERS.

(2) The ageing of meat by hanging in a cool place for several days results in softening of the muscle tissue, which stiffens after death (rigor mortis), due to anaerobic metabolism leading to the formation of lactic acid.

(3) Ageing of wheat flour for bread making is due to oxidation, either by storage for some weeks after milling or by chemical action. Freshly milled flour produces a weaker and less resilient dough, and hence a less 'bold' loaf, than flour that has been aged. Chemicals used to age (improve) flour include ammonium persulphate, ascorbic acid, chlorine, SULPHUR DIOXIDE, potassium bromate and CYSTEINE. In addition, nitrogen peroxide or benzoyl peroxide may be used to bleach flour, and chlorine dioxide both to bleach and age.

agene Nitrogen trichloride, used at one time as a bleaching and improving agent for wheat flour in bread making. It can react with the AMINO ACID METHIONINE in proteins to form the toxic compound methionine sulphoximine, and is no longer used.

ageusia Loss or impairment of the sense of TASTE.

agglomeration The process of producing a free-flowing, dust-free powder from substances such as dried milk powder and wheat flour, by moistening the powder with droplets of water and then redrying in a stream of air. The resulting agglomerates can readily be wetted.

agglutinins See LECTINS.

Aginomoto Trade name for the FLAVOUR ENHANCER MONOSODIUM GLUTAMATE.

AI Adequate Intake, level of intake of a micronutrient that is more than adequate to meet requirements; based on observed levels of intake, used when there is inadequate information to derive REFERENCE INTAKES.

air classification A way of separating the particles of powdered materials in a current of air, on the basis of their weight and size or density. Particularly applied to the fractionation of the ENDOSPERM of milled wheat flour; smaller particles are richer in protein. Various fractions range from 3–25% protein.

air cycle See HEAT PUMP.

airfuge Air-driven bench-top ultra-CENTRIFUGE using frictionless magnetic suspension of the rotor; can achieve $160\,000\,g$ in 30 s.

akee See ACKEE.

ala See BULGUR.

alactasia Partial or complete deficiency of the enzyme LACTASE in the small intestine, resulting in an inability to digest the sugar LACTOSE in milk, and hence intolerance of milk and milk products.
See also DISACCHARIDE INTOLERANCE.

alanine A non-essential AMINO ACID; abbr Ala (A), M_r 89.1, pK_a 2.35, 9.87, CODONS GCNu.

β-alanine An ISOMER of alanine in which the amino group is attached to carbon-3 rather than carbon-2 as in alanine; it is important as part of PANTOTHENIC ACID, CARNOSINE and ANSERINE, M_r 89.1, pK_a 3.55, 10.24.

alant starch See INULIN.

albacore A long-finned species of tunny fish, *Thunnus alalunga*, usually canned as TUNA fish.

albedo The white pith (mesocarp) of the inner peel of citrus fruits, accounting for some 20–60% of the whole fruit. It consists of sugars, CELLULOSE and PECTINS, and is used as a commercial source of pectin.

albumin (albumen) A specific class of relatively small PROTEINS which are soluble in water and readily coagulated by heat. Oval-bumin is the main protein of egg white, lactalbumin occurs in milk, and plasma or serum albumin is one of the major blood proteins. Serum albumin concentration is sometimes measured as an index of PROTEIN–ENERGY MALNUTRITION. Often used as a non-specific term for proteins (e.g. albuminuria is the excretion of proteins in the urine).

albumin index   A measure of the quality or freshness of an egg – the ratio of the height:width of the albumin when the egg is broken onto a flat surface. As the egg deteriorates, so the albumin spreads further, i.e. the albumin index decreases.

albumin milk   See PROTEIN MILK.

albuminoids   Fibrous proteins that have a structural or protective rather than enzymic rôle in the body. Also known as scleroproteins. The main proteins of the CONNECTIVE TISSUES of the body. There are three main types:

(1) Collagens in skin, tendons and bones are resistant to enzymic digestion with TRYPSIN and PEPSIN, and can be converted to soluble GELATINE by boiling with water;

(2) Elastins in tendons and arteries, which are not converted to gelatine on boiling;

(3) Keratins, the proteins of hair, feathers, scales, horns and hooves, which are insoluble in dilute acid or alkali, and resistant to digestive enzymes.

albumin water   Beverage made from lightly whisked egg white and cold water, seasoned with lemon juice and salt.

alcaptonuria (alkaptonuria)   A GENETIC DISEASE of phenylalanine and TYROSINE metabolism, due to lack of the enzyme homogentisic acid oxidase (EC 1.13.11.5). As a result, homogentisic acid accumulates and is excreted in the urine; it oxidises in air and turns the urine black. The defect does not appear to be harmful.

alcohol   Chemically alcohols are compounds with the general formula $C_nH_{(2n+1)}OH$. The alcohol in ALCOHOLIC BEVERAGES is ethanol (ethyl alcohol, C_2H_5OH); pure ethyl alcohol is also known as absolute alcohol. The ENERGY yield of alcohol is 7 kcal (29 kJ)/g.

The strength of alcoholic beverages is most often shown as the percentage of alcohol by volume (sometimes shown as % v/v or ABV). This is not the same as the percentage of alcohol by weight (% w/v) since alcohol is less dense than water (density 0.79): 5% v/v alcohol = 3.96% by weight (w/v); 10% v/v = 7.93% w/v and 40% v/v = 31.7% w/v.

See also PROOF SPIRIT.

alcohol, denatured   Drinkable alcohol is subject to tax in most countries and for industrial use it is denatured to render it unfit for consumption by the addition of 5% methanol CH_3OH, which is poisonous. This is industrial rectified spirit. For domestic use a purple dye and pyridine (which has an unpleasant odour) are also added; this is methylated spirit.

alcoholic beverages   Made by fermenting sugars in fruit juices with YEAST to form ALCOHOL. These include BEER, CIDER and PERRY, 4–6% alcohol by volume; WINES, 9–13% alcohol; SPIRITS (e.g. BRANDY, GIN, RUM, VODKA, WHISKY) made by distilling fermented liquor, 37–45% alcohol; LIQUEURS made from distilled spirits, sweetened and flavoured, 20–40% alcohol; and fortified wines (APÉRITIF WINES, MADEIRA, PORT, SHERRY) made by adding spirit to wine, 18–25% alcohol.

See also ALCOHOL; PROOF SPIRIT.

alcoholism Physiological addiction to ALCOHOL, associated with persistent heavy consumption of ALCOHOLIC BEVERAGES. In addition to the addiction, there may be damage to the liver (cirrhosis), stomach (gastritis) and pancreas (pancreatitis), as well as behavioural changes and peripheral nerve damage.

See also WERNICKE–KORSAKOFF SYNDROME.

alcohol units For convenience in calculating intakes of alcohol, a unit of alcohol is defined as 8 g (10 mL) of absolute alcohol; this is the amount in $\frac{1}{2}$ pint (300 mL) beer, a single measure of spirit (25 mL) or a single glass of wine (100 mL). The upper limit of prudent consumption of alcohol is 21 units (168 g alcohol) per week for men and 14 units (112 g alcohol) for women.

aldehydes Compounds containing a carbonyl (C=O) group, in which one valency of the carbon is occupied by hydrogen and the other by an aliphatic or aromatic group. Formed by oxidation of ALCOHOLS; further oxidation yields carboxylic acids.

alderman's walk The name given in London to the longest and finest cut from the haunch of venison or lamb.

aldosterone A MINERALOCORTICOID STEROID hormone secreted by the zona glomerulosa of the adrenal cortex (see ADRENAL GLAND); acts to regulate sodium and potassium transport by stimulating the renal tubule resorption of sodium. Synthesis and secretion stimulated by ANGIOTENSIN. Aldosteronism is overproduction of aldosterone leading to HYPERTENSION.

ale See BEER.

alecost An aromatic herbaceous plant, *Tanacetum (Chrysanthemum) balsamita*, related to TANSY, used in salads and formerly used to flavour ale.

aleurone layer The single layer of large cells under the bran coat and outside the endosperm of CEREAL grains. About 3% of the weight of the grain, and rich in protein, as well as containing about 20% of the VITAMIN B_1, 30% of the VITAMIN B_2 and 50% of the NIACIN of the grain. Botanically the aleurone layer is part of the endosperm, but in milling it remains attached to the inner layer of the BRAN.

alewives River herrings, *Pomolobus pseudoharengus*, commonly used for canning after salting.

alexanders A herb, black lovage (*Smyrnium olisatrum*) with a celery-like flavour.

alfacalcidiol   1α-Hydroxycholecalciferol; synthetic VITAMIN D analogue used in treatment of conditions associated with failure of the renal 1-hydroxylation of calcidiol to active CALCITRIOL. Undergoes 25-hydroxylation to CALCITRIOL in the liver.

alfalfa   Or lucerne, *Medicago sativa*, commonly grown for animal feed or silage.

Sprouted seeds, composition per 100 g: 100 kJ (24 kcal), protein 4 g, fat 0.7 g, carbohydrate 0.4 g (0.3 g sugars), nsp 1.7 g, Na 6 mg, K 79 mg, Ca 32 mg, Mg 27 mg, P 70 mg, Fe 1 mg, Cu 0.16 mg, Zn 0.9 mg, vitamin A 16 µg (96 µg carotene), B_1 0.04 mg, B_2 0.06 mg, niacin 1.1 mg, B_6 0.03 mg, folate 36 µg, pantothenate 0.6 mg, C 2 mg. Serving 20 g.

See also BEAN SPROUTS.

algae   Simple plants that do not show differentiation into roots, stems and leaves. They are mostly aquatic, either seaweeds or pond and river-weeds. Some seaweeds, such as DULSE and IRISH MOSS, have long been eaten, and a number of unicellular algae, including *Chlorella*, *Scenedesmus* and SPIRULINA spp have been grown experimentally as novel sources of food (50–60% of the dry weight is protein), but are only used as dietary supplements.

alginates   Salts of alginic acid found in many seaweeds as calcium salts or the free acid. Chemically, alginic acid is a non-starch POLYSACCHARIDE of mannuronic acid. Iron, magnesium and ammonium salts of alginic acid form viscous solutions and hold large amounts of water.

Used as thickeners, stabilisers and gelling, binding and emulsifying agents in food manufacture, especially ICE-CREAM and synthetic CREAM. Trade name Manucol.

Used in combination with magnesium and aluminium hydroxides in ANTACIDS; alginate-containing antacids form a 'raft' floating on the gastric contents, so reducing oesophageal reflux.

alimentary canal   See GASTROINTESTINAL TRACT.

alimentary pastes   See PASTA.

aliphatic   ORGANIC compounds with (branched or straight) open chain structure, as distinct from cyclic compounds which contain rings of carbon atoms.

alkali formers   See ACID FOODS.

alkaline phosphatase   Enzyme (EC 3.1.3.1) that hydrolyses a variety of phosphate esters; has alkaline pH optimum. Serum enzyme comes from a variety of tissues, but especially bone, and elevated serum levels indicate metabolic bone disease or VITAMIN D deficiency, hence a sensitive index of preclinical RICKETS or OSTEOMALACIA.

alkali reserve   See BUFFERS.

alkaloids Term proposed by Meissner (1819) for naturally occurring nitrogen-containing organic bases that have pharmacological actions in man and other animals. Many are found in plant foods, including potatoes and tomatoes (the *Solanum* alkaloids), or as the products of fungal action (e.g. ERGOT), although they also occur in animal foods (e.g. tetrodotoxin in PUFFER FISH, tetramine in shellfish). Alkylamines, CHOLINE, PURINES and PYRIMIDINES are not usually considered as alkaloids.

alkalosis Increase in blood pH above pH 7.45; may be caused by excessive loss of carbon dioxide (e.g. in hyperventilation), excessive intake of bases, as in antacid drugs, loss of gastric juice by vomiting, high intake of sodium and potassium salts of weak organic acids.

See also ACID–BASE BALANCE; ACIDOSIS.

alkannet (alkanet, alkannin, alkanna) A colouring obtained from the root of *Anchusa (Alkanna) tinctoria* which is insoluble in water but soluble in alcohol and oils. Blue in alkali (or in the presence of lead), crimson with tin and violet with iron. Used for colouring fats, cheese, essences etc. Also known as orcanella.

allantoin Oxidation product of URIC ACID; excretory end-product of PURINE metabolism in most animals other than man and other primates, which lack the enzyme uric acid oxidase (EC 1.7.3.3) and therefore excrete uric acid. Some allantoin is formed non-enzymically by reaction of uric acid with oxygen RADICALS, and uric acid may be considered to be part of the body's antioxidant defence.

allergen A chemical compound, commonly a protein, which causes the production of antibodies, and hence an allergic reaction.

See also ADVERSE REACTIONS TO FOODS.

allergy Often used indiscriminately to cover a number of ADVERSE REACTIONS TO FOOD, true allergy is an immune response to a food leading to the formation of immunoglobulin E (IgE) which results in the release of histamine and leucotrienes, among other substances, into the tissues. They are released from mast cells in eyes, skin, respiratory system and intestinal system. Allergy requires an initial sensitisation; reactions may range from relatively short-lived discomfort to anaphylactic shock which can be fatal.

Over 170 foods have been shown to cause allergic reactions. The main serious food allergens include milk and eggs (and their products), wheat, soya, nuts, shellfish and fruits, also, to a lesser extent, sunflower and cottonseeds, molluscs, and certain beans. Allergens are usually active in extremely small amounts so that contamination from offending foodstuffs can result from traces left on processing machinery and utensils.

allicin   A sulphur-containing compound partially responsible for the flavour of GARLIC.

alligator pear   See AVOCADO.

Allinson bread   A wholewheat BREAD named after Allinson, who advocated its consumption in England at the end of the nineteenth century, as did Graham in the USA (hence GRAHAM bread). Now trade name for a wholemeal loaf.

alloisoleucine   Isomer of ISOLEUCINE.

allolactose   An isomer of LACTOSE, β1,6-galactosyl-glucose.

allotriophagy   An unnatural desire for abnormal foods; also known as cissa, cittosis and pica.

alloxan   Pyrimidine derivative used experimentally to induce insulin-dependent DIABETES mellitus; specifically cytotoxic to β-cells of the pancreatic islets of Langerhans, which secrete INSULIN. Now largely superseded by STREPTOZOTOCIN.

alloxazine   The tricyclic structure that is the central part of the molecule of riboflavin (VITAMIN B_2).

allspice   Dried fruits of the evergreen plant *Pimenta officinalis*, also known as pimento (as distinct from PIMIENTO) or Jamaican pepper. The name allspice derives from the aromatic oil, which has an aroma similar to a mixture of CLOVES, CINNAMON and NUTMEG.

allysine   Semi-aldehyde of amino-adipic acid in connective tissue proteins; forms cross-links with lysine in COLLAGEN, and complex links between three or four peptide chains in elastin (DESMOSINES and isodesmosines). It is formed by oxidative deamination of peptide-bound lysine by the enzyme lysyl oxidase (EC 1.4.3.13), which is copper-dependent, and its activity is impaired in dietary COPPER deficiency and by β-aminopropionitrile, one of the toxins in *Lathyrus* spp (see odoratism).

almond   A nut, the seed of *Prunus amygdalus* var. *dulcis*. All varieties contain the GLYCOSIDE AMYGDALIN, which forms hydrogen cyanide when the nuts are crushed. The bitter almond, used for ALMOND OIL (*P. amygdalus* var. *amara*), may yield dangerous amounts of cyanide.

Composition per 100 g: 2561 kJ (612 kcal), protein 21.1 g, fat 55.8 g (8.8% saturated, 64.5% mono-, 26.6% polyunsaturated), carbohydrate 6.9 g (4.2 g sugars, 2.7 g starch), dietary fibre 12.9 g, nsp 7.4 g, Na 14 mg, K 780 mg, Ca 240 mg, Mg 270 mg, P 550 mg, Fe 3 mg, Cu 1 mg, Zn 3.2 mg, Se 4 µg, I 2 µg, vitamin E 24 mg, B_1 0.21 mg, B_2 0.75 mg, niacin 6.5 mg, B_6 0.15 mg, folate 48 µg, pantothenate 0.4 mg, biotin 64 µg. A 20 g serving (20 kernels) is a source of Mg; good source of Cu; rich source of vitamin E.

almond oil   Essential oil from the seeds of either the almond tree (*Prunus amygdalis*) or more commonly the apricot tree (*Prunus armeniaca*), containing benzaldehyde, hydrogen cyanide and benzaldehyde cyanohydrin. After removal of the hydrogen cyanide, used as a flavour and in perfumes and cosmetics.

almond paste   Ground almonds mixed with powdered sugar, bound with egg, used to decorate cakes and make petits fours. Also known as marzipan.

Composition per 100 g: 1691 kJ (404 kcal), protein 5.3 g, fat 14.4 g (8.6% saturated, 64.4% mono-, 26.8% polyunsaturated), carbohydrate 67.6 g (67.6 g sugars), dietary fibre 3.2 g, nsp 1.9 g, Na 20 mg, K 160 mg, Ca 66 mg, Mg 68 mg, P 130 mg, Fe 0.9 mg, Cu 0.24 mg, Zn 0.8 mg, Se 1 µg, vitamin E 6.2 mg, B$_1$ 0.05 mg, B$_2$ 0.19 mg, niacin 1.6 mg, B$_6$ 0.04 mg, folate 12 µg, pantothenate 0.1 mg, biotin 16 µg.

aloe vera   See LAXATIVES.

Alpha–Laval centrifuge   A continuous bowl centrifuge for separating liquids of different densities and for clarifying. Widely used for cream separation.

aluminium   The third most abundant element in the earth's crust (after oxygen and silicon) but with no known biological function. Present in small amounts in many foods but only a small proportion (0.01%) is absorbed. Aluminium is used in cooking vessels and as foil for wrapping food, as well as in cans and tubes.

The 'silver' beads used to decorate confectionery are coated with either silver foil or an alloy of aluminium and COPPER. BAKING POWDERS containing sodium aluminium sulphate as the acid agent were used at one time (alum baking powders), and aluminium hydroxide and silicates are commonly used in ANTACID medications.

Aluminium salts are found in the abnormal nerve tangles in the brain in Alzheimer's disease, and it has been suggested that aluminium poisoning may be a factor in the development of the disease, although there is little evidence.

ALV   Available lysine value, see AVAILABLE LYSINE.

alveographe   A device for measuring the stretching quality of DOUGH as an index of its protein quality for baking. A standard disc of dough is blown into a bubble and the pressure curve and bursting pressure are measured to give the stability, extensibility and strength of the dough.

alverine citrate   Bulking agent and antispasmodic used to treat IRRITABLE BOWEL SYNDROME and other colon disorders.

amaranth   A Burgundy red colour (E-123), stable to light; trisodium salt of 1-(4-sulpho-1-naphthylazo)-2-naphthol-3,6-disulphonic acid.

Amaranthus Genus of plants of which some (*A. paniculatus*) are cultivated for their leaves (a good source of carotene) and seeds and others only for their leaves (*A. polygamus* and *A. gracilis*).

ambergris A waxy concretion obtained from the intestine of the sperm whale, containing CHOLESTEROL, ambrein and benzoic acid. Used in drugs and perfumery.

Amberlite Group of polystyrene ION-EXCHANGE RESINS. Sulphonic acid derivatives are used for cation exchange, basic types for anion exchange.

amblyopia Poor sight not due to any detectable disease of the eye. May occur in VITAMIN B_2 deficiency.

amenorrhoea Cessation of menstruation, normally occurring between the ages of 45–55 (the menopause), but sometimes at an early age, especially as a result of severe undernutrition (as in ANOREXIA NERVOSA) when body weight falls below about 45 kg.

Amer Picon Trade name; pungent BITTERS invented in 1830 by Gaston Picon; contains quinine, gentian and orange.

Ames test An *in vitro* test for the ability of chemicals, including potential food ADDITIVES, to cause mutation in bacteria (the mutagenic potential). Commonly used as a preliminary screening method to detect substances likely to be carcinogenic. The test is based on treating bacteria that are already mutant at an easily detectable locus for reversal of the mutation (e.g. a strain of bacteria that cannot grow in the absence of histidine to a form that can do so).

amines Formed by the decarboxylation of AMINO ACIDS. Physiologically active amines with vasoconstrictor (pressor) activity present in foods or formed by intestinal bacteria include tyramine, tryptamine, phenylethylamine and histamine.

Have been proposed as triggers for diet-induced MIGRAINE, and in patients taking monoamine oxidase (EC 1.4.3.4) inhibitors as antidepressant medication, intake of foods such as cheese, chocolate and fermented foods that are rich in these amines may provoke a potentially lethal hypertensive crisis.

amino acids The basic units from which PROTEINS are made. Chemically compounds with an amino group ($-NH_2$) and a carboxyl group ($-COOH$) attached to the same carbon atom.

Thirteen of the amino acids involved in proteins can be synthesised in the body, and so are called non-essential or dispensable amino acids, since they do not have to be provided in the diet. They are alanine, arginine, aspartic acid, asparagine, cysteine, cystine, glutamic acid, glutamine, glycine, hydroxyproline, proline, serine and tyrosine.

Nine amino acids cannot be synthesised in the body at all and so must be provided in the diet; they are called the essential or

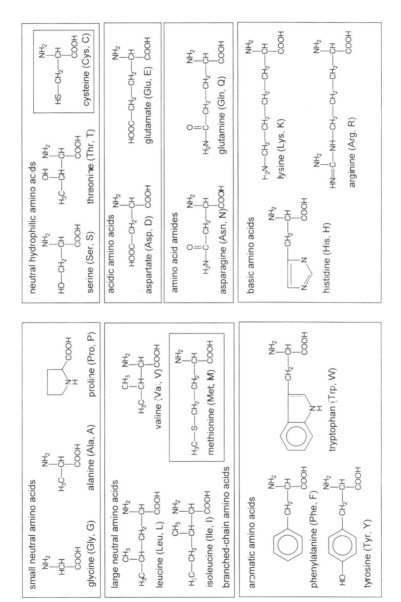

indispensable amino acids: histidine, isoleucine, leucine, lysine, methionine, phenylalanine, threonine, tryptophan and valine. Arginine may be essential for infants, since their requirement is greater than their ability to synthesise it.

Two of the non-essential amino acids are made in the body from essential amino acids: cysteine (and cystine) from methionine, and tyrosine from phenylalanine.

A number of other amino acids also occur in proteins, including hydroxyproline, hydroxylysine, γ-carboxyglutamate and methylhistidine, but are nutritionally unimportant since they cannot be reutilised for protein synthesis. Other amino acids occur as intermediates in metabolic pathways, but are not required for protein synthesis and are nutritionally unimportant, although they may occur in foods. These include HOMOCYSTEINE, citrulline and ornithine. Some of the non-protein amino acids that occur in plants are toxic.

The amino acids are sometimes classified by the chemical nature of the side chain. Two are acidic: glutamic acid (glutamate) and aspartic acid (aspartate) with a carboxylic acid (−COOH) group in the side chain. Three, lysine, arginine and histidine, have basic groups in the side chain. Three, phenylalanine, tyrosine and tryptophan, have an aromatic group in the side chain. Three, leucine, isoleucine and valine, have a branched chain structure. Two, methionine and cysteine, contain sulphur in the side chain; although cysteine is not an essential amino acid, it can only be synthesised from methionine, and it is conventional to consider the sum of methionine plus cysteine (the sulphur amino acids) in consideration of PROTEIN QUALITY.

An alternative classification of the amino acids is by their metabolic fate; whether they can be utilised for glucose synthesis or not. Those that can give rise to glucose are termed glucogenic (or sometimes antiketogenic); those that give rise to KETONES or acetyl CoA when they are metabolised are termed ketogenic. Only leucine and lysine are purely ketogenic. Isoleucine, phenylalanine, tyrosine and tryptophan give rise to both ketogenic and glucogenic fragments; the remainder are purely glucogenic.

amino acids, acidic Two of the amino acids, GLUTAMIC ACID and ASPARTIC ACID, which have a carboxylic acid (−COOH) group in the side chain.

amino acids, antiketogenic See AMINO ACIDS, GLUCOGENIC.

amino acids, aromatic Three of the amino acids, PHENYLALANINE, TYROSINE and TRYPTOPHAN, which have an aromatic group in the side chain. HISTIDINE is technically also aromatic, but is not generally grouped with the aromatic amino acids.

amino acids, basic   Three of the amino acids, LYSINE, ARGININE and HISTIDINE, which have basic groups in the side chain.

amino acids, branched chain   Three of the amino acids, LEUCINE, ISOLEUCINE and VALINE, which have a branched aliphatic side chain.

See also MAPLE SYRUP URINE DISEASE.

amino acids disorders   A number of extremely rare GENETIC DISEASES, occurring between 1–80 per million live births, which affect the metabolism of individual AMINO ACIDS; if untreated many result in mental retardation. Screening for those conditions that can be treated is carried out shortly after birth in most countries. Treatment is generally by feeding specially formulated diets providing minimal amounts of the amino acid involved.

See also ARGININAEMIA; ARGININOSUCCINIC ACIDURIA; CITRULLI-NAEMIA; CYSTINURIA; CYSTATHIONINURIA; HARTNUP DISEASE; HOMO CYSTINURIA; HYPERAMMONAEMIA; MAPLE SYRUP URINE DISEASE; PHENYLKETONURIA.

amino acids, glucogenic   Those amino acids which can give rise to glucose when they are metabolised. Sometimes known as anti-ketogenic, since the glucose formed in their metabolism reduce the rate of production of KETONE bodies. All except LYSINE and LEUCINE can be used for glucose synthesis in the body, although some are also KETOGENIC.

amino acids, ketogenic   Those amino acids which give rise to KETONES or acetyl CoA when they are metabolised. LEUCINE is purely ketogenic, and ISOLEUCINE, PHENYLALANINE, TYROSINE and TRYPTOPHAN give rise to both ketogenic and glucogenic fragments.

amino acids, limiting   The essential AMINO ACID present in a protein in the lowest amount relative to the requirement for that amino acid. The ratio between the amount of the limiting amino acid in a protein and the requirement for that amino acid provides a chemical estimate of the nutritional value (PROTEIN QUALITY) of that protein (CHEMICAL SCORE). Most cereal proteins are limited by LYSINE, and most animal and other vegetable proteins by the sum of METHIONINE + CYSTEINE (the sulphur amino acids). In complete diets it is usually the sulphur amino acids that are limiting.

amino acids, non-protein   A number of amino acids occur as metabolic intermediates, but are not involved in protein synthesis and are nutritionally unimportant, although they may occur in foods. These include ornithine and citrulline. Some in higher plants are toxic to animals and potentially so to man, e.g. mimosine (in LUCERNE), djenkolic acid (Djenkola bean), hypoglycin (unripe ACKEE FRUIT), oxalylaminoalanine (*Lathyrus* pea).

amino acids profile   Amino acid composition of a protein.

amino acids, sulphur   Three amino acids, METHIONINE, CYSTEINE and CYSTINE, contain sulphur in the side chain; although cysteine is not an essential amino acid, it can only be synthesised from methionine, and it is conventional to consider the sum of methionine + cysteine in determinations of PROTEIN QUALITY.

aminoaciduria   Excretion of abnormally large amounts of an AMINO ACID or a group of metabolically related amino acids. Overflow aminoaciduria occurs when the plasma concentration exceeds the renal threshold, as a result of impaired metabolism; renal aminoaciduria occurs with normal or lower than normal plasma concentrations, as a result of impaired renal resorption of a group of amino acids that share a common transport system. In either case aminoaciduria may be due to a genetic defect or acquired (i.e. secondary to toxicity or disease).

aminoacylase   Enzyme (EC 3.5.1.14) which catalyses esterification specifically of D-amino acids; used in resolution of RACEMIC mixtures of amino acids resulting from chemical synthesis.

aminogram   A diagrammatic representation of the amino acids in a protein or peptide. A plasma aminogram represents the amounts of free amino acids in blood plasma.

amino group   Chemically the $-NH_2$ group of AMINO ACIDS and amines, etc.

aminopeptidase   Enzyme (EC 3.4.11.1) secreted in the intestinal juice which removes amino acids sequentially from the free amino terminal of a peptide or protein, i.e. an EXOPEPTIDASE.

aminopterin   Aminopteroylglutamic acid; specific antagonist (antivitamin) of FOLIC ACID.

aminosalicylates   5-Aminosalicylate and its derivatives (balsalazide, mesalazine, olsalazine, sulphasalazine) used in treatment of ulcerative COLITIS.

aminotransferase   See TRANSAMINASE.

amla   Indian gooseberry, *Emblica officinalis* Gaertn., important in Ayurvedic medicine and reported to reduce HYPERCHOLESTEROLAEMIA. An extremely rich source of vitamin C (600 mg/100 g).

amoebiasis (amoebic dysentery)   Infection of the intestinal tract with pathogenic amoeba (commonly *Entamoeba histolytica*) from contaminated food or water, causing profuse diarrhoea, intestinal bleeding, pain, jaundice, anorexia and weight loss.

amomum   A group of tropical plants including CARDAMOM and melegueta PEPPER, which have pungent and aromatic seeds.

AMP   Adenosine monophosphate, see ADENINE.

amphetamine   A chemical at one time used as an APPETITE

SUPPRESSANT, addictive and a common drug of abuse ('speed'), its use is strictly controlled by law.

amphoteric   See ISOELECTRIC POINT.

amydon   A traditional starchy material made by steeping wheat flour in water, then drying the starch sediment in the sun, used for thickening broths, etc.

amygdalin   (1) A GLYCOSIDE in ALMONDS and apricot and cherry stones which is hydrolysed by the enzyme EMULSIN to yield glucose, cyanide and benzaldehyde. It is therefore highly poisonous, although it has been promoted, with no evidence, as a nutrient, laetrile or so-called vitamin B_{17}. Unfounded claims have been made for its value in treating cancer.

(2) French name for cakes and sweets made with almonds.

amylases   Enzymes that hydrolyse STARCH. α-Amylase (dextrinogenic amylase or diastase, EC 3.2.1.1) acts randomly on α-1,4-glucoside bonds in the molecule, and produces small DEXTRIN fragments. β-Amylase (maltogenic or glucoamylase, EC 3.2.1.2) acts at the non-reducing end of the molecule to liberate maltose plus some free glucose, and isomaltose from the branch points in AMYLOPECTIN.

Salivary amylase (sometimes called by its obsolete name of ptyalin) and pancreatic amylase are both α-amylases. Major sources of α-amylase in the baking and brewing industries are *Aspergillus oryzae* and *Bacillus subtilis*, in addition to malted (sprouted) cereals added to increase the hydrolysis of starch to fermentable sugars.

See also DEBRANCHING ENZYMES; Z-ENZYME.

amyli   Dried TAMARIND.

amylo-amylose   Old name for AMYLOSE.

amylodyspepsia   An inability to digest starch.

amyloglucosidase   See DEBRANCHING ENZYMES.

amylograph   A device to measure the viscosity of flour paste as it is heated from 25°C to 90°C (as occurs in baking), which serves as a measure of the DIASTATIC ACTIVITY of the flour.

amyloins   Carbohydrates that are complexes of dextrins with varying proportions of maltose.

amylopectin   The branched chain form of STARCH, about 75% of the total, the remainder being straight chain AMYLOSE. Consists of chains of glucose units linked α-1,4, with 5% of the glucose linked α-1,6 at branch points; gives purplish colour with iodine.

amylopeptic   A general term for enzymes that are able to hydrolyse STARCH to soluble products.

amyloplasts   Organelles in the ENDOSPERM of cereal grains in which starch granules are synthesised.

amylopsin   Alternative name for pancreatic AMYLASE.

amylose   The straight chain form of STARCH, 25% of the total, consisting of glucose units linked α-1,4; gives blue colour with iodine. See also AMYLOPECTIN.

anabiosis   Suspended animation with stoppage of respiration and heart beat caused by freeze drying, e.g. of insects during cold spells.

anabolic hormones   Those HORMONES (and hormone-like drugs) that stimulate growth and the development of muscle tissue.

anabolism   The process of building up or synthesising. See METABOLISM.

anaemia   Shortage of HAEMOGLOBIN in blood (less than 85% of the reference range; <130 g/L in adult men, or 120 g/L in women) leading to chronic pallor and shortness of breath on exertion. Most commonly due to dietary deficiency of iron or chronic blood loss resulting in a reduced number of smaller red blood cells (microcytic) which also include less haemoglobin (hypochromic anaemia).

Other dietary deficiencies can lead to anaemia: VITAMIN B_6 deficiency impairs haemoglobin synthesis; VITAMIN C deficiency impairs iron absorption; FOLIC ACID and VITAMIN B_{12} deficiencies result in megaloblastic anaemia, the release of immature precursors of red blood cells into the circulation.

anaemia, haemolytic   ANAEMIA caused by premature and excessive destruction of red blood cells, commonly in response to a toxic stress (see FAVISM). Rarely due to nutritional deficiency, but may be a result of vitamin E deficiency in premature infants. Measurement of haemolysis *in vitro*, induced by dialuronic acid or hydrogen peroxide, provides an index of VITAMIN E status.

anaemia, megaloblastic   Release into the circulation of immature precursors of red BLOOD CELLS, due to deficiency of either FOLIC ACID or VITAMIN B_{12}.

See also ANAEMIA, PERNICIOUS; FIGLU TEST; dUMP SUPPRESSION TEST; SCHILLING TEST.

anaemia, pernicious   ANAEMIA due to deficiency of VITAMIN B_{12}, most commonly as a result of failure to absorb the vitamin from the diet. There is release into the circulation of immature precursors of red BLOOD CELLS, the same type of megaloblastic anaemia as is seen in FOLIC ACID deficiency. There is also progressive irreversible damage to the spinal cord (subacute combined degeneration). The underlying cause of the condition may be the production of ANTIBODIES against either the INTRINSIC FACTOR that is required for absorption of the vitamin, or the cells of the gastric mucosa that secrete intrinsic factor. Atrophy of the gastric mucosa with ageing also impairs vitamin

B_{12} absorption, and causes pernicious anaemia. Dietary deficiency of vitamin B_{12} may occur in strict VEGETARIANS (Vegans).

See also dUMP SUPPRESSION TEST; INTRINSIC FACTOR; SCHILLING TEST.

anaerobes See AEROBIC.

anaerobic threshold The level of exercise at which the rate of oxygen uptake into muscle becomes limiting and there is an increasing proportion of anaerobic GLYCOLYSIS to yield lactate.

See also AEROBIC (2).

analysis, gastric See FRACTIONAL TEST MEAL.

analysis, proximate See PROXIMATE ANALYSIS.

analyte A compound that is analysed or assayed.

ananas See PINEAPPLE.

anaphylactic (anaphylaxic) shock Abnormally severe allergic reaction to an antigen in which HISTAMINE is released from mast cells, causing widespread symptoms.

anatto See ANNATTO.

anchovy Small oily FISH, *Engraulis* spp, usually semipreserved with 10–12% salt and sometimes BENZOIC ACID.

Composition/100 g (canned in oil): 1172 kJ (280 kcal), protein 25.2 g, fat 19.9 g, carbohydrate 0 g, Na 3930 mg, K 230 mg, Ca 300 mg, Mg 56 mg, P 300 mg, Fe 4.1 mg, Cu 0.17 mg, Zn 3.2 mg, vitamin A 62 µg, B_2 0.1 mg, niacin 8.5 mg, folate 18 µg, B_{12} 11 µg. A 50 g serving (small tin) is a source of Ca, Fe, Cu, Zn; good source of protein, niacin; rich source of vitamin B_{12}.

Anchovy butter is prepared from pounded fillets of anchovy mixed with butter as a savoury spread; anchovy paste from pounded fillets of anchovy mixed with vinegar and spices.

ancyclostomiasis Infestation with HOOKWORM.

androgens Male sex hormones (STEROIDS), testosterone, dihydrotestosterone and androsterone. Sometimes used as ANABOLIC AGENTS.

aneurine Obsolete name for VITAMIN B_1.

aneurysm Local dilatation (swelling and weakening) of the wall of a blood vessel, usually the result of ATHEROSCLEROSIS and HYPERTENSION; especially serious in the aorta, where rupture may prove fatal.

angelica Crystallised young stalks of the umbelliferous herb *Angelica archangelica*, which grows in southern Europe. They are bright green in colour, and are used to decorate and flavour confectionery goods. The roots are used together with JUNIPER BERRIES to flavour GIN, and the seeds are used in VERMOUTH and CHARTREUSE. ESSENTIAL OILS are distilled from the root, stem and leaves.

angels on horseback   Shelled oysters wrapped in bacon, skewered on a toothpick and then grilled.

See also DEVILS ON HORSEBACK.

angina (angina pectoris)   Paroxysmal thoracic pain and choking sensation, especially during exercise or stress, due to partial blockage of the coronary artery (the blood vessel supplying the heart), as a result of ATHEROSCLEROSIS.

angiotensin   Peptide hormone formed in the circulation by the action of RENIN (EC 3.4.23.15) on α-globulin; converted to the active vasoconstrictor angiotensin II by angiotensin converting enzyme (ACE, EC 3.4.15.1) in the lungs. Angiotensin II also stimulates secretion of ALDOSTERONE and vasopressin, so increasing blood pressure.

angiotensinogenase   See RENIN.

Angostura   The best known of the BITTERS, widely used in cocktails; a secret blend of herbs and spices, including the bitter aromatic bark of either of two trees of the orange family (*Galipea officinalis*, *Cusparia felorifuga*). Invented in 1824 by Dr Siegert in the town of Angostura in Bolivia, originally as a medicine, and now made in Trinidad. A few drops of Angostura in GIN makes a 'pink gin'.

Ångstrom   A unit of length equal to 10^{-8} cm (10^{-10} m) and hence = 10 nm; not an official SI unit, but still commonly used in structural chemistry and crystallography.

angular stomatitis   A characteristic cracking and fissuring of the skin at the angles of the mouth, a symptom of VITAMIN B_2 deficiency, but also seen in other conditions.

anhydrovitamin A   Isomer of retinol in which the –OH group has been removed by treatment with hydrochloric acid, with corresponding shift in the double bonds. Once incorrectly called cyclised or spurious VITAMIN A, it has very slight biological activity.

animal charcoal   See BONE CHARCOAL.

animal protein factor   A name given to a growth factor or factors which were found to be present in animal but not vegetable proteins, one of which was identified as VITAMIN B_{12}.

anion   A negatively charged ION.

aniseed (anise)   The dried fruit of *Pimpinella anisum*, a member of the parsley family, which is used to flavour baked goods, meat dishes and drinks, including ANISE, ANISETTE and OUZO. Chief component of the volatile oil is anethole (methoxypropenyl benzene).

See also ANISE, STAR.

anise pepper   A pungent spice from the Sichuan region of China (the fruit of *Zanthoxylum piperitum*); the flavour develops gradually after biting into the pepper.

anise, star   A spice, the seeds of *Illicium verum*, widely used in Chinese cooking. Distinct from ANISEED.

annatto (anatto)   Also known as bixin, butter colour or rocou; a yellow colouring (E-160b) extracted from the pericarp of the fruit of the tropical shrub *Bixa orellana*. The main component is the CAROTENOID BIXIN, which is fat-soluble. It is used to colour cheese, dairy produce and baked goods. The seeds are used for flavouring in Caribbean foods.

anomers   A pair of stereo-ISOMERS related in the same way as α- and β-glucose are related to one another.

anona   See CUSTARD APPLE.

anorectic drugs (anorexigenic drugs)   Drugs that depress the appetite, used as an aid to weight reduction. The most commonly used are diethylpropion, FENFLURAMINE (and dexfenfluramine), phenmetrazine hydrochloride and mazindol. AMPHETAMINES were used at one time, but are addictive and subject to special control.

anorexia   Lack of appetite.

anorexia nervosa   A psychological disturbance resulting in a refusal to eat, possibly with restriction to a very limited range of foods, and often accompanied by a rigid programme of vigorous physical exercise, to the point of exhaustion. Anorectic subjects generally do not feel sensations of hunger. The result is a very considerable loss of weight, with tissue atrophy and a fall in BASAL METABOLIC RATE. It is especially prevalent among adolescent girls; when body weight falls below about 45 kg there is a cessation of menstruation.

See also BULIMIA NERVOSA.

anosmia   Lack or impairment of the sense of smell.

anserine   A DIPEPTIDE of β-ALANINE and METHYLHISTIDINE found in MUSCLE, of unknown function.

Antabuse   Trade name for the drug disulfiram (tetraethyl thiuramdisulphide), used in the treatment of ALCOHOLISM. It inhibits the further metabolism of acetaldehyde arising from the metabolism of alcohol, and so causes headache, nausea, vomiting and palpitations if alcohol is consumed.

antacids   BASES or BUFFERS that neutralise acids, used generally to counteract excessive GASTRIC ACIDITY and treat INDIGESTION. Antacid preparations generally contain such compounds as SODIUM BICARBONATE, aluminium hydroxide, magnesium carbonate or magnesium hydroxide.

anthelmintic   Drugs used to treat infestation with parasitic worms (helminths).

See also FLUKES; HOOKWORM; TAPEWORM.

anthocyanidins   The aglycones of ANTHOCYANINS.

anthocyanins   Violet, red and blue water-soluble pigments in many flowers, fruits and leaves, used in food colours (E-163).

Relatively stable to heat, light and oxygen. They can react with iron or tin, giving rise to discoloration in canned foods.

anthoxanthins   Alternative name for FLAVONOIDS.

anthrone method   See CLEGG ANTHRONE METHOD.

anthropometry   Measurement of the physical dimensions and gross composition of the body as an index of development and nutritional status; a non-invasive way of assessing body composition.

Weight-for-age provides information about the overall nutritional status of children; weight-for-height is used to detect acute malnutrition (wasting); height-for-age to detect chronic malnutrition (stunting). Mid-upper arm circumference provides an index of muscle wastage in undernutrition.

SKINFOLD THICKNESS is related to the amount of subcutaneous fat as an index of over- or undernutrition.

Head circumference for age provides an index of chronic undernutrition during intrauterine development or the first two years of life.

See also BODY COMPOSITION; BODY MASS INDEX; CRISTAL HEIGHT; KNEE HEIGHT; STUNTING; TUXFORD'S INDEX; WETZEL GRID.

antibiotics   Substances produced by living organisms which inhibit the growth of other organisms. The first antibiotic to be discovered was PENICILLIN, which is produced by the MOULD *Penicillium notatum* and inhibits the growth of sensitive bacteria. Many antibiotics are used to treat bacterial infections in human beings and animals; different compounds affect different bacteria.

Small amounts of antibiotics may be added to animal feed (a few grams per tonne), resulting in improved growth, possibly by controlling mild infections or changing the population of intestinal bacteria and so altering the digestion and absorption of food. To prevent the development of antibiotic-resistant strains of disease-causing bacteria, only those antibiotics that are not used clinically are permitted in animal feed (e.g. NISIN, which is also used as a food preservative (E-234)).

See also PENICILLIN; TETRACYCLINES.

antibodies   A class of proteins formed in the body in response to the presence of ANTIGENS (foreign proteins and other compounds), which bind to the antigen, so inactivating it. Immunity to infection is due to the production of antibodies against specific proteins of bacteria, viruses or other disease-causing organisms, and immunisation is the process of giving these marker proteins, generally in an inactivated form, to stimulate the production of antibodies. ADVERSE REACTIONS TO FOODS (food allergies) may be due to the production of antibodies against specific food proteins. Chemically the antibodies form a class of proteins known as the γ-globulins or immunoglobulins; there are five types, classified as IgA, IgD, IgE, IgG and IgM.

A monoclonal antibody consists of a single protein species. They are produced by fusing sensitised B-lymphocytes from the spleen of an animal immunised with the ANTIGEN with myeloma cells, *in vitro*. The hybrid cells are selected by use of appropriate culture media, diluted so that individual colonies can be raised from a single cell, and therefore produce a single antibody. Theoretically permits very much more specific IMMUNOASSAY than mixed antisera raised *in vivo*, which are polyclonal antibodies.

anticaking agents Substances added in small amounts to powdered foodstuffs such as salt, icing sugar and baking powder to prevent caking, e.g. polyphosphates (E-544, 545), aluminium calcium silicate (E-556), calcium silicate (E-55(?)), magnesium carbonate (E-50(4)), calcium carbonate (E-170).

anticoagulants Compounds that prevent or slow the process of blood clotting or coagulation, either in samples of blood taken for analysis or in the body. One of the most commonly used such substances is HEPARIN, which is formed in the lungs and liver. People at risk of thrombosis are often treated with WARFARIN and similar compounds as an anticoagulant, to reduce the risk of intravenous blood clotting. These act as antagonists of VITAMIN K in the synthesis of blood clotting proteins. Oxalate and citrate function as anticoagulants *in vitro* because they remove calcium from the blood clotting system; hirudin (from leeches) inactivates prothrombin.

See also BLOOD CLOTTING.

antidiarrhoeal agents Two groups of compounds are used to treat diarrhoea: adsorbants such as attapulgite (hydrated aluminium magnesium silicate) and kaolin (hydrated aluminium silicate), and compounds that decrease intestinal motility, such as codeine, diphenoxylate and loperamide.

See also ANTIMOTILITY AGENTS.

antidiuretic Drug used to reduce the formation of urine and so conserve fluid in the body.

See also WATER BALANCE.

antidiuretic hormone (ADH) See VASOPRESSIN.

antiemetics A variety of compounds may be used to treat persistent vomiting, including dopamine, serotonin and muscarinic cholinergic antagonists, antihistamines, cannabinoids, corticosteroids and some of the neuroleptic agents.

antienzymes Substances that specifically inhibit the action of enzymes. Many specifically inhibit digestive enzymes and are present in raw legumes (antitrypsin and antiamylase), anticholinesterase (solanine), anti-invertase. Most are proteins and are therefore inactivated by heat. Many intestinal parasites are protected by antienzymes.

antifoaming agents Octanol, sulphonated oils, silicones, etc used to reduce foaming caused by the presence of dissolved protein.

antigalactic Drug that reduces or prevents the secretion of milk in women after parturition.

antigen Any compound that is foreign to the body (e.g. bacterial, food or pollen protein, or some complex carbohydrates) which, when introduced into the circulation, stimulates the formation of an ANTIBODY.

See also ADVERSE REACTIONS TO FOODS.

anti-grey hair factor Deficiency of the VITAMIN PANTOTHENIC ACID causes loss of hair colour in black and brown rats, and at one time the vitamin was known as the anti-grey hair factor. It is not related to the loss of hair pigment in human beings.

antihaemorrhagic vitamin See VITAMIN K.

antihistamine Drug that antagonises the actions of HISTAMINE; those that block histamine H_1 receptors are used to treat allergic reactions; those that block H_2 receptors are used to treat peptic ULCERS.

antihypertensive Drug, diet or other treatment used to treat HYPERTENSION by lowering blood pressure.

antilipidaemic Drug, diet or other treatment used to treat HYPERLIPIDAEMIA by lowering blood lipids.

antimetabolite Compound that inhibits a normal metabolic process, acting as an analogue of a normal metabolite. Some are useful in chemotherapy of cancer, others are naturally occurring toxins in foods, frequently causing vitamin deficiency diseases by inhibiting the normal metabolism of the vitamin.

See also ANTIVITAMINS.

antimony Toxic metal of no known metabolic function, and therefore not a dietary essential. Antimony compounds are used in treatment of some parasitic diseases.

antimotility agents Drugs used to reduce gastrointestinal motility, and hence reduce the discomfort associated with DIARRHOEA: codeine phosphate, co-phenotrope (diphenoxylate plus ATROPINE SULPHATE), loperamide, morphine.

antimycotics (antimould agents) Substances that inhibit the growth of MOULDS and FUNGI. Sorbates (E-200–203), benzoates (E-210–213), propionates (E-280–283), hydroxybenzoates (E-214–219) are used in foods.

antioxidant (1) A substance that retards the oxidative RANCIDITY of fats in stored foods. Many fats, and especially vegetable oils, contain naturally occurring antioxidants, including VITAMIN E (E-306–309), which protect them against rancidity for some time. Synthetic antioxidants include propyl, octyl and dodecyl gallates (E-310–312), butylated hydroxyanisole (BHA, E-320) and butylated hydroxytoluene (BHT, E-321).

See also INDUCTION PERIOD.

(2) Highly reactive oxygen RADICALS are formed both during normal oxidative METABOLISM and in response to infection, radiation and some chemicals. They cause damage to FATTY ACIDS in cell membranes, and the products of this damage can then cause damage to proteins and DNA. The most widely accepted theory of the biochemical basis of much CANCER, and also of ATHEROSCLEROSIS and possibly KWASHIORKOR, is that the key factor in precipitating the condition is tissue damage by radicals.

A number of different mechanisms are involved in protection against, or repair after, oxygen radical damage, involving a number of nutrients, especially VITAMIN E, CAROTENE, VITAMIN C and SELENIUM. Collectively these are known as antioxidant nutrients.

antiscorbutic vitamin   See VITAMIN C.

antisialagogues   Substances that reduce the flow of SALIVA.

antispasmodic   Drugs that relieve spasm of smooth muscle (e.g. intestinal muscle).

antispattering agents   Compounds such as lecithin (E-322), sucrose esters of fatty acids (E-473) and esters of mono- and diglycerides (E-472) which are added to frying oils and fats to prevent potentially dangerous spattering. They function by preventing the coalescence of water droplets.

antistaling agents   Substances that soften the crumb and retard STALING of baked products; e.g. sucrose stearate (E-473), polyoxyethylene monostearate (E-430, 431), glyceryl monostearate (E-472), stearoyl tartrate (E-483).

antivitamins   Substances that interfere with the normal metabolism or function of VITAMINS, or destroy them. Dicoumarol in spoiled sweet clover inhibits the metabolism of VITAMIN K, thiaminase in raw fish hydrolyses VITAMIN B_1, the drug methotrexate antagonises folic acid action (this is part of its mechanism of action in treating cancer), the drug isoniazid forms an inactive adduct with VITAMIN B_6.

antixerophthalmic vitamin   See VITAMIN A.

antral chalone   Peptide hormone secreted by the stomach; decreases gastric secretion.

antralectomy   Surgical removal of the ANTRUM of the STOMACH, for treatment of peptic ULCERS that are resistant to other therapy.

antrum   The region of the STOMACH adjacent to the pylorus; it secretes most of the gastric acid, PEPSIN and GASTRIN.

aortic aneurysm   See ANEURYSM.

apastia   Refusal to take food, as an expression of a psychiatric disturbance.

See also ANOREXIA NERVOSA.

aperient   Any mild LAXATIVE.

APF   See ANIMAL PROTEIN FACTOR.

aphagia   Inability to swallow. Difficulty in swallowing is dysphagia.

aphagosis   Inability to eat.

aphtha   Small ulcers occurring singly or in groups in the mouth as small red or white spots. Cause unknown.

apo-carotenals   See CAROTENALS.

apoenzyme   The protein part of an enzyme which requires a COENZYME for activity, and is therefore inactive if the coenzyme is absent.

See also ENZYME ACTIVATION ASSAYS; PROSTHETIC GROUP.

apoferritin   The protein part of FERRITIN. See IRON STORAGE.

apolipoprotein   The protein part of LIPOPROTEINS, without the associated lipid. See LIPIDS, PLASMA.

Apollinaris water   An alkaline, highly aerated, MINERAL WATER containing sodium chloride and calcium, sodium and magnesium carbonates, from a spring in the valley of Ahr (in Germany).

aporrhegma   Any of the toxic substances formed from AMINO ACIDS during the bacterial decomposition of a protein.

aposia   Absence of sensation of thirst.

apositia   Aversion to food.

appendix (vermiform appendix)   A residual part of the intestinal tract, a small sac-like process extending from the caecum, some 4–8 cm long. Acute inflammation, caused by an obstruction (appendicitis) can lead to perforation and peritonitis if surgery is not performed in time.

See also GASTROINTESTINAL TRACT.

appertisation   French term for the process of destroying all the microorganisms of significance in food, i.e. 'commercial sterility'; a few organisms remain alive but quiescent. Named after Nicholas Appert (1752–1841), a Paris confectioner who invented the process of CANNING.

appestat   See APPETITE CONTROL.

appetite control   Hunger centres found in the lateral hypothalamus initiate feeding; satiety centres found in the ventromedial hypothalamus signal satiety. Centres found in the temporal lobe (amygdala) control learnt food behaviour.

See also LEPTIN.

apple   Fruit of the tree *Malus sylvestris* and its many cultivars and hybrids; there are more than 2000 varieties in the British

National Fruit Collection. Crab apples are grown mainly for decoration and for pollination of fruit-bearing trees, although the sour fruit can be used for making jelly. Cooking apples are generally sourer varieties than dessert apples and normally have flesh which crumbles on cooking; cider apples are sour varieties especially suited to the making of CIDER.

Composition/100 g: 108–175 kJ (26–42 kcal), protein 0.2–0.4 g, fat 0.1 g, carbohydrate 6–10 g (6–10 g sugars), dietary fibre 1.6–1.8 g, nsp 1.1–1.6 g, Na 2 mg, K 63–110 mg, Ca 3–4 mg, Mg 2–4 mg, P 5–10 mg, Fe 0.1 mg, Cu 0.01 mg, vitamin A 2 µg (16 µg carotene), E 0.2–0.5 mg, B_1 0.03 mg, B_2 0.01–0.02 mg, niacin 0.2–1.0 mg, B_6 0.04 mg, folate 1–4 µg, biotin 1 µg, C 5–10 mg. A 110 g serving (one apple) is a good source of vitamin C.

apple brandy   SPIRIT made by distillation of CIDER, known in France as calvados.

See also APPLE JACK.

apple butter   Apple that has been boiled in an open pan to a thick consistency; similar to apple sauce, but darker in colour due to the prolonged boiling.

apple jack   American name for APPLE BRANDY, normally distilled, but traditionally prepared by leaving cider outside in winter, when the water froze out as ice crystals, leaving the alcoholic spirit.

apple nuggets   Crisp granules of apple of low moisture content, used commercially for manufacture of apple sauce.

apple-pear   Not a cross between apple and pear but a distinctive type of pear-shaped fruit with apple texture. Also called Japanese pear, pear-apple, and shalea or chalea.

apricot   Fruit of the tree *Prunus armeniaca*.

Composition/100 g: 121 kJ (29 kcal), protein 0.8 g, fat 0.1 g, carbohydrate 6.6 g (6.6 g sugars), dietary fibre 1.7 g, nsp 1.6 g, Na 2 mg, K 250 mg, Ca 14 mg, Mg 10 mg, P 18 mg, Fe 0.5 mg, Cu 0.05 mg, Zn 0.1 mg, Se 1 µg, vitamin A 62 µg (375 µg carotene), B_1 0.04 mg, B_2 0.05 mg, niacin 0.6 mg, B_6 0.07 mg, folate 5 µg, pantothenate 0.2 mg, C 5 mg. Serving (one apricot) 40 g.

Apricot kernels are used to prepare ALMOND OIL.

aquamiel   See PULQUE.

aquavit (akvavit or akavit)   Scandinavian; spirit flavoured with herbs (commonly caraway, cumin, dill or fennel). Also known as snaps, and in Germany as schnapps.

aquocobalamin   See VITAMIN B_{12}.

araboascorbic acid   See ERYTHORBIC ACID.

arachidonic acid   Polyunsaturated FATTY ACID (C20:4 ω 6). Not strictly essential, since it can be formed from LINOLEIC ACID, but three times more potent than linoleic acid in curing the signs of essential fatty acid deficiency.

arachin   One of the GLOBULIN proteins from the PEANUT.

arachis oil   See PEANUT OIL.

Arbroath smokie   Smoked haddock; unlike FINNAN HADDOCK not split but smoked whole to a dull copper colour.

arbute   Fruit of the South European strawberry tree (*Arbutus unedo*); resembles strawberries in appearance but with little taste and a grainy texture.

areca nut   See BETEL.

arginase   Enzyme (EC 3.5.3.1) that hydrolyses arginine to urea and ornithine, the last stage of UREA synthesis.

argininaemia   A GENETIC DISEASE due to lack of ARGINASE affecting the formation of urea and elimination of nitrogenous waste. Depending on the severity of the condition, affected infants may become comatose and die after a moderately high intake of protein. Treatment is by severe restriction of protein intake.

Sodium benzoate may be given to increase the excretion of nitrogenous waste as hippuric acid.

See also BENZOIC ACID.

arginine   A basic AMINO ACID; abbr Arg (R), M_r 174.2, pK_a 1.83, 8.99, 12.48 (guanido), CODONS CGNu, AGPu. Not a dietary essential for adult human beings, but infants may not be able to synthesise enough to meet the high demands of growth so some may be required in infant diets.

argininosuccinic aciduria   A GENETIC DISEASE due to lack of argininosuccinase (EC 4.32.2.1) affecting the formation of urea and elimination of nitrogenous waste. Depending on the severity of the condition, affected infants may become comatose and die after a moderately high intake of protein. Treatment is by restriction of protein intake and feeding supplements of the amino acid arginine, which permits elimination of nitrogenous waste as argininosuccinic acid.

Sodium benzoate may be given to increase the excretion of nitrogenous waste as hippuric acid.

See also BENZOIC ACID.

argol   Crust of crude CREAM OF TARTAR (potassium acid tartrate) which forms on the sides of wine vats, also called wine stone. It consists of 50–85% potassium hydrogen tartrate and 6–12% calcium tartrate, and will be coloured by the grapes, so white argol comes from white grapes and red argol from red grapes. Used in VINEGAR fermentation, in the manufacture of TARTARIC ACID and as a mordant in dyeing.

ariboflavinosis   Deficiency of riboflavin (VITAMIN B$_2$) characterised by swollen, cracked, bright red lips (cheilosis), an enlarged, tender magenta-red tongue (glossitis), cracking at the corners of the mouth (angular stomatitis), congestion of the blood vessels of the conjunctiva and a characteristic dermatitis with filiform (wire-like) excrescences.

arkshell See COCKLES.

armagnac BRANDY made from white wine from one of three defined areas of France: Bas-Armagnac, Haut-Armagnac or Ténarèze.

See also COGNAC.

Armenian bole Ferric oxide (iron oxide), either occurring naturally as haematite or prepared by heating ferrous sulphate and other iron salts. Used in metallurgy, polishing compounds, paint pigment and as a food colour (E-172).

Arogel Trade name for a potato starch preparation which is stable to heating and is used as a thickener in gravies, sauces and canned foods.

Aros See P. 4000.

arrowroot Tuber of the Caribbean plant *Maranta arundinacea*, mainly used to prepare arrowroot starch, a pure starch containing only a trace of protein (0.2%) and free from vitamins. Used to thicken sauces and in bland, low-salt and protein-restricted diets.

arsenic A toxic metal, with no known metabolic function. Organic arsenic derivatives (arsenicals) have been used as pesticides and in treatment of diseases such as syphilis, leprosy and yaws. Arsenic can accumulate in crops treated with arsenical pesticides, and in fish and shellfish living in arsenic-polluted water.

arteriolsclerosis Thickening of the walls of the arterioles due to ageing or HYPERTENSION.

arteriosclerosis Thickening and calcification of the arterial walls, leading to loss of elasticity, occurring with ageing and especially in HYPERTENSION.

See also ATHEROMA; ATHEROSCLEROSIS.

artichoke, Chinese Tubers of *Stachys affinis*, similar to Jerusalem ARTICHOKE but smaller.

artichoke, globe Young flower heads of *Cynara scolymus*; the edible part is the fleshy bracts and the base; the choke is the inedible filaments.

Composition/100g: 33 kJ (8 kcal), protein 1.2 g, fat 0.1 g, carbohydrate 1.2 g (0.6 g sugars), Na 6 mg, K 140 mg, Ca 19 mg, Mg 12 mg, P 17 mg, Fe 0.2 mg, Cu 0.04 mg, Zn 0.2 mg, vitamin A 6 µg (39 µg carotene), E 0.1 mg, B_2 0.01 mg, niacin 0.6 mg, B_6 0.01 mg, folate 21 µg, pantothenate 0.2 mg, biotin 1.8 µg. Serving 50 g.

artichoke, Japanese Tubers of the perennial plant *Stachys sieboldi*, similar to Jerusalem ARTICHOKE.

artichoke, Jerusalem Tubers of *Helianthus tuberosus* introduced into Europe from Canada in the seventeenth century; the origin

34

of the name Jerusalem is from the Italian *girasole* (sunflower). Much of the carbohydrate is the NON-STARCH POLYSACCHARIDE INULIN.

Composition/100 g: 171 kJ (41 kcal), protein 1.6 g, fat 0.1 g, carbohydrate 10.6 g (1.6 g sugars), nsp 3.5 g, Na 3 mg, K 420 mg, Ca 30 mg, Mg 11 mg, P 33 mg, Fe 0.4 mg, Cu 0.12 mg, Zn 0.1 mg, vitamin A 3 µg (20 µg carotene), E 0.2 mg, B$_1$ 0.1 mg, niacin 1.3 mg, C 2 mg. A 120 g serving is a source of Cu.

artificial sweeteners   See SWEETENERS, INTENSE.

asafoetida   A resin extracted from the oriental umbelliferous plant *Narthex asafoetida*, with a bitter flavour and strong garlic-like odour, used widely in oriental and middle-eastern cooking, and in small amounts in sauces and pickles. (The strength of its aroma is suggested by its French and German names: *merde du diable* Fr, *Teufelsdreck* Ger.)

ascariasis   Intestinal infestation with the parasitic nematode worm *Ascaris lumbricoides*.

ascites   Abnormal accumulation of fluid in the peritoneal cavity, occurring as a complication of cirrhosis of the liver, congestive heart failure, cancer and infectious diseases. Depending on the underlying cause, treatment may sometimes consist of a high-energy, high-protein, low-sodium diet, together with diuretic drugs and fluid restriction.

ascorbic acid   VITAMIN C, chemically L-xyloascorbic acid, to distinguish it from the ISOMER D-araboascorbic acid (isoascorbic acid or erythorbic acid), which has only slight vitamin C activity. Both ascorbic acid and erythorbic acid have strong chemical reducing properties, and are used as ANTIOXIDANTS in foods and to preserve the red colour of fresh and preserved meats, and in the curing of hams.

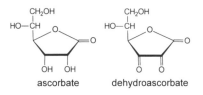

ascorbate   dehydroascorbate

ascorbic acid oxidase   An enzyme (EC 1.10.3.3) in plant tissues that oxidises ASCORBIC ACID to dehydroascorbic acid. In the intact fresh plant the enzyme is separated from the ascorbic acid, and is only released when the plant wilts or is cut; in addition to the loss of vitamin C, this is important in BROWNING REACTIONS.

ascorbic acid, monodehydro   Or semidehydro, a free RADICAL which is the intermediate stage in the oxidation of ASCORBIC ACID to dehydroascorbic acid; it has a relatively long half-life compared with other radicals, and can undergo enzymic or non-enzymic reaction to yield ascorbic acid and dehydroascorbic acid.

ascorbin stearate An ester of ASCORBIC ACID and STEARIC ACID; a fat-soluble form of the vitamin used as an ANTIOXIDANT.

ascorbyl palmitate An ester of ASCORBIC ACID and PALMITIC ACID used as an ANTISTALING compound in bakery goods (E-304).

aseptic filling See CANNING.

ash The residue left behind after all organic matter has been burnt off, a measure of the total content of mineral salts in a food.

asparagine A non-essential AMINO ACID, chemically the β-amide of ASPARTIC ACID; abbr Asn (N), M_r 132.1, pK_a 2.1, 8.84, CODONS AAPy.

asparagus The young shoots of the plant *Asparagus officinalis*.

Composition/100 g: 108 kJ (26 kcal), protein 3.4 g, fat 0.8 g, carbohydrate 1.4 g (1.4 g sugars), dietary fibre 1.4 g, nsp 1.4 g, Na 60 mg, K 220 mg, Ca 25 mg, Mg 13 mg, P 50 mg, Fe 0.6 mg, Cu 0.08 mg, Zn 0.7 mg, Se 1 μg, vitamin A 88 μg (530 μg carotene), E 1.2 mg, B_1 0.12 mg, B_2 0.06 mg, niacin 1.4 mg, B_6 0.07 mg, folate 155 μg, pantothenate 0.2 mg, biotin 0.4 μg, C 10 mg. A 125 g serving (five spears) a source of vitamin A, E, B_1, Cu; good source of vitamin C; rich source of folate.

aspartame An artificial SWEETENER, β-aspartyl-phenylalanine methyl ester, some 200 times as sweet as sucrose. Stable for a few months in solution, then gradually breaks down. Used in soft drinks, dessert mixes and as a 'table top sweetener'.

Trade names Canderel, Equal, Nutrasweet, Sanecta.

Because aspartame contains PHENYLALANINE, it is specifically recommended that children with PHENYLKETONURIA avoid consuming it, although the amounts that would be consumed are extremely small.

aspartic acid (aspartate) A non-essential AMINO ACID; abbr Asp (D), M_r 133.1, pK_a 1.99, 3.90, 9.90, CODONS GAPy.

aspartyl-phenylalanine methyl ester See ASPARTAME.

Aspergillus A family of moulds, important in the spoiling of stored nuts and grains because *A. flavus* produces AFLATOXINS. *A. oryzae* is grown commercially as a source of TAKADIASTASE.

aspic jelly A clear jelly made from fish, chicken or meat stock, sometimes with added GELATINE, flavoured with lemon, tarragon, vinegar, sherry, peppercorns and vegetables, used to glaze foods such as meat, fish and game. The name may be derived from the herb espic or spikenard.

astaxanthin A CAROTENOID, the pink colour of salmon and trout muscle; not VITAMIN A active.

astringency   The action of unripe fruits and cider apples, among other foods, to cause a contraction of the epithelial tissues of the tongue (literally astringency means 'a drawing together'). It is believed to result from a destruction of the lubricant properties of SALIVA because of precipitation by TANNINS.

atheroma   The fatty deposit composed of lipids, complex carbohydrates and fibrous tissue which forms on the inner wall of blood vessels in ATHEROSCLEROSIS.

atherosclerosis   Degenerative disease of the arteries in which there is accumulation on the inner wall of lipids together with complex carbohydrates and fibrous tissue, called ATHEROMA. This leads to narrowing of the lumen of the arteries. When it occurs in the coronary artery it can lead to failure of the blood supply to the heart muscle (ischaemia).

See also ARTERIOSCLEROSIS.

atholl brose   Scottish beverage made from malt whisky, honey, cream and oatmeal.

atomic absorption spectrometry   Technique for measurement of a variety of metals in a flame or heated gas, in the atomic state, by absorption of light at a wavelength specific for each element.

ATP   Adenosine triphosphate, the coenzyme that acts as an intermediate between energy-yielding (catabolic) METABOLISM (the oxidation of metabolic fuels) and ENERGY EXPENDITURE as physical work and in synthetic (anabolic) reactions. ADP (adenosine diphosphate) is phosphorylated to ATP linked to oxidations; in energy expenditure ATP is hydrolysed to ADP and phosphate ions.

See also ADENINE; PURINES.

atrophy   Wasting of normally developed tissue or muscle as a result of disuse, ageing or undernutrition.

atropine   One of the belladonna ALKALOIDS; anticholinergic compound acting on muscarinic receptors. Acts as a smooth muscle relaxant, used as the sulphate in treatment of DYSPEPSIA, IRRITABLE BOWEL SYNDROME and DIVERTICULAR DISEASE. Synthetic compounds with similar action and uses, but fewer central nervous system actions, include dicyclomine, dicycloverine, propantheline and hyoscine.

See also ANTIMOTILITY AGENTS.

attapulgite   See ANTIDIARRHOEAL AGENTS.

Atwater factors   See ENERGY CONVERSION FACTORS.

aubergine   The fruit of *Solanum melongena*, a native of SE Asia, widely cultivated and eaten as a vegetable, also known as eggplant and (in W Africa) field egg.

Composition/100 g: 62 kJ (15 kcal), protein 0.9 g, fat 0.4 g, carbohydrate 2.2 g (2 g sugars, 0.2 g starch), dietary fibre 2.3 g, nsp

2 g, Na 2 mg, K 210 mg, Ca 10 mg, Mg 11 mg, P 16 mg, Fe 0.3 mg, Cu 0.01 mg, Zn 0.2 mg, Se 1 µg, I 1 µg, vitamin A 11 µg (70 µg carotene), B_1 0.02 mg, B_2 0.01 mg, niacin 0.3 mg, B_6 0.08 mg, folate 18 µg, pantothenate 0.1 mg, C 4 mg. A 130 g serving ($^1/_2$ aubergine) is a source of folate.

audit ale Strong BEER originally brewed at Oxford and Cambridge Universities to be drunk on 'audit days'.

aurantiamarin A GLUCOSIDE present in the ALBEDO of the bitter orange which is partly responsible for its flavour.

aureomycin Oxytetracycline, one of the TETRACYCLINE ANTI-BIOTICS.

autoclave A vessel in which high temperatures can be achieved by using high pressure; the domestic pressure cooker is an example.

At atmospheric pressure water boils at 100°C; at 5 lb (35 kPa) above atmospheric pressure the boiling point is 109°C; at 10 lb (70 kPa), 115°C; at 15 lb (105 kPa), 121°C and at 20 lb (140 kPa), 126°C.

Autoclaves have two major uses. In cooking, the higher temperature reduces the time needed. At these higher temperatures, and under moist conditions, bacteria are destroyed more rapidly, so permitting sterilisation of foods, surgical dressings and instruments, etc.

autocrine Production by a cell of hormones or growth factors that influence the growth of the cell producing them.

See also ENDOCRINE GLANDS; PARACRINE.

autoimmune disease Condition in which ANTIBODIES are produced against normal body tissues (autoantibodies). May be a cause of pernicious ANAEMIA, some forms of HYPOTHYROIDISM and perhaps insulin-dependent DIABETES mellitus.

autolysis Process of self-digestion catalysed by the hydrolytic enzymes normally contained in lysosomes. Responsible for the softening of meat when hung, as a result of hydrolysis of CONNECTIVE TISSUE proteins. YEAST EXTRACT is produced by autolysis of yeast.

autotrophes Organisms that can synthesise all the compounds required for growth from simple inorganic salts, as distinct from heterotrophes, which must be supplied with complex organic compounds. Plants are autotrophes, whereas animals are heterotrophes. Bacteria may be of either type; heterotrophic bacteria are responsible for food spoilage and disease.

auxin A plant hormone produced by shoot tips, responsible for controlling cell growth and differentiation, and frequently used as a rooting hormone for cuttings. Chemically indoleacetic acid and related compounds.

auxotrophe Mutant strain of microorganism that requires one or more nutrients for growth that are not required by the parent organism. Commonly used for microbiological assay of vitamins, amino acids, etc.

availability Also known as bioavailability or biological availability. In some foodstuffs, nutrients that can be demonstrated to be present chemically may not be available, or only partially so, when they are eaten. This is because the nutrients are chemically bound in a form that is not susceptible to enzymic digestion, although it is susceptible to the strong acid or alkali HYDROLYSIS used in chemical analysis. For example, the NIACIN in cereal grains, CALCIUM bound to PHYTATE and LYSINE combined with sugars in the Maillard complex (see MAILLARD REACTION), are all biologically unavailable.

See also AVAILABLE LYSINE.

available carbon dioxide See BAKING POWDER; FLOUR, SELF-RAISING.

available lysine Not all of the LYSINE in proteins is biologically available, since some is linked through the ε-amino group, either to sugars in the Maillard complex (see MAILLARD REACTION), or to other AMINO ACIDS. These linkages are not HYDROLYSED by digestive enzymes, and so the lysine cannot be absorbed.

Available lysine is that proportion of the protein-bound lysine in which the ε-amino group is free, so that it can be absorbed after digestion of the protein.

avenalin, avenin PROTEINS present in oats. Avenalin is a globulin, avenin a PROLAMIN, and the major storage protein in the cereal.

avern jelly Scottish; jelly made from wild strawberries.

aversion to foods See ADVERSE REACTIONS TO FOODS.

Avicel Trade name for microcrystalline α-cellulose. It is natural CELLULOSE which has been partially HYDROLYSED with ACID, and reduced to a fine powder. It disperses in water and has the properties of a GUM. Used in oily foods such as CHEESE and PEANUT BUTTER, as well as in SYRUPS and HONEY, sauces and dressings.

avidin Protein in white of eggs that binds BIOTIN with very high affinity.

avitaminosis The absence of a VITAMIN; may be used specifically, as, for example, avitaminosis A, or generally, to mean any vitamin deficiency disease.

avocado Fruit of the tree *Persica americana*, also known as the avocado pear or alligator pear, because of its rough skin and pear shape, although it is not related to the PEAR. It is unusual among fruits for its high fat content, of which 12% is LINOLEIC ACID, and also for the fact that it does not ripen until after it has been removed from the tree.

Composition/100g: 560kJ (134kcal), protein 1.3g, fat 13.8g (22.1% saturated, 65.6% mono-, 12.2% polyunsaturated), carbohydrate 1.3g (0.4g sugars), nsp 2.4g, Na 4mg, K 320mg, Ca 8mg, Mg 18mg, P 28mg, Fe 0.3mg, Cu 0.13mg, Zn 0.3mg, I 1μg, vitamin A 1μg (11μg carotene), E 2.3mg, B_1 0.07mg, B_2 0.13mg, niacin 1mg, B_6 0.26mg, folate 8μg, pantothenate 0.8mg, biotin 2.6μg, C 4mg. A 75g serving ($^1/_2$ fruit) is a source of vitamin E, Cu.

avron See CLOUDBERRY.

axerol, axerophthol Early names for vitamin A.

azlon Textile fibres produced from proteins such as CASEIN and ZEIN.

azo dyes Synthetic chemicals used as dyestuffs and food colours, made by reacting a diazonium salt with a phenol or aromatic AMINE. Also known as diazo or diazonium compounds.

azorubin(e) A red colour, carmoisine (E-122).

Azotobacter Genus of free-living soil bacteria of family Bacteriaceae which can reduce nitrogen gas to ammonia, and hence fix nitrogen for incorporation into amino acids, etc.

See also NITROGENASE.

B

baba A French cake supposedly invented by King Stanislas I of Poland and named after Ali Baba. 'Rum baba' is flavoured with rum; a French modification using a 'secret' syrup was called brillat-savarin or savarin.

babaco The seedless fruit of the tree *Carica pentagona*, related to the PAWPAW, discovered in Ecuador in the 1920s, introduced into New Zealand in 1973, and more recently into the Channel islands.

Composition/100g: 71kJ (17kcal), protein 1.1g, fat 0.1g, carbohydrate 3.1g (3.1g sugars), Na 2mg, K 140mg, Ca 11mg, Mg 6mg, P 14mg, Fe 0.4mg, Zn 0.1mg, vitamin A 29μg (175μg carotene), B_1 0.03mg, B_2 0.04mg, niacin 0.7mg, C 26mg. A 140g serving (one slice) is a rich source of vitamin C.

babassu oil Edible oil from the Brazilian palm nut, similar in fatty acid composition to COCONUT OIL, and used for food and in soaps and cosmetics.

Babcock test For fat in milk; the sample is mixed with sulphuric acid in a long-necked Babcock bottle, centrifuged, diluted and recentrifuged. The amount of fat is read off the neck of the bottle.

bacalao See KLIPFISH.

Bacillus cereus SPORE-forming bacterium in cereals (especially rice), cause of food poisoning by production of ENTEROTOXINS in the food (emetic type TX 1.3.6.1) or in the gut (diarrhoeal type TX 2.1.1.1–2). Infective dose 10^5–10^7 organisms, emetic type onset 1–6 h, duration 6–24 h; diarrhoeal type onset 6–12 h, duration 12–24 h.

bacon Cured (and sometimes smoked) meat from the back, sides and belly of a pig; variety of cuts with differing fat contents. Gammon is bacon made from the top of the hind legs; green bacon has been cured but not smoked.

Composition/100 g: 1734 kJ (414 kcal), protein 24.9 g, fat 35 g (41.2% saturated, 47.6% mono-, 11% polyunsaturated), cholesterol 130 mg, carbohydrate 0 g, Na 2000 mg, K 290 mg, Ca 12 mg, Mg 16 mg, P 160 mg, Fe 1.5 mg, Cu 0.16 mg, Zn 2.9 mg, Se 4 µg, I 10 µg, vitamin E 0.1 mg, B_1 0.41 mg, B_2 0.16 mg, niacin 9 mg, B_6 0.26 mg, folate 1 µg, pantothenate 0.5 mg, biotin 2 µg. A 60 g serving (two rashers) is a source of vitamin B_1, Cu, Zn; good source of protein, niacin.

bacteria Unicellular microorganisms, ranging between 0.5–5 µm in size. They may be classified on the basis of their shape: spherical (coccus); rodlike (bacilli); spiral (spirillum); comma-shaped (vibrio); corkscrew-shaped (spirochaetes) or filamentous.

Other classifications are based on whether or not they are stained by Gram stain, AEROBIC or anaerobic, and autotrophic (see AUTOTROPHES) or heterotrophic (see HETEROTROPHES).

Some bacteria form spores which are relatively resistant to heat and sterilising agents. Bacteria are responsible for much food spoilage, and for disease (pathogenic bacteria which produce toxins), but they are also made use of, for example in the PICKLING process and FERMENTATION of milk, as well as in the manufacture of VITAMINS and AMINO ACIDS and a variety of enzymes and HORMONES.

Between 45–85% of the dry matter of bacteria is protein, and some can be grown on petroleum residues, methane or methanol, for use in animal feed.

bacterial count See PLATE COUNT.

bacterial filter A filter 0.5–5 µm in diameter (fine enough to prevent the passage of BACTERIA); permits removal of bacteria and hence sterilisation of solutions. Viruses are considerably smaller, and will pass through a bacterial filter.

bactericidal Conditions or compounds that are capable of killing bacteria.

See also BACTERIOSTATIC.

bacteriophage VIRUSES that attack bacteria, commonly known as phages. They pass through BACTERIAL FILTERS, and can be a cause of considerable trouble in bacterial cultures (e.g. milk starter cultures). Each phage acts specifically against a particular species of bacterium; this can be exploited in phage typing as a means of identifying bacteria.

bacteriostatic Conditions or compounds that are capable of inhibiting growth of bacteria, but not BACTERICIDAL.

Bacterium aceti See ACETOBACTER.

bactofugation Belgian process for removing bacteria from milk by high speed CENTRIFUGATION.

bactometer A device for the rapid estimation of bacterial contamination (within a few hours) based on measuring the early stages of breakdown of nutrients by the bacteria through changes in the electrical impedance of the medium.

badderlocks Edible seaweed (*Alaria esculenta*) found on northern British coasts and around Faroe Islands. Known as honeyware in Scotland.

bagasse The residues from sugar-cane milling, consisting of the crushed stalks from which the juice has been expressed; it consists of 50% CELLULOSE, 25% HEMICELLULOSES and 25% LIGNIN. It is used as a fuel, for cattle feed and in the manufacture of paper and fibre board. The name is sometimes also applied to the residues of other plants, such as sugar beet, which is sometimes incorporated into foods as a source of DIETARY FIBRE.

bagel A circular BREAD roll with a hole in the middle, made from fermented wheat flour dough with egg, which is boiled before being baked. Traditionally a Jewish speciality.

baguette A French BREAD, a long thin loaf about 60 cm long, weighing 250 g, with a crisp crust.

bain marie A double saucepan (from the French for *water bath*).

bajoa See MILLET.

baked apple berry See CLOUDBERRY.

baker's cheese See CHEESE, COTTAGE.

baking additives Materials added to flour products for a variety of purposes, including bleaching the flour, AGEING, slowing the rate of staling and improving the texture of the finished product.

baking blind A pastry case for a tart or flan, baked empty and then filled.

baking powder A mixture that liberates carbon dioxide when moistened and heated. The source of carbon dioxide is sodium bicarbonate, and an acid is required. This may be CREAM OF TARTAR (in fast-acting baking powders which liberate carbon dioxide in the dough before heating) or calcium acid phosphate, sodium pyrophosphate or sodium aluminium sulphate (in slow-acting powders, which liberate most of the carbon dioxide during heating).

Legally baking powder must contain not less than 8% available, and not more than 1.5% residual, carbon dioxide.

Golden raising powder is similar, but is coloured yellow (formerly known as egg substitute), and must contain not less than 6% available, and not more than 1.5% residual, carbon dioxide.

baking soda   See SODIUM BICARBONATE.

balance   (1) With reference to diet, positive balance is a net gain to the body and negative balance a net loss from the body. When intake equals excretion the body is in equilibrium or balance with respect to the nutrient in question. Used in reference to nitrogen (protein), mineral salts and energy.

(2) A balanced diet is one containing all nutrients in appropriate amounts.

(3) A weighing device.

balantidiasis   Infestation of the large intestine with the parasitic protozoan *Balantidum coli*. A rare cause of DYSENTERY.

Balling   A table of specific gravity of sugar solutions published by von Balling in 1843, giving the weight of cane sugar in 100 g of a solution for the specific gravity determined at 17.5°C. It is used to calculate the percentage extract in BEER WORT. The original table was corrected for slight inaccuracies by Plato in 1900, and extracts are referred to as per cent Plato.

balm   A herb (*Melissa officinalis*) with hairy leaves and a lemon scent, therefore often known as lemon balm. Used for its flavour in fruit salads, sweet or savoury sauces, etc, as well as for preparation of herb teas. Claimed to have calming medicinal properties, and promoted at one time as an elixir of life and a cure for impotence; it is rich in tannins.

balsalazide   See AMINOSALICYLATES.

bambarra groundnut   Also known as the Madagascar peanut or earth pea, *Voandseia subterranea*. It resembles the true GROUNDNUT, but the seeds are low in oil. They are hard and require soaking or pounding before cooking.

bamboo shoots   Thick pointed young shoots of *Bambusa vulgaris* and *Phyllostachys pubescens* eaten in E Asia.

bamies, bamya   See OKRA.

banana   Fruit of the genus *Musa*; cultivated kinds are sterile hybrids, and so cannot be given species names. Dessert bananas have a high sugar content (17–19%) and are eaten raw; PLANTAINS (sometimes known as green bananas) have a higher starch and lower sugar content and are picked when too hard to be eaten raw.

Composition/100 g: 259 kJ (62 kcal), protein 0.8 g, fat 0.2 g, carbohydrate 15.3 g (13.8 g sugars, 1.5 g starch), dietary fibre 2 g, nsp 0.7 g, Na 1 mg, K 270 mg, Ca 4 mg, Mg 22 mg, P 18 mg, Fe 0.2 mg, Cu 0.66 mg, Zn 0.1 mg, Se 1 µg, I 5 µg, vitamin A 2 µg (14 µg carotene), E 0.2 mg, B_1 0.03 mg, B_2 0.04 mg, niacin 0.6 mg, B_6 0.19 mg, folate

9 μg, pantothenate 0.2 mg, biotin 1.7 μg, C 7 mg. A 100 g serving (one fruit) is a source of vitamin C; rich source of Cu.

banana, baking   American name for PLANTAIN.

banana, false   The fruit of *Ensete ventricosum*, related to the banana. The fruits are small and, unlike bananas, contain seeds. The rhizome and inner tissue of the stem are eaten after cooking, a major part of the diet in southern Ethiopia.

banana figs   Bananas that have been split longitudinally and sun-dried without treating with SULPHUR DIOXIDE. The product is dark in colour and sticky.

banian days   Days on which no meat was served; named after Banian (Hindu) merchants who abstained from eating meat. An obsolete term for 'days of short commons'.

bannock   A flat round cake made from oat, rye or barley meal and baked on a hearth or griddle. Pitcaithly bannock is a type of almond shortbread containing CARAWAY seeds and chopped peel.

Bantu beer   See BEER.

bap   Traditionally a soft, white, flat, flour-coated Scottish break-fast roll. Now also used for any relatively large soft-crusted roll, made from white, brown or wholemeal flour.

bara brith   See BARM BRACK.

bara lawr   See LAVER.

Barbados cherry   See CHERRY, WEST INDIAN.

Barbados sugar   See SUGAR.

barbecue   Originally native American name for a wooden frame used to smoke and dry meat over a slow smoky fire; the whole animal was placed on a spit over burning coals. Now outdoor cooking of meat, sausages, etc, on a charcoal or gas fire; also the fire on which they are cooked.

barberry   Fruits of *Berberis* spp.

barberry fig   See PRICKLY PEAR.

Barcelona nut   Spanish variety of HAZEL NUT (*Corylus avellana*).
  Composition/100 g: 2674 kJ (639 kcal), protein 10.9 g, fat 64 g, carbohydrate 5.2 g (3.4 g sugars, 1.8 g starch), dietary fibre 9.3 g, Na 3 mg, K 940 mg, Ca 170 mg, Mg 200 mg, P 300 mg, Fe 3 mg, Cu 0.96 mg, vitamin B_1 0.11 mg. A 25 g serving (30 kernels) is a source of Mg; rich source of Cu.

barium   A metal of no known metabolic function and hence not a dietary essential. Barium sulphate is opaque to X-rays and a suspension is used (a barium meal) to allow examination of the shape and movements of the stomach for diagnostic purposes, and as a barium enema for X-ray investigation of the lower intestinal tract.

barley   Grain of *Hordeum vulgare*, one of the hardiest of the CEREALS; mainly used as animal feed and for malting and brewing. The whole grain with only the outer husk removed (pot, Scotch or hulled barley) requires several hours cooking; the commercial product is usually pearl barley, where most of the husk and germ is removed. Barley flour is ground pearl barley; barley flakes are the flattened grain.

Composition of pearl barley/100 g: 1506 kJ (360 kcal), protein 7.9 g, fat 1.7 g, carbohydrate 83.6 g (83.6 g starch), dietary fibre 5.9 g, Na 3 mg, K 270 mg, Ca 20 mg, Mg 65 mg, P 210 mg, Fe 3 mg, Cu 0.4 mg, Zn 2.1 mg, Se 1 µg, vitamin E 0.4 mg, B_1 0.12 mg, B_2 0.05 mg, niacin 4.8 mg, B_6 0.22 mg, folate 20 µg, pantothenate 0.5 mg.

barleycorn An obsolete measure of length; the size of a single grain of barley, 0.85 cm.

barley, malted See MALT.

barley sugar SUGAR confectionery made by melting and cooling sugar, originally made by boiling with a decoction of barley.

barley water A drink made by boiling pearl barley with water, commonly flavoured with orange or lemon.

barley wine Fermented malted barley, stronger than BEER (8–10% ALCOHOL by volume), bottled under pressure, so sparkling.

Barlow's disease Infantile SCURVY, also known as Moeller's disease or Cheadle's disease.

barm An alternative name for YEAST or leaven, or the froth on fermenting malt liquor. Spon (short for spontaneous) or virgin barm is made by allowing wild yeast to fall into sugar medium and multiply.

barm brack Irish; yeast cake made with butter, egg, buttermilk and dried fruit, flavoured with caraway seed. Similar Welsh cake is bara brith.

Barmene Trade name for YEAST EXTRACT, prepared from autolysed brewer's yeast, plus vegetable juices, used for flavouring.

baron of beef The pair of sirloins of BEEF, left uncut at the bone.

barquette Small boat-shaped pastry cases, used for savoury or sweet mixtures.

barrel A standard barrel contains 36 gallons. (36 Imperial gallons (UK) = 163.6 L; 36 US gallons = 113.7 L.)

basal metabolic rate (BMR) The ENERGY cost of maintaining metabolic integrity of the body, nerve and muscle tone, respiration and circulation. For children the BMR also includes the energy cost of growth.

It depends on the amount of metabolically active body tissue, and hence can be calculated from body weight, height and age:

MJ/day = $0.0418 \times$ weight (kg) + $0.026 \times$ height (cm) – $0.0209 \times$ age (y) – 0.674 (for males) or – 0.0291 (for females).

kcal/day = 9.99 × weight (kg) + 6.25 × height (cm) − 5 × age (y) − 161 (males) or + 5 (females).

Experimentally, BMR is measured as the heat output from the body, or the rate of oxygen consumption, under strictly standardised conditions, 12–14 h after the last meal, completely at rest (but not asleep) and at an environmental temperature of 26–30°C, to ensure thermal neutrality. Measurement of metabolic rate under less rigorously controlled conditions gives the resting metabolic rate (RMR).

For people with a sedentary lifestyle and relatively low physical activity, BMR accounts for about 70% of total energy expenditure. The energy costs of different activities are generally expressed as the physical activity ratio, the ratio of energy expenditure in the activity to BMR.

Basedow's disease   See THYROTOXICOSIS.

basic foods   See ACID FOODS.

basic foods plan   A grouping of foods used for public health education with a recommendation to eat some food from each group every day; foods may be divided into four, five or seven groups. For the seven group plan, the groups are: (1) green and yellow vegetables; (2) oranges, grapefruit, tomatoes and raw salads; (3) potatoes and other vegetables and fruits; (4) milk and cheese; (5) meat, poultry, fish and eggs; (6) bread, pasta, flour and other cereal products; (7) butter, margarine, oils and fats.

basil   An aromatic herb *Ocimum basilicum* and *O. minimum*; other members of the genus *Ocimum* are also used as seasoning.

Composition/100 g: 167 kJ (40 kcal), protein 3.1 g, fat 0.8 g, carbohydrate 5.1 g, Na 9 mg, K 300 mg, Ca 250 mg, Mg 11 mg, P 37 mg, Fe 5.5 mg, Zn 0.7 mg, vitamin A 658 µg (3950 µg carotene), B_1 0.08 mg, B_2 0.31 mg, niacin 1.1 mg, C 26 mg.

basmati   Long-grain Indian variety of rice; much prized for its delicate flavour (the name means 'fragrant' in Hindi).

bass   A white fish, *Dicentrarchus labrax*.

Composition/100 g: 418 kJ (100 kcal), protein 19.3 g, fat 2.5 g (25% saturated, 37.5% mono-, 37.5% polyunsaturated), cholesterol 80 mg, carbohydrate 0 g, Na 69 mg, Ca 130 mg, P 410 mg, Fe 2.2 mg, Zn 0.3 mg, vitamin niacin 3.6 mg, B_{12} 4 µg. A 120 g serving is a source of Ca, Fe; good source of niacin; rich source of protein, vitamin B_{12}.

baste   To ladle hot fat (or other liquid) over meat, poultry, etc, at intervals while it is baking or roasting, in order to improve the texture, flavour and appearance.

batata   See POTATO, SWEET.

Bath bun   A small English cake made from milk-based yeast dough, with dried fruit and a topping of sugar crystals, attributed to Dr W Oliver of Bath (eighteenth century).

Bath chap   The cheek and jawbones of the pig, salted and smoked. Originated in Bath.

Bath cheese   A small English CHEESE, made from cow's milk with the subsequent addition of cream.

Bath Oliver   A biscuit made with yeast, attributed to Dr W Oliver of Bath (eighteenth century).

Baudouin test   A colour test for the presence of sesame oil. In some countries sesame oil is added to all food oils except olive oil, hence permitting detection of the adulteration of olive oil with cheaper vegetable oils.

Baumé   A scale used to measure the density of liquids. For all liquids heavier than water, the density at 15.5°C corresponds to degrees Baumé.

bavarois(e)   (1) A hot drink made from eggs, milk and tea, sweetened and flavoured with a liqueur; seventeenth-century Bavarian.

(2) French; (*crème bavarois*) a cold dessert made from egg custard with gelatine and cream.

(3) Hollandaise sauce with CRAYFISH garnish.

bay (bay leaf)   A herb, the leaf of the Mediterranean sweet bay tree (*Lauris nobilis*) with a strong characteristic flavour. Rarely used alone, but an important component of BOUQUET GARNI, and used with other herbs in MARINADES, pickles, stews and stuffing.

Baycovin   Trade name for DIETHYL PYROCARBONATE.

bay lobster   Or Moreton Bay bug, a variety of sand lobster found in Australia.

bdelygmia   An extreme loathing for food.

bean, adzuki   Also known as aduki or feijoa bean, the seed of the Asian adzuki plant *Phaseolus (Vigna) angularis*. Sweet tasting, the basis of Cantonese red bean paste used to fill DIM-SUM. Also ground to a flour and used in bread, pastry and sweets or eaten after sprouting as BEAN SPROUTS.

Composition/100 g: 514 kJ (123 kcal), protein 9.3 g, fat 0.2 g, carbohydrate 22.5 g (0.5 g sugars, 20.8 g starch), nsp 5.5 g, Na 2 mg, K 570 mg, Ca 39 mg, Mg 60 mg, P 180 mg, Fe 1.9 mg, Cu 0.51 mg, Zn 2.3 mg, Se 1 µg, vitamin A 1 µg (6 µg carotene), B_1 0.14 mg, B_2 0.08 mg, niacin 2.4 mg. A 60 g serving is a source of protein, Mg; rich source of Cu.

bean, black eyed   Also known as black eyed pea or cow pea, *Vigna sinensis*; creamy white bean with a black mark on one edge.

Composition/100 g: 485 kJ (116 kcal), protein 8.8 g, fat 0.7 g, carbohydrate 19.9 g (1.1 g sugars, 18 g starch), nsp 3.5 g, Na 5 mg, K 320 mg, Ca 21 mg, Mg 45 mg, P 140 mg, Fe 1.9 mg, Cu 0.22 mg, Zn

1.1 mg, Se 3 μg, vitamin A 2 μg (13 μg carotene), B_1 0.19 mg, B_2 0.05 mg, niacin 2.4 mg, B_6 0.1 mg, folate 210 μg, pantothenate 0.3 mg, biotin 7 μg. A 60 g serving is a source of protein, Cu; rich source of folate.

bean, borlotti   Italian variety of *Phaseolus vulgaris*. See BEAN, HARICOT.

bean, broad   Also known as fava or horse bean, *Vicia faba*.

Composition/100 g: 339 kJ (81 kcal), protein 7.9 g, fat 0.6 g, carbohydrate 11.7 g (1.3 g sugars, 10 g starch), nsp 6.5 g, Na 8 mg, K 280 mg, Ca 56 mg, Mg 36 mg, P 150 mg, Fe 1.6 mg, Cu 0.32 mg, Zn 1 mg, I 6 μg, vitamin A 37 μg (225 μg carotene), E 0.6 mg, B_1 0.03 mg, B_2 0.06 mg, niacin 4.3 mg, B_6 0.08 mg, folate 32 μg, pantothenate 3.8 mg, biotin 2.1 μg, C 8 mg. A 120 g serving is a source of protein, folate, vitamin C, Mg, Fe; good source of niacin; rich source of pantothenate, Cu.

bean, butter   Several large varieties of *Phaseolus vulgaris*, also known as Lima, curry, Madagascar and sugar bean.

Composition/100 g: 322 kJ (77 kcal), protein 5.9 g, fat 0.5 g, carbohydrate 13 g (1.1 g sugars, 10.9 g starch), nsp 4.6 g, Na 420 mg, K 290 mg, Ca 15 mg, Mg 27 mg, P 68 mg, Fe 1.5 mg, Cu 0.14 mg, Zn 0.6 mg, vitamin E 0.3 mg, B_1 0.05 mg, B_2 0.03 mg, niacin 1.1 mg, B_6 0.05 mg, folate 12 μg. A 60 g serving is a source of Cu.

bean curd   See TOFU.

bean, French   Unripe seeds and pods of *Phaseolus vulgaris*; ripe seeds are HARICOT BEANS.

Composition/100 g: 100 kJ (24 kcal), protein 1.9 g, fat 0.5 g, carbohydrate 3.2 g (2.3 g sugars, 0.9 g starch), dietary fibre 3 g, nsp 2.2 g, K 230 mg, Ca 36 mg, Mg 17 mg, P 38 mg, Fe 1.2 mg, Cu 0.01 mg, Zn 0.2 mg, vitamin A 55 μg (330 μg carotene), E 0.2 mg, B_1 0.05 mg, B_2 0.07 mg, niacin 1.4 mg, B_6 0.05 mg, folate 80 μg, pantothenate 0.1 mg, biotin 1 μg, C 12 mg. A 90 g serving is a source of vitamin C; rich source of folate.

bean, haricot.   Ripe seed of small variety of *Phaseolus vulgaris* (the unripe seed is the FRENCH BEAN). Also known as navy, string, pinto or snap bean.

Composition/100 g: 397 kJ (95 kcal), protein 6.6 g, fat 0.5 g, carbohydrate 17.2 g (0.8 g sugars, 15.8 g starch), dietary fibre 6.7 g, nsp 6.1 g, Na 15 mg, K 320 mg, Ca 65 mg, Mg 45 mg, P 120 mg, Fe 2.5 mg, Cu 0.14 mg, Zn 1 mg, Se 4 μg, vitamin E 0.1 mg, B_1 0.1 mg, B_2 0.04 mg, niacin 1.7 mg, B_6 0.12 mg, pantothenate 0.2 mg. A 60 g serving is a source of Fe, Cu.

bean, Lima   See BEAN, BUTTER.

bean, mung   Whole or split seed of *Vigna radiata* (*Phaseolus aureus, P. radiatus*), green gram.

Composition/100 g: 380 kJ (91 kcal), protein 7.6 g, fat 0.4 g, carbohydrate 15.3 g (0.5 g sugars, 14.1 g starch), dietary fibre 4.8 g, nsp 3 g, Na 2 mg, K 270 mg, Ca 24 mg, Mg 43 mg, P 81 mg, Fe 1.4 mg, Cu 0.19 mg, Zn 0.9 mg, Se 5 μg, vitamin A 2 μg (12 μg carotene), B_1 0.09 mg, B_2 0.07 mg, niacin 1.7 mg, B_6 0.07 mg, folate 35 μg, pantothenate 0.4 mg. A 60 g serving is a source of folate, Cu.

bean, red kidney Ripe seed of large variety of *Phaseolus vulgaris*.
Composition/100 g: 431 kJ (103 kcal), protein 8.4 g, fat 0.5 g, carbohydrate 17.4 g (1 g sugars, 14.5 g starch), dietary fibre 9 g, nsp 6.7 g, Na 2 mg, K 420 mg, Ca 37 mg, Mg 45 mg, P 130 mg, Fe 2.5 mg, Cu 0.23 mg, Zn 1 mg, Se 6 μg, vitamin E 0.2 mg, B_1 0.17 mg, B_2 0.05 mg, niacin 1.9 mg, B_6 0.12 mg, folate 42 μg, pantothenate 0.2 mg, C 1 mg. A 60 g serving is a source of protein, folate, Fe, Cu.

See also LECTINS.

bean, runner *Phaseolus multiflorus*.
Composition/100 g: 75 kJ (18 kcal), protein 1.2 g, fat 0.5 g, carbohydrate 2.3 g (2 g sugars, 0.3 g starch), dietary fibre 3.1 g, nsp 1.9 g, Na 1 mg, K 130 mg, Ca 22 mg, Mg 14 mg, P 21 mg, Fe 1 mg, Cu 0.01 mg, Zn 0.2 mg, vitamin A 20 μg (120 μg carotene), E 0.2 mg, B_1 0.05 mg, B_2 0.02 mg, niacin 0.3 mg, B_6 0.04 mg, folate 42 μg, biotin 0.5 μg, C 10 mg. A 90 g serving is a source of folate, vitamin C.

beans, baked Usually mature haricot beans, cooked in sauce; often canned with tomato sauce and starch with added sugar (or sweetener) and salt.

bean, soya See SOYA.

bean sprouts A number of peas, beans and seeds can be germinated and the sprouts eaten raw or cooked. The sprouting causes the synthesis of vitamin C. One of the commonest sprouts is that of the MUNG BEAN, but ALFALFA and ADZUKI BEANS are also used.
Composition/100 g: 129 kJ (31 kcal), protein 2.9 g, fat 0.5 g, carbohydrate 4 g (2.2 g sugars, 1.8 g starch), dietary fibre 5.6 g, nsp 1.5 g, Na 5 mg, K 74 mg, Ca 20 mg, Mg 18 mg, P 48 mg, Fe 1.7 mg, Cu 0.08 mg, Zn 0.3 mg, vitamin A 6 μg (40 μg carotene), B_1 0.11 mg, B_2 0.04 mg, niacin 1 mg, B_6 0.1 mg, folate 61 μg, pantothenate 0.4 mg, C 7 mg. Serving 20 g.

bean, string Either RUNNER BEANS or FRENCH BEANS which have a climbing habit rather than growing as small bushes. The name derives from the method of growing them up strings.

béarnaise sauce A thick French sauce made with egg yolk, butter, wine vinegar or white wine and chopped SHALLOTS, named after Béarn in SW France.

béchamel sauce Also known as white sauce. One of the basic

French sauces, made with milk, butter and flour. Named after Louis de Béchamel, of the court of Louis XIV of France.

bêche-de-mer The sea slug, *Stichopus japonicus*, an occasional food in many parts of the world; also called trepang.

beechwood sugar See XYLOSE.

beef Flesh of the ox (*Bos taurus*); flesh from young calves is VEAL.

Composition/100 g (depending on joint of meat): 650–960 kJ (160–230 kcal), protein 23–31 g, fat 4.4–15.2 g (44.2% saturated, 52% mono-, 3.8% polyunsaturated), cholesterol 82 mg, carbohydrate 0 g, Na 139 mg, K 307 mg, Ca 11 mg, Mg 22 mg, P 184 mg, Fe 2.8 mg, Cu 0.19 mg, Zn 6.3 mg, Se 3 μg, I 6 μg, vitamin E 0.3 mg, B_1 0.06 mg, B_2 0.33 mg, niacin 11 mg, B_6 0.31 mg, folate 16 μg, B_{12} 2 μg, pantothenate 0.8 mg. A 100 g serving is a source of vitamin B_6, pantothenate, Fe; good source of vitamin B_2, Cu; rich source of protein, niacin, vitamin B_{12}, Zn.

beefalo A cross between the domestic cow (*Bos taurus*) and the buffalo (*Bubalus* spp) which can be fattened on range grass, rather than requiring cereal and protein supplements.

beefburger See HAMBURGER.

beef, corned See CORNED BEEF.

beef, pressed (Salt beef); boned brisket beef that has been salted, cooked and pressed. Known as CORNED BEEF in USA.

beefsteak fungus Large edible fungus (*Fistulina hepatica*) with a stringy, meat-like texture and deep red juice. See MUSHROOMS.

beer ALCOHOLIC BEVERAGE made by the fermentation of CEREALS; traditionally barley, but also maize, rice or sorghum. The first step is the malting of barley; it is allowed to sprout, when the enzyme AMYLASE hydrolyses some of the starch to dextrins and maltose. The sprouted (malted) barley is dried, then extracted with hot water (the process of mashing) to produce wort. After the addition of HOPS for flavour, the wort is allowed to ferment. Two types of YEAST are used in brewing: top fermenting yeasts which float on the surface of the wort and bottom or deep fermenters.

Most traditional British beers (ale, bitter, stout and porter) are brewed with top fermenting yeasts. UK beers, brown ale and stout, around 3–4% alcohol by volume; strong ale is 6.6% alcohol. Ale is a light-coloured beer, relatively high in alcohol content, and relatively heavily hopped. Bitter beers are darker and contain more hops. Lager is the traditional mainland European type of beer, sometimes called Pilsner lager or Pils, since the original lager was brewed in Pilsen in Bohemia. It is brewed by deep fermentation.

Composition/100 g bitter or lager: 120–33 kJ (29–32 kcal), protein 0.3 g, fat 0 g, carbohydrate 1.5–2.3 g (1.5–2.3 g sugars), Na

4–12 mg, K 36 mg, Ca 4–11 mg, Mg 6–9 mg, P 13 mg, Cu 0.08 mg, Zn 0.1 mg, I 8 µg, vitamin B_2 0.02–0.04 mg, niacin 0.6 mg, B_6 0.02 mg, folate 4–9 µg, B_{12} 0.1–0.2 µg, pantothenate 0.1 mg, biotin 0.5 µg. A 570 mL serving (one pint) is a source of niacin, folate, Mg; good source of vitamin B_{12}.

Porter and stout are almost black in colour; they are made from wort containing some partly charred malt; milk stout is made from wort containing added LACTOSE.

Composition/100 g stout: 154 kJ (37 kcal), protein 0.3 g, fat 0 g, carbohydrate 4.2 g (4.2 g sugars), Na 23 mg, K 45 mg, Ca 8 mg, Mg 8 mg, P 17 mg, Fe 0.1 mg, Cu 0.08 mg, vitamin B_2 0.03 mg, niacin 0.5 mg, B_6 0.01 mg, folate 4 µg, B_{12} 0.1 µg, pantothenate 0.1 mg, biotin 0.5 µg. A 570 mL serving (one pint) is a source of vitamin B_2, niacin, folate, Mg; rich source of vitamin B_{12}, Cu.

Lite beer is beer which has been allowed to ferment until virtually all of the carbohydrate has been converted to alcohol and so lower in carbohydrate and higher in alcohol.

Low alcohol beer may be made either by fermentation of a low carbohydrate wort, or by removal of much of the alcohol after fermentation (de-alcoholised beer).

Sorghum beer (African, made also from millet, maize or plantain) is a thick sour beverage consumed while still fermenting. Also known by numerous local names, kaffir beer, bouza, pombé, Bantu beer. 3–8% alcohol, 3–10% carbohydrate.

bees' royal jelly See ROYAL JELLY.

beestings The first milk given by the cow after calving, the COLOSTRUM, rich in immunoglobulins.

beet sugar See SUGAR; SUGAR BEET.

beet, leaf, silver, spinach See SWISS CHARD.

beetroot The root of *Beta vulgaris*, eaten cooked or pickled. Known simply as beet in N America. The violet-red pigment, betanin, is used as a food colour (E-162).

Composition/100 g: 192 kJ (46 kcal), protein 2.3 g, fat 0.1 g, carbohydrate 9.5 g (8.8 g sugars, 0.7 g starch), dietary fibre 2.3 g, nsp 1.9 g, Na 110 mg, K 510 mg, Ca 29 mg, Mg 16 mg, P 87 mg, Fe 0.8 mg, Cu 0.03 mg, Zn 0.5 mg, vitamin A 4 µg (27 µg carotene), B_1 0.01 mg, B_2 0.01 mg, niacin 0.4 mg, B_6 0.04 mg, folate 110 µg, pantothenate 0.1 mg, C 5 mg. A 35 g serving is a source of folate.

beeturia Excretion of red-coloured urine after eating BEETROOT, due to excretion of the pigment betanin. It occurs, not consistently, in about one person in eight.

bee wine Wine produced by fermentation of sugar, using a clump of yeast and lactic bacteria which rises and falls with the bubbles of carbon dioxide formed during fermentation, hence the name 'bee'.

belching See ERUCTATION.

bell pepper See PEPPER.

beluga Russian name for the white sturgeon (*Acipenser huro*), whose roe forms the most prized CAVIAR.

Bénédictine A French LIQUEUR invented in about 1510 by the monks of the Benedictine Abbey of Fécamp in France. The Abbey was closed, and the recipe lost after the French revolution, then rediscovered about 1863. It is based on double-distilled BRANDY, flavoured with some 75 herbs and spices; it contains 40% alcohol by volume and 30% sugar; 1.3 MJ (300 kcal)/100 mL.

Benedict–Roth spirometer See SPIROMETER.

Benedict's reagent Alkaline copper reagent (sodium citrate, sodium carbonate and copper sulphate) used for detection and semi-quantitative determination of GLUCOSE and other reducing sugars. Benedict's quantitative reagent also includes potassium thiocyanate and potassium ferrocyanide. The colour of the precipitate on boiling gives an indication of the concentration of glucose between 0.05–2%.

See also FEHLING'S REAGENT; SOMOGYI–NELSON REAGENT.

benniseed See SESAME.

Benn's index Ratio of weight divided by height^p, where p is derived from weight/height ratio and the regression coefficient of log(weight) on log(height) for the population group. Values of p range between 1.60–1.83.

bentonite See FULLER'S EARTH.

benzidine test Very sensitive test for blood; a green colour is developed when the sample is treated with a saturated solution of benzidine in glacial acid, followed by hydrogen peroxide.

benzoic acid A preservative normally used as the sodium, potassium or calcium salts and their derivatives (E-210–E-219), especially in acid foods such as pickles and sauces.

Occurs naturally in a number of fruits, including CRANBERRIES, PRUNES, GREENGAGES, CLOUDBERRIES and CINNAMON. Cloudberries contain so much benzoic acid that they can be stored for long periods of time without any precautions being taken against bacterial or fungal spoilage.

Benzoic acid and its derivatives are excreted conjugated with the AMINO ACIDS glycine (forming hippuric acid) and alanine. Because of this, benzoic acid is sometimes used in the treatment of ARGININAEMIA, ARGININOSUCCINIC ACIDURIA and CITRULLINAEMIA, permitting excretion of nitrogenous waste as these conjugates.

bergamot (1) A pear-shaped orange, *Citrus bergamia*, grown mainly in Calabria, Italy, for its peel oil.

(2) An ornamental herb, *Monarda didyma*, the dried leaves of which were used to make Oswego tea.

(3) A type of PEAR, *Pyrus persica*.

beriberi   The result of severe and prolonged deficiency of VITAMIN B_1, still a problem in parts of SE Asia where the diet is high in carbohydrate (polished RICE) and poor in vitamin B_1. In developed countries vitamin B_1 deficiency is associated with alcohol abuse; while it may result in beriberi, more commonly the result is central nervous system damage, the WERNICKE–KORSAKOFF SYNDROME.

In beriberi there is degeneration of peripheral nerves, starting in the hands and feet and ascending the arms and legs, with a loss of sensation and deep muscle pain. There is also enlargement of the heart, which may lead to OEDEMA (wet beriberi), and death results from heart failure. Fatal heart failure may develop without the nerve damage being apparent (Shoshin or sudden beriberi).

The name is derived from the Bahasa-Malay word for sheep, to describe the curious sheep-like gait adopted by sufferers.

berry   Botanical term for fleshy juicy fruits with one or more seeds not having a stone, e.g. grape, gooseberry, tomato, banana, blackcurrant, cranberry.

best before   See DATE MARKING.

beta-carotene (β-carotene)   See CAROTENE.

betacyanins   See BETALAINS.

betaine   *N*-Trimethyl glycine, a source of methyl groups in various reactions, especially the methylation of HOMOCYSTEINE to METHIONINE in tissues other than the brain; an intermediate in the metabolism of CHOLINE. Occurs in beetroot and cottonseed. (Obsolete names lycine, oxyneurine.)

betalains   Red and yellow N-containing pigments (chromoalkaloids) in plants. Betacyanins (e.g. betanin and isobetanin in beetroot) are red, betaxanthins yellow. Unlike ANTHOCYANINS the colour is little affected by pH.

betanin   Red-purple ANTHOCYANIN pigment in beetroot; permitted food colour E-162.

betaxanthins   See BETALAINS.

betel   Leaves of the creeper *Piper betel*, chewed in some parts of the world for its stimulating effect, due to the presence of the ALKALOIDS arecoline and guvacoline. The leaves are chewed with the nuts of the areca palm, *Arecha catechu*, which is therefore often called the betel palm, and the nut is called betel nut.

The Indian delicacy *pan* is based on betel leaf and areca nut, together with aromatic spices and herbs.

beurre manié   Butter with an equal amount of flour blended in, used for thickening sauces.

bezafibrate   See FIBRIC ACID.

bezoar   A hard ball of undigested food, sometimes together with hair, which forms in the stomach or intestine and can cause obstruction. Foods with a high content of PECTIN can form bezoars if swallowed without chewing. The name is derived from the Arabic meaning *protection against poison*, since bezoars were formerly believed to have protective properties.

See also GASTROLITH; TRICHOBEZOAR.

BHA   See BUTYLATED HYDROXYANISOLE.

bhaji   (1) Chinese spinach (*Amaranthus gangeticus*) also known as callaloo.

(2) Also bhajia, Indian vegetable fritters, normally made with gram (lentil) flour.

bhindi   See OKRA.

BHT   See BUTYLATED HYDROXYTOLUENE.

BIE   See BIOELECTRICAL IMPEDANCE.

biffins   Apples that have been peeled, partly baked, then pressed and dried.

Bifidobacterium   See PROBIOTICS.

bifidus factor   A carbohydrate in human milk which contains nitrogen and stimulates the growth of *Lactobacillus bifidus* in the intestine. In turn, this organism lowers the pH of the intestinal contents and suppresses the growth of *E. COLI* and other pathogenic BACTERIA.

See also LACTULOSE; PREBIOTICS.

bigarade (bigaradier)   See ORANGE, BITTER.

biguanides   See HYPOGLYCAEMIC AGENTS.

bilberry   The berry of wild shrubs of the genus *Vaccinium*, not generally cultivated. Variously known as whortleberry, blaeberry, whinberry, huckleberry.

Composition/100 g: 125 kJ (30 kcal), protein 0.6 g, fat 0.2 g, carbohydrate 6.9 g (6.9 g sugars), dietary fibre 2.5 g, nsp 1.8 g, Na 3 mg, K 88 mg, Ca 12 mg, Mg 5 mg, P 14 mg, Fe 0.5 mg, Cu 0.08 mg, Zn 0.2 mg, vitamin A 5 µg (30 µg carotene), B_1 0.03 mg, B_2 0.03 mg, niacin 0.5 mg, B_6 0.05 mg, folate 6 µg, pantothenate 0.3 mg, biotin 1.1 µg, C 17 mg. A 110 g serving is a source of Cu; rich source of vitamin C.

bile   Fluid produced by the liver and stored in the gall bladder before secretion into the small intestine (duodenum) via the bile duct. It contains the BILE SALTS, bile pigments (BILIRUBIN and biliverdin) and CHOLESTEROL. Alkaline, and neutralises the ACID from the stomach as the food reaches the small intestine.

Relatively large amounts of VITAMIN B_{12} and FOLIC ACID are

54

secreted in the bile and then reabsorbed from the small intestine (enterohepatic circulation). Most of the cholesterol and bile salts are also reabsorbed from the small intestine.

See also GASTROINTESTINAL TRACT.

bile salts (bile acids)   Salts of cholic and chenodeoxycholic acids, secreted in the bile as glycine and taurine conjugates; act as emulsifying agents in the absorption of fats. Also important as the cofactor of CAROTENE DIOXYGENASE (EC 1.13.11.21).

Bacterial metabolism in the colon leads to hydrolysis of the conjugates and formation of the secondary bile salts, lithocholic and deoxycholic acids, which are absorbed and then resecreted in the bile, again as glycine and taurine conjugates. Total secretion of bile salts is about 30 g/day; faecal output 1–2 g/day.

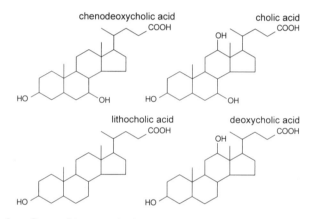

bilharzia   See *schistosomiasis*.

bilirubin, biliverdin   The BILE pigments, formed by catabolism of HAEMOGLOBIN. Blood bilirubin is normally <17 μmol/L; when it rises above 20–30 μmol/L there is visible jaundice.

biltong   South African; strips of dried meat, salted, spiced and dried in air for 10–14 days.

binge–purge syndrome   A feature of the eating disorder BULIMIA NERVOSA, characterised by the ingestion of excessive amounts of food and the excessive use of LAXATIVES.

Bingham plastic   COLLOIDAL SUSPENSION in which there is an initial resistance to flow which must be overcome before there is a normal increase in flow in response to shear stress.

bioassay   Biological assay; measurement of biologically active compounds (e.g. vitamins and essential amino acids) by their ability to support growth of microorganisms or animals.

biocytin   BIOTIN bound to the ε-amino group of lysine. The form in which biotin is present in enzymes; normally hydrolysed to release free biotin by the enzyme biotinidase (EC 3.5.1.12).

bioelectrical impedance (BIE) A method of measuring the proportion of fat in the body by the difference in the resistance to passage of an electric current between fat and lean tissue.

Correctly measures the impedance, since a 50 MHz alternating current (800 μA) is passed between electrodes attached to the hand and foot, and the fall in voltage is measured.

See also TOTAL BODY ELECTRICAL CONDUCTIVITY.

bioflavonoids See FLAVONOIDS.

biological oxygen demand (BOD) A way of assessing bacterial contamination of water, milk, etc by microorganisms which take up oxygen for their metabolism.

biological value (BV) A measure of PROTEIN QUALITY.

biopterin Pterin coenzyme required by PHENYLALANINE (EC 1.14.16.1), TYROSINE (EC 1.14.16.2) and TRYPTOPHAN (EC 1.14.16.4) hydroxylases. Not a dietary requirement, but synthesised from cGMP.

Rare patients with a variant form of PHENYLKETONURIA cannot synthesise biopterin, and have to receive supplements.

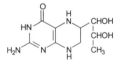

bios A name given to a factor in cell-free extract of yeast which was essential for the growth of yeast, by Wildiers in 1901. Three components were subsequently identified: INOSITOL, β-ALANINE and BIOTIN. Of these, only biotin is a VITAMIN and essential for human beings.

biotin A VITAMIN, sometimes known as vitamin H, required as coenzyme for carboxylation reactions in synthesis of fatty acids and glucose. Widely distributed in foods; dietary deficiency is unknown. There is no evidence on which to base REFERENCE INTAKES other than to state that current average intakes (between 15–70 μg/day) are obviously more than adequate to prevent deficiency.

The protein, avidin, in raw egg white, binds biotin strongly, preventing its absorption, and individuals who consume abnormally large amounts of uncooked egg (several dozen eggs per week) have been reported to show biotin deficiency. Avidin is denatured (see DENATURATION) on cooking, and does not combine with biotin; indeed cooked egg is a rich source of available biotin.

See also BIOCYTIN.

56

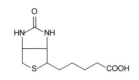

biotinidase   See BIOCYTIN.
biphenyl   See DIPHENYL.
birch beer   A non-alcoholic carbonated beverage flavoured with oil of wintergreen or oils of sweet birch and SASSAFRAS.
bisacodyl   A stimulant LAXATIVE.
biscuit   A baked flour confectionery dried down to low moisture content. The name is derived from the Latin *bis coctus*, meaning cooked twice. Known as cookie in the USA, where 'biscuit' means a small cake-like bun.
biscuit check   The development of splitting and cracking in BISCUITS immediately after baking.
Biskoids   Trade name for SACCHARIN.
Bismarck herring   Pickled and spiced whole HERRING.
bismuth   Mineral of no known metabolic function. A variety of bismuth salts are used as ANTACIDS and astringents in treating gastrointestinal disorders; the carbonate is used in treatment of peptic ULCER, especially when *HELICOBACTER PYLORI* is the causative agent.
bisque   Thick rich soup, generally made from FISH or SHELLFISH stock.
Bitot's spots   Irregular shaped foam-like plaques on the conjunctiva of the eye, characteristically seen in VITAMIN A deficiency, but not considered to be a diagnostic sign without other evidence of deficiency.
bitters   Extracts of herbs, spices, roots and bark, steeped in, or distilled with, SPIRITS. Originally prepared for medicinal use (tinctures or alcoholic extracts of the natural products); now used mainly to flavour spirits and cocktails, or as aperitifs.
  See also ANGOSTURA; WINE, APERITIF.
biuret reaction   Method for colorimetric determination of protein using an alkaline copper sulphate plus tartrate reagent which forms a coordination complex with four —NH groups in peptide bonds; sensitivity 1 mg/mL, maximum absorbance 540–560 nm.
bixin   A CAROTENOID pigment found in the seeds of the tropical plant *Bixa orellana*; the crude extract is the colouring agent ANNATTO (E-160).
blackberry   Berry of the bramble, *Rubus fruticosus*.
  Composition/100 g: 104 kJ (25 kcal), protein 0.9 g, fat 0.2 g, carbohydrate 5.1 g (5.1 g sugars), dietary fibre 6.6 g, nsp 3.1 g, Na

2 mg, K 160 mg, Ca 41 mg, Mg 23 mg, P 31 mg, Fe 0.7 mg, Cu 0.11 mg, Zn 0.2 mg, vitamin A 13 µg (80 µg carotene), E 2.4 mg, B_1 0.02 mg, B_2 0.05 mg, niacin 0.6 mg, B_6 0.05 mg, folate 34 µg, pantothenate 0.3 mg, biotin 0.4 µg, C 15 mg. A 110 g serving is a source of folate, Cu; good source of vitamins E, C.

blackcock See GROUSE.

blackcurrant Fruit of the bush *Ribes nigra*, of special interest because of its high vitamin C content. The British National Fruit Collection has 120 varieties.

Composition/100 g: 117 kJ (28 kcal), protein 0.9 g, fat 0 g, carbohydrate 6.6 g (6.6 g sugars), dietary fibre 7.8 g, nsp 3.6 g, Na 3 mg, K 370 mg, Ca 60 mg, Mg 17 mg, P 43 mg, Fe 1.3 mg, Cu 0.14 mg, Zn 0.3 mg, vitamin A 16 µg (100 µg carotene), E 1 mg, B_1 0.03 mg, B_2 0.06 mg, niacin 0.4 mg, B_6 0.08 mg, pantothenate 0.4 mg, biotin 2.4 µg, C 200 mg. A 110 g serving is a source of vitamin E, Fe, Cu; rich source of vitamin C.

Black Forest mushroom Or shiitake, *Lentinula (Lentinus) edodes*, see MUSHROOMS.

black fungus Or woodears, edible wild fungus, *Auriculia polytricha*; see MUSHROOMS.

black jack See CARAMEL.

black PN A black food colour (E-151), also known as brilliant black BN.

black pudding Also known as blood pudding. Traditional European dish made with sheep or pig blood and suet, originally together with oatmeal, liver and herbs, stuffed into membrane casings shaped like a horseshoe. Although it is already cooked, it is usually sliced and fried. German *Blutwurst* and French *boudin noir* are made without cereal.

Composition/100 g: 1276 kJ (305 kcal), protein 12.9 g, fat 21.9 g (42% saturated, 40% mono-, 17.8% polyunsaturated), cholesterol 68 mg, carbohydrate 15 g (15 g starch), dietary fibre 0.5 g, Na 1210 mg, K 140 mg, Ca 35 mg, Mg 16 mg, P 110 mg, Fe 20 mg, Cu 0.37 mg, Zn 1.3 mg, vitamin A 41 µg, E 0.2 mg, B_1 0.09 mg, B_2 0.07 mg, niacin 3.8 mg, B_6 0.04 mg, folate 5 µg, B_{12} 1 µg, pantothenate 0.6 mg, biotin 2 µg. An 85 g serving is a source of niacin, a good source of protein; rich source of vitamin B_{12}, Fe, Cu.

blackthorn See SLOE.

black tongue disease A sign of NIACIN deficiency in dogs, the canine equivalent of PELLAGRA, historically important in isolation of the VITAMIN.

blaeberry See BILBERRY.

blanching Partial precooking by treating food with hot gas, hot water, steam, super-heated steam, microwave, for a short time.

Fruits and vegetables are blanched before dehydrating or freezing, to soften the texture, shrink the food or remove air, destroy enzymes that may cause spoilage when frozen, and remove undesirable flavours. Blanching is also performed to remove excess salt from preserved meat, and to aid the removal of skin, e.g. from almonds and tomatoes.

There can be a loss of 10–20% of the sugars, salts and protein, as well as some of the vitamins B_1, B_2 and niacin, and up to one third of the vitamin C.

blancmange powder   Usually a cornflour base with added flavour and colour, mixed with hot milk to make a dessert.

bland diet   A diet that is non-irritating, does not overstimulate the digestive tract and is soothing to the intestines, generally avoiding alcohol, strong tea or coffee, pickles, spices and high intake of DIETARY FIBRE.

blawn fish   Scottish (Orkney); fresh fish, rubbed with salt and hung in a windy passage for a day, then grilled.

bleach figure (for flour)   A measure of the extent of bleaching of the flour from the relative paleness of the extracted (yellow) pigments.

bleaching   The removal or destruction of colour. In the context of food it usually refers to the bleaching of flour. It also refers to the bleaching of oils, a stage in the purification by which dispersed impurities and natural colouring materials are removed by activated CHARCOAL or FULLER'S EARTH.

See also AGEING (3).

bleeding bread   A bacterial infection with *Bacillus prodigiosus* or *Serratia marcescens*, which stains the bread bright red. Under warm and damp conditions the infection can appear overnight, and contamination of the shewbread in churches has led to accusations and riots against religious minorities over the centuries.

blewits   Edible wild fungus, *Tricholoma (Lepista) saevum*, also known as bluetail; also wood blewits, *T. nudum*, see MUSHROOMS.

blind loop syndrome   Or stagnant loop syndrome; stasis of the small intestine, permitting bacterial overgrowth and causing malabsorption and STEATORRHOEA. Usually the result of chronic obstruction or surgical by-pass operations producing a stagnant length of bowel.

blind staggers   Acute VITAMIN B_1 deficiency in horses and other animals, caused by eating bracken, which contains THIAMINASE.

bloaters   Salted, cold-smoked HERRINGS.

blood   Various BLOOD CELLS suspended in plasma; carries nutrients and oxygen to tissues, and removes waste metabolic products from the tissues. Oxygenated blood travels from the lungs in arteries, while deoxygenated blood returns to the lungs in veins; in the tissues the blood from the arteries enters smaller vessels, the arterioles, then capillaries, which then drain into venules, then the veins.

Average blood volume is 5.3 L (78 mL/kg body weight) in males and 3.8 L (56 mL/kg body weight) in females.

blood cells Three main types of cell are present in blood: erythrocytes or red cells, LEUCOCYTES or white cells and platelets. Red blood cells contain HAEMOGLOBIN, which is responsible for the transport of oxygen from the lungs to tissues, and of carbon dioxide from tissues. White blood cells are generally concerned with protection against invading microorganisms, and platelets with the process of BLOOD CLOTTING.

blood clotting The process by which the soluble protein fibrinogen in BLOOD PLASMA is converted to insoluble fibrin, thus preventing blood loss through cuts, etc. VITAMIN K is required and deficiency is characterised by excessive bleeding.

See also ANTICOAGULANTS; THROMBOSIS.

blood plasma The liquid component of blood, accounting for about half the total volume of the blood. Plasma is a solution of nutrients and proteins, mainly albumin and globulins, including the immunoglobulins which are responsible for defence against infection, as well as some ADVERSE REACTIONS TO FOODS. When blood has clotted (see BLOOD CLOTTING), the resultant fluid is known as serum.

See also LIPIDS, PLASMA.

blood pressure Blood pressure (bp) is measured as millimetres of mercury (Hg) at systole (when the heart contracts) and diastole (when the heart relaxes), and increases with age due to loss of elasticity of the arteries.

Normal systolic bp is 120 mm Hg at the age of 12 rising to 160 (men) or 175 (women) at 70. Normal diastolic bp 70 mm Hg at age 12, rising to 85 (men) or 95 (women) at age 70.

Diastolic bp above 105 is moderate, and above 115 severe, HYPERTENSION.

blood sausage See BLACK PUDDING.

blood serum See BLOOD PLASMA.

blood sugar GLUCOSE; normal concentration is about 3.5–5 mmol (60–90 mg)/L, and maintained in the fasting state by mobilisation of tissue reserves of GLYCOGEN and gluconeogenesis (synthesis from AMINO ACIDS). Only in prolonged starvation does it fall below about 3.5 mmol (60 mg)/L. If it falls to 2 mmol (35 mg)/L there is loss of consciousness (hypoglycaemic coma, see HYPOGLYCAEMIA).

After a meal the concentration of glucose rises, but this rise is limited by the hormone INSULIN, which is secreted by the pancreas to stimulate the uptake of glucose into tissues. DIABETES mellitus is the result of failure of the insulin mechanism.

See also GLUCOSE TOLERANCE TEST.

bloom Fat bloom is the whitish appearance on the surface of chocolate which sometimes occurs on storage. It is due either to a change in the form of the fat at the surface or to fat diffusing outwards and being deposited as crystals on the surface. Sugar bloom is due to the deposition of sugar crystals on the surface, but is less common than fat bloom.

See also TEMPERING.

Bloom gelometer An instrument for measuring the strength of jellies, and also for any test of firmness, e.g. the staleness of bread.

blotting A series of techniques involving the transfer of DNA, RNA or protein after gel ELECTROPHORESIS onto an inert nitrocellulose membrane, under denaturing conditions, so that it remains bound to the membrane. Southern blotting uses fragments of DNA produced using RESTRICTION ENZYMES, and they are identified by annealing with radioactive cDNA. Northern blotting is essentially similar, for identification of RNA fragments. Western blotting is for proteins, which are identified using labelled antibodies.

blueberry Fruit of *Vaccinium corymbosum* (the high-bush blueberry) or *V. augustifolium* (low-bush blueberry) grown mainly in N America.

Composition/100 g: 125 kJ (30 kcal), protein 0.6 g, fat 0.2 g, carbohydrate 6.9 g (6.9 g sugars), dietary fibre 2.5 g, nsp 1.8 g, Na 3 mg, K 88 mg, Ca 12 mg, Mg 5 mg, P 14 mg, Fe 0.5 mg, Cu 0.08 mg, Zn 0.2 mg, vitamin A 5 µg (30 µg carotene), B_1 0.03 mg, B_2 0.03 mg, niacin 0.5 mg, B_6 0.05 mg, folate 6 µg, pantothenate 0.3 mg, biotin 1.1 µg, C 17 mg. A 110 g serving is a source of Cu; rich source of vitamin C.

BMI See BODY MASS INDEX.

BMR See BASAL METABOLIC RATE.

boar, wild Meat of *Sus scrofa*. Hunted in parts of Europe, farmed on small scale in UK.

BOD See BIOLOGICAL OXYGEN DEMAND.

body composition Various methods are used to assess gross body composition, including ANTHROPOMETRY, BIOELECTRICAL IMPEDANCE, TOTAL BODY ELECTRICAL CONDUCTIVITY, SKINFOLD THICKNESS and BODY DENSITY.

body density Body fat has a density of 0.90, while fat-free body mass is 1.10. Direct determination of density by weighing in air and in water, or by determination of body volume by PLETHYS-

MOGRAPHY, therefore permits calculation of the proportions of fat and lean body tissue.

body mass index (BMI)   An index of fatness and obesity. The weight (in kg) divided by the square of height (in m). The acceptable (desirable) range is 20–25. Above 25 is overweight, and above 30 is OBESITY. BMI below the lower end of the acceptable range indicates undernutrition and wasting.

Also called Quetelet's index.

body surface area   Heat loss from the body is related to surface area; BASAL METABOLIC RATE and energy expenditure are sometimes expressed per unit body surface area. It is commonly calculated according to the formulae of Du Bois or Meeh:

Du Bois: area $(cm^2) = 71.84 \times weight^{0.425} (kg) \times height^{0.725} (cm)$
Meeh: area $(cm^2) = 11.9 \times weight^{2/3} (kg)$

The surface area of adults is about $18000 cm^2$ (men) or $16000 cm^2$ (women).

bog butter   Norsemen, Finns, Scots and Irish used to bury firkins of butter in bogs to ripen and develop a strong flavour.

bog myrtle   A wild plant (*Myrica gale*) with a strong resinous flavour. The leaves and seeds are used to flavour soups and stews.

bole   See ARMENIAN BOLE.

boletus   Edible wild MUSHROOM, *Boletus edulis* or *B. granulatus*, also known as the yellow mushroom or cep (cèpe).

bologna   Italian smoked pork and veal SAUSAGE, also known as polony.

bolus   Soft mass of chewed food that is ready to be swallowed.

bomb calorimeter   See CALORIMETER.

Bombay duck   Bombil, a fish found in Indian waters, *Harpodon nehereus* or *Saurus ophiodon*, eaten either fresh or after salting and curing.

Bombay mix   See CHEVDA.

bombil   See BOMBAY DUCK.

bone   Bones consist of an organic matrix composed of COLLAGEN and other proteins and crystalline mineral, mainly HYDROXY-APATITE (calcium phosphate and hydroxide), together with magnesium phosphate, fluorides and sulphates.

Cortical (compact) bone forms the outer shell of bones; it is a solid mass of bony tissue.

Spongy (cancellous) bone beneath the cortical bone consists of a meshwork of trabeculae with interconnecting spaces containing bone MARROW.

Bone density can be assessed as an index of calcium and VITAMIN D status by X-ray, photon absorptiometry or NEUTRON ACTIVATION.

See also CALCIUM; MARROW (1); OSTEOMALACIA; OSTEOPOROSIS; RICKETS.

bone broth Prepared by prolonged boiling of bones to break down the COLLAGEN and extract it as GELATINE. Of little nutritive value, consisting of 2–4% gelatine, with little calcium.

bone charcoal Animal charcoal, produced by heating pieces of bone sufficiently to burn off the organic matter, leaving the carbon deposited on a framework of calcium carbonate. It is used to purify solutions because it will absorb colouring matter and other impurities.

bone meal Prepared from degreased bones and used as a supplement in both animal and human foods as a source of calcium and phosphate. Also used as a plant fertiliser; a slowly released source of phosphate.

Bontrae Trade name for TEXTURED VEGETABLE PROTEIN prepared by spinning or extrusion.

boracic acid See BORIC ACID.

borage A herb, *Borago officinalis*. The flowers and leaves have a cucumber-like flavour and are used to flavour drinks.

borborygmos (Plural borborygmi); audible abdominal sound produced by excessive intestinal motility.

borderline substances Foods that may have characteristics of medication in certain circumstances, and which may then be prescribed under the National Health Service in UK, e.g. nutritional supplements for treatment of short bowel disease, lactose-free milk for children with LACTOSE INTOLERANCE, GALACTOSAEMIA and GALACTOKINASE DEFICIENCY, GLUTEN-FREE foods for patients with COELIAC DISEASE, specially formulated foods for treatment of a variety of GENETIC DISEASES.

borecole See KALE.

boric acid Chemically H_3BO_4; has been used in the past as a preservative in bacon and margarine, but BORON accumulates in the body. Formerly used as an anti-infective agent and eye-wash (boracic acid) but there was a high incidence of toxic reactions.

Borneo tallow See VEGETABLE BUTTERS.

boron An element, known to be essential for plant growth, but not known to have any physiological function in animals. Suggested to modify the actions and metabolism of OESTROGENS, and sometimes used in preparations to alleviate premenstrual syndrome, although there is little evidence of efficacy; toxic in excess. Occurs mainly as salts of BORIC ACID.

Boston brown bread An American spiced pudding, steamed in the can.

bottle The traditional wine bottle holds 700, 720 or 750 mL of wine, depending on the variety. A two-bottle size is a magnum;

four a Jeroboam or double magnum, six a Methuselah, 12 a Salmanazar and 20 a Nebuchadnezzar.

bottled sweat See SPORTS DRINKS.

bottlers' sugar See SUGAR.

botulinum cook The degree of heat required to ensure destruction of (virtually) all spores of *Clostridium botulinum*, the causative organism of BOTULISM, the most resistant of bacterial spores.

botulism A rare form of food poisoning caused by the extremely potent neurotoxins (TX1.2.5.1–7) produced by *Clostridium botulinum*. At least seven different toxins have been identified; they can be inactivated by heating. Although rare, it is often fatal unless the antitoxin is given.

The name is derived from *botulus*, for sausage, since the disease was originally associated with sausages in Germany. A wide range of foods have been involved, including meat, fish, milk, fruits and vegetables which have been incorrectly preserved or treated, so that competing microorganisms have been destroyed; spores of *C. botulinum* are extremely resistant to heat, and dangerous amounts of toxins can accumulate in contaminated foods without apparent spoilage.

boucanning A Caribbean process by which meat was preserved by sun-drying and smoking while resting on a wooden grid known as a boucan.

bouillabaisse French; fish stew or soup flavoured with saffron, spices and herbs; speciality of the Mediterranean region.

bouquet garni A small bundle of parsley, thyme, marjoram and bay leaves, tied together with cotton and added to the dish being cooked. Now also the same mixture of herbs in a porous paper sack. Also known as a faggot.

bourbon American WHISKEY made by distilling fermented MAIZE mash. Sour mash bourbon is made from mash that has yeast left in it from a previous fermentation.

bourbonal Ethylvanillin, see VANILLA.

Bournvita Trade name for a preparation of malt, milk, sugar, cocoa, eggs and flavouring, to make a beverage when mixed with milk.

bovine somatotrophin (BST) See SOMATOTROPHIN, BOVINE.

bovine spongiform encephalopathy See BSE.

Bovril Trade name for a preparation of MEAT EXTRACT, hydrolysed beef, beef powder and yeast extract, used as a beverage, flavouring agent and for spreading on bread.

Composition/100 g: 707 kJ (169 kcal), protein 38 g, fat 0.7 g, carbohydrate 2.9 g (2.9 g starch), Na 4800 mg, K 1200 mg, Ca 40 mg, Mg 61 mg, P 590 mg, Fe 14 mg, Cu 0.45 mg, Zn 1.8 mg, vitamin B_1

9.1 mg, B_2 7.4 mg, niacin 85 mg, B_6 0.53 mg, folate 1040 µg, B_{12} 8.3 µg. A 4 g serving is a source of vitamin B_2, niacin; good source of vitamin B_1, folate; rich source of vitamin B_{12}.

boysenberry   Similar to LOGANBERRY.

brachyose   See ISOMALTOSE.

bracken   Young unopened leaves (fronds) of bracken (*Pteridium* spp), eaten as a vegetable and regarded as a delicacy in the Far East. Known as fiddleheads in Canada.

Contain THIAMINASE, which cleaves VITAMIN B_1; cattle and horses eating large amounts suffer from BLIND STAGGERS due to acute vitamin B_1 deficiency; also contain a number of known or suspected CARCINOGENS.

Bradford method   See COOMASSIE BRILLIANT BLUE.

bradycardia   An unusually slow heart beat, less than 60 beats/min; may be normal in trained athletes.

bradyphagia   Eating very slowly.

brain sugar   Obsolete name for GALACTOSE.

bramble   Wild BLACKBERRY.

bran   The outer layers of cereal grain, which are largely removed when the grain is milled (i.e. in the preparation of white flour or white rice). The germ is discarded at the same time, and there is a considerable loss of iron and other minerals, and particularly of the B vitamins, as well as of dietary fibre.

See also FLOUR, EXTRACTION RATE; WHEATFEED.

branched-chain amino acids   See AMINO ACIDS.

brander   Scottish name for gridiron or grill.

brandy   A SPIRIT distilled from wine, and containing 37–45% (most usually 40%) alcohol by volume. The name is derived from the German *brandtwein*, meaning burnt wine, corrupted to brandy wine. Most wine-producing countries also make brandy.

The age of brandy is generally designated as three-star (3–5 years old before bottling); VSOP (very special old pale, aged 4–10 or more years, the name indicating that it has not been heavily coloured with caramel); Napoleon (premium blend aged 6–20 years); XO, extraordinary old (extra or grand reserve, possibly 50 years old).

COGNAC and ARMAGNAC are brandies made in defined regions of France. Fruit brandies are either distilled from fruit wines (e.g. plum and apple brandies) or are prepared by soaking fruit in brandy (e.g. cherry and apricot brandies).

See also MARC.

Brassica   Genus of vegetables that includes broccoli, Brussels sprouts, cabbage, cauliflower, kale, kohlrabi, mustard, swede.

brawn   Made from pig meat, particularly the head, boiled with peppercorns and herbs, minced and pressed into a mould. Mock brawn (head cheese) differs in that other meat by-products are used.

Brazil nuts   Fruit of the tree *Bertholletia excelsa*.

Composition/100 g: 2854 kJ (682 kcal), protein 14.1 g, fat 68.2 g (25.1% saturated, 39.5% mono-, 35.2% polyunsaturated), carbohydrate 3.1 g (2.4 g sugars, 0.7 g starch), dietary fibre 8.1 g, nsp 4.3 g, Na 3 mg, K 660 mg, Ca 170 mg, Mg 410 mg, P 590 mg, Fe 2.5 mg, Cu 1.76 mg, Zn 4.2 mg, Se 1530 µg, I 20 µg, vitamin E 7.2 mg, B_1 0.67 mg, B_2 0.03 mg, niacin 3.3 mg, B_6 0.31 mg, folate 21 µg, pantothenate 0.4 mg, biotin 11 µg. A 10 g serving (three nuts) is a source of Mg; good source of Cu; rich source of Se.

bread   Baked dough made from cereal flour, usually wheat, although rye, barley and other cereals are also used. Normally leavened by fermentation of the dough with yeast, or addition of sodium bicarbonate. Soda bread is an Irish speciality, made with whey or buttermilk, and leavened with SODIUM BICARBONATE and acid in place of yeast, although yeast may also be used.

Unleavened bread is flat bread made by baking dough which has not been leavened with yeast or baking powder. MATZO is baked to a crisp texture, while PITTA and CHAPATTIS have a softer texture.

Aerated bread is made from dough which is prepared with water saturated with carbon dioxide under pressure, rather than being leavened with yeast. The aim was to produce an aerated loaf without the loss of carbohydrate involved in a yeast fermentation (7% of the total ingredients). The resultant loaf was insipid in flavour and the method went out of use.

Wholemeal bread is baked with 100% extraction flour, i.e. containing the whole of the cereal grain. White bread is made from 72% extraction flour. Brown bread is made with flour of extraction rate intermediate between that of white bread and wholemeal. A loaf may not legally be described as brown unless it contains at least 0.6% FIBRE on a dry weight basis. Black bread is a coarse wholemeal wheat or rye bread leavened with sourdough (*sauerteig*).

The white loaf in UK has added iron, vitamin B_1 and niacin, but not to the level of wholemeal bread, and white but not wholemeal is enriched with calcium. Some bakers also enrich bread with FOLIC ACID. In some countries RIBOFLAVIN but not calcium is added.

Composition/100 g white bread: 983 kJ (235 kcal), protein 8.4 g, fat 1.9 g, carbohydrate 49.3 g (2.6 g sugars, 46.7 g starch), dietary fibre 3.8 g, nsp 1.5 g, Na 520 mg, K 110 mg, Ca 110 mg, Mg 24 mg, P 91 mg, Fe 1.6 mg, Cu 0.19 mg, Zn 0.6 mg, Se 28 µg, I 6 µg, vitamin B_1 0.21 mg, B_2 0.06 mg, niacin 3.4 mg, B_6 0.07 mg, folate 29 µg, pantothenate 0.3 mg, biotin 1 μg. A 120 g serving (four slices) is a source of vitamin B_1, folate, Ca, Fe; good source of protein, niacin, Cu; rich source of Se.

Composition/100 g brown bread: 912 kJ (218 kcal), protein 8.5 g, fat 2 g, carbohydrate 44.3 g (3 g sugars, 41.3 g starch), dietary fibre 5.9 g, nsp 3.5 g, Na 540 mg, K 170 mg, Ca 100 mg, Mg 53 mg, P 150 mg, Fe 2.2 mg, Cu 0.16 mg, Zn 1.1 mg, vitamin B_1 0.27 mg, B_2 0.09 mg, niacin 4.2 mg, B_6 0.13 mg, folate 40 μg, pantothenate 0.3 mg, biotin 3 μg. A 120 g serving (four slices) is a source of Ca, Fe; good source of protein, vitamin B_1, niacin, folate, Mg, Cu.

Composition/100 g wholemeal bread: 899 kJ (215 kcal), protein 9.2 g, fat 2.5 g, carbohydrate 41.6 g (1.8 g sugars, 39.8 g starch), dietary fibre 7.4 g, nsp 5.8 g, Na 550 mg, K 230 mg, Ca 54 mg, Mg 76 mg, P 200 mg, Fe 2.7 mg, Cu 0.26 mg, Zn 1.8 mg, Se 35 μg, vitamin E 0.2 mg, B_1 0.34 mg, B_2 0.09 mg, niacin 5.9 mg, B_6 0.12 mg, folate 39 μg, pantothenate 0.6 mg, biotin 6 μg. A 120 g serving (four slices) is a source of pantothenate, Zn; good source of protein, vitamin B_1, folate, Fe; rich source of niacin, Mg, Cu, Se.

Rye bread is baked wholly or partly with rye flour, of varying extraction rate, so that it can vary from very light to grey or black. It is commonly a sourdough bread and may contain caraway seeds. A 100 g portion (four slices from a small loaf) is a good source of vitamin B_1, niacin; a source of protein, Ca, Fe; contains 4.5 g dietary fibre; supplies 220 kcal (925 kJ).

Sourdough bread is commonly wholemeal wheat or rye bread, but may also be white bread, that has been leavened with sourdough (*sauerteig*), dough that has been left to ferment overnight, and contains a mixture of fermenting microorganisms, including peptonising bacteria that turn the dough to a more plastic state, yeast and lactic or acetic bacteria that produce the sour flavour.

There is a wide variety of different types of bread, with loaves baked in different shapes, or with various additions to the dough. For batch bread, the moulded pieces of dough touch each other in the oven, so that when baked and separated only the top and bottom of the loaf have crusts. Traditional French bread is made with soft-wheat flour, and has a more open texture and crisp crust. Focaccia is Italian white bread made with olive oil (9%) and herbs; ciabatta (also Italian) is a flat white bread with large holes, made with olive oil (5%), literally *old slipper*. Bank holiday bread is made with extra fat to soften the crumb so that it will last over a long (Bank holiday) weekend. Cornell bread was originally developed at Cornell University, with increased nutritional value from the addition of 6% soya flour and 8% skim milk solids. Lactein bread has added milk, usually about 6%

milk solids, (3–4% milk solids are often added to the ordinary loaf in the USA).

See also CHORLEYWOOD BREAD PROCESS; FLOUR, EXTRACTION RATE; HOVIS; QUICKBREADS.

breadfruit Large spherical, starchy fruit of the tree *Artocarpus communis* or *A. incisa* (fig family). Seasonal staple food in the Caribbean, eaten roasted whole when ripe, or boiled in pieces when green.

Composition/100 g: 498 kJ (119 kcal), protein 1.6 g, fat 0.4 g, carbohydrate 29 g (1.5 g sugars, 27.5 g starch), Na 1 mg, K 350 mg, Ca 18 mg, Mg 23 mg, P 28 mg, Fe 0.9 mg, Cu 0.05 mg, Zn 0.1 mg, vitamin A 5 μg (30 μg carotene), B_1 0.08 mg, B_2 0.05 mg, niacin 0.7 mg, pantothenate 0.4 mg, C 20 mg. A 200 g serving is a source of vitamin B_1, pantothenate, Mg, Fe, Cu; rich source of vitamin C.

breadspreads General term for fats used to spread on bread, including BUTTER, MARGARINE and low-fat spreads that may not legally be called margarine.

bread, starch-reduced Bread is normally 9–10% protein and about 50% starch; if the starch is reduced, either by washing some of it out of the dough or by adding extra protein, the bread is referred to as starch-reduced, and is often claimed to be of value in slimming and diabetic diets (see DIABETIC FOODS). Legally, the name 'starch-reduced bread' may be applied only to bread containing less than 50% carbohydrate, and any claims for its value as a slimming aid are strictly controlled.

breadstick See GRISSINI.

breakfast cereal (breakfast food) Legally defined as any food obtained by the swelling, roasting, grinding, rolling or flaking of any cereal.

break middlings See DUNST.

break rolls See MILLING.

bream White fish, *Abramis brama* (N American bluegill bream is *Leponis macrochinus*).

Composition/100 g: 401 kJ (96 kcal), protein 17.5 g, fat 2.9 g, cholesterol 38 mg, carbohydrate 0 g, Na 110 mg, K 270 mg, Ca 40 mg, Mg 23 mg, P 230 mg, Fe 0.5 mg, Cu 0.05 mg, Zn 0.3 mg, vitamin B_1 0.08 mg, B_2 0.1 mg, niacin 8.7 mg, B_6 0.46 mg, B_{12} 2 μg, pantothenate 0.2 mg. A 120 g serving is a good source of vitamin B_6; rich source of protein, niacin, vitamin B_{12}.

Bredsoy Trade name for an unheated (i.e. enzyme active) full-fat SOYA FLOUR.

bretzels See PRETZELS.

brewers' grains Cereal residue from brewing, containing about 25% protein; used as animal feed.

brewnzyme Mixture of bacterial PROTEASES and AMYLASES with barley β-amylase, used to mash unmalted starch for BEER making.

Brillat-Savarin A French gourmet (1755–1826) whose name is given to a CONSOMMÉ, BABA and several other dishes.

brilliant acid green BS See GREEN S.

brine Salt solutions of varying concentrations used in PICKLING. 'Fresh' brine may have added nitrite; 'live' brine contains microorganisms that convert nitrate to nitrite (pickling salts).

brining The process of soaking vegetables in BRINE before pickling in vinegar, in order to remove some of the water, and retain a crisp texture. Dry brining is when the vegetables are covered with dry salt, rather than immersed in a salt solution.

brisling Young SPRAT, *Clupea sprattus*.

Brix A table of specific gravity based on the BALLING tables, calculated in grams of cane sugar in 100 g of solution at 20°C; degree Brix = percentage sugar. It is used to refer to the concentration of sugar syrups used in canned fruits.

broasting A cooking method in which the food is deep fried under pressure, which is quicker than without pressure, and the food absorbs less fat.

broccoli, Chinese (Chinese kale) *Brassica oleracea* var *alboglabra*; similar to CALABRESE and sprouting BROCCOLI.

broccoli, sprouting Member of the cabbage family, *Brassica oleracea italica* group with purple and white clusters of flower buds (which turn green when boiled) with smaller heads than CALABRESE (broccoli = *little shoots*, It).

Composition/100 g: 100 kJ (24 kcal), protein 3.1 g, fat 0.8 g, carbohydrate 1.1 g (0.9 g sugars), nsp 2.3 g, Na 13 mg, K 170 mg, Ca 40 mg, Mg 13 mg, P 57 mg, Fe 1 mg, Cu 0.02 mg, Zn 0.4 mg, I 2 µg, vitamin A 79 µg (475 µg carotene), E 1.1 mg, B_1 0.05 mg, B_2 0.05 mg, niacin 1.3 mg, B_6 0.11 mg, folate 64 µg, C 44 mg. An 85 g serving is a good source of folate; rich source of vitamin C.

broiling Cooking by direct heat over a flame, as in a barbecue; American term for grilling. Pan broiling is cooking through hot dry metal over direct heat.

bromatology The science of foods, from the Greek *broma*, food.

bromelains Enzymes (EC 3.4.22.32 and 33) in the PINEAPPLE and related bromelids, which hydrolyse proteins. They are available as by-products from commercial pineapple production, usually from the stems, and are used to tenderise meat, treat sausage casings and CHILLPROOF beer.

See also TENDERISERS.

brominated oils Oils from a variety of sources, including peach and apricot kernels, olive and soya oils which have been reacted with BROMINE to add across the carbon–carbon double bonds.

They are used to help to stabilise emulsions of flavouring substances in soft drinks. Also known as weighting oils.

brose A Scottish dish made by pouring boiling water onto oatmeal or barley meal; fish, meat and vegetables may be added.

brown adipose tissue (brown fat) Metabolically highly active adipose tissue, which may be involved in heat production to maintain body temperature as a result of partial uncoupling of electron transport (see ELECTRON TRANSPORT CHAIN) and OXIDATIVE PHOSPHORYLATION. Colour comes from its high content of MITOCHONDRIA.

See also UNCOUPLING PROTEINS.

brown colours Three brown colours are used in foods: Brown FK (E-154), synthetic, which is used to colour KIPPERS; chocolate brown HT (E-155), synthetic, and CARAMEL (E-150).

brown fat See BROWN ADIPOSE TISSUE.

brownie American cake made with chocolate.

browning reactions Chemical reactions in foods which result in the formation of a brown colour. See MAILLARD REACTION; PHENOL OXIDASES; STRECKER DEGRADATION.

brugnon Hybrid fruit, a cross between plum and peach. Resembles nectarine, and name sometimes used in France for nectarines.

brûlé Literally burnt; food grilled or otherwise heated sufficiently to give it a brown colour.

Brunner's glands MUCUS-secreting glands embedded in the submucosa of the duodenum and upper jejunum.

brush border See MICROVILLI.

Brussels sprouts Leaf buds of *Brassica oleracea gemmifera*.
Composition/100g: 146 kJ (35 kcal), protein 2.9 g, fat 1.3 g, carbohydrate 3.5 g (3 g sugars, 0.3 g starch), dietary fibre 2.6 g, nsp 3.1 g, Na 2 mg, K 310 mg, Ca 20 mg, Mg 13 mg, P 61 mg, Fe 0.5 mg, Cu 0.03 mg, Zn 0.3 mg, I 1 µg, vitamin A 53 µg (320 µg carotene), E 0.9 mg, B_1 0.07 mg, B_2 0.09 mg, niacin 0.5 mg, B_6 0.19 mg, folate 110 µg, pantothenate 0.3 mg, biotin 0.3 µg, C 60 mg. A 90 g serving (9 sprouts) is a rich source of folate, vitamin C.

BS 5750 British Standard of excellence in quality management; originally an engineering standard but applicable to food companies, hospitals, etc; incorporates the EU equivalent IS0 9002.

BSE Bovine spongiform encephalopathy; a degenerative brain disease, transmitted between animals by feeding slaughter-house waste from infected animals. Commonly known as 'mad cow disease'. The infective agent is believed to be a PRION, and can be transmitted to human beings, causing a form of Creutzfeldt–Jakob disease.

BST See SOMATOTROPHIN, BOVINE.

bubble and squeak   English, originally cold boiled beef fried with cooked potatoes and cabbage (the name comes from the sound made as it cooks). More commonly a fried mixture of left-over cabbage and potatoes. Colcannon is a similar Irish dish.

buccal glands   Small glands in the mucous membrane of the mouth that secrete material that mixes with saliva.

buck rarebit   See WELSH RAREBIT.

buckling   A hot-smoked HERRING (the KIPPER is cold-smoked).

buck's fizz   Sparkling wine mixed with orange juice; known in USA as a mimosa.

buckwheat   A cereal, the grains of *Fagopyrum esculentum* and other spp, also known as Saracen corn, and, when cooked, as kasha (Russian). It is unsuitable for breadmaking, and is eaten as the cooked grain, a porridge or baked into pancakes.

buffalo currant   Two varieties of N American currant: *Ribes odoratum*, which has a distinctive smell, and *R. aureum*, the golden or Missouri currant.

buffer   Substance that prevents a change in the pH when acid or alkali is added. Salts of weak acids and bases are buffers and are commonly used to control the acidity of foods. Amino acids and proteins also act as buffers.

   The pH of blood (see ACID–BASE BALANCE) is maintained by physiological buffers including phosphates, bicarbonate and proteins.

bulbogastrone   Peptide hormone secreted by the duodenum; decreases gastric secretion.

bulgur   The oldest processed food known, originally from the Middle East. Wheat is soaked, cooked and dried, then lightly milled to remove the outer bran and cracked. It is eaten in soups and cooked with meat (when it is known as kibbe). Also called ala, burghul, cracked wheat and American rice.

bulimia nervosa   An eating disorder, especially of women aged between 15–30, characterised by powerful and intractable urges to overeat, followed by self-induced vomiting and the excessive use of purgatives.

   See also ANOREXIA NERVOSA.

bulking agents   Non-nutritive substances (commonly NON-STARCH POLYSACCHARIDES) added to foods to increase the bulk and hence sense of SATIETY, especially in foods designed for weight reduction.

bulk sweeteners   See SUGAR ALCOHOLS.

bullace   Fruit of the wild DAMSON, *Prunus insititia*; similar to SLOE, very acidic.

bullnose pepper   See PEPPER.

bullock's heart   See CUSTARD APPLE.

bully beef The name given by troops during the first World War to CORNED BEEF (canned salted beef).

bulrush A wild plant common in ponds and marshes (correctly the false bulrush or common reedmace, *Typha latifolia*). The young sprouts and shoots can be eaten in salads, the pollen is used as a flavouring, and the roots and unripe flower heads may be boiled as a vegetable.

buni Coffee beans left in the field to dry; generally hard and of poor quality.

bunt See SMUT.

burger See HAMBURGER.

burghul See BULGUR.

burnet Salad burnet, a wild plant (*Poterium sanguisorba*) growing in grassland on chalky soil. The leaves have the flavour of cucumber, and can be used to flavour fruit wines, vinegar and butter, and are used in salads. Also called pimpernel.

burning foot syndrome Nutritional melalgia (neuralgic pain); severe aching, throbbing and burning pain in the feet, associated with nerve damage, observed in severely undernourished prisoners of war in the Far East. It results from long periods on a diet poor in protein and B VITAMINS, and may (doubtfully) be due specifically to a deficiency of PANTOTHENIC ACID.

busa See MILK, FERMENTED.

bushel A traditional dry measure of volume, equivalent to the volume of 80 lb of distilled water at 17°C with a barometer reading of 30 inches, i.e. 8 Imperial gallons (36.4 L); used as a measure of corn, potatoes, etc. The American (Winchester) bushel is 3% larger.

The weight of a bushel varies with the product: wheat 27 kg, maize and rye 25 kg, barley 22 kg, paddy rice 20 kg, oats 14.5 kg.

butt A cask for beer or wine, containing 108 Imperial gallons (491 L).

butter Made from separated CREAM by churning (sweet cream butter); legally not less than 80% fat (and not more than 16% water). Lactic butter is made by first ripening the cream with a bacterial culture to produce lactic acid and increase the flavour (due to diacetyl). This is normally unsalted or up to 0.5% salt added. Sweet cream butter may be salted up to 2%.

Composition/100 g: 3085 kJ (737 kcal), protein 0.5 g, fat 81.7 g (70.6% saturated, 25.9% mono-, 3.4% polyunsaturated), cholesterol 230 mg, carbohydrate 0 g, Na 750 mg, K 15 mg, Ca 15 mg, Mg 2 mg, P 24 mg, Fe 0.2 mg, Cu 0.03 mg, Zn 0.1 mg, I 38 μg, vitamin A 886 μg (430 μg carotene), D 0.76 μg, E 2 mg, B_2 0.02 mg, niacin 0.1 mg. A 15 g serving is a source of vitamin A.

Clarified butter is butter fat, prepared by heating butter and separating the fat from the water. It does not become RANCID as rapidly as butter. Also known as ghee or ghrt (India) and samna (Egypt).

Process or renovated butter has been melted and rechurned with the addition of milk, cream or water.

Drawn butter is melted butter used as a dressing for cooked vegetables. Devilled butter is mixed with lemon juice, cayenne and black pepper and curry powder. Ravigote butter is creamed with chopped fresh aromatic herbs (tarragon, parsley, chives, chervil), usually served with grilled meat. Green butter is mixed with chopped herbs and other seasonings to produce a savoury spread. Black butter is browned by heating, then vinegar, salt, pepper or other seasonings are added.

See also VEGETABLE BUTTERS.

butterine   US term for MARGARINE.

buttermilk   The residue left after churning butter, 0.1–2% fat, with the other constituents of milk increased proportionally. Slightly acidic, with a distinctive flavour due to the presence of DIACETYL and other substances. Usually made by adding lactic bacteria to skim milk; 90–92% water, 4% lactose with acidic flavour from lactic acid.

butterscotch   See TOFFEE.

butter, whey (serum butter)   Butter made from the small amount of fat left in WHEY; it has a slightly different FATTY ACID composition from ordinary butter.

butylated hydroxyanisole (BHA)   An ANTIOXIDANT (E-320) used in fats and fatty foods; stable to heating, and so is useful in baked products.

butylated hydroxytoluene (BHT)   An ANTIOXIDANT (E-321) used in fats and fatty foods.

butyric acid   Short-chain saturated FATTY ACID containing four carbon atoms. It occurs as 5–6% of butter fat, and in small amounts in other fats and oils.

BV   Biological value, a measure of PROTEIN QUALITY.

C

CA   Controlled atmosphere. See GAS STORAGE, CONTROLLED.

cabbage   Leaves of *Brassica oleracea capitata*.

Composition/100g: 108kJ (26kcal), protein 1.7g, fat 0.4g, carbohydrate 4.1g (4g sugars, 0.1g starch), dietary fibre 2.9g, nsp 2.4g, Na 5mg, K 270mg, Ca 52mg, Mg 8mg, P 41mg, Fe 0.7mg, Cu 0.02mg, Zn 0.3mg, Se 1µg, I 2µg, vitamin A 64µg (385µg carotene) in green cabbage, 2–6µg (15–40µg carotene) in white and red cabbage, E 0.2 mg, B_1 0.15 mg, B_2 0.02 mg, niacin 0.8 mg, B_6 0.17 mg, folate 75 µg, pantothenate 0.2 mg, biotin 0.1 µg, C 49 mg. A 95 g serving is a source of vitamin B_1; rich source of folate, vitamin C.

cabbage, Chinese Name given to two oriental vegetables: *Brassica pekinensis* (pe-tsai, Pekin cabbage, snow cabbage); pale green compact head resembling lettuce, and *B. chinensis* (pak choi, Chinese greens, Chinese chard); loose bunch of dark green leaves and thick stalks.

cabbie-claw Scottish (Shetland); fresh codling, salted and hung in open air for 1–2 days, then simmered with horseradish. The name derives from the Shetland dialect name for COD, kabbilow.

cacao butter See COCOA BUTTER.

cacen-gri Welsh; soda scones made with currants and BUTTERMILK.

cachectin (cachexin) See CACHEXIA; TUMOUR NECROSIS FACTOR.

cachexia The condition of extreme emaciation and wasting seen in patients with advanced diseases such as cancer and AIDS. Due to both an inadequate intake of food and the effects of the disease in increasing METABOLIC RATE (hypermetabolism) and the breakdown of tissue protein.

See also PROTEIN–ENERGY MALNUTRITION; TUMOUR NECROSIS FACTOR.

cachou Small scented tablets for sweetening the breath.

cadmium A mineral of no known function in the body and there-fore not a dietary essential. It accumulates in the body through-out life, reaching a total body content of 20–30 mg (200–300 µmol). It is toxic and cadmium poisoning is a recognised industrial disease.

In Japan cadmium poisoning has been implicated in itai-itai disease, a severe and sometimes fatal loss of calcium from the bones; the disease occurred in an area where rice was grown on land irrigated with contaminated waste water.

Accidental contamination of drinking water with cadmium salts also leads to kidney damage, and enough cadmium can leach out from cooking vessels with cadmium glaze to pose a hazard.

caecum The first part of the large intestine, separated from the small intestine by the ileocolic sphincter. It is small in carnivo-rous animals and very large in herbivores, since it is involved in the digestion of cellulose. In omnivorous animals, including man, it is of intermediate size.

See also GASTROINTESTINAL TRACT.

caffeine A PURINE, trimethylxanthine, an ALKALOID found in coffee and tea, also known as theine. It raises blood pressure, acts as a DIURETIC and temporarily averts fatigue, so has a stimulant action.

Acts to potentiate the action of hormones and neurotransmitters that act via cAMP, since it inhibits phosphodiesterase (EC 3.1.4.17). It can also be a cause of insomnia in some people, and decaffeinated coffee and tea are commonly available.

COFFEE beans contain about 1% caffeine, and the beverage contains about 70 mg/100 mL. Tea contains 1.5–2.5% caffeine, about 50–60 mg/100 mL of the beverage. COLA DRINKS contain 12–18 mg/100 mL.

See also THEOBROMINE; XANTHINE.

caffeol A volatile oil in coffee beans, giving the characteristic flavour and aroma.

calabasa West Indian or green pumpkin, with yellow flesh.

calabash See GOURD.

calabrese An annual plant (*Brassica oleracea italica*), a variety of BROCCOLI which yields a crop in the same year as it is sown. Also called American, Italian or green sprouting broccoli.

calamondin A CITRUS fruit resembling a small tangerine, with a delicate pulp and a lime-like flavour.

calandria A heat exchanger consisting of a closed cylindrical vessel with a number of tubes passing through.

calbindin An intracellular calcium binding protein induced by VITAMIN D; involved in CALCIUM transport.

calcidiol 25-Hydroxycholecalciferol, 25-hydroxy derivative of VITAMIN D, the main storage and circulating form of the vitamin in the body.

See also CALCITRIOL.

calciferol Used at one time as a name for ercalciol (ergocalciferol or vitamin D_2) made by ultraviolet irradiation of ergosterol. Also used as a general term to include both VITAMERS of VITAMIN D (vitamins D_2 and D_3).

calcinosis Abnormal deposition of CALCIUM salts in tissues. May be due to excessive intake of VITAMIN D.

calciol Official name for cholecalciferol, the naturally occurring form of VITAMIN D (vitamin D_3).

calcipotriol VITAMIN D analogue used as ointment for treatment of psoriasis.

calcitonin-gene related peptide Peptide hormone secreted throughout gut; decreases gastric acid secretion.

calcitriol 1,25-Dihydroxycholecalciferol, the active metabolite of VITAMIN D in the body.

calcium The major inorganic component of bones and teeth; the total body content of an adult is about 1–1.5 kg (15–38 mol). The small amounts in blood plasma (2.1–2.6 mmol/L, 85–105 mg/L) and in tissues play a vital rôle in the excitability of nerve tissue, the control of muscle contraction and the integration and regulation of metabolic processes. An unacceptably high plasma concentration of calcium is HYPERCALCAEMIA.

The absorption of calcium from the intestinal tract requires VITAMIN D, and together with parathyroid hormone, vitamin D also controls the body's calcium balance, mobilising it from the bones to maintain the plasma concentration within a very narrow range.

Although a net loss of calcium from bones occurs as a normal part of the ageing process, and may lead to OSTEOPOROSIS, there is little evidence that higher intakes of calcium in later life will affect the process.

calcium acid phosphate   Also known as monocalcium phosphate and acid calcium phosphate or ACP, $Ca(H_2PO_4)_2$. Used as the acid ingredient of BAKING POWDER and self-raising FLOUR, since it reacts with bicarbonate to liberate carbon dioxide. Calcium phosphates are permitted food additives (E-341).

calculi (calculus)   Stones formed in tissues such as the gall bladder (biliary calculus or GALLSTONE), kidney (renal calculus) or ureters. Renal calculi may consist of URIC ACID and its salts (especially in GOUT) or of OXALIC ACID salts. Oxalate calculi may be of metabolic or dietary origin and people at metabolic risk of forming oxalate renal calculi are advised to avoid dietary sources of oxalic acid and its precursors. Rarely, renal calculi may consist of the amino acid CYSTINE.

See also TARTAR.

calf's foot jelly   GELATINE, stock made by boiling calves' feet in water; it sets to a stiff jelly on cooling.

calmodulin   Small intracellular calcium-binding protein that acts to regulate adenylate cyclase (EC 4.6.1.1) and protein kinases in response to changes in intracellular calcium concentrations.

calorie   A unit of ENERGY used to express the energy yield of foods and energy expenditure by the body. One calorie (cal) is the amount of heat required to raise the temperature of 1 g of water through 1°C (from 14.5–15.5°C).

Nutritionally the kilocalorie (1000 calories) is used, the amount of heat required to raise the temperature of 1 kg of water through 1°C, and is abbreviated as either kcal or Cal.

The calorie is not an SI unit, and correctly the JOULE is used as the unit of energy, although kcal are widely used. 1 kcal = 4.18 kJ; 1 kJ = 0.24 kcal.

See also ENERGY; ENERGY CONVERSION FACTORS.

calorimeter (bomb calorimeter)   An instrument for measuring the amount of oxidisable energy in a substance, by burning it in oxygen and measuring the heat produced.

The energy yield of a foodstuff in the body is equal to that obtained in a bomb calorimeter only when the metabolic end-products are the same as those obtained by combustion. Thus, proteins liberate 5.65 kcal (23.64 kJ)/g in a calorimeter, when the nitrogen is oxidised to the dioxide, but only 4.4 kcal (18.4 kJ)/g in the body, when the nitrogen is excreted as urea (which has a heat of combustion equal to the 'missing' 1.25 kcal (5.23 kJ)).

See also ENERGY CONVERSION FACTORS.

calorimetry   The measurement of energy expenditure by the body.

Direct calorimetry is the measurement of heat output from the body, as an index of energy expenditure, and hence energy requirements. The subject is placed inside a small thermally insulated room, and the heat produced is measured. Few such difficult studies have been performed, and only a limited range of activities can be studied under these confined conditions.

Indirect calorimetry is a means of estimating energy expenditure indirectly, rather than by direct measurement of heat production. Two methods are in use:

(1) Measurement of the rate of oxygen consumption, using a SPIROMETER, permits calculation of energy expenditure. Most studies of the energy cost of activities have been performed by this method.

(2) Estimation of the total production of carbon dioxide over a period of 7–10 days, after consumption of dual isotopically labelled water (i.e. water labelled with both ^{2}H and ^{18}O). See DOUBLE-LABELLED WATER.

caltrops   See CHESTNUT, WATER.

Camembert   French soft CHEESE made from cows' milk, originating from Auge in Normandy. Covered with a white mould (*Penicillium candidum* or *P. camembertii*) which participates in the ripening process.

camomile   Either of two herbs, *Anthemis nobilis* or *Matricaria recutica*. The essential oil is used to flavour LIQUEURS; camomile tea is a TISANE prepared by infusion of the dried flower heads and the whole herb can be used to make a herb beer.

Campden process   The preservation of food by the addition of sodium bisulphite (E-222), which liberates sulphur dioxide. Also known as cold preservation, since it replaces heat STERILISATION.

Campden tablets   Tablets of sodium bisulphite (E-222), used for sterilisation of bottles and other containers and in the preservation of foods.

Campylobacter A genus of pathogenic organisms which are the most commonly reported cause of gastroenteritis in UK, although it is not known what proportion of cases are foodborne. Campylobacteriosis has been associated with the consumption of undercooked meats, milk that has been inadequately pasteurised or contaminated by birds, and contaminated water. *C. jejuni* (*C. coli*, TX 4.1.2.1) invades intestinal epithelial cells. Infective dose 10^3 organisms, onset 3–8 days, duration weeks. HELICOBACTER PYLORI was formerly classified as a *Campylobacter*.

camu-camu Fruit of the Peruvian bush *Myrciaria paraensis*; burgundy red in colour, weighing 6–14 g and about 3 cm in diameter; contains 3000 mg vitamin C/100 g.

canbra oil Oil extracted from selected strains of RAPESEED containing not more than 2% ERUCIC ACID.

cancer A wide variety of diseases characterised by uncontrolled growth of tissue. Dietary factors may be involved in the initiation of some forms of cancer, and a high fat diet has been especially implicated. There is some evidence that ANTIOXIDANT nutrients such as CAROTENE, VITAMINS C and E and the mineral SELENIUM may be protective, as may NON-STARCH POLYSACCHARIDE.

See also CARCINOGEN; CACHEXIA.

Canderel Trade name for tablets of the SWEETENER ASPARTAME.

Candida Genus of yeasts that inhabit the gut. *C. albicans* can, under some circumstances, cause candidiasis (thrush) in the vagina, mouth and skin folds.

candy (1) Crystallised sugar made by repeated boiling and slow evaporation.

(2) USA, general term for SUGAR confectionery.

candy doctor See SUGAR DOCTOR.

cane sugar SUCROSE extracted from the sugar cane *Saccharum officinarum*; identical to sucrose prepared from any other source, such as sugar beet. See SUGAR.

canihua Seeds of *Chenopodium pallidicaule*, grown in the Peruvian Andes; nutritionally similar to cereals.

cannelloni See PASTA.

canner's alkali A mixture of sodium hydroxide (and sometimes also sodium carbonate) used to remove the skin from fruit before canning.

canners' sugar See SUGAR.

canning The process of preserving food by sterilisation and cooking in a sealed metal can, which destroys bacteria and protects from recontamination. If foods are sterilised and cooked in glass jars which are then closed with hermetically sealed lids, the process is known as bottling.

Canned foods are sometimes known as tinned foods, because the cans were originally made using tin-plated steel. Usually now they are made of lacquered steel or aluminium.

In aseptic canning, foods are presterilised at a very high temperature (150–175°C) for a few seconds and then sealed into cans under sterile (aseptic) conditions. The flavour, colour and retention of vitamins are superior with this short-time high-temperature process compared with conventional canning.

canola   A variety of RAPE which is low in glucosinolates.

cantaloup   See MELON.

canthaxanthin   A red CAROTENOID pigment, not a precursor of VITAMIN A. It is used as a food colour (E-161g), and can be added to the diet of broiler CHICKENS to colour the skin and shanks, and to the diet of farmed TROUT to produce the same bright colour as is seen in wild fish.

Cape gooseberry   Fruit of the Chinese lantern *Physalis peruviana*, *P. pubescens* or *P. edulis*; herbaceous perennial resembling small cherry, surrounded by dry, bladder-like calyx, also known as golden berry, physalis, Chinese lantern, Peruvian cherry and ground tomato.

Composition/100 g: 221 kJ (53 kcal), protein 1.8 g, fat 0.2 g, carbohydrate 11.1 g (11.1 g sugars), Na 1 mg, K 320 mg, Ca 10 mg, Mg 31 mg, P 67 mg, Fe 2 mg, Cu 0.19 mg, vitamin A 238 μg (1430 μg carotene), B_1 0.05 mg, B_2 0.02 mg, niacin 0.6 mg, C 49 mg.

caper   Unopened flower buds of the subtropical shrub *Capparis spinosa* or *C. inermis* with a peppery flavour; commonly used in pickles and sauces. Unripe seeds of the nasturtium (*Tropaeolum majus*) may be pickled and used as a substitute.

capercaillie (capercailzie)   A large GAME bird (*Tetrao urogallus*), also known as wood grouse or cock of the wood.

capillary fragility   A measure of the resistance to rupture of the small blood vessels (capillaries), which would lead to leakage of red blood cells into tissue spaces. Deficiency of VITAMIN C can lead to increased capillary fragility.

See also FLAVONOIDS.

capon   A castrated cockerel (male chicken), which has a faster rate of growth, and more tender flesh, than the cockerel. Surgery has generally been replaced by chemical caponisation, the implantation of pellets of female sex hormone.

caprotil   An ACE inhibitor.

capsicum   See PEPPER.

carambola   Or star fruit, star apple; 8–12 cm long ribbed fruit of *Averrhoa carambola* and *A. bilimbi*.

Composition/100 g: 133 kJ (32 kcal), protein 0.5 g, fat 0.3 g, carbohydrate 7.3 g (7.1 g sugars, 0.2 g starch), dietary fibre 1.7 g, nsp 1.3 g, Na 2 mg, K 150 mg, Ca 5 mg, Mg 6 mg, P 15 mg, Fe 0.6 mg, Cu 0.12 mg, Zn 0.1 mg, vitamin A 6 μg (37 μg carotene), B_1 0.03 mg, B_2 0.03 mg, niacin 0.4 mg, C 31 mg.

caramel Brown material formed by heating carbohydrates in the presence of acid or alkali; also known as burnt sugar. It can be manufactured from various sugars, starches and starch hydrolysates and is used as a flavour and colour (E-150) in a wide variety of foods.

caramels Sweets similar to TOFFEE but boiled at a lower temperature; may be soft or hard.

caraway Dried ripe fruit of *Carum carvi*, an aromatic spice.

carbachol Parasympathomimetic drug used to restore the function of inactive bowels or bladder after surgery.

carbenoxolone Synthetic derivative of GLYCYRRHIZINIC acid (from LIQUORICE) used in combination with ANTACIDS for treatment of gastric ULCERS and gastro-oesophageal reflux; stimulates secretion of protective mucus.

carbohydrate Sugars and starches, which provide 50–70% of energy intake. Chemically they are composed of carbon, hydrogen and oxygen in the ratio $C_n : H_{2n} : O_n$. The basic carbohydrates are the MONOSACCHARIDE SUGARS, of which glucose, fructose and galactose are nutritionally the most important.

Disaccharides are composed of two monosaccharides: nutritionally the important disaccharides are SUCROSE, LACTOSE, MALTOSE and TREHALOSE. A number of oligosaccharides occur in foods, consisting of 3–5 monosaccharide units; in general these are not digested, and should be considered among the unavailable carbohydrates.

Larger polymers of carbohydrates are known as polysaccharides or complex carbohydrates. Nutritionally two classes of polysaccharide can be distinguished: (a) starches, polymers of glucose, either as a straight chain (AMYLOSE) or with a branched structure (AMYLOPECTIN); (b) a variety of other polysaccharides which are collectively known as NON-STARCH POLYSACCHARIDES (nsp) and are not digested by human digestive enzymes. The carbohydrate reserve in liver and muscles is glycogen, a glucose polymer with the same branched structure as amylopectin.

The metabolic energy yield of carbohydrates is 17 kJ (4 kcal)/g. More precisely, monosaccharides yield 15.7 kJ (3.74 kcal), disaccharides 16.6 kJ (3.95 kcal) and starch 17.6 kJ (4.18 kcal)/g. GLYCEROL is a three-carbon sugar alcohol, and is classified as a carbohydrate; it yields 18.1 kJ (4.32 kcal)/g.

See also STARCH; SUGAR; SUGAR ALCOHOLS.

80

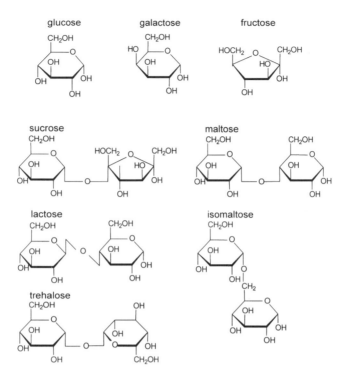

carbohydrate by difference It is relatively difficult to determine the various carbohydrates present in foods, and an approximation is often made by subtracting the measured PROTEIN, FAT, ASH and water from the total weight. It is the sum of: nutritionally available carbohydrates (dextrins, starches and sugars); nutritionally unavailable carbohydrate (pentosans, pectins, hemicelluloses and cellulose) and non-carbohydrates such as organic acids and LIGNINS.

carbohydrate loading Practice of some endurance athletes (e.g. marathon runners) in training for a major event; it consists of exercising to exhaustion, so depleting muscle GLYCOGEN, then eating a large carbohydrate-rich meal so as to replenish glycogen reserves, with a higher than normal proportion of straight-chain glycogen.

carbohydrate metabolism See GLUCOSE METABOLISM.

carbohydrate, unavailable A general term for those carbohydrates present in foods that are not digested, and are therefore excluded from calculations of energy intake, although they may be fermented by intestinal bacteria and yield some energy. The term includes both indigestible oligosaccharides and the various NON-STARCH POLYSACCHARIDES.

See also FATTY ACIDS, VOLATILE; STARCH, RESISTANT.

carbon dioxide, available See BAKING POWDER; FLOUR, SELF-RAISING.

carbon dioxide storage See GAS STORAGE.

γ-carboxyglutamate A derivative of the AMINO ACID glutamate (abbr Gla, M_r 191.1) which is found in PROTHROMBIN and other calcium-binding proteins involved in BLOOD CLOTTING. Its formation requires VITAMIN K. Also occurs in the protein osteocalcin in BONE, where it has a function in ensuring the correct crystallisation of bone mineral.

carboxymethylcellulose See CELLULOSE DERIVATIVES.

carboxypeptidases Enzymes (EC 3.4.17.1 and 2) secreted in the pancreatic juice that remove amino acids sequentially from the free carboxyl end of a peptide or protein, i.e. EXOPEPTIDASES.

carcinogen Any compound that is capable of inducing cancer, commonly by interaction with DNA.

carcinoid syndrome Condition in which there are metastases to the liver of a carcinoid tumour of the enterochromaffin cells of the small intestine. The tumour produces a variety of physiologically active AMINES, including HISTAMINE (which causes flushing reactions) and 5-HYDROXYTRYPTAMINE. The depletion of TRYPTOPHAN to form 5-hydroxytryptamine can be severe enough to lead to the development of PELLAGRA.

cardamom The dried, nearly ripe, fruit and seeds of *Elettaria cardamomum*, a member of the ginger family. An aromatic spice used as a flavouring in sausages, bakery goods, SUGAR confectionery and whole in mixed pickling spice. It is widely used in Indian cooking (the Hindi name is elaichi), and as one of the ingredients of CURRY POWDER. Arabic coffee (similar to Turkish coffee) is flavoured with ground cardamom seeds.

cardiomyopathy Any chronic disorder affecting the muscle of the heart. May be associated with ALCOHOLISM and VITAMIN B_1 deficiency.

cardoon Leafy vegetable (*Cynara cardunculus*); both the fleshy root and the ribs and stems of the inner (blanched) leaves are eaten. Sometimes called chard, although distinct from true CHARD or spinach beet.

caries Dental decay caused by attack on the tooth enamel by acids produced by bacteria that are normally present in the mouth. Sugars in the mouth promote bacterial growth and acid production; SUCROSE specifically promotes PLAQUE-forming bacteria, which cause the most damage. A moderately high intake of FLUORIDE increases the resistance of tooth enamel to acid attack.

See also TOOTHFRIENDLY SWEETS.

cariogenic Causing tooth decay (CARIES) by stimulating the growth of acid-forming bacteria on the teeth; the term is applied to sucrose and other fermentable carbohydrates.

carmine Brilliant red colour derived from COCHINEAL (E-120).

carminic acid See COCHINEAL.

carmoisine A red colour, also known as azorubine, synthetic azo-dye (E-122).

carnitine γ-Amino-β-hydroxybutyric acid trimethylbetaine, required for the transport of fatty acids into MITOCHONDRIA for oxidation. There is no evidence that it is a dietary essential for human beings, since it can readily be formed from lysine, although there is some evidence that increased intake may enhance the work capacity of muscles. A dietary essential for some insects, at one time called vitamin B_T.

carnosine A dipeptide, β-alanylhistidine, found in the muscle of most animals, function not known.

carob Seeds and pod of the tree *Ceratonia siliqua*, also known as locust bean and St John's bread. It contains a sweet pulp which is rich in sugar and gums, as well as containing 21% protein and 1.5% fat. It is used as animal feed, and to make confectionery (as a substitute for chocolate).

Carob GUM (locust bean gum) is extracted from the carob, used as an emulsifier and stabiliser (E-410) as well as in cosmetics and as a size for textiles.

Carophyll Trade name for apo-8-carotenal, a CAROTENE derivative.

carotenals Also known as apo-carotenals. Aldehydes formed by asymmetric oxidative cleavage of CAROTENE by carotene dioxygenase (EC 1.13.11.21); RETINALDEHYDE is the carotenal formed by 15-15′ cleavage of carotene. Depending on where the carotene molecule was split, the products are variously 8′-, 10′- and 12′-apo-carotenal, which may be oxidised to yield RETINOIC ACID, but cannot form RETINOL.

See also VITAMIN A.

carotene The red and orange pigments of many plants, obvious in carrots, red palm oil and yellow maize, but masked by CHLOROPHYLL in leaves. Three main carotenes in foods are important as precursors of VITAMIN A: α-, β- and γ-carotene, which are also used as food colours (E-160a). Plant foods contain a considerable number of other carotenes, most of which are not precursors of vitamin A.

Carotene is converted into vitamin A (RETINOL) in the intestinal mucosa, or is absorbed unchanged. 6 µg of β-carotene, and 12 µg of other provitamin A carotenoids, are nutritionally equivalent to 1 µg of preformed vitamin A. About 30% of the vitamin A in western diets, and considerably more in diets in less developed countries, comes from carotene.

In addition to their rôle as precursors of vitamin A, carotenes are important as ANTIOXIDANT nutrients.

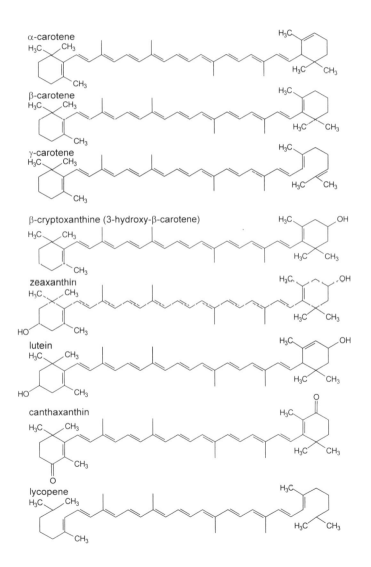

carotenoids   A general term for the wide variety of red and yellow compounds chemically related to CAROTENE that are found in plant foods, some of which are precursors of VITAMIN A, and hence known as provitamin A carotenoids.

carotenols   Hydroxylated carotenoids, including xanthophyll.

carotinaemia   Presence of excessive amounts of CAROTENE in blood plasma. Also known as xanthaemia.

carp   Freshwater FISH, *Cyprinus carpio*.
   Composition/100 g: 468 kJ (112 kcal), protein 17.5 g, fat 4.7 g (27.2% saturated, 48.4% mono-, 24.2% polyunsaturated), cholesterol 67 mg, carbohydrate 0 g, Na 43 mg, K 360 mg, Ca 47 mg, Mg 36 mg, P 240 mg, Fe 0.9 mg, Cu 0.06 mg, Zn 1 mg, Se 28 μg, vitamin E 0.6 mg, B_1 0.09 mg, B_2 0.07 mg, niacin 5.8 mg, B_6 0.17 mg, B_{12} 2 μg, pantothenate 0.2 mg. A 100 g serving is a source of Mg; a rich source of protein, niacin, vitamin B_{12}, Se.

carrageen   Edible seaweeds, *Chondrus crispus*, also known as Iberian moss or Irish sea moss, and *Gigartina stellata*; stewed in milk to make a jelly or blancmange. A source of CARRAGEENAN.

carrageenan   A POLYSACCHARIDE extracted from red algae, especially *Chondrus crispus* (Irish moss) and *Gigartina stellata*. One of the plant GUMS, it binds water to form a gel, increases viscosity and reacts with proteins to form emulsions. It is used as an emulsifier and stabiliser in milk drinks, processed cheese, low-energy foods, etc (E-407).

carrot   The root of *Daucus carota*, commonly used as a vegetable.
   Composition/100 g: 100 kJ (24 kcal), protein 0.6 g, fat 0.4 g, carbohydrate 4.9 g (4.6 g sugars, 0.2 g starch), dietary fibre 2.8 g, nsp 2.5 g, Na 50 mg, K 120 mg, Ca 24 mg, Mg 3 mg, P 17 mg, Fe 0.4 mg, Cu 0.01 mg, Zn 0.1 mg, Se 1 μg, I 2 μg, vitamin A 1260 μg (7560 μg carotene), E 0.6 mg, B_1 0.09 mg, niacin 0.1 mg, B_6 0.1 mg, folate 16 μg, pantothenate 0.2 mg, biotin 0.4 μg, C 2 mg. A 60 g serving is a rich source of vitamin A.

Carr–Price reaction   Colorimetric assay for VITAMIN A, based on the development of a blue colour after reaction with antimony trichloride in chloroform. The Neeld–Pearson method uses trifluoroacetic acid in place of antimony trichloride.

cartilage   The hard connective tissue of the body, composed mainly of COLLAGEN, together with chondromucoid (a protein combined with chondroitin sulphate) and chondroalbuminoid (a protein similar to ELASTIN). New BONE growth consists of cartilage on which calcium salts are deposited as it develops.

Cartose   Trade name for a steam hydrolysate of maize starch, used as a carbohydrate modifier in milk preparations for infant feeding. It consists of a mixture of DEXTRIN, MALTOSE and GLUCOSE.

carubinose   See MANNOSE.

cascara   See LAXATIVES.

casein   About 75% of the proteins of milk are classified as caseins; a group of 12–15 small hydrophobic proteins, in four main classes (α-, β-, γ- and κ-caseins). They occur in milk as coarse colloidal particles (micelles) some 100 mm in diameter. Often used as a protein supplement, since the casein fraction from milk is more than 90% protein.

Hammarsten's casein is prepared by diluting fat-free milk with water and precipitating the protein with acetic acid. The precipitate is washed three times with water, dissolved in ammonium hydroxide and reprecipitated; this is repeated twice. The final precipitate is washed with alcohol and ether and finally extracted with ether.

caseinogen   An obsolete name for the form in which CASEIN is present in solution in milk; when it was precipitated it was then called casein.

cashew nut   Fruit of the tropical tree *Anacardium occidentale*, generally eaten roasted and salted. The nut hangs from the true fruit, a large fleshy but sour apple-like fruit, which is very rich in vitamin C.

Composition/100 g (unsalted): 2398 kJ (573 kcal), protein 17.7 g, fat 48.2 g (20.6% saturated, 60.3% mono-, 19% polyunsaturated), carbohydrate 18.1 g (4.6 g sugars, 13.5 g starch), nsp 3.2 g, Na 15 mg, K 710 mg, Ca 32 mg, Mg 270 mg, P 560 mg, Fe 6.2 mg, Cu 2.11 mg, Zn 5.9 mg, Se 29 µg, I 11 µg, vitamin A 1 µg (6 µg carotene), E 0.9 mg, B_1 0.69 mg, B_2 0.14 mg, niacin 5.7 mg, B_6 0.49 mg, folate 67 µg, pantothenate 1.1 mg, biotin 12.7 µg. A 25 g serving is a source of vitamin B_1, Fe, Se; good source of Mg; rich source of Cu.

Casilan   Trade name for a CASEIN preparation used as a protein concentrate.

cassareep   Caribbean; boiled-down juice from grated CASSAVA root, flavoured with cinnamon, cloves and brown sugar; used as a base for sauces. It can also be fermented with MOLASSES.

cassava (manioc)   The tuber of the tropical plant *Manihot utilissima*. It is the dietary staple in many tropical countries, although it is an extremely poor source of protein; the plant grows well even in poor soil, and is extremely hardy, withstanding considerable drought. It is one of the most prolific crops, yielding up to 13 million kcal/acre, compared with YAM 9 million, and SORGHUM or MAIZE 1 million.

Cassava root contains cyanide, and before it can be eaten it must be grated and left in the open to allow the cyanide to evaporate. The leaves can be eaten as a vegetable, and the tuber is the source of TAPIOCA.

Composition/100 g: 648 kJ (155 kcal), protein 0.7 g, fat 0.2 g, carbohydrate 40.1 g (1.6 g sugars, 38.5 g starch), dietary fibre 1.9 g, nsp 1.7 g, Na 5 mg, K 350 mg, Ca 19 mg, Mg 26 mg, P 36 mg, Fe 0.5 mg, Cu 0.09 mg, Zn 0.7 mg, vitamin B_1 0.04 mg, B_2 0.02 mg, niacin 0.4 mg, folate 11 µg, C 17 mg. A 100 g serving is a source of Cu; good source of vitamin C.

Cassava meal (gari) composition/100 g: 1498 kJ (358 kcal), protein 1.3 g, fat 0.5 g, carbohydrate 92.9 g (1 g sugars, 91.9 g starch), dietary fibre 2.9 g, Ca 37 mg, P 67 mg, Fe 3.1 mg, Cu 1.4 mg, Zn 1.5 mg, vitamin E 0.1 mg, B_1 0.03 mg, B_2 1 mg, niacin 0.3 mg, C 7 mg. A 100 g serving is a source of vitamin C, Zn; good source of Fe; rich source of vitamin B_2, Cu.

See also CASSAREEP.

cassia   The inner bark of a tree grown in the Far East (*Cinnamomium cassia*), used as a flavouring, similar to CINNAMON.

cassina   A tea-like beverage made from cured leaves of a holly bush, *Ilex cassine*, containing 1–1.6% CAFFEINE and 8% TANNIN.

castor oil   Oil from the seeds of the castor oil plant, *Ricinus* spp. The oil itself is not irritating, but in the small intestine it is hydrolysed by LIPASE to release ricinoleic acid, which is irritant to the intestinal mucosa and therefore acts as a purgative. The seeds also contain the toxic LECTIN ricin.

catabolism   Those pathways of METABOLISM concerned with the breakdown and oxidation of fuels and hence provision of metabolic energy. People who are undernourished or suffering from CACHEXIA are sometimes said to be in a catabolic state, in that they are catabolising their body tissues, without replacing them.

catadromous fish   Fish that live in fresh water and go to sea to spawn, such as eels.

catalase   HAEM-containing enzyme (EC 1.11.1.6) which catalyses the decomposition of HYDROGEN PEROXIDE to water and oxygen. Its main function *in vivo* is removal of hydrogen peroxide formed by a variety of OXYGENASES. Used in food processing to remove hydrogen peroxide used as a sterilant, and together with GLUCOSE oxidase (EC 1.1.3.4) to remove traces of oxygen.

catchup   See KETCHUP.

catecholamines   General term for dihydroxyphenylamines, including DOPAMINE, ADRENALINE and NORADRENALINE.

catechol oxidase   See PHENOL OXIDASES.

catharsis   Purging or cleansing out of the bowels by giving a LAXATIVE (cathartic) to stimulate intestinal activity.

cathepsins   (Also kathepsins); a group of intracellular enzymes in animal tissues which hydrolyse proteins. They are involved in the normal turnover of tissue protein, and the softening of meat when GAME is hung.

CAT scanning   Computerised axial tomography, an X-ray technique that permits a three-dimensional X-ray image to be generated. Used nutritionally to determine ADIPOSE TISSUE distribution and BONE mass.

catsup   See KETCHUP.

caudle   Hot spiced wine, MULLED WINE.

caul   Membrane enclosing the foetus; that from sheep or pig used to cover meat while roasting.

cauliflower   The edible flower of *Brassica oleracea botrytis*, normally creamy-white in colour, although some cultivars have green or purple flowers. Horticulturally, varieties that mature in summer and autumn are called cauliflower, and those that mature in winter BROCCOLI, but commonly both are called cauliflower.

Composition/100 g: 117 kJ (28 kcal), protein 2.9 g, fat 0.9 g, carbohydrate 2.1 g (1.8 g sugars, 0.2 g starch), dietary fibre 1.6 g, nsp 1.6 g, Na 4 mg, K 120 mg, Ca 17 mg, Mg 12 mg, P 52 mg, Fe 0.4 mg, Cu 0.02 mg, Zn 0.4 mg, vitamin A 10 µg (60 µg carotene), E 0.1 mg, B_1 0.07 mg, B_2 0.04 mg, niacin 1.1 mg, B_6 0.15 mg, folate 51 µg, pantothenate 0.4 mg, biotin 1 µg, C 27 mg. A 90 g serving is a good source of folate; rich source of vitamin C.

caviar(e)   The salted hard ROE of the sturgeon, *Acipenser* spp; three main types, sevruga, asetra (ocietre) and BELUGA, the prime variety. Mock caviare (also known as German, Danish or Norwegian caviare) is the salted hard roe of the lumpfish (*Cyclopterus lumpus*).

cayenne pepper   See PEPPER.

CCK   See CHOLECYSTOKININ.

cDNA   Copy or complementary DNA; a single-stranded DNA copy of mRNA, synthesised using REVERSE TRANSCRIPTASE (EC 2.7.7.49), which can then be inserted into a PLASMID or other vector, for the introduction of new DNA into a bacterial or other cell.

Celacol   Trade name for methyl, hydroxyethyl and other CELLULOSE derivatives.

celeriac   A variety of CELERY with a thick root which is eaten grated in salads or cooked as a vegetable, *Apium graveolens* var *rapaceum*, also known as turnip-rooted or knob celery.

Composition/100 g: 75 kJ (18 kcal), protein 1.2 g, fat 0.4 g, carbohydrate 2.3 g (1.8 g sugars, 0.5 g starch), dietary fibre 5.1 g, nsp 3.7 g, Na 91 mg, K 460 mg, Ca 40 mg, Mg 21 mg, P 63 mg, Fe 0.8 mg, Cu 0.04 mg, Zn 0.3 mg, vitamin A 4 µg (26 µg carotene), B_1 0.18 mg, B_2 0.02 mg, niacin 0.4 mg, B_6 0.08 mg, folate 51 µg, C 14 mg. A 50 g serving is a source of folate, vitamin C.

celery Edible stems of *Apium graveolens* var *dulce*.
Composition/100 g: 29 kJ (7 kcal), protein 0.5 g, fat 0.2 g, carbo-
hydrate 0.9 g (0.9 g sugars), dietary fibre 1.6 g, nsp 1.1 g, Na 60 mg,
K 320 mg, Ca 41 mg, Mg 5 mg, P 21 mg, Fe 0.4 mg, Cu 0.01 mg,
Zn 0.1 mg, Se 3 μg, vitamin A 8 μg (50 μg carotene), E 0.2 mg, B_1
0.06 mg, B_2 0.01 mg, niacin 0.4 mg, B_6 0.03 mg, folate 16 μg, pan-
tothenate 0.4 mg, biotin 0.1 μg, C 8 mg. Serving 30 g (one stick).
See also CELERIAC.

celiac disease See COELIAC DISEASE.

cellobiose A disaccharide of glucose linked β-1,4; formed by
hydrolysis of CELLULOSE by CELLULASE, and not hydrolysed by
mammalian digestive enzymes.

Cellofas Trade name for derivatives of CELLULOSE: Cellofas A is
methylethylcellulose, Cellofas B is sodium carboxymethylcellulose.

Cellophane Trade name for the first of the transparent, non-
porous films, made from wood pulp (CELLULOSE) (1925). Still
widely used for wrapping foods and other commodities.

celluflour Powdered CELLULOSE, used in experimental diets to
provide indigestible bulk.

cellulase Enzymes that hydrolyse CELLULOSE. Present in the
digestive juices of some wood-boring insects and various
microorganisms, but not mammals.
1 : 4-β-glucan cellobiohydrolase (EC 3.2.9.1) is an endohydro-
lase, yielding soluble cellulose fragments. 1 : 4-β-glucan glu-
canohydrolase (EC 3.2.1.4) is an exohydrolase, yielding
CELLOBIOSE. β-Glucosidase (EC 3.7.1.21) catalyses the hydrolysis
of cellobiose to glucose.
Cell-free preparations of cellulase from *Trichoderma* spp
(especially the mesophilic fungus *T. resie*) are used to liquefy
fruit pulps, and to prepare glucose SYRUPS from waste cellulose
from pulp mills, etc.

cellulose A POLYSACCHARIDE of GLUCOSE units linked β-1,4 which
is not hydrolysed by mammalian digestive enzymes. The main
component of plant cell walls, but does not occur in animal
tissues. It is digested by bacterial CELLULASE, and hence only
RUMINANTS and animals that have a large CAECUM have an adequate population of intestinal bacteria to permit them to digest
cellulose to any significant extent. There is little digestion of cellulose in the human large intestine; nevertheless, it serves a valuable purpose in providing bulk to the intestinal contents, and is
one of the major components of DIETARY FIBRE or NON-STARCH
POLYSACCHARIDES.
See also CELLULOSE, MICROCRYSTALLINE.

cellulose derivatives A number of chemically modified forms of cellulose are used in food processing for their special properties, including:

(1) Carboxymethylcellulose (E-466), which is prepared from the pure cellulose of cotton or wood. It absorbs up to 50 times its own weight of water to form a stable colloidal mass. It is used, together with stabilisers, as a whipping agent, in ice-cream, confectionery, jellies, etc, and as an inert filler in 'slimming aids'.

(2) Methylcellulose (E-461), which differs from carboxymethylcellulose (and other GUMS) since its viscosity increases with increasing temperature rather than decreasing. Hence it is soluble in cold water and forms a gel on heating. Used as a thickener and emulsifier, and in foods formulated to be low in GLUTEN.

(3) Other cellulose derivatives used as emulsifiers and stabilisers are hydroxypropylcellulose (E-463), hydroxypropylmethylcellulose (E-464) and ethylmethylcellulose (E-465).

cellulose, microcrystalline Partially hydrolysed CELLULOSE used as a filler in slimming and other foods (E-460).

celtuce Stem lettuce, *Lactuca sativa*; enlarged stem eaten raw or cooked, with a flavour between celery and lettuce; leaves are not palatable.

centrifuge A machine that exerts a force many thousand times that of gravity, by spinning. Commonly used to clarify liquids by settling the heavier solids or separate liquids of different density, e.g. cream from milk. High speed centrifuges run up to 60000 g; preparative and analytical ultracentrifuges at 500000–600000 g.

cereal Any grain or edible seed of the grass family which may be used as food; e.g. WHEAT, RICE, OATS, BARLEY, RYE, MAIZE and MILLET. Cereals are collectively known as corn in UK, in USA corn is specifically maize. Cereals provide the largest single foodstuff in most diets; in some less developed countries up to 90% of the total diet may be cereal; in UK BREAD and FLOUR provide 25–30% of the total energy and protein of the average diet.

cerebrose Obsolete name for GALACTOSE.

cerebrosides Glycolipids containing no phosphate, but with a polar head region consisting of neutral oligosaccharides of GALACTOSE. Especially important in nerve membranes and the myelin sheath of nerves. The fatty acids may be esterified to either GLYCEROL or sphingosine (SPHINGOLIPIDS).

See also GANGLIOSIDES.

cerelose A commercial preparation of GLUCOSE containing about 9% water.

ceruloplasmin A copper-containing protein in BLOOD PLASMA, the main circulating form of copper in the body. Has ferrioxidase (EC 1.16.3.1) activity and is important in IRON metabolism. Not useful for assessment of copper status since levels are elevated in pregnancy, lactation, inflammatory diseases and in response to oral contraceptive agents.

cestode See TAPEWORM.

CF See CITROVORUM FACTOR.

cfu Colony forming units, a measure of the bacterial content of foods, etc.

chalasia Abnormal relaxation of the cardiac sphincter muscle of the stomach so that gastric contents reflux into the oesophagus, leading to regurgitation.

chamomile Either of two herbs, *Anthemis nobilis* or *Matricaria recutica*. The essential oil is used to flavour LIQUEURS; chamomile tea is a TISANE prepared by infusion of the dried flower heads and the whole herb can be used to make a herb beer.

champagne Sparkling wine from the Champagne region of north-eastern France, made by a second fermentation in the bottle. Sparkling wine from other regions, even when made in the same way, cannot legally be called champagne, but is known as méthode champenoise.

chanterelle Edible wild fungus, *Cantharellus cibarius*, see MUSHROOMS.

chappati (chapati, chuppati) Indian; unleavened whole-grain wheat or millet bread, baked on an ungreased griddle. Phulka are small chappatis; roti are chappatis prepared with maize flour.

Composition/100 g, made with fat: 1373 kJ (328 kcal), protein 8.1 g, fat 12.8 g, carbohydrate 48.3 g (1.8 g sugars, 46.5 g starch), dietary fibre 7 g; made without fat: 845 kJ (202 kcal), protein 7.3 g, fat 1 g (16.6% saturated, 16.6% mono-, 66.6% polyunsaturated), carbohydrate 43.7 g (1.6 g sugars, 42.1 g starch), dietary fibre 6.4 g; Na 130 mg, K 160 mg, Ca 66 mg, Mg 41 mg, P 130 mg, Fe 2.3 mg, Cu 0.2 mg, Zn 1.1 mg, vitamin B_1 0.26 mg, B_2 0.04 mg, niacin 3.4 mg, B_6 0.2 mg, folate 15 μg, pantothenate 0.2 mg, biotin 2 μg. A 60 g serving (1 chappati) is a source of vitamin B_1, niacin, Cu.

chaptalisation Addition of sugar to grape must during fermentation to increase the alcohol content of the WINE.

charcoal Finely divided carbon, obtained by heating bones (BONE CHARCOAL) or wood in a closed retort to carbonise the organic matter. Used to purify solutions because it will absorb colouring matter and other impurities.

charlotte Dessert made from stewed fruit encased in, or layered alternately with, bread or cake crumbs, e.g. apple charlotte. In charlotte russe there is a centre of a cream mixture surrounded by cake.

charqui (charki) S American; dried meat, normally prepared from beef, but may also be made from sheep, llama and alpaca. Strips of meat cut lengthways and pressed after salting, then air-dried. The final form is flat, thin, flaky sheets, so differing from the long strips of BILTONG. Also called jerky or jerked beef.

chartreuse (1) A LIQUEUR invented in 1605 and still made by the Carthusian monks, named for the great charterhouse (la grande chartreuse), the mother house of the order, near Grenoble in southern France. It is reputed to contain more than 200 ingredients. There are three varieties: green Chartreuse is 55%, yellow 43% and white 30% ALCOHOL.

(2) A dish turned out of a mould; more usually fruit enclosed in jelly.

Chastek paralysis Acute deficiency of vitamin B_1 in foxes and mink fed on diets high in raw fish, which contains THIAMINASE.

chateaubriand Thick steak cut from BEEF fillet. Originally named in 1822 in honour of the Comte de Chateaubriand.

CHD Coronary heart disease, see HEART DISEASE.

cheddar Hard CHEESE dating from sixteenth century prepared by a particular method (CHEDDARING); originally from the Cheddar area of Somerset, England; matured for several months or even years. Red Cheddar is coloured with ANNATTO.

Composition/100 g: 1724 kJ (412 kcal), protein 25.5 g, fat 34.4 g (66.7% saturated, 28.9% mono-, 4.3% polyunsaturated), cholesterol 100 mg, carbohydrate 0.1 g (0.1 g sugars); reduced fat varieties 1092 kJ (261 kcal), protein 31.5 g, fat 15 g (66.1% saturated, 30.9% mono-, 2.8% polyunsaturated), cholesterol 43 mg, Na 670 mg, K 77 mg, Ca 720 mg, Mg 25 mg, P 490 mg, Fe 0.3 mg, Cu 0.03 mg, Zn 2.3 mg, Se 12 µg, I 39 µg, vitamin A 362 µg (225 µg carotene), D 0.26 µg, E 0.5 mg, B_1 0.03 mg, B_2 0.4 mg, niacin 6.1 mg, B_6 0.1 mg, folate 33 µg, B_{12} 1.1 µg, pantothenate 0.4 mg, biotin 3 µg. A 40 g serving is a source of vitamin A, niacin, I, Se; good source of protein; rich source of vitamin B_{12}, Ca.

cheddaring In the manufacture of CHEESE, after coagulation of the milk, heating of the curd and draining, the curds are piled along the floor of the vat, when they consolidate to a rubbery sheet of curd. This is the cheddaring process; for cheeses with a more crumbly texture the curd is not allowed to settle so densely.

cheese Prepared from the curd precipitated from milk by RENNET, purified CHYMOSIN or lactic acid. Cheeses other than cottage and cream cheeses are cured by being left to mature with salt, under various conditions that produce the characteristic flavour of that type of cheese.

Although most cheeses are made from cow's milk, goat's milk and sometimes ewe's milk can be used to make speciality cheeses. These are generally soft cheeses. There is a very wide variety of different types of cheese. There are numerous variants (over 800) including more than 100 from England and Wales alone (nine major regional cheeses: Caerphilly, Derby, Double Gloucester, CHEDDAR, Lancashire, Red Leicester, STILTON and Wensleydale).

Some varieties are regional specialities, and legally may only be made in a defined geographical area; others are defined by the process rather than the region of production. The strength of flavour of cheese increases as it ages; mild or mellow cheeses are younger, and less strongly flavoured, than mature or extra mature cheeses. The flavour that develops on ripening is due to the activity of PROTEINASES and LIPASES, with further metabolism of free fatty acids to a variety of products.

Cheeses differ in their water and fat content and hence their nutrient and energy content, ranging from 50–80% water in soft cheeses (mozzarella, quark, boursin, cottage) to less than 20% in hard cheese (PARMESAN, Emmental, Gruyère, CHEDDAR) with semi-hard cheeses around 40% water (Caerphilly, Gouda, Edam, Stilton). They contain much of the calcium of the milk and many contain a relatively large amount of sodium from the added salt.

Blue-veined cheeses (Gorgonzola, Stilton, Roquefort, etc) derive the colour (and flavour) from the growth of the mould *Penicillium roquefortii*, during ripening.

Traditionally, hard cheeses must contain not less than 40% fat on a dry weight basis, and that fat must be milk fat. However, a number of low-fat variants of traditional hard cheeses, and vegetarian cheeses, are now made.

Cottage cheese is soft uncured white cheese made from pasteurised skim milk (or milk powder) by lactic acid starter (with or without added rennet), heated, washed and drained (salt may be added). Contains more than 80% water. Also known as pot cheese, Schmierkäse and, in USA, as Dutch cheese. Baker's or hoop cheese is made in the same way as cottage cheese, but the curd is not washed, and it is drained in bags, giving it a finer grain. It contains more water and acid than cottage cheese.

Composition/100 g: 410 kJ (98 kcal), protein 13.8 g, fat 3.9 g (66.6% saturated, 30.5% mono-, 2.7% polyunsaturated), cholesterol 13 mg, carbohydrate 2.1 g (2.1 g sugars); reduced fat varieties 326 kJ (78 kcal), protein 13.3 g, fat 1.4 g (69.2% saturated, 30.7% mono-, 0% polyunsaturated), cholesterol 5 mg, carbohydrate 3.3 g (3.3 g sugars), Na 380 mg, K 89 mg, Ca 73 mg, Mg 9 mg, P 160 mg, Fe 0.1 mg, Cu 0.04 mg, Zn 0.6 mg, Se 4 µg, vitamin

A 45 µg (10 µg carotene), D 0.03 µg, E 0.1 mg, B_1 0.03 mg, B_2 0.26 mg, niacin 3.3 mg, B_6 0.08 mg, folate 27 µg, B_{12} 0.7 µg, pantothenate 0.4 mg, biotin 3 µg. A 112 g serving (small pot) is a source of vitamin B_2, folate, Ca, Se; good source of niacin; rich source of protein, vitamin B_{12}.

Cream cheese is unripened soft cheese made from cream with varying fat content (20–25% fat or 50–55% fat).

Composition/100 g: 1837 kJ (439 kcal), protein 3.1 g, fat 47.4 g (66.2% saturated, 30.5% mono-, 3.1% polyunsaturated), cholesterol 95 mg, carbohydrate 0 g, Na 300 mg, K 160 mg, Ca 98 mg, Mg 10 mg, P 100 mg, Fe 0.1 mg, Cu 0.04 mg, Zn 0.5 mg, Se 1 µg, vitamin A 421 µg (220 µg carotene), D 0.27 µg, E 1 mg, B_1 0.03 mg, B_2 0.13 mg, niacin 0.8 mg, B_6 0.04 mg, folate 11 µg, B_{12} 0.3 µg, pantothenate 0.3 mg, biotin 1.6 µg. A 30 g serving is a source of vitamin A.

Processed cheese is made by milling various hard cheeses with emulsifying salts (phosphates and citrates), whey and water, then pasteurising to extend the shelf life. Typically 40% water, a 30 g portion contains 5 g protein, 8 g fat; provides 100 kcal (410 kJ). Soft version with 50% water is used as a spread.

Feta is Balkan (especially Greek), white, soft, crumbly, salted cheese made from goat's or ewe's milk.

Swiss cheese is an American name for any hard cheese that contains relatively large bubbles of air, like the Swiss Emmentaler and Gruyère. The holes arise during ripening from gases produced by bacteria.

cheese analogues   Cheese-like products made from CASEIN or SOYA and vegetable fat.

cheese, vegetarian   Cheese in which animal RENNET has not been used to precipitate the curd. Precipitation is achieved using lactic acid alone, or a plant enzyme or biosynthetic CHYMOSIN. Truly vegetarian cheese is made from vegetable protein rather than milk.

cheese, whey   Made from WHEY by heat coagulation of the proteins (lactalbumin and lactoglobulin).

cheilosis   Cracking of the edges of the lips, one of the clinical signs of VITAMIN B_2 (riboflavin) deficiency.

chelating agents   Chemicals that combine with metal ions and remove them from their sphere of action, also called sequestrants. Used in food manufacture to remove traces of metal ions which might otherwise cause foods to deteriorate and clinically to alter absorption of a mineral, or to increase its excretion in cases of metal poisoning, e.g. EDTA, citrates, DESFERRIOXAMINE, tartrates, penicillamine, phosphates.

See also IRON OVERLOAD.

chemical caponisation See CAPON.

chemical ice Ice containing a preservative, e.g. a solution of ANTIBIOTIC or other chemicals; used to preserve fish.

chemical score A measure of PROTEIN quality based on chemical analysis. See AMINO ACIDS.

chenodeoxycholic acid One of the primary BILE salts synthesised in the liver and secreted in the bile as a GLYCINE or TAURINE conjugate.

chenopods Seeds of *Chenopodium* spp eaten in the Peruvian Andes: *C. quinoa* (QUINOA) and *C. pallidicaule* (CANIHUA). Other *Chenopodium* spp have been considered for poultry feed, including Russian thistle, summer cypress and garden orache.

cherimoya See CUSTARD APPLE.

cherry Fruits of *Prunus* spp.

Composition/100 g: 163 kJ (39 kcal), protein 0.7 g, fat 0.1 g, carbohydrate 9.5 g (9.5 g sugars), dietary fibre 1.2 g, nsp 0.7 g, Na 1 mg, K 170 mg, Ca 11 mg, Mg 8 mg, P 17 mg, Fe 0.2 mg, Cu 0.06 mg, Zn 0.1 mg, Se 1 μg, vitamin A 3 μg (21 μg carotene), E 0.1 mg, B_1 0.02 mg, B_2 0.02 mg, niacin 0.3 mg, B_6 0.04 mg, folate 4 μg, pantothenate 0.2 mg, biotin 0.3 μg, C 9 mg. An 80 g serving is a source of vitamin C.

Peruvian cherry is CAPE GOOSEBERRY, Surinam cherry is PITANGA.

cherry, ground Fruit of *Physalis pruinosa*, similar to CAPE GOOSE-BERRY, grows wild, eaten raw but more usually boiled or as preserve; also called strawberry tomato, and dwarf Cape gooseberry.

cherry, West Indian The fruit of a small bush native to the tropical and subtropical regions of America, *Malpighia punicifolia*. It is the richest known source of vitamin C; the edible portion of the ripe fruit contains 1000 mg, and the green fruit 3000 mg/100 g. Also known as acerola, Barbados or Antilles cherry.

chervil (1) A herb, *Anthriscus cerefolium*, with parsley-like leaves, used in the fresh green state as a garnish and fresh or dried to flavour salads and soups.

(2) The turnip-rooted chervil, *Chaerophyllum bulbosum*, a hardy biennial vegetable cultivated for its roots.

(3) Sweet chervil is a wild plant (*Myrrhis odorata*) with a smell of aniseed. The leaves are used to flavour fruit cups, fruit salads and cooked fruit; the main root can be boiled, sliced and used in salads. Also known as sweet cecily.

Cheshire cat An old English cheese measure.

chestnut (1) Spanish or sweet chestnut from trees of *Castanea* spp. Unlike other common nuts it contains very little fat, being largely starch and water.

Composition/100 g (weighed with shells): 586 kJ (140 kcal),

protein 1.6g, fat 2.2g, carbohydrate 30.4g (5.8g sugars, 24.6g starch), dietary fibre 5.1g, nsp 3.4g, Na 9mg, K 410mg, Ca 38mg, Mg 27mg, P 61mg, Fe 0.7mg, Cu 0.19mg, Zn 0.4mg, vitamin E 1mg, B_1 0.12mg, B_2 0.02mg, niacin 0.7mg, B_6 0.28mg, pantothenate 0.4mg, biotin 1.2µg. A 50g serving (five nuts) is a source of Cu.

(2) Water chestnut, seeds of *Trapa natans*, also called caltrops or sinharanut; eaten raw or roasted.

(3) Chinese water chestnut, also called matai or waternut; tuber of the sedge, *Eleocharis tuberosa* or *E. dulcis*; white flesh on a black horned shell.

chestnut mushroom See MUSHROOMS.

chest sweetbread The thymus of an animal, as distinct from the gut sweetbread (sometimes called simply sweetbread), which is the PANCREAS.

chevda (chewda) A dry and highly spiced mixture of deep fried rice, DHAL, CHICKPEAS and small pieces of chickpea batter, with peanuts and raisins, seasoned with sugar and salt, a common N Indian snack food, also known as Bombay mix.

Composition/100g: 2105kJ (503kcal), protein 18.8g, fat 32.9g (12.6% saturated, 51.4% mono-, 35.8% polyunsaturated), carbohydrate 35.1g (2.3g sugars, 32.8g starch), nsp 6.2g, Na 770mg, K 770mg, Ca 58mg, Mg 100mg, P 290mg, Fe 3.8mg, Cu 0.62mg, Zn 2.5mg, vitamin E 4.7mg, B_1 0.38mg, B_2 0.1mg, niacin 7.8mg, B_6 0.54mg, pantothenate 1.2mg, biotin 24µg. A 30g serving is a source of protein, vitamin E, niacin, Mg; good source of Cu.

chewing gum Based on CHICLE with sugar or other sweetener, balsam of Tolu and various flavours.

chicken Domestic fowl, *Gallus domesticus*. There are differences between the white (breast) and dark (leg) meat, the former being lower in fat but also lower in iron and vitamin B_2. Poussin or spring chicken is a young bird, 4–6 weeks old, weighing 250–300g.

Average composition/100g: 590–900kJ (140–216kcal), protein 22.6–26.5g, fat 4–14g (31.5% saturated, 50% mono-, 18.4% polyunsaturated), cholesterol 56–103mg, carbohydrate 0g, Na 79mg, K 300mg, Ca 9mg, Mg 23mg, P 197mg, Fe 0.5–1.0mg, Cu 0.12mg, Zn 1.5mg, Se 6.5µg, I 5µg, vitamin E 0.1mg, B_1 0.06mg, B_2 0.14mg, niacin 10mg, B_6 0.19mg, folate 7.5µg, B_{12} 0.25µg, pantothenate 0.9mg, biotin 2µg. A 100g serving is a source of pantothenate, Cu, Se, Zn; good source of vitamin B_{12}; rich source of protein, niacin.

chicken, mountain See CRAPAUD.

chickling pea or vetch *Lathyrus sativus*, see LATHYRISM.

chickpea   Also known as garbanzo; seeds of *Cicer arietinum*, widely used in Mediterranean and Middle Eastern stews and casseroles. Puréed chickpea is the basis of HUMMUS and deep fried balls of chickpea batter are FELAFEL.

Composition/100 g: 506 kJ (121 kcal), protein 8.4 g, fat 2.1 g, carbohydrate 18.2 g (1 g sugars, 16.6 g starch), dietary fibre 5.1 g, nsp 4.3 g, Na 5 mg, K 270 mg, Ca 46 mg, Mg 37 mg, P 83 mg, Fe 2.1 mg, Cu 0.28 mg, Zn 1.2 mg, Se 1 µg, vitamin A 3 µg (23 µg carotene), E 1.1 mg, B_1 0.1 mg, B_2 0.07 mg, niacin 1.8 mg, B_6 0.14 mg, folate 54 µg, pantothenate 0.3 mg. A 90 g serving is a source of protein, Mg, Fe; good source of folate; rich source of Cu.

chicle   The partially evaporated milky latex of the evergreen sapodilla tree (*Achra sapota*); it contains gutta (which has elastic properties) and resin, together with carbohydrates, waxes and tannins. Used in manufacture of chewing gum. The same tree also produces the SAPODILLA plum.

chicory   Witloof or Belgian chicory (Belgian endive in USA), *Cichorium intybus*; the root is harvested and grown in the dark to produce bullet-shaped heads of young white leaves (chicons). Also called succory; red variety is radicchio. The leaves are eaten as a salad or braised as a vegetable and the bitter root, dried and partly caramelised, is often added to coffee as a diluent to cheapen the product.

Composition/100 g: 46 kJ (11 kcal), protein 0.5 g, fat 0.6 g, carbohydrate 2.8 g (0.7 g sugars, 0.2 g starch), nsp 0.9 g, Na 1 mg, K 170 mg, Ca 21 mg, Mg 6 mg, P 27 mg, Fe 0.4 mg, Cu 0.05 mg, Zn 0.2 mg, vitamin A 20 µg (120 µg carotene), B_1 0.14 mg, niacin 0.3 mg, B_6 0.01 mg, folate 14 µg, C 5 mg. Serving 20 g.

chilled foods   Foods stored at −1 to +1°C (fresh fish and meats); at 0–5°C (baked goods, milk, salads); 0 to +8°C (cooked meats, butter, margarine, soft fruits). Often combined with controlled GAS STORAGE.

chill haze   See HAZE.

chilli (chili)   See PEPPER.

chillproofing   A treatment to prevent the development of haziness or cloudiness due to precipitation of proteins when BEER is chilled. Treatments include the addition of TANNINS to precipitate proteins, materials such as BENTONITE to adsorb them and proteolytic enzymes to hydrolyse them.

chimche   Korean; fermented cabbage with garlic, red peppers and pimientos.

chine   A joint of meat containing the whole or part of the backbone of the animal.

See also CHINING.

Chinese cabbage (Chinese leaves)   See CABBAGE, CHINESE.

Chinese cherry See LYCHEE.

Chinese eggs Known as pidan, houeidan and dsaoudan, depending on variations in the method of preparation. Prepared by covering fresh duck eggs with a mixture of sodium hydroxide, burnt straw ash and slaked lime, then storing for several months (sometimes referred to as 'hundred year old eggs'). The white and yolk coagulate and become discoloured, with partial decomposition of the protein and PHOSPHOLIPIDS.

Chinese gooseberry See KIWI.

Chinese lantern See CAPE GOOSEBERRY.

Chinese restaurant syndrome Flushing, palpitations and numbness associated at one time with the consumption of MONOSODIUM GLUTAMATE, and then with HISTAMINE, but the cause of these symptoms after eating various foods is not known.

chining To sever the rib bones from the backbone by sawing through the ribs close to the spine.
    See also CHINE.

chips Chipped potatoes; pieces of potato deep fried in fat or oil. Known in French as *pommes frites* or just *frites*; in USA chips are potato crisps and chips are called French fries or fries. Fat content depends on size of chip and the process, commonly about 25% but can be 40% in fine-cut chips and as little as 4–8% in frozen oven-baked chips.

chitin Poly-N-acetylglucosamine, the organic matrix of the exoskeleton of insects and crustaceans, and present in small amounts in mushrooms. An insoluble NON-STARCH POLYSACCHARIDE. Partial deacetylation results in the formation of chitosans, which are used as protein-flocculating agents.

chitosan See CHITIN.

chitterlings The (usually fried) small intestine of ox, calf or pig.

chives Small member of the onion family (*Allium schoenoprasum*); the leaves are used as a garnish or dried as a herb; mild onion flavour.
    Composition/100 g: 96 kJ (23 kcal), protein 2.8 g, fat 0.6 g, carbohydrate 1.7 g (1.7 g sugars), nsp 1.9 g, Na 5 mg, K 230 mg, Ca 85 mg, Mg 30 mg, P 50 mg, Fe 1.6 mg, Zn 0.4 mg, vitamin A 383 µg (2300 µg carotene), E 1.6 mg, B_1 0.1 mg, B_2 0.18 mg, niacin 1.4 mg, B_6 0.2 mg, pantothenate 0.2 mg, C 45 mg. Serving 10 g.

chlonorchiasis Infestation with the liver FLUKE *Chlonorchis sinensis* in the BILE ducts. Acquired by eating undercooked freshwater fish harbouring the larval stage.

chlorella See ALGAE.

chlorine An element found in biological tissues as the chloride ION; the body contains about 100 g (3 mol) of chloride and the average diet contains 6–7 g (0.17–0.2 mol), mainly as sodium chloride. Free chlorine is used as a sterilising agent, e.g. for drinking water.

chlorine dioxide A bread improver, see AGEING.

chlorophyll The green pigment of leaves, etc; a substituted PORPHYRIN ring chelating a Mg^{2+} ion. The essential pigment in PHOTOSYNTHESIS, responsible for the trapping of light energy for the formation of carbohydrates from carbon dioxide and water. Both α- and β-chlorophylls occur in leaves, together with the CAROTENOIDS xanthophyll and carotene.

Chlorophyll has no nutritional value, although it does contain MAGNESIUM as part of its molecule, and although it is used in breath fresheners and toothpaste, there is no evidence that it has any useful action.

chlorophyllide The dull green pigment found in the water after cooking some vegetables; it is a water-soluble derivative of CHLOROPHYLL, the product of hydrolysis of the phytol sidechain, by either enzymic action (chlorophyllase, EC 3.1.1.14) in the vegetables or alkaline hydrolysis. Also formed enzymically by degradation of chlorophyll as fruit and vegetables ripen or age.

See also PHEOPHORBIDE; PHEOPHYTIN.

chlorothiazide DIURETIC drug used to treat OEDEMA and HYPERTENSION.

chlorpropamide See HYPOGLYCAEMIC AGENTS.

chlortetracycline An ANTIBIOTIC.

chlorthalidone DIURETIC drug used to treat OEDEMA and HYPERTENSION.

chocolate Made from cocoa nibs (husked, fermented and roasted COCOA beans) by refining and the addition of sugar, COCOA BUTTER, flavouring, LECITHIN and, for milk chocolate, milk solids. It may also contain vegetable oils other than cocoa butter.

Cocoa beans grow in pods contained in a soft, starchy pulp. This is allowed to ferment to a liquid that drains away leaving the beans. They are roasted, broken into small pieces and dehusked leaving 'nibs'; this is finely ground to 'cocoa mass' and some of the fat removed, leaving cocoa powder. The powder is mixed with sugar, cocoa butter (and milk powder for milk chocolate) in a MELANGUER, then subjected to severe mechanical treatment (CONCHING). The fats can solidify in six polymorphs melting at different temperatures and require cooling and reheating (TEMPERING) before being moulded into a bar.

Composition/100 g milk chocolate: 2214 kJ (529 kcal), protein 8.4 g, fat 30.3 g (61.8% saturated, 32.9% mono-, 5.2% polyunsaturated), cholesterol 30 mg, carbohydrate 59.4 g (56.5 g sugars, 2.9 g starch), Na 120 mg, K 420 mg, Ca 220 mg, Mg 55 mg,

P 240 mg, Fe 1.6 mg, Cu 0.3 mg, Zn 0.2 mg, Se 4 µg, vitamin A 6 µg (40 µg carotene), E 0.7 mg, B_1 0.1 mg, B_2 0.23 mg, niacin 1.6 mg, B_6 0.07 mg, folate 10 µg, pantothenate 1.1 mg, biotin 3 µg. A 50 g serving (small bar) is a source of Ca, Cu.

Composition/100 g plain chocolate: 2197 kJ (525 kcal), protein 4.7 g, fat 29.2 g (61.6% saturated, 33.9% mono-, 4.3% polyunsaturated), cholesterol 9 mg, carbohydrate 64.8 g (59.5 g sugars, 5.3 g starch), Na 11 mg, K 300 mg, Ca 38 mg, Mg 100 mg, P 140 mg, Fe 2.4 mg, Cu 0.7 mg, Zn 0.2 mg, Se 2 µg, vitamin A 6 µg (40 µg carotene), E 0.9 mg, B_1 0.07 mg, B_2 0.08 mg, niacin 1.2 mg, B_6 0.07 mg, folate 10 µg, pantothenate 1.1 mg, biotin 3 µg. A 50 g serving (small bar) is a source of Mg; rich source of Cu.

See also COCOA; COCOA BUTTER (substitutes).

chocolate, drinking   Partially solubilised COCOA powder for preparation of a chocolate-flavoured milk drink, containing about 75% sucrose.

Composition/100 g: 1532 kJ (366 kcal), protein 5.5 g, fat 6 g (61.4% saturated, 35% mono-, 3.5% polyunsaturated), carbohydrate 77.4 g (73.8 g sugars, 3.6 g starch), Na 250 mg, K 410 mg, Ca 33 mg, Mg 150 mg, P 190 mg, Fe 2.4 mg, Cu 1.1 mg, Zn 1.9 mg, vitamin E 0.2 mg, B_1 0.06 mg, B_2 0.04 mg, niacin 1.7 mg, B_6 0.02 mg, folate 10 µg. An 18 g serving (for one mug) is a good source of Cu.

cholagogue   A substance that stimulates the secretion of BILE from the GALL BLADDER.

cholangitis   Inflammation of the BILE ducts.

cholecalciferol   See vitamin D.

cholecystectomy   Surgical removal of the GALL BLADDER.

cholecystitis   Inflammation of the GALL BLADDER.

cholecystography   X-ray examination of the gall bladder after administration of a radio-opaque compound that is excreted in the BILE. Cholangiography is similar examination of the bile ducts.

cholecystokinin (CCK)   Peptide hormone secreted by the I-cells of the duodenum in response to partially digested food entering from the stomach. Stimulates contraction of the GALL BLADDER, secretion of BILE, secretion of pancreatic enzymes. Also stimulates contraction of the pyloric sphincter, and so controls the rate of gastric emptying. Also known as pancreozymin.

cholelithiasis   See GALLSTONES.

choleretic   An agent that stimulates the secretion of BILE.

cholestasis   Failure of normal amounts of BILE to reach the intestine, resulting in obstructive jaundice. May be caused by bile stones or liver disease.

See also BILIRUBIN, BILIVERDIN.

cholesterol   The principal sterol in animal tissues, an essential component of cell membranes and the precursor for the formation of the STEROID hormones. Not a dietary essential, since it is synthesised in the body.

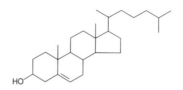

Transported in the plasma LIPOPROTEINS. An elevated plasma concentration of cholesterol in low density lipoprotein is a risk factor for ATHEROSCLEROSIS. The synthesis of cholesterol in the body is increased by a high intake of saturated FATS, but apart from people with a rare genetic defect in the regulation of cholesterol synthesis, a high dietary intake of cholesterol does not affect the plasma concentration, since there is normally strict control over the rate of synthesis.

See also HMG COA REDUCTASE inhibitors; HYPERCHOLESTERO-LAEMIA; HYPERLIPIDAEMIA; LIPIDS, PLASMA.

cholestyramine   Ion-exchange resin used to treat HYPERLIPIDAEMIA by complexing BILE SALTS in the intestinal lumen and increasing their excretion, so increasing the metabolic clearance of CHOLESTEROL.

cholic acid   One of the primary BILE SALTS synthesised in the liver and secreted in the bile as a GLYCINE or TAURINE conjugate.

choline   N-Trimethylethanolamine, a derivative of the amino acid SERINE; an important component of cell membranes.

Phosphatidylcholine is also known as LECITHIN, and preparations of mixed phospholipids rich in phosphatidylcholine are generally called lecithin, although they also contain other phospholipids; lecithin from PEANUTS and SOYA BEANS is widely used as an emulsifying agent (E-322).

Choline released from membrane phospholipids is important for the formation of the neurotransmitter ACETYLCHOLINE, and choline is also important in the metabolism of methyl groups. Synthesised in the body, and a ubiquitous component of cell membranes, therefore occurs in all foods; dietary deficiency is unknown. Deficiency has been observed in patients on long-term total PARENTERAL NUTRITION, suggesting that the ability to synthesise choline is inadequate to meet requirements without some intake. There is no evidence on which to base estimates of requirements; the average intake is between 0.25–0.5 g/day.

cholla (challa)   A loaf of white bread made in a twisted form by plaiting together a large and small piece of dough, the Biblical beehive coil. The dough is made from white flour, enriched with eggs and a pinch of saffron, and the loaf is decorated with poppyseed. It is mentioned in the Bible, translated as 'loaves' and is traditionally used for benediction of the Jewish sabbath and festivals.

chondroitin A polysaccharide, classified as a mucopolysaccharide, a polymer of galactosamine and glucuronic acid. Chondroitin sulphate is a component of cartilage and the organic matrix of bone.

chondrometer An instrument used to determine the specific weight of wheat. A wet English wheat may weigh 68 kg, and a dry American wheat 84 kg/hectolitre.

Chondrus crispus A seaweed, the source of CARRAGEENAN.

chopsuey Chinese dishes based on bean sprouts and shredded vegetables, cooked with shredded quick-fried meat, capped with a thin omelette. Not authentically Chinese, but an invention of Chinese restaurateurs in western countries. Unlike true Chinese food, the flavours of a chopsuey are all mixed together; one translation is 'savoury mess'.

Chorleywood process A method of preparing dough for breadmaking by submitting it to intense mechanical working, so that together with the aid of oxidising agents, the need for bulk fermentation of the dough is eliminated. This is a so-called 'no-time' process and saves $1^1/_2$–2 h in the process; permits use of an increased proportion of weaker flour, and produces a softer, finer loaf, which stales more slowly. Named after the British Baking Industries Research Association at Chorleywood.

choux (chou) pastry Light airy pastry, invented by the French chef Carême, used in éclairs and profiteroles. The batter is pre-cooked in a saucepan, then baked. The name comes from the French *chou* for cabbage, the characteristic shape of the cream-filled puffs.

chowder Thick soup made from shellfish (especially clams) or other fish, with pork or bacon. Originally French, now mainly New England and Newfoundland.

chromatography Technique for separation of solutes by partition between adsorption onto a stationary phase and solution in a mobile phase. The mobile phase may be gas or liquid; the stationary phase may be solid (paper, a thin layer of adsorbent or a column of adsorbent) or liquid.

High performance liquid chromatography (HPLC) uses a column of extremely uniform particles of stationary phase and a solvent under high pressure; in reverse phase chromatography the stationary phase is more lipophilic than the mobile phase.

In ion-exchange chromatography the stationary phase is an ion-exchange resin, so achieving separation on the basis of ionic charge.

In gel exclusion chromatography the stationary phase is a gel that permits molecules up to a given size to penetrate the gel matrix, so achieving separation on the basis of molecular size and shape.

chromium   A metallic element that is a dietary essential. It forms an organic complex, the GLUCOSE TOLERANCE FACTOR, and deficiency results in impaired GLUCOSE TOLERANCE. There is little evidence on which to base estimates of requirements; deficiency has been observed at intakes below 6 μg (0.12 μmol)/day, and the SAFE AND ADEQUATE INTAKE level is estimated at about 25 μg (0.5 μmol)/day.

High intakes of inorganic chromium salts (in excess of 1–2 g/day) are associated with kidney and liver damage.

chromoproteins   Proteins conjugated with a metal-containing group, such as the haem group of HAEMOGLOBIN, which contains iron.

chuck   See BEEF.

chufa   See TIGER NUT.

chuño   Traditional dried potato prepared in the highlands of Peru and Bolivia. The tubers are crushed, pressed, frozen during the night then dried in the sunshine during the day.

chyle   See LYMPH.

chylomicrons   Large plasma lipoproteins, assembled in the small intestinal mucosa, and containing mainly triacylglycerol synthesised from the products of intestinal lipid hydrolysis. Absorbed into the lymphatic system, then enter the bloodstream at the thoracic duct. Tissues take up triacylglycerol by the action of lipoprotein LIPASE, and chylomicron remnants are cleared by the liver.

See also LIPIDS, PLASMA.

chymase   Alternative name for CHYMOSIN.

chyme   The partly digested mass of food as it exists in the stomach.

chymosin   Also known as rennin, an enzyme (EC 3.4.23.4) in the abomasum of calves and the stomach of human infants which clots milk; it hydrolyses the κ-casein surrounding the CASEIN micelles, so permitting coagulation and precipitation. No evidence that it plays any part in digestion in the adult. Biosynthetic chymosin is used in cheese-making (vegetable RENNET).

See also CHEESE; RENNET.

chymotrypsin   An enzyme (EC 3.4.21.1) involved in the DIGESTION of proteins; secreted as the inactive precursor chymotrypsinogen in the pancreatic juice. It is activated by TRYPSIN, and is an ENDOPEPTIDASE, with a different specificity from TRYPSIN and PEPSIN.

chytridiomycetes   Anaerobic fungi with a motile zoospore phase resembling the flagellate protozoa of the RUMEN flora; they make a significant contribution to ruminant digestion of lignocellulose. The vegetative phase colonises lignified regions of the leaves of a variety of tropical grasses.

ciabatta   See BREAD.

cibophobia   Dislike of food.

cider, cyder   An ALCOHOLIC BEVERAGE; fermented APPLE juice (in UK may include not more than 25% PEAR juice). In USA the term cider or fresh cider is used for unfermented apple juice; the fermented product is hard or fermented cider.

   Dry cider, 2.6% sugars, 3.8% alcohol, 460 kJ (110 kcal);. sweet cider, 4.3% sugars, 525 kJ (125 kcal); vintage cider 7.3% sugars, 10.5% alcohol, 1260 kJ (300 kcal)/300 mL (half pint).

cieddu   See MILK, FERMENTED.

ciguatera   Poisoning from eating fish feeding in the region of coral reefs in the Caribbean, Indian and Pacific Oceans. The species of fish are normally edible, and appear to derive the toxins, ciguatoxins, from their diet. Reported in seafarers' tales in the sixteenth century.

ciguatoxins   See CIGUATERA.

cimetidine   See HISTAMINE RECEPTOR ANTAGONISTS.

cinnamon   The aromatic bark of *Cinnamomum* spp; it is split off the shoots, cured and dried. During drying the bark shrinks and curls into a cylinder or quill. It is used as a flavour in meat products, bakery goods and confectionery, and may be available either as the whole quill or powdered ready for use.

   Ceylon or true cinnamon (*C. zeylican*) differs from other types and the oil contains mostly cinnamic aldehyde, together with some eugenol. Saigon cinnamon also contains cineol; Chinese cinnamon has no eugenol.

cis-   Chemical description of arrangement about a carbon–carbon double bond when groups are arranged on the same side of the bond; in the *trans*-isomer they are on opposite sides of the double bond. See ISOMERS.

cissa   An unnatural desire for foods; alternative words, cittosis, allotriophagy and pica.

citral   An important constituent of many essential oils, especially lemon. Used as the starting material for the synthesis of ionone (the synthetic perfume with an odour of violets), which is an intermediate in the chemical synthesis of RETINOL.

citrange   A hybrid CITRUS fruit.

citric acid   A tricarboxylic ACID, widely distributed in plant and animal tissues and an important metabolic intermediate, yielding 10.9 kJ (2.47 kcal)/g. Used as a flavouring and acidifying agent (E-330). Citrates are used as acidity regulators (E-331–333). Commercially prepared by the fermentation of sugars by *Aspergillus niger* or extracted from CITRUS fruits, lemon juice contains 5–8% citric acid.

citrin   A mixture of two flavonones found in citrus pith, hesperidin and eriodictin. See FLAVONOIDS.

citron   A CITRUS fruit.

citronella   Lemon scented tropical grass *Cymbopogon nardus* used in salads and dressings; the essential oil is also used as an insect repellent.

citronin   A flavonone GLYCOSIDE from the peel of immature Ponderosa lemons. See FLAVONOIDS.

citrovorum factor   The name given to a growth factor for the microorganism *Leuconostoc citrovorum*, now known to be formyltetrahydropteroylglutamic acid. See FOLIC ACID.

citrullinaemia   A GENETIC DISEASE caused by lack of argininosuccinate synthetase (EC 6.3.4.5) affecting the synthesis of urea, and hence the elimination of nitrogenous waste. The defect may be mild, or so severe that affected infants become comatose and may die after a moderately high intake of protein. Treatment is usually by restriction of protein intake and feeding supplements of the AMINO ACID ARGININE, so as to permit excretion of nitrogenous waste as CITRULLINE.

Sodium benzoate (see BENZOIC ACID) may be given to increase the excretion of nitrogenous waste as hippuric acid.

citrulline   An AMINO ACID formed as a metabolic intermediate, but not involved in proteins, and of no nutritional importance.

citrus   Genus of trees with fleshy, juicy fruits; there is considerable confusion over the names because of hybridisation and mutations.

Sweet orange *Citrus sinensis*; various cultivars including Valencia, Washington navel, Shamouti. Sour, bitter, or Seville orange *C. aurantium*; too bitter to eat, used for marmalade.

Lemon *C. limon*. Lime *C. aurantifolia*. Citron *C. medica,* thick, white inner skin; used mainly to make candied peel. Pomelo (shaddock) *C. grandis*, parent of the grapefruit. Grapefruit *C. paradisi* (hybrid of pomelo and sweet orange).

Tangerine or satsuma, mandarin, calamondin, naartje (S Africa), small citrus fruit with loose skin. Clementine is a hybrid of tangerine and bitter orange, sometimes regarded as variety of tangerine. Mineola is a hybrid of grapefruit and tangerine. Ortanique is a hybrid of orange and tangerine, unique to

Jamaica. Citrange is a hybrid of citron and orange. Tangors are hybrids of tangerine and sweet orange. Ugli fruit is a hybrid of grapefruit and tangerine. Tangelo is a hybrid of tangerine and pomelo.

All are a rich source of vitamin C and contain up to 10% sugars.

cittosis An unnatural desire for foods; alternative words, cissa, allotriophagy, pica.

clabbered milk Unpasteurised milk that has soured naturally, becoming thick and curdy. Clabber cheese is curd or cottage cheese.

clams Various marine bivalve molluscs, including SCALLOP, *Tridacna gigas*, quahog, *Mya arenaria* and *Venus mercenaria*.

claret Name given in UK to red wines from the Bordeaux region of France.

clarification The process of clearing a liquid of suspended particles. It may be carried out by filtration, centrifugation (see CENTRIFUGE), the addition of enzymes to hydrolyse and solubilise particulate matter (proteolytic or pectolytic enzymes) or the addition of flocculating agents.

clarifixation A method of homogenising milk in which the cream is separated, homogenised and remixed with the milk in one machine, the clarifixator.

clarifying Of fats; freeing the fat of water so that it can be used for frying, pastry-making, etc. Clarified fats are less susceptible to RANCIDITY on storage; GHEE is clarified butter fat. Also the process of filtering juices before making jellies, etc.

Clarke degrees A measure of WATER HARDNESS.

Clegg anthrone method For determination of total available carbohydrate. The sample is digested with perchloric acid to yield monosaccharides which are determined colorimetrically using anthrone in sulphuric acid (maximum absorbance 630 nm).

clementine A CITRUS fruit, *Citrus nobilis* var. *deliciosa*; regarded by some as a variety of tangerine and by others as a cross between the tangerine and a wild N African orange.

Composition/100 g: 117 kJ (28 kcal), protein 0.7 g, fat 0.1 g, carbohydrate 6.5 g (6.5 g sugars), dietary fibre 1.3 g, nsp 0.9 g, Na 3 mg, K 97 mg, Ca 23 mg, Mg 7 mg, P 13 mg, Fe 0.1 mg, Cu 0.01 mg, Zn 0.1 mg, vitamin A 9 µg (57 µg carotene), B_1 0.07 mg, B_2 0.03 mg, niacin 0.3 mg, B_6 0.05 mg, folate 25 µg, pantothenate 0.2 mg, C 41 mg. An 80 g serving (one fruit) is a source of folate; rich source of vitamin C.

climacteric (1) Post-harvesting increase in metabolic rate and production of carbon dioxide and ETHYLENE associated with ripening in some (but not all) fruits, e.g. apple, apricot, avocado, banana, mango, peach, pear, plum and tomato. Stimulated by low concentrations of ethylene (1 ppm). Non-climacteric fruits include cherry, cucumber, fig, grapefruit, lemon, pineapple, strawberry and vegetables.

(2) Clinically, the menopause in women, or declining sexual drive and fertility in men after middle age.

clofibrate   See FIBRIC ACID.

clone   A colony of microorganisms, or a plant or animal produced by vegetative (asexual) reproduction from a single cell, so that all cells have identical genetic composition.

cloning vector   The DNA of a PLASMID or virus into which a segment of foreign DNA can be inserted in order to introduce a new gene into the cells of another organism.

Clostridium   Genus of spore-forming bacteria responsible for food poisoning.

Cl. botulinum causes BOTULISM, a rare but often fatal form of food poisoning where the exotoxins are present in the food. The spores are the most heat-resistant food poisoning organism encountered, and their thermal death time is used as a minimum standard for processing foods with pH above 4.5.

Cl. perfringens produces an ENTEROTOXIN in the gut. Infective dose 10^7–10^8 organisms, onset 8–16 h, duration 16–24 h, TX2.1.1.3.

cloudberry   An orange-yellow fruit resembling the raspberry in shape; *Rubus chamaemorus*, known as avron in Scotland, and baked-apple berries in Canada. An extremely rich natural source of BENZOIC ACID and will not ferment; remains fresh for many months without preservation.

clove   A spice, the dried aromatic flower buds of *Caryophyllus aromaticus*; mother of clove is the ripened fruit, which is inferior in flavour.

clupeine   See PROTAMINES.

CMC   Carboxymethylcellulose, see CELLULOSE DERIVATIVES.

Co I, Co II   Abbreviations of coenzymes I and II, now known as nicotinamide adenine dinucleotide (NAD) and nicotinamide adenine dinucleotide phosphate (NADP), respectively.

CoA   Coenzyme A, see COENZYMES.

coacervation   The heat-reversible aggregation of the AMYLOPECTIN form of STARCH, which is believed to be one of the mechanisms involved in the staling of bread.

coagulase   The name given to an enzyme said to be present in milk and to account for the ability of milk to clot a solution of fibrinogen.

coagulation   (1) A process involving the denaturation of proteins, loss of their native, soluble, structure, so that they become insoluble; it may be effected by heat, strong acids and alkalis, metals and various other chemical agents. Some proteins are coagulated by specific enzymic action. Denaturation is due to the breaking of hydrogen bonds which maintain the protein in its native structure. As the process continues, there is considerable unfolding of the protein, and interaction between adjacent molecules, forming aggregates which reach such a size that they precipitate.

(2) The final stage in BLOOD CLOTTING is the precipitation of fibrils of insoluble fibrin, formed from the soluble plasma protein fibrinogen, an example of coagulation caused by enzymic action. The enzyme responsible is prothrombin (EC 3.4.21.5), which is normally inactive, and is activated by a cascade of events in response to injury. VITAMIN K is required for the synthesis of prothrombin, and clotting requires calcium ions.

coalfish See SAITHE.

cob nut See HAZEL NUT.

cobalamin See VITAMIN B_{12}.

cobalt A mineral whose main function is in VITAMIN B_{12}, although there are a few cobalt-dependent enzymes. There is no evidence of cobalt deficiency in human beings, and no evidence on which to base estimates of requirements for inorganic cobalt. 'Pining disease' in cattle and sheep is due to cobalt deficiency (their rumen microorganisms synthesise vitamin B_{12}). Cobalt salts are toxic in excess, causing degeneration of the heart muscle, and habitual intakes in excess of 300 mg/day are considered undesirable.

cobamide Obsolete term for coenzymes derived from VITAMIN B_{12}: adenosyl and methyl cobalamin.

Coca Cola Trade name for a COLA DRINK.
See also COCA LEAVES.

coca leaves From the S American plant, *Erythroxylon coca*; they contain the narcotic alkaloid cocaine, and are traditionally chewed by the natives of Peru as a stimulant. Originally the beverage COCA COLA contained coca leaf extract, although this was removed from the formulation many years ago.
See also COLA DRINKS.

cocarboxylase An obsolete name for thiamin diphosphate, the metabolically active COENZYME form of VITAMIN B_1.

cocarcinogen A substance that does not itself induce cancer, but potentiates the action of a CARCINOGEN.
See also PROMOTER.

cochineal A water-soluble red colour obtained from the female conchilla, *Dactilopius coccus (Coccus cactus)*, an insect found in Mexico, Central America and the Caribbean. Colour due to anthroquinones such as kermesic and carminic acids. 1 kg of the colour is obtained from about 150 000 insects. Legally permitted in foods in most countries (E-120). Cochineal red A is an alternative name for PONCEAU 4R (E-124), often used to replace cochineal. Carmine is produced from cochineal.

cockles (arkshell)   Several types of marine bivalve molluscs of genus *Cardium*, often sold preserved in brine or vinegar.

Composition/100 g: 200 kJ (48 kcal), protein 11.3 g, fat 0.3 g, cholesterol 53 mg, carbohydrate 0 g, Na 3520 mg, K 43 mg, Ca 130 mg, Mg 51 mg, P 200 mg, Fe 26 mg, Cu 0.28 mg, Zn 1.2 mg, Se 45 µg, I 160 µg, vitamin A 1 µg (11 µg carotene), niacin 2.4 mg. A 25 g serving is a good source of I, Se; rich source of Fe.

cock of the wood   See CAPERCAILLIE.

cocoa   Originally known as cacao, introduced into Europe from Mexico by the Spaniards in the early sixteenth century. The powder prepared from the seed embedded in the fruit of the cocoa plant, *Theobroma cacao*, also a milk drink prepared with cocoa powder. Used to prepare CHOCOLATE. Contains the ALKALOIDS THEOBROMINE and CAFFEINE.

Composition/100 g: 1306 kJ (312 kcal), protein 18.5 g, fat 21.7 g (62.1% saturated, 34.9% mono-, 2.9% polyunsaturated), carbohydrate 11.5 g (11.5 g starch), nsp 12.1 g, Na 950 mg, K 1500 mg, Ca 130 mg, Mg 520 mg, P 660 mg, Fe 10.5 mg, Cu 3.9 mg, Zn 6.9 mg, vitamin A 6 µg (40 µg carotene), E 0.7 mg, B_1 0.16 mg, B_2 0.06 mg, niacin 5.6 mg, B_6 0.07 mg, folate 38 µg. A 6 g serving (one tsp) is a source of Mg; good source of Cu.

cocoa butter   The fat from the cocoa bean, used in chocolate manufacture and in pharmaceuticals; it has a sharp melting point, between 31–35°C, so melts in the mouth; mostly 2-oleopalmitostearin.

Various mixtures of vegetable fats with physical and chemical properties similar to those of cocoa butter (e.g. illipe and shea nut butter) are used as cocoa butter substitutes in the preparation of chocolate to avoid the difficulties of TEMPERING necessary with cocoa butter.

cocoa, Dutch   Cocoa treated with a dilute solution of alkali (carbonate or bicarbonate) to improve its colour, flavour and solubility. The process is known as 'Dutching'.

cocolait   A form of coconut 'milk' made by pressing COCONUTS under high pressure and homogenising the oil and water emulsion obtained. Bottled and used (e.g. in Philippines) in place of cow's milk.

coconut   Fruit of the tropical palm, *Cocos nucifera*. The dried nut is copra which contains 60–65% oil. The residue after extraction of the oil is used for animal feed. The hollow unripe nut contains a watery liquid known as coconut milk, which is gradually absorbed as the fruit ripens.

Composition/100 g: 1469 kJ (351 kcal), protein 3.2 g, fat 36 g (91.7% saturated, 5.9% mono-, 2.3% polyunsaturated), carbohydrate 3.7 g (3.7 g sugars), dietary fibre 12.2 g, nsp 7.3 g, Na 17 mg, K 370 mg, Ca 13 mg, Mg 41 mg, P 94 mg, Fe 2.1 mg, Cu 0.32 mg, Zn 0.5 mg, Se 1 μg, I 1 μg, vitamin E 0.7 mg, B_1 0.04 mg, B_2 0.01 mg, niacin 1.1 mg, B_6 0.05 mg, folate 26 μg, pantothenate 0.3 mg, C 3 mg. A 50 g serving is a source of Cu.

cocoyam W African; new cocoyam is TANNIA, old cocoyam is TARO.

cod A white FISH, *Gadus morrhua* and other species.

Composition/100 g: 334 kJ (80 kcal), protein 18.3 g, fat 0.7 g, cholesterol 46 mg, carbohydrate 0 g, Na 60 mg, K 340 mg, Ca 9 mg, Mg 22 mg, P 180 mg, Fe 0.1 mg, Cu 0.02 mg, Zn 0.4 mg, Se 28 μg, I 110 μg, vitamin A 2 μg, E 0.4 mg, B_1 0.04 mg, B_2 0.05 mg, niacin 5.8 mg, B_6 0.18 mg, folate 12 μg, B_{12} 1 μg, pantothenate 0.3 mg, biotin 1 μg. A 120 g serving is a source of vitamin B_6; rich source of protein, niacin, vitamin B_{12}, I, Se.

codeine See ANTIDIARRHOEAL AGENTS.

Codes of Practice In the area of food production these refer to standards of procedure which cannot be covered by exact specifications and serve as agreed guide lines. They may originate from government departments, trade organisations, professional institutes or individual companies.

Codex Alimentarius Originally Codex Alimentarius Europaeus; since 1961 part of the United Nations FAO/WHO Commission on Food Standards to simplify and integrate food standards for adoption internationally.

cod liver oil The oil from codfish liver; the classical source of vitamins A and D, used for its medicinal properties long before the vitamins were discovered. An average sample contains 120–1200 μg vitamin A and 1–10 μg vitamin D per gram. British Pharmacopoeia standard: minimum 180 μg vitamin A and 2 μg vitamin D per gram.

codon A sequence of three bases (PURINES or PYRIMIDINES) in DNA or MRNA that codes for an amino acid. Where codons for amino acids are shown in this book, Pu is used to indicate either purine, Py either pyrimidine, and Nu any nucleotide.

coeliac disease (celiac disease) Intolerance of the proteins of wheat, rye and barley; specifically, the gliadin fraction of the protein GLUTEN. The villi of the small intestine are severely affected and absorption of food is poor. Stools are bulky and fermenting from unabsorbed carbohydrate, and contain a large amount of unabsorbed fat (steatorrhoea). As a result of the malabsorption, affected people are malnourished and children suffer from growth retardation.

Treatment is by exclusion of wheat, rye and barley proteins

(the starches are tolerated); rice, oats and maize are generally tolerated. Manufactured foods that are free from gluten, and hence suitable for consumption by people with coeliac disease are usually labelled as 'gluten-free'. Also known as gluten-induced enteropathy, and sometimes as non-tropical sprue.

coenzymes   Organic compounds required for the activity of some enzymes; most are derived from vitamins. Coenzymes that remain tightly bound to the enzyme at all times are sometimes known as prosthetic groups, non-protein components of the enzyme molecule.

Other coenzymes act to transfer groups from one enzyme to another, e.g. coenzyme A transfers acetyl groups between enzymes, NAD transfers hydrogen between enzymes in oxidation and reduction reactions.

An enzyme that requires a tightly bound coenzyme is inactive in the absence of its coenzyme; this can be exploited to assess VITAMIN B_1, B_2 and B_6 NUTRITIONAL STATUS, by measuring the activity of enzymes that require coenzymes derived from these vitamins (see ENZYME ACTIVATION ASSAYS).

Coenzyme A (CoA) is derived from the VITAMIN PANTOTHENIC ACID; it is required for the transfer and metabolism of acetyl groups (and other fatty acyl groups). Coenzyme I and coenzyme II are obsolete names for nicotinamide adenine dinucleotide (NAD) and nicotinamide adenine dinucleotide phosphate (NADP). Coenzyme Q is UBIQUINONE; coenzyme R is obsolete name for BIOTIN.

coffee   A beverage produced from the roasted beans from the berries of two principal types of shrub: *Coffea arabica* (arabica coffee) and *C. canephora* (robusta coffee). NIACIN is formed from trigonelline during the roasting process, and the coffee can contain 10–40 mg niacin/100 g, making a significant contribution to average intakes.

Instant coffee is dried coffee extract which can be used to make a beverage by adding hot water or milk. It may be manufactured by spray drying (see SPRAY DRYER) or FREEZE DRYING. Coffee essence is an aqueous extract of roasted coffee; usually about 400 g of coffee/L.

Coffee contains CAFFEINE; decaffeinated coffee is coffee beans (or instant coffee) from which the caffeine has been extracted with solvent (e.g. methylene or ethylene chloride), carbon dioxide under pressure (supercritical CO_2) or water. Coffee decaffeinated by water extraction is sometimes labelled as 'naturally' decaffeinated.

coffee whitener   See CREAMER, NON-DAIRY.

cognac   BRANDY made in the Charentes region of NW France, around the town of Cognac, from special varieties of grape grown on shallow soil and claimed to be distilled only in pot, not continuous, stills. Sometimes used (incorrectly) as a general name for brandy.

See also ARMAGNAC.

cohort study Systematic follow-up of a group of people for a defined period of time or until a specified event, also known as longitudinal or prospective study.

cola drinks Carbonated drinks containing extract of cola bean, the seed of the tree *Cola acuminata*, and a variety of other flavouring ingredients. Cola seed contains CAFFEINE, and the drink contains 10–15 mg caffeine/100 mL, unless decaffeinated.

colcannon (1) Irish; potato mashed with kale or cabbage, often fried. See also BUBBLE AND SQUEAK.

(2) Scottish; cabbage, carrots, potatoes and turnips mashed together.

colchicine An ALKALOID isolated from the meadow saffron, or autumn crocus (*Colchicum* spp). An old remedy for GOUT, it inhibits cell division, and is used in experimental horticulture to produce plants with an abnormal number of chromosomes.

cold preservation See CAMPDEN PROCESS.

cold-shortening (of meat) When the temperature of muscle is reduced below 10°C while the pH remains above 6–6.2 (early in the post-mortem conversion of glycogen to lactic acid) the muscle contracts in reaction to cold and, when cooked, the meat is tough.

cold sterilisation See IRRADIATION; STERILISATION, COLD.

cold store bacteria See PSYCHROPHILIC BACTERIA.

cole, coleseed See RAPE.

colectomy Surgical removal of all or part of the colon, to treat cancer or severe ulcerative COLITIS.

colestipol Drug used to treat hypercholesterolaemia; it binds BILE salts in the gut, preventing their reabsorption and reutilisation, so forcing *de novo* synthesis from cholesterol.

coley See SAITHE.

colic Severe abdominal pain, of fluctuating severity, with waves of pain a few minutes apart.

coliform bacteria A group of aerobic, lactose-fermenting bacteria, *Escherichia coli* is the most important member. Many coliforms are not harmful, but since they arise from faeces, they are useful as a test of faecal contamination particularly as a test for water pollution. Some strains of E. COLI produce toxins, or are otherwise pathogenic, and are associated with FOOD POISONING.

colipase Small protein secreted in pancreatic juice; obligatory activator of pancreatic LIPASE (EC 3.1.1.3).

colitis Inflammation of the large intestine, with pain, diarrhoea and weight loss; there may be ulceration of the large intestine (ulcerative colitis).

See also CROHN'S DISEASE; GASTROINTESTINAL TRACT; IRRITABLE BOWEL SYNDROME.

collagen Insoluble protein in CONNECTIVE TISSUE, bones, tendons and skin of animals and fish; converted into soluble GELÁTINE, by moist heat. The quantity and quality of collagen in meat affects its texture, and hence toughness.

See also MUSCLE.

collagen sugar Old name for GLYCINE.

collard (collard greens) American name for varieties of cabbage (*Brassica oleracea*) which do not form a compact head. Generally known in UK as greens or SPRING GREENS.

colloid (colloidal suspension) A two phase system consisting of a solvent or dispersant medium and a separate dispersed phase. Main types are: EMULSION; FOAM; GEL; SOL.

Lyophilic colloids are those in which there is a high affinity between the particles of the dispersed phase and the dispersion medium. They include proteins and higher carbohydrates. Very viscous; electrically charged; require large amounts of electrolyte for precipitation, which is reversible. Also known as emulsions.

Lyophobic colloids are those in which there is no affinity between the particles of the dispersed phase and the dispersion medium. The particles carry an electric charge and are flocculated irreversibly by electrolytes. Also called suspensoids. For example, colloids of metals and inorganic salts.

See also EMULSIFYING AGENTS; STABILISERS.

colocasia See TARO.

cologel Alternative name for methylcellulose, see CELLULOSE DERIVATIVES.

Colombo Plan A co-operative effort to develop the resources and living standards of the peoples of S and SE Asia, started at meeting held in Colombo in 1950.

colon Also known as the large intestine or bowel, consisting of three anatomical regions: the ascending, the transverse and the descending colon. The colon normally has a considerable population of bacteria, while it is rare to find a significant bacterial population in the small intestine. The colon terminates at the rectum, where faeces are compacted and stored before voiding.

See also GASTROINTESTINAL TRACT; IRRITABLE BOWEL SYNDROME.

colostomy Surgical creation of an artificial conduit in the abdominal wall for voiding of intestinal contents following surgical removal of much of the COLON and/or rectum.

colostrum The milk produced by mammals during the first few days after parturition; compared with mature human milk, human colostrum contains more protein (2 g/100 mL compared with 1.3); slightly less lactose (6.6 g/100 mL compared with 7.2), considerably less fat (2.6 g/100 mL compared with 4.1) and overall slightly less energy, 235 kJ (56 kcal)/100 mL compared with 290 kJ (69 kcal).

Colostrum is a valuable source of antibodies for the new-born infant. Animal colostrum is sometimes known as beestings.

colours Widely used in foods to increase their aesthetic appeal; may be natural, NATURE-IDENTICAL or synthetic. Natural colours include CAROTENOIDS (red, yellow and orange colours), some of which are VITAMIN A precursors; CHLOROPHYLL (green pigments in all leaves and stems); ANTHOCYANINS (red, blue and violet pigments in beetroot, raspberries, red cabbage); FLAVONES (yellow pigments in most leaves and flowers).

There are twenty permitted synthetic colours (mainly azo dyes).

CARAMEL is used both for flavour and as a brown colour made by heating sugar.

In addition to all these there are various ingredients such as paprika, saffron, turmeric that also provide colour.

See Table 6.

colza See RAPE.

COMA Committee on Medical Aspects of Food Policy; permanent Advisory Committee to the UK Department of Health.

co-magaldrox Mixture of aluminium and magnesium hydroxides, used as an ANTACID.

combining diet See HAY DIET.

commensal Microorganisms that live in close association with another species without either harming or benefiting it, e.g. many of the intestinal bacteria, which find nutrition and a habitat in the gut, but neither harm nor benefit the host.

See also PATHOGEN; SYMBIOTIC.

comminuted Finely divided; used with reference to minced meat products and fruit drinks made from crushed whole fruit including the peel.

comparator See LOVIBOND COMPARATOR.

competitive radioassay See RADIOIMMUNOASSAY.

Complan Trade name for a mixture of dried skim milk, arachis oil, casein, maltodextrins, sugar, and vitamins, used as a nutritional supplement.

complementation Used with respect to proteins when a relative deficiency of an AMINO ACID in one is compensated by a relative surplus from another protein consumed at the same time. The

PROTEIN QUALITY is higher than the average of the individual values.

conalbumin One of the proteins of egg-white, comprising 12% of the total solids. It binds iron in a pink-coloured complex; this accounts for the pinkish colour resulting when eggs are stored in rusty containers.

conching Part of the process of making CHOCOLATE in which the mixture is subjected to severe mechanical treatment with heavy rollers to produce a uniform smooth consistency.

conditioning (of meat) After slaughter, muscle GLYCOGEN is broken down to LACTIC ACID, and this acidity gradually improves the texture and keeping qualities of the meat. When all the changes have occurred, the meat is 'conditioned'.

See also RIGOR MORTIS.

confabulation Invention of circumstantial fictitious detail about events supposed to have occurred. May occur with any form of memory loss, but especially associated with Korsakoff's psychosis in VITAMIN B$_1$ deficiency.

confectioner's glucose See SYRUP.

congee (1) Chinese soft rice soup or gruel, may be sweet or savoury.

(2) Also congie or conje, water from cooking rice; used as a drink and contains much of the thiamin and niacin from the rice.

Conge machine Used, in the manufacture of CHOCOLATE blend, for coating, to obtain smoothness by kneading the material.

congeners Flavour substances in alcoholic SPIRITS that distil over with the alcohol, a mixture of higher alcohols and esters. Said to be responsible for many of the symptoms of HANGOVER after excessive consumption.

See also FUSEL OIL.

conidendrin Substance isolated from a number of coniferous woods whose derivatives, norconidendrin and α- and β-conidendrol, are antioxidants. Chemically similar to NORDIHYDROGUAIARETIC ACID.

conjugase Intestinal enzyme, poly-γ-glutamyl hydrolase (EC 3.4.19.9) that hydrolyses the γ-glutamyl side-chain of FOLIC ACID conjugates for absorption.

conjugated linolenic acid An isomer of LINOLENIC ACID in which the double bonds are conjugated, rather than methylene-interrupted.

conjunctival impression cytology Microscopic examination of conjunctival epithelial cells to detect morphological changes due to VITAMIN A deficiency.

connective tissue Consists of the proteins COLLAGEN and ELASTIN; in fish collagen is found between the muscle segments (myotomes); in meat it is spread through the muscle, uniting the muscle fibres into bundles and supporting the blood vessels, and consists of both collagen and elastin. A high content of connective tissue results in tougher meat; collagen is softened to some extent by stewing, but roasting or frying have little effect. Elastin is unaffected by heating, and remains tough, elastic and insoluble.

constipation Difficulty in passing stools or infrequent passage of hard stools. In the absence of intestinal disease, frequently a result of a diet low in NON-STARCH POLYSACCHARIDE, and treated by increasing the intake of fruits, vegetables and especially whole grain cereal products. Severe cases may be treated by CATHARTICS, LAXATIVES or PURGATIVES.

contaminants Undesirable compounds found in foods, as a result of residues of agricultural chemicals (pesticides, fungicides, herbicides, fertilisers, etc), through the manufacturing process or as a result of pollution. For many such compounds there are limits to the amount that may legally be present in the food.

See also ACCEPTABLE DAILY INTAKE.

controlled atmosphere storage See GAS STORAGE, CONTROLLED.

convicine One of the toxins in broad beans, responsible for the acute haemolytic anaemia of FAVISM.

cook-chill A method of catering involving cooking followed by fast chilling and storage at −1 to +5°C, giving a storage time of only a few days.

cooker, fireless See HAYBOX COOKING.

cook-freeze A method of catering involving cooking followed by rapid freezing and storage below −18°C, giving a storage time of several months.

cookie See BISCUIT.

cooking Required to make food more palatable, more digestible and safer. There is breakdown of the CONNECTIVE TISSUE in meat, softening of the CELLULOSE in plant tissues, and proteins are denatured by heating, so increasing their digestibility.

In general, water-soluble vitamins and minerals are lost in the cooking water, the amount depending on the surface area–volume ratio, i.e. greater losses take place from finely cut or minced foods. Fat-soluble vitamins are little affected except at frying temperatures. Proteins suffer reduction of available lysine when they are heated in the presence of reducing substances, and further loss at high temperature. Dry heat, as in baking, results in some loss of vitamin B_1 and available lysine. The most sensitive nutrients are vitamins C and B_1.

cooler shrink Surface dehydration of meat and poultry kept under refrigeration.

Coomassie brilliant blue Dye used for detection and determination of proteins (the Bradford method), especially in electrophoretic gels; sensitivity 20 μg/mL, maximum absorbance 595 nm; dye binding capacity of proteins depends on the content of basic amino acids.

co-phenotrope See ANTIMOTILITY AGENTS.

copper A dietary essential trace metal, which forms the PROSTHETIC GROUP of a number of enzymes. The REFERENCE NUTRIENT INTAKE is 1.2 mg/day. Toxic in excess, and it is recommended that not more than 2–10 mg/day should be consumed habitually.

copra Dried COCONUT used for production of oil for MARGARINE and soap manufacture.

coprolith Mass of hard faeces in colon or rectum due to chronic CONSTIPATION.

coprophagy Eating of faeces. Since B vitamins are synthesised by intestinal bacteria, animals that eat their faeces can make use of these vitamins, which are not absorbed from the large intestine, the site of bacterial action.

CoQ See UBIQUINONE.

coquille St Jacques See SCALLOP.

coracan See MILLET.

coral The ovaries of female LOBSTERS, used as the basis for sauces; red coloured when cooked.

cordial, fruit Originally a fruit LIQUEUR, and still used in this sense in USA; in UK a cordial is now used to mean any fruit drink, usually a concentrate to be diluted. See SOFT DRINKS.

coriander *Coriandrum sativum* (a member of the parsley family); the leaf is used fresh or dried as a herb, and the dried ripe fruit (also called dhanyia) as a spice.

Composition/100 g leaves: 83 kJ (20 kcal), protein 2.4 g, fat 0.6 g, carbohydrate 1.8 g (1.5 g sugars, 0.3 g starch), Na 28 mg, K 540 mg, Ca 98 mg, Mg 26 mg, P 36 mg, Fe 1.9 mg, Cu 0.1 mg, Zn 0.2 mg, vitamin A 101 μg (610 μg carotene), B_1 0.07 mg, B_2 0.12 mg, niacin 1.1 mg, B_6 0.18 mg, folate 18 μg, C 63 mg. A 10 g serving is a source of vitamin C.

corked Of wines, the development of an unpleasant flavour due to fungal contamination of the cork.

corm The thickened, underground base of the stem of plants, often called bulbs, as, for example, TARO and ONION.

corn The seed of a cereal plant, especially that of the chief cereal of the district, thus in England WHEAT, in Scotland OATS, in USA MAIZE.

corned beef In UK a canned product made from low quality beef that has been partially extracted with hot water to make MEAT EXTRACT. In USA and elsewhere corned beef is pickled beef (in UK this is salt beef).

Composition/100 g: 908 kJ (217 kcal), protein 26.9 g, fat 12.1 g (55.2% saturated, 42.1% mono-, 2.6% polyunsaturated), cholesterol 93 mg, carbohydrate 0 g, Na 950 mg, K 140 mg, Ca 14 mg, Mg 15 mg, P 120 mg, Fe 2.9 mg, Cu 0.24 mg, Zn 5.6 mg, Se 8 µg, I 14 µg, vitamin E 0.8 mg, B_2 0.23 mg, niacin 9 mg, B_6 0.06 mg, folate 2 µg, B_{12} 2 µg, pantothenate 0.4 mg, biotin 2 µg. A 50 g serving (one thick slice) is a source of Fe, Cu, Se, Zn; good source of protein, niacin; rich source of vitamin B_{12}.

Cornell bread See BREAD.

cornflour Purified starch from maize; in the USA called corn starch. Used in custard, blancmange and baking powders and for thickening sauces and gravies.

corn grits See HOMINY.

corn, Guinea, kaffir See SORGHUM.

Cornish pastie Traditional Cornish pastry turnover with a variety of fillings, commonly seasoned meat and cooked vegetables. Historically meat baked in a pastry crust without a dish.

corn oil (maize oil) Extracted from maize germ, *Zea mays*; 13% saturated, 27% mono-, 60% polyunsaturated fatty acids.

corn pone Small corn (maize) cakes, a speciality of Alabama, USA.

corn salad Winter salad vegetable, *Valeriana olitoria*, also known as lamb's lettuce.

corn starch See CORNFLOUR.

corn starch hydrolysate, corn syrup See SYRUP.

corn sugar See GLUCOSE.

coronary heart disease See ISCHAEMIC HEART DISEASE.

coronary thrombosis See ATHEROSCLEROSIS.

corrinoids Compounds with the corrin ring structure of VITAMIN B_{12}; some have vitamin activity.

corticosteroids Steroid HORMONES synthesised in the adrenal cortex. Two main groups: glucocorticoids (e.g. cortisol, cortisone, corticosterone) involved in glucose homeostasis, and mineralo-corticoids (e.g. aldosterone) involved in salt and water balance.

cossettes Thin chips of sugar beet shredded for hot-water extraction of the sugar.

cottonseed Seed of *Gossypium* spp; of double use in the food field because the oil is valuable as cooking oil, or for margarine manufacture when hardened, and the protein residue is a valuable animal feedingstuff. The oil is 25% saturated and 50% polyunsaturated.

coulis Also cullis; originally the juices that run out of meat when it is cooked, now used to mean rich sauce or gravy made from meat juices, puréed shellfish, vegetables or fruit. Most usually now a sauce made from puréed and sieved fruit.

coumarin   See DICOUMAROL.

courgette   Variety of MARROW developed to be harvested when small; also known as Italian marrow, Italian squash or zucchini.

Composition/100 g: 79 kJ (19 kcal), protein 2 g, fat 0.4 g, carbohydrate 2 g (1.9 g sugars, 0.1 g starch), nsp 1.2 g, Na 1 mg, K 210 mg, Ca 19 mg, Mg 17 mg, P 36 mg, Fe 0.6 mg, Cu 0.01 mg, Zn 0.2 mg, Se 1 µg, vitamin A 73 µg (440 µg carotene), B_1 0.08 mg, B_2 0.02 mg, niacin 0.5 mg, B_6 0.09 mg, folate 31 µg, pantothenate 0.1 mg, C 11 mg. A 100 g serving is a source of folate, vitamin C.

Courlose   Trade name for sodium carboxymethylcellulose. See CELLULOSE DERIVATIVES.

couscous   N African; millet flour or fine semolina, steamed until fluffy and traditionally served with mutton stew.

Composition/100 g: 950 kJ (227 kcal), protein 5.7 g, fat 1 g, carbohydrate 51.3 g, Ca 19 mg, P 240 mg, Fe 5 mg, vitamin B_1 0.2 mg, B_2 0.06 mg, niacin 1.9 mg. A 150 g serving is a source of protein, niacin; good source of vitamin B_1; rich source of Fe.

cow-heel   Dish made from heel of ox or cow, stewed to a jelly; also known as neat's-foot.

cow manure factor   See VITAMIN B_{12}.

cow pea   See BEAN, BLACK EYED.

C-peptide   The linking region between the A- and B-chains of PRO-INSULIN, cleaved in the conversion of pro-insulin to INSULIN. Useful as an index of pancreatic β-islet cell function since it is cleared from the circulation more slowly than is insulin.

crab   SHELLFISH; *Cancer* and *Carcinus* spp; king crab is *Limulus polyphemus*.

Composition/100 g: 104 kJ (25 kcal), protein 4 g, fat 1 g, cholesterol 11 mg, carbohydrate 0 g, Na 73 mg, K 54 mg, Ca 6 mg, Mg 10 mg, P 70 mg, Fe 0.3 mg, Cu 1 mg, Zn 1.1 mg, Se 3 µg, vitamin B_1 0.02 mg, B_2 0.03 mg, niacin 1.3 mg, B_6 0.07 mg, folate 4 µg, pantothenate 0.1 mg. A 325 g serving ($^1/_2$ dressed crab) a source of vitamin B_6, Mg; good source of protein, niacin, Se, Zn; rich source of Cu.

crab stick   See SEAFOOD STICK.

crackers   Plain thin biscuits such as water biscuits, cream crackers and wholemeal crackers, made from wheat flour, fat and bicarbonate as a raising agent.

cran   A traditional measure for herrings containing $37^1/_2$ gallons (167 L) or about 800 fish.

cranberry   The fleshy, acid fruit of *Vaccinium oxycoccus* or *V. macrocarpon*, resembling a cherry; commonly used to make sauce and juice.

Composition/100 g: 62 kJ (15 kcal), protein 0.4 g, fat 0.1 g, carbohydrate 3.4 g (3.4 g sugars), dietary fibre 3.8 g, nsp 3 g, Na 2 mg,

K 95 mg, Ca 12 mg, Mg 7 mg, P 11 mg, Fe 0.7 mg, Cu 0.05 mg, Zn 0.2 mg, vitamin A 3 μg (22 μg carotene), B_1 0.03 mg, B_2 0.02 mg, niacin 0.2 mg, B_6 0.07 mg, folate 2 μg, pantothenate 0.2 mg, C 13 mg. An 80 g serving is a source of vitamin C.

crapaud Large edible Caribbean frogs, also known as mountain chicken.

crawfish Crustaceans (without claws), family Palinuridae, also called spiny lobster, rock lobster, sea crayfish. See LOBSTER.

crayfish Crustaceans; freshwater crayfish are members of the families Astacidae, Parasiticidae and Austroastacidae. Sea crayfish (CRAWFISH) are Palinuridae.

Composition/100 g: 280 kJ (67 kcal), protein 14.9 g, fat 0.8 g, cholesterol 105 mg, carbohydrate 0 g, Na 150 mg, K 260 mg, Ca 33 mg, Mg 25 mg, P 240 mg, Fe 2.2 mg, Cu 0.44 mg, Zn 1.3 mg, Se 70 μg, I 100 μg, vitamin B_1 0.05 mg, B_2 0.04 mg, niacin 4.7 mg, B_6 0.07 mg, folate 30 μg, B_{12} 2 μg, pantothenate 0.6 mg. A 40 g serving is a source of protein, niacin; good source of Cu, I; rich source of vitamin B_{12}, Se.

See also LOBSTER.

cream Fatty part of milk; 4% of ordinary milk, 4.8% Channel Islands milk. Half cream is similar to 'top of the milk', 12% fat, cannot be whipped or frozen; single cream, 18% fat, will not whip and cannot be frozen unless included in a frozen dish; extra thick single cream is also 18% fat, but has been homogenised to a thick spoonable consistency; whipping cream, will whip to double volume, 34% fat; double cream, will whip and can be frozen, 48% fat; clotted, Devonshire and Cornish, 55% fat.

Composition/100 g single cream: 828 kJ (198 kcal), protein 2.6 g, fat 19.1 g (66.4% saturated, 30.7% mono-, 2.7% polyunsaturated), cholesterol 55 mg, carbohydrate 4.1 g (4.1 g sugars), Na 49 mg, K 120 mg, Ca 91 mg, Mg 9 mg, P 76 mg, Fe 0.1 mg, Zn 0.5 mg, vitamin A 335 μg (125 μg carotene), D 0.14 μg, E 0.4 mg, B_1 0.04 mg, B_2 0.17 mg, niacin 0.7 mg, B_6 0.05 mg, folate 7 μg, B_{12} 0.3 μg, pantothenate 0.3 mg, biotin 1.8 μg, C 1 mg.

Composition/100 g double cream: 1879 kJ (449 kcal), protein 1.7 g, fat 48 g (66.2% saturated, 30.6% mono-, 3% polyunsaturated), cholesterol 130 mg, carbohydrate 2.7 g (2.7 g sugars), Na 37 mg, K 65 mg, Ca 50 mg, Mg 6 mg, P 50 mg, Fe 0.2 mg, Zn 0.2 mg, vitamin A 654 μg (325 μg carotene), D 0.27 μg, E 1.1 mg, B_1 0.02 mg, B_2 0.16 mg, niacin 0.4 mg, B_6 0.03 mg, folate 7 μg, B_{12} 0.2 μg, pantothenate 0.2 mg, biotin 1.1 μg, C 1 mg. A 30 g serving (one tablespoon) is a good source of vitamin A.

Composition/100 g clotted cream: 2452 kJ (586 kcal), protein 1.6 g, fat 63.5 g (66.2% saturated, 30.7% mono-, 3% polyunsaturated), cholesterol 170 mg, carbohydrate 2.3 g (2.3 g sugars),

Na 18 mg, K 55 mg, Ca 37 mg, Mg 5 mg, P 40 mg, Fe 0.1 mg, Cu 0.09 mg, Zn 0.2 mg, vitamin A 819 µg (685 µg carotene), D 0.28 µg, E 1.5 mg, B_1 0.02 mg, B_2 0.16 mg, niacin 0.4 mg, B_6 0.03 mg, folate 6 µg, B_{12} 0.1 µg, pantothenate 0.1 mg, biotin 1 µg. A 25 g serving is a good source of vitamin A.

Soured cream is made from single cream; crème fraîche is soured double cream; 'extra thick double cream' is also 48% fat, but has been homogenised to be spoonable, and will not whip or freeze successfully.

cream, artificial   A name given to
(1) emulsion of vegetable oil, milk or milk powder, egg yolk and sugar,
(2) emulsion of water with methyl CELLULOSE, MONOGLYC-ERIDES, and other materials.

cream, bitty   Cream on the surface of milk appears as particles of fat released from fat globules when the membrane is broken down by LECITHINASE from *Bacillus cereus*, the spores of which have resisted destruction during PASTEURISATION.

creamer, non-dairy   Milk substitute used in tea and coffee (coffee whitener or creamer) made with glucose, fat and emulsifying salts. A stable product dry or as liquid. May be made with CASEIN, in which case it is not technically (or by US law) non-dairy.

creaming   Beating together fat and sugar to give a fluffy mixture, for making cakes with a high fat content. The creaming quality of a fat is its ability to take up air during mixing.

cream line index   The cream line or layer usually forms about 6% of the total depth of milk. The cream line index is the ratio between the percentage cream layer and the percentage of fat in the milk; in bulk pasteurised milk it is about 1.7.

cream of tartar   Potassium hydrogen tartrate, used with SODIUM BICARBONATE as BAKING POWDER because it acts more slowly than TARTARIC ACID and gives a more prolonged evolution of carbon dioxide. This is tartrate baking powder. Also used to invert SUGAR in making boiled sweets.

cream, plastic   A term used for a cream containing as much fat as butter (80–83%) but as an emulsion of fat in water, while butter is water in fat. Prepared by intense centrifugal treatment of cream; crumbly, not greasy, in texture; used for preparation of cream cheese and whipped cream.

cream, sleepy   Cream that will not churn to butter in the normal time.

cream, synthetic   See CREAM, ARTIFICIAL.

creatine   Amino-iminomethyl-*N*-methyl glycine, important in muscle as a store of phosphate for resynthesis of ATP during muscle contraction and work.

Synthesised in the body from the AMINO ACIDS glycine and argi-nine, and no evidence that a dietary intake is essential, nor that additional intake has any effect on muscle work output.

Meat extract contains a mixture of creatine and CREATININE derived from the creatine that was present in the fresh muscle. Creatine plus creatinine is used as an index of quality of com-mercial meat extract, and as a measure of meat extract present in manufactured products, such as soups.

Urinary excretion of creatine occurs only when there is muscle loss.

creatinine The anhydride of creatine, formed non-enzymically from CREATINE and creatine phosphate, and not usable.

Urinary excretion of creatinine can be used to estimate total muscle mass, 1 g of creatinine excreted/24 h represents 18–20 kg of fat-free muscle tissue. The creatinine/height index is the ratio of urinary creatinine excretion over 24 h/that expected for height. It provides an index of protein depletion.

creatorrhoea Excessive loss of nitrogenous compounds in faeces as a result of impaired intestinal digestion of proteins or absorp-tion of amino acids.

creeping sickness OSTEOMALACIA in livestock due to phosphate deficiency.

crème (1) Term used for cream, custards and desserts. Crème brûlée is cream and egg custard with sugar sprinkled on top and caramelised under a hot grill; a traditional speciality of Trinity College Cambridge, and also known as burnt cream or Cambridge cream. Crème caramel is topped with caramel. Crème Chantilly is whipped cream sweetened and flavoured with VANILLA.

(2) Various liqueurs, including: crème de bananes (banana); crème de cacao (chocolate); crème de café (coffee); crème de menthe (peppermint); crème de mûres (wild blackberries); crème de myrtilles (wild bilberries); crème de noix (green walnuts and honey); crème de violettes (violet petals).

crème fraîche Double CREAM that has been thickened and slightly soured by lactic fermentation.

cress Garden cress, pepper grass, *Lepidium sativum*. Seed leaves eaten raw with mustard seed leaves: mustard and cress or salad rape (*Brassica napus* var. *napus*). American or land cress is *Barbarea verna*, the leaves have a peppery flavour. Unlike WATERCRESS it can be grown in soil without running water.

Creta Praeparata British Pharmacopoeia name for prepared chalk, made by washing and drying naturally occurring calcium carbonate. The form in which calcium is added to flour (14 oz per 280 lb sack, or approximately 3 g/kg).

cretinism Severe underactivity of the thyroid (see THYROID HORMONES) gland (hypothyroidism) in children, resulting in poor growth, deafness and severe mental retardation. Hypothyroidism in adults is myxoedema. Commonly the result of a dietary deficiency of IODINE; may be congenital if the mother's iodine intake was severely inadequate during pregnancy.

crevettes See SHRIMPS.

crispbread Name given to a flour and water wafer, originally Swedish and made from rye flour, but may be made from wheat flour. They have a much lower water content than bread and some brands are richer in protein because of added wheat GLUTEN.

crisps See CHIPS; POTATO CRISPS.

cristal height A measure of leg length taken from the floor to the summit of the iliac crest. As a proportion of height it increases with age in children, and a reduced rate of increase indicates undernutrition.

See also ANTHROPOMETRY.

crocin See SAFFRON.

Crohn's disease Chronic inflammatory disease of the bowel, commonly the terminal ileum, of unknown aetiology, treated with antibiotics to prevent infection and anti-inflammatory agents. Sufferers may be malnourished as a result of both loss of appetite due to illness and also malabsorption. Also known as regional enteritis, since only some regions of the gut are affected.

See also GASTROINTESTINAL TRACT.

cromoglycate 1,2-Bis(2-carboxychromon-5-yloxy)-2-hydropropane, used in treatment of vomiting, colic and diarrhoea associated with food ALLERGY and IRRITABLE BOWEL SYNDROME; also used in treatment of other allergic reactions. Trade name Cromlyn.

cropadeau Scottish; oatmeal dumpling with haddock liver in the middle.

crowdie Scottish; soft cheese made from buttermilk or soured milk curd, also a dish of buttermilk and oatmeal.

crowdies See MILK, FERMENTED.

Cruciferae Family of plants with flowers with four equal petals; most vegetables in this family belong to the genus BRASSICA.

crude fibre See FIBRE, CRUDE.

crude protein See PROTEIN, CRUDE.

crumb softeners Derivatives of mono-acylglycerols (monoglycerides) added to bread as emulsifiers to give a softer crumb and retard staling (E-430–436); also called polysorbates.

See also SUPERGLYCINERATED FATS.

crustacea Zoological class of hard-shelled marine arthropods (SHELLFISH) including CRABS, CRAYFISH, LOBSTER, PRAWNS, SCAMPI, SHRIMPS.

cryodesiccation See FREEZE DRYING.

cryogenic freezing Effected by substances that change phase by absorbing LATENT HEAT such as solid or liquid carbon dioxide, liquid nitrogen.

Cryovac Trade name of thermoplastic resin wrapping film which can be heat-shrunk onto foods.

cryptoxanthin Hydroxylated CAROTENOID found in a few foods such as yellow MAIZE and the seeds of *PHYSALIS*. VITAMIN A active.

crystal boiling Chinese method of cooking; food is heated in a pan of boiling water, then removed from the heat and cooking continued by the retained heat.

crystallin The protein of the lens of the eye. Uniquely among body proteins, there is no turnover of crystallin, and while the amount increases with growth, crystallin formed before birth remains in the lens until death.

CSM Corn-soya-milk; a protein-rich baby food (20% protein) made in the USA from 68% precooked maize (corn), 25% defatted soya flour and 5% skim milk powder, with added vitamins and calcium carbonate.

CTC machine A device consisting of two contrarotating toothed rollers that rotate at different speeds and provide a crushing, tearing and curling action, used in breaking up leaves of tea to form small particles.

cubeb Grey pepper (*Piper cubeba*) native to SE Asia; pungent flavour akin to camphor.

cucumber Fruit of *Cucumis sativus*, a member of the GOURD family, eaten as a salad vegetable.

Composition/100 g: 41 kJ (10 kcal), protein 0.7 g, fat 0.1 g, carbohydrate 1.5 g (1.4 g sugars, 0.1 g starch), dietary fibre 0.7 g, nsp 0.6 g, Na 3 mg, K 140 mg, Ca 18 mg, Mg 8 mg, P 49 mg, Fe 0.3 mg, Cu 0.01 mg, Zn 0.1 mg, I 3 µg, vitamin A 10 µg (60 µg carotene), E 0.1 mg, B_1 0.03 mg, B_2 0.01 mg, niacin 0.3 mg, B_6 0.04 mg, folate 9 µg, pantothenate 0.3 mg, biotin 0.9 µg, C 2 mg. Serving 25 g.

See also GHERKIN.

cucurbit A term used for vegetables of the family Cucurbitaceae, see GOURDS.

cultivar A plant variety that has arisen in cultivation.

cumin (cummin) Pungent herb, the crescent-shaped seed of *Cuminum cyminum* (parsley family). Black cumin is the seed of *Nigella sativa* (fennel flower) and sweet cumin is ANISE (*Pimpinella anisum*).

cumquat See KUMQUAT.

cup N American and Australian measure for ingredients in cooking; the standard American cup contains 250 mL (8 fl oz).

curcumin Yellow pigment extracted from the rhizomes of turmeric, *Curcuma longa*.

curds Clotted protein formed when milk is treated with RENNET; the fluid left is WHEY.

curd tension A measure of the toughness of the curd formed from milk by the digestive enzymes, and used as an index of the digestibility of the milk. The sample is coagulated with CHYMOSIN and the force needed to pull a knife-blade through the curd is measured under standardised conditions.

Ideal score is zero, below 20 g satisfactory; cow's milk 46; diluted with equal volume of water 20; reconstituted spray-dried milk 10; reconstituted roller-dried milk 5; evaporated milk 3; human milk 1.

curing, of meat A method of preservation by treating with SALT and sodium nitrate (and nitrite), which serves to inhibit the growth of pathogenic organisms while salt-tolerant bacteria develop. During the PICKLING process the nitrate is converted into nitrite, which reacts with myoglobin, to form nitrosomyoglobin, the characteristic red colour of pickled meat products.

currants Fruit of *Ribes* spp; See BLACKCURRANTS; RED CURRANTS; WHITE CURRANTS.

currants, dried Made by drying the small seedless black grapes grown in Greece and Australia; usually dried in bunches on the vine or after removal from the vine on supports. The name is derived from *raisins of Corauntz* (Corinth).

Composition/100 g: 1117 kJ (267 kcal), protein 2.3 g, fat 0.4 g, carbohydrate 67.8 g (67.8 g sugars), dietary fibre 5.9 g, nsp 1.9 g, Na 14 mg, K 720 mg, Ca 93 mg, Mg 30 mg, P 71 mg, Fe 1.3 mg, Cu 0.81 mg, Zn 0.3 mg, vitamin A 1 μg (6 μg carotene), B_1 0.16 mg, B_2 0.05 mg, niacin 1.1 mg, B_6 0.23 mg, folate 4 μg, pantothenate 0.1 mg, biotin 4.8 μg. A 30 g serving (one tablespoon) is a rich source of Cu.

See also RAISINS; SULTANAS.

curry Name given by the British (it means *sauce* in Tamil) to an Indian dish of stewed meat or vegetables. It is served with a pungent sauce whose components and pungency vary.

See also CURRY POWDER; VINDALOO.

curry plant (curry leaves) An aromatic herb, *Murraya koenigii*.

curry powder A mixture of turmeric with spices including cardamom, cinnamon, cloves, coriander, cumin and fenugreek, made pungent with mustard, chilli and pepper. A 10 g portion can contain 7.5–10 mg iron, but much of this is probably the result of contamination during the milling of the spices.

cushion   The cut nearest the udder in lamb or beef.

custard   Sweet sauce, traditionally made by cooking milk with eggs; more commonly using custard powder (coloured and flavoured CORNFLOUR) and milk.

Composition/100 g custard powder: 1481 kJ (354 kcal), protein 0.6 g, fat 0.7 g (20% saturated, 20% mono-, 60% polyunsaturated), carbohydrate 92 g (92 g starch), nsp 0.1 g, Na 320 mg, K 61 mg, Ca 15 mg, Mg 7 mg, P 39 mg, Fe 1.4 mg, Cu 0.05 mg, Zn 0.3 mg, vitamin niacin 0.1 mg. Serving 30 g (one tablespoon).

custard apple   The fruit of one of a number of tropical American trees, *Anona* spp. Sour sop, *A. muricata*, has white fibrous flesh and is less sweet than the others; the fruit may weigh up to 4 kg (8 lb). The sweet sop (*A. squamosa*) is also known as the 'true' custard apple, or sugar apple.

Composition/100 g: 288 kJ (69 kcal), protein 1.6 g, fat 0.3 g, carbohydrate 16.1 g (14.9 g sugars, 1.2 g starch), Na 7 mg, K 290 mg, Ca 21 mg, Mg 34 mg, P 35 mg, Fe 0.6 mg, Cu 0.15 mg, Zn 0.2 mg, vitamin B_1 0.11 mg, B_2 0.11 mg, niacin 0.9 mg, B_6 0.2 mg, pantothenate 0.2 mg, C 36 mg. A 100 g serving is a source of vitamin B_6, Mg, Cu; rich source of vitamin C.

The bullock's heart (*A. reticulata*) has buff-coloured flesh.

Composition/100 g: 293 kJ (70 kcal), protein 1.5 g, fat 0.4 g, carbohydrate 16.1 g (14.9 g sugars, 1.2 g starch), Na 5 mg, K 440 mg, Ca 24 mg, Mg 21 mg, P 25 mg, Fe 0.6 mg, Cu 0.15 mg, Zn 0.2 mg, vitamin A 4 µg (29 µg carotene), B_1 0.09 mg, B_2 0.08 mg, niacin 0.6 mg, B_6 0.22 mg, pantothenate 0.1 mg, C 21 mg. A 100 g serving is a source of vitamin B_6, Cu; rich source of vitamin C.

cyamopsis gum   See GUAR GUM.

cyanocobalamin   See VITAMIN B_{12}.

cyanogen(et)ic glycosides   Organic compounds of cyanide found in a variety of plants; chemically cyanhydrin glycosides. Toxic through liberation of the cyanide when the plants are cut or chewed.

See also ALMOND; AMYGDALIN.

cycasin   Methylazoxymethanol β-glucoside, a toxin in seeds of *Cycas* spp.

cyclamate   Cyclohexylsulphamate, a non-nutritive SWEETENER, 30 times as sweet as sugar, used as the sodium or calcium salt; first synthesised in 1937. Useful in low-calorie foods; unlike SACCHARIN, it is stable to heat and can be used in cooking. Trade name Sucaryl.

cyclitols   Cyclic SUGAR ALCOHOLS such as inositol, quercitol and tetritol.

Cymogran   Trade name for a protein-rich food low in PHENYL-ALANINE for feeding patients with PHENYLKETONURIA.

cystathioninuria   A GENETIC DISEASE due to lack of cystathionase (EC 4.4.1.1) affecting the metabolism of the AMINO ACID METHIONINE and its conversion to CYSTEINE. May result in mental retardation if untreated. Treatment is by feeding a diet low in methionine and supplemented with cysteine, or, in some cases, by administration of high intakes of VITAMIN B_6 (about 100–500 times the normal requirement).

cysteine   A non-essential AMINO ACID, abbr Cys (C), M_r 121.2, pK_a 1.92, 8.35, 10.46 (–SH), CODONS UGPy. Nutritionally important since it is synthesised from the essential amino acid METHIONINE. In addition to its rôle in protein synthesis, cysteine is important as the precursor of TAURINE, in formation of COENZYME A from the VITAMIN PANTOTHENIC ACID and in formation of the tripeptide GLUTATHIONE. It is used as a dough 'improver' in baking.
See also CYSTINE.

cysticercosis   Infection by the larval stage of TAPEWORMS caused by ingestion of their eggs in food and water contaminated by human faeces. Normally the larval form develops in the animal host, and human beings are infected with the adult form by eating undercooked infected meat.

cystic fibrosis   A GENETIC DISEASE due to a failure of the normal transport of chloride ions across cell membranes. This results in abnormally viscous mucus, affecting especially the lungs and secretion of pancreatic juice, hence impairing digestion.

cystine   The dimer of CYSTEINE produced when the sulphydryl group (–SH) is oxidised to form a disulphide (–S–S–) bridge. Such disulphide bridges are especially important in maintaining the structure of proteins, and also in the rôle of the tripeptide GLUTATHIONE as an ANTIOXIDANT. Hair protein (keratin) is especially rich in cystine, which accounts for about 12% of its total amino acid content.

cystinuria   A GENETIC DISEASE in which there is abnormally high excretion of the amino acids CYSTEINE and CYSTINE, resulting in the formation of kidney stones. Treatment is by feeding a diet low in the sulphur AMINO ACIDS methionine, cysteine and cystine.

cytochromes   HAEM-containing proteins. Some react with oxygen directly; others are intermediates in the oxidation of reduced COENZYMES. Unlike HAEMOGLOBIN, the iron in the haem of cytochromes undergoes oxidation and reduction.

cytochromes P450.   A family of CYTOCHROMES involved in the DETOXICATION system of the body (see PHASE I METABOLISM). They act on a wide variety of (potentially toxic) compounds, both endogenous metabolites and foreign compounds (XENOBIOTICS), rendering them more water-soluble, and more readily conjugated for excretion in the urine.

The CYP26 group of cytochromes P450 are specific for RETINOIC ACID, leading to a variety of metabolites that may be physiologically active (especially in cell differentiation), including 4-hydroxy-, 4-oxo-, 5,6-epoxy- and 18-hydroxy-retinoic acid.

cytokines A number of proteins secreted by cells in response to various stimuli that act to regulate proliferation and differentiation, immune and inflammatory responses, etc.

Cytokines produced by lymphocytes are sometimes known as lymphokines; those from monocytes as monokines.

cytokinins Plant hormones derived from isopentenyl adenosine; produced by root tips, seed embryos, developing fruits and buds; they stimulate cell division (cytokinesis) and regulate development of the plant.

See also AUXINS.

cytosine One of the PYRIMIDINE bases of NUCLEIC ACIDS.

D

D-, L- and DL- Prefixes to chemical names for compounds that have a centre of asymmetry in the molecule, and which can therefore have two forms.

Most naturally occurring sugars have the D-conformation; apart from a few microbial proteins and some invertebrate peptides, all the naturally occurring amino acids have the L-configuration. Chemical synthesis yields a mixture of the D- and L-isomers (the racemic mixture), generally shown as DL-.

See also ISOMERS; *R*- and *S*-; OPTICAL ACTIVITY.

d- **and** *l*- An obsolete way of indicating dextrorotatory and laevorotatory OPTICAL ACTIVITY, now replaced by (+) and (−).

dabberlocks Edible seaweed, *Alaria esculenta*.

dadhi See MILK, FERMENTED.

dahl See LEGUMES.

dahlin See INULIN.

daily value Reference amounts of energy, fat, saturated fat, carbohydrate, fibre, sodium, potassium and cholesterol, as well as protein, vitamins and minerals, introduced for food labelling in USA in 1994. The nutrient content of a food must be declared as percentage of the daily value provided by a standard serving.

Daltose Trade name for a carbohydrate preparation consisting of maltose, glucose and dextrin for infant feeding.

damson Small dark purple PLUM (*Prunus damascena*); very acid, mainly used to make jam.

Composition/100g: 142kJ (34kcal), protein 0.5g, fat 0g,

carbohydrate 8.6 g (8.6 g sugars), dietary fibre 3.3 g, nsp 1.6 g, Na 2 mg, K 260 mg, Ca 22 mg, Mg 10 mg, P 14 mg, Fe 0.4 mg, Cu 0.07 mg, Zn 0.1 mg, vitamin A 44 μg (265 μg carotene), E 0.6 mg, B_1 0.09 mg, B_2 0.03 mg, niacin 0.4 mg, B_6 0.05 mg, folate 3 μg, pantothenate 0.2 mg, biotin 0.1 μg, C 5 mg. Serving 80 g.

dandelion The leaves of the weed *Taraxacum officinale* may be eaten as a salad or cooked. In French dandelion greens are known as *pis-en-lit* because of their diuretic action. The root can be cooked as a vegetable, or may be roasted and used as a substitute for COFFEE.

Danish agar See FURCELLARAN.

dansyl reagent 5-Dimethylamino naphthalene sulphonic acid; reacts with amino terminal amino acid of a peptide to give a fluorescent derivative which can be identified by thin-layer CHROMATOGRAPHY after hydrolysis of the peptide.

danthron An anthroquinone stimulant LAXATIVE.

dark adaptation In the eye, the visual pigment rhodopsin is formed by reaction between VITAMIN A aldehyde (retinaldehyde) and the protein opsin, and is bleached by exposure to light, stimulating a nerve impulse (this is the basis of VISION). At an early stage of vitamin A deficiency it takes considerably longer than normal to adapt to see in dim light after exposure to normal bright light, because of the limitation of the amount of rhodopsin that can be reformed. Measuring the time taken to adapt to dim light (the dark adaptation time) provides a sensitive index of early vitamin A deficiency. More severe vitamin A deficiency results in NIGHT BLINDNESS, and eventually complete blindness.

dasheen See TARO.

date Fruit of date palm, *Phoenix dactylifera*. Three types: 'soft' (about 80% of the dry matter is INVERT SUGAR); semi-dry (about 40% invert sugar, 40% sucrose); and dry (20–40% invert sugar, 40–60% is sucrose).

Composition/100 g (fresh dates): 447 kJ (107 kcal), protein 1.3 g, fat 0.1 g, carbohydrate 26.9 g (26.9 g sugars), dietary fibre 3.1 g, nsp 1.5 g, Na 6 mg, K 350 mg, Ca 21 mg, Mg 21 mg, P 24 mg, Fe 0.3 mg, Cu 0.1 mg, Zn 0.2 mg, Se 1 μg, vitamin A 2 μg (15 μg carotene), B_1 0.05 mg, B_2 0.06 mg, niacin 1.2 mg, B_6 0.1 mg, folate 21 μg, pantothenate 0.2 mg, C 12 mg. A 150 g serving (six dates) is a source of niacin, folate, Mg, Cu; rich source of vitamin C.

date, Chinese Fruit of *Zisiphus jujuba* (also called jujube), smaller than the true date.

DATEM Diacetyl tartaric esters of mono- and diglycerides used as EMULSIFIERS to strengthen bread dough and delay staling (E-472e).

date marking 'Best before' is the date up until when the food will remain in optimum condition, i.e. will not be stale. Foods with a shelf life up to 12 weeks are marked 'best before day, month, year'; foods with a longer shelf life are marked 'best before end of month, year'.

Perishable foods with a shelf life of less than a month may have a 'sell-by' date instead. 'Use by' date is given for foods that are microbiologically highly perishable and could become a danger to health; it is the date up to and including which the food may safely be used if stored properly.

Frozen foods and ice-cream carry star markings which correspond to the star marking on freezers and frozen food compartments of refrigerators. One star (*) $-4°C$ ($25°F$) will keep for one week; two star (**) $-11°C$ ($12°F$), 1 month; three star (***) $-18°C$ ($0°F$), 3 months. Corresponding times for ice-cream are 1 day, 1 week, 1 month, after which they are fit to eat but the texture changes.

date plum See PERSIMMON.

DBD process See DRY-BLANCH-DRY PROCESS.

db **gene** See LEPTIN.

DCPIP See DICHLOROPHENOLINDOPHENOL.

DE See DEXTROSE EQUIVALENT VALUE.

debranching enzymes Enzymes that hydrolyse the α-1,6 glycoside bonds that form the branch points in AMYLOPECTIN. Amyloglucosidase (EC 3.2.1.3) and glucoamylase (EC 3.2.1.20) also hydrolyse α-1,4 links; pullulanase (EC 3.2.1.41) and isoamylase (EC 3.2.1.68) hydrolyse only α-1,6 links.

See also AMYLASE; Z-ENZYME.

decimal reduction time (*D* value) Term used in sterilising canned food, etc; the duration of heat treatment required to reduce the number of microorganisms to one-tenth of the initial value, with the temperature shown as a subscript, e.g. D_{121} is time at $121°C$.

deglutition Swallowing.

degumming Removal of proteins, phospholipids, gum, resin, etc in the refining of oils and fats by the addition of dilute hydrochloric or phosphoric acid, brine or alkaline phosphate solution. Permits recovery of LECITHIN from the aqueous phase.

dehydroascorbic acid The oxidised form of VITAMIN C which is readily reduced back to the active form in the body, and therefore has vitamin activity. Not measured by all methods for vitamin C estimation.

See also ASCORBIC ACID.

dehydrocanning A process in which 50% of the water is removed from a food before canning. The advantages are that the texture is retained by the partial dehydration and there is a saving in bulk and weight.

7-dehydrocholesterol   Intermediate in the synthesis of CHOLESTEROL, and precursor for the synthesis of VITAMIN D in the skin.

dehydrofreezing   A process for preservation of fruits and vegetables by evaporation of 50–60% of the water before freezing. The texture and flavour are claimed to be superior to those resulting from either dehydration or freezing alone, and rehydration is more rapid than with dehydrated products.

dehydroretinol   An analogue of VITAMIN A found in freshwater fish, which has about half the biological activity of RETINOL. Formerly termed vitamin A_2.

Delaney Amendment   Clause in the US Federal Food, Drug and Cosmetic Act (1958) which states that no food additive shall be deemed safe (and therefore may not be used) after it is found to induce cancer when ingested by man or animals, at any dose level.

demerara sugar   See SUGAR.

demersal fish   Those fish found living on or near the bottom of the sea, including cod, haddock, whiting and halibut. They contain little oil (1–4%). See WHITE FISH.

denaturation   A normally irreversible change in the structure of protein by heat, acid, alkali or other agents which results in loss of solubility and COAGULATION. Denatured proteins lose biological activity (e.g. as enzymes), but not nutritional value. Indeed, digestibility is improved compared with the native structure, which is relatively resistant to enzymic hydrolysis.

denatured alcohol   See ALCOHOL, DENATURED.

dendritic salt   A form of ordinary table SALT, sodium chloride, with the crystals branched or star-like (dendritic) instead of the normal cubes. This is claimed to have a number of advantages: lower bulk density, more rapid solution, and an unusually high capacity to absorb moisture before becoming wet.

dental fluorosis   See FLUORIDE; mottled enamel.

dental plaque   See PLAQUE, dental.

dent corn   See MAIZE.

deodorisation   The removal of an undesirable flavour or odour. Fats are deodorised during refining by bubbling superheated steam through the hot oil under vacuum, when most of the flavoured substances are distilled off.

deoxycholic acid   One of the secondary BILE SALTS, formed by intestinal bacterial metabolism of CHOLIC ACID.

4-deoxypyridixine   Antimetabolite of VITAMIN B_6 used in experimental studies of vitamin B_6 deficiency.

deoxyribonucleic acid   See DNA; NUCLEIC ACIDS.

deoxyuridine suppression test   See dUMP SUPPRESSION TEST.

depectinisation   The removal of PECTIN from fruit juice to produce a clear thin juice instead of a viscous, cloudy liquid, by enzymic hydrolysis.

Derbyshire neck   See GOITRE.

dermatitis   A lesion or inflammation of the skin caused by outside agents (unlike eczema, which is an endogenous disease); many nutritional deficiency diseases include more or less specific skin lesions (e.g. ARIBOFLAVINOSIS, KWASHIORKOR, PELLAGRA, SCURVY), but most cases of dermatitis are not associated with nutritional deficiency, and do not respond to nutritional supplements. Dermatitis herpetiformis is an uncommon itchy and blistering rash associated with COELIAC DISEASE.

desferrioxamine   Chelating agent used in treatment of IRON overload; the iron chelate is excreted in the urine. Given by 8–12 h subcutaneous perfusion 3–7 times a week.

desmosine   The cross-linkage compound between chains of the CONNECTIVE TISSUE protein ELASTIN, formed by reaction of two or three lysine residues in adjacent polypeptide chains.

detoxication   The metabolism of (potentially) toxic compounds to yield less toxic derivatives which are more soluble in water and can be excreted in the urine or BILE. A wide variety of 'foreign compounds' (i.e. compounds that are not normal metabolites in the body), sometimes referred to as xenobiotics, and some hormones and other normal body metabolites, are metabolised in the same way.
 See also CYTOCHROMES; PHASE I METABOLISM.

devils on horseback   Bacon wrapped around stoned prunes, skewered with a toothpick and then grilled.
 See also ANGELS ON HORSEBACK.

devitalised gluten   See GLUTEN.

dewberry   A hybrid fruit, a large variety of BLACKBERRY; rather than climbing, the plant trails on the ground.

dewpoint   A measure of the humidity of air; the temperature at which it becomes saturated and deposits dew when cooled.

dexedrine   Anorectic (appetite suppressing, see APPETITE CONTROL) drug used in the treatment of OBESITY.

dexfenfluramine   See FENFLURAMINE.

dextrins   A mixture of soluble compounds formed by the partial breakdown of STARCH by heat, acid or enzymes (AMYLASES). Formed when bread is toasted. Nutritionally equivalent to starch; industrially used as adhesives, in the sizing of paper and textiles, and as gums.
 Limit dextrin is the product of enzymic hydrolysis of branched polysaccharides such as GLYCOGEN or AMYLOPECTIN, when glucose

units are removed one at a time until the branch point is reached, when the DEBRANCHING ENZYME is required for further hydrolysis.

dextronic acid   See GLUCONIC ACID.

dextrose   Alternative name for GLUCOSE. Commercially the term 'glucose' is often used to mean CORN syrup (a mixture of glucose with other sugars and DEXTRINS) and pure glucose is called dextrose.

dextrose equivalent value (DE)   A term used to indicate the degree of hydrolysis of starch into GLUCOSE syrup. It is the percentage of the total solids that have been converted to reducing sugars; the higher the DE, the more sugars and less dextrins are present. Liquid glucoses are commercially available ranging from 2 DE to 65 DE. Complete acid hydrolysis converts all the starch into glucose but produces bitter degradation products.

Glucose syrups above 55 DE are termed 'high conversion' (of starch); 35–55, regular conversion; below 20 the products of hydrolysis are maltins or maltodextrins.

DFD meat   Dark, firm, dry; the condition of meat when the pH remains high through lack of GLYCOGEN (which would form LACTIC ACID). It poses a microbiological hazard.

See also MEAT CONDITIONING; RIGOR MORTIS.

DHA   Docosohexaenoic acid, a long chain polyunsaturated FATTY ACID (C22:6 ω3). See FISH OILS.

dhal   Indian term for split peas of various kinds, e.g. the pigeon pea (*Cajanus indicus*), khesari (*Lathyrus sativus*); red dhal or Massur dhal is the lentil (*Lens esculenta*).

dhanyia   See CORIANDER.

dhool   The name given to leaves of TEA up to the stage of drying.

diabetes   Two distinct conditions: diabetes insipidus and diabetes mellitus. The latter condition is more common, and is generally referred to simply as diabetes or sugar diabetes. Diabetes insipidus is a metabolic disorder characterised by extreme thirst, excessive consumption of liquids and urination, due to failure of secretion of the antidiuretic hormone.

Diabetes mellitus is a metabolic disorder involving impaired metabolism of GLUCOSE due to either failure of secretion of the HORMONE INSULIN (Type I, insulin-dependent diabetes) or impaired responses of tissues to insulin (Type II, non-insulin-dependent diabetes).

If untreated, the blood concentration of glucose rises to abnormally high levels (hyperglycaemia) after a meal and glucose is excreted in the urine (glucosuria). Prolonged hyperglycaemia may damage nerves, blood vessels and kidneys, and lead to development of cataracts, so effective control of blood glucose levels is important.

Type I diabetes develops in childhood (sometimes called juvenile-onset diabetes) and is due to failure to secrete INSULIN. Treatment is by injection of insulin, either purified from beef or pig pancreas or, more commonly now, biosynthetic human insulin, together with restriction of the intake of sugars.

Type II diabetes generally arises in middle age (maturity-onset diabetes) and is due to resistance of the tissues to insulin action, probably as a result of reduced insulin receptor activity; secretion of insulin by the pancreas may be normal or higher than normal. It can sometimes be treated by restricting the consumption of sugars and reducing weight, or by the use of oral drugs which stimulate insulin secretion and/or enhance the insulin responsiveness of tissues (sulphonylureas and biguanides). It is also treated by injection of insulin to supplement secretion from the pancreas and overcome the resistance.

Impairment of GLUCOSE TOLERANCE similar to that seen in diabetes mellitus sometimes occurs in late pregnancy, when it is known as gestational diabetes. Sometimes pregnancy is the stress that precipitates diabetes, but more commonly the condition resolves when the child is born.

Renal diabetes is the excretion of glucose in the urine without undue elevation of the blood glucose concentration. It is due to a reduction of the renal threshold which allows the blood glucose to be excreted.

See also GLUCOKINASE; GLUCOSE TOLERANCE.

diabetic foods   Loose term for foods that are specially formulated to be suitable for consumption by people with DIABETES mellitus; generally low in carbohydrate (and especially sugar), and frequently containing SORBITOL, XYLULOSE or sugar derivatives that are slowly or incompletely absorbed.

diacetyl   Acetyl methyl carbonyl ($CH_3.CO.CO.CH_3$), the main flavour in butter, formed during the ripening stage by the organism *Streptococcus lactis cremoris*. Synthetic diacetyl is added to margarine as 'butter flavour'.

dialysis   A process for separating small solutes (e.g. salts and sugars) from larger ones (e.g. proteins) in solution. Small molecules can pass through a SEMIPERMEABLE MEMBRANE, while large molecules cannot. The membrane may be natural, such as pig bladder, or artificial, such as cellulose derivatives or collodion.

diaminopimelic acid   Intermediate in synthesis of lysine in bacteria; also important in sporulating bacteria for formation of spore coat. M_r 190.2, pK_a 1.8, 2.2, 8.8, 9.9.

diaphysis   The shaft of a long BONE.
   See also EPIPHYSIS; METAPHYSIS.

diarrhoea   Frequent passage of loose watery stools, commonly the result of intestinal infection; rarely as a result of ADVERSE REACTION TO FOODS or DISACCHARIDE INTOLERANCE. Severe diarrhoea in children can lead to dehydration and death; it is treated by feeding a solution of salt and sugar to replace fluid and electrolyte losses.

   Osmotic diarrhoea is associated with retention of water in the bowel as a result of an accumulation of nonabsorbable water-soluble compounds; especially associated with excessive intake of SORBITOL and MANNITOL. Also occurs in DISACCHARIDE INTOLERANCE.

   See also ANTIMOTILITY AGENTS.

diastase   See AMYLASE.

diastatic activity   Of flour. A measure of the ability of flour to produce maltose from its own starch by the action of its own AMYLASE (diastase). This sugar is needed for the growth of the yeast during fermentation.

   See also AMYLOGRAPH.

diazoxide   7-Chloro-3-methyl-1,2,4-benzothiadiazone 1,1-dioxide, used in treatment of chronic hypoglycaemia associated with excessive secretion of INSULIN due to pancreatic β-islet cell hyperplasia or cancer.

dichlorophenolindophenol (DCPIP)   Purple-blue dye used in titrimetric assay of VITAMIN C; reduced to a colourless leuco dye by ascorbic acid, but not by dehydroascorbate, so does not measure total vitamin C.

dicoumarol (dicoumarin, coumarin)   Naturally occurring VITAMIN K antagonist, found in spoilt hay containing sweet clover (*Melilotus alba* or *M. officinalis*); leads to haemorrhagic disease in cattle as a result of impaired synthesis of prothrombin and other vitamin K-dependent blood clotting proteins.

dicyclomine   See ATROPINE.

didronel   Drug used to enhance bone mineralisation in women with post-menopausal OSTEOPOROSIS.

dielectric heating   Similar principle to microwave heating but at lower frequencies. Food is passed between capacitor plates and high frequency energy applied by using alternating electrostatic fields, which changes the orientation of the dipoles. The use of the process is limited by the space between the plates; used for thawing blocks of frozen food, melting fats and drying biscuits.

   See also IRRADIATION.

dietary fibre   Material mostly derived from plant cell walls which is not digested by human digestive enzymes but is partially broken down by intestinal bacteria to volatile FATTY ACIDS that can be used as a source of energy. A large proportion consists of NON-STARCH POLYSACCHARIDES (nsp); these include soluble fibre that reduces levels of blood cholesterol and increases the viscosity of the intestinal contents and insoluble fibre (cellulose and cell walls) that acts as a laxative. Earlier known as roughage or bulk.

dietary folate equivalents (DFE) Method for calculating FOLIC ACID intake taking into account the lower availability of mixed folates in food compared with synthetic tetrahydrofolate used in food enrichment and supplements. $1\,\mu g$ DFE = $1\,\mu g$ food folate or $0.6\,\mu g$ synthetic folate; total DFE = μg food folate + $1.7 \times \mu g$ synthetic folate.

Dietary reference intakes (DRI) US term for DIETARY REFERENCE VALUES. In addition to average requirement and RDA, include tolerable upper levels (UL) of intake from supplements. See REFERENCE INTAKES.

Dietary reference values (DRV) A UK set of standards of the amounts of each nutrient needed to maintain good health. See REFERENCE INTAKES.

dietetic foods Foods prepared to meet the particular nutritional needs of people whose assimilation and metabolism of foods are modified, or for whom a particular effect is obtained by a controlled intake of foods or individual nutrients. They may be formulated for people suffering from physiological disorders or for healthy people with additional needs.

See also PARNUTS.

dietetics The study or prescription of diets under special circumstances (e.g. metabolic or other illness) and for special physiological needs such as pregnancy, growth, weight reduction.

See also DIETITIAN.

diethylpropion Anorectic (appetite suppressant, see APPETITE CONTROL) drug with amphetamine-like action, used in the treatment of obesity.

diethyl pyrocarbonate A preservative for wines, soft drinks and fruit juice at a level of 50–300 ppm; it does not inhibit the growth of moulds. It breaks down within a few days to alcohol and carbon dioxide. Also known as pyrocarbonic acid diethyl, trade name Baycovin.

diet-induced thermogenesis The increase in heat production by the body after eating. It is due to both the metabolic energy cost of digestion (the secretion of digestive enzymes, active transport of nutrients from the gut and gut motility) and the energy cost of forming tissue reserves of fat, glycogen and protein. It can be up to 10–15% of the energy intake. Also known as the specific dynamic action (SDA), *luxus konsumption* or thermic effect of foods.

dietitian, dietician According to the US Department of Labor Dictionary of Occupational Titles, one who applies the principles of nutrition to the feeding of individuals and groups; plans menus and special diets; supervises the preparation and serving of meals; instructs in the principles of nutrition as applied to selection of foods. In UK the training and state registration of dietitians (i.e. legal permission to practise) is controlled by law.

See also NUTRITIONIST.

differential cell count See LEUCOCYTES.

digester See AUTOCLAVE.

digestibility The proportion of a foodstuff absorbed from the digestive tract into the bloodstream, normally 90–95%. It is measured as the difference between intake and faecal output, with allowance being made for that part of the faeces that is not derived from undigested food residues (such as shed cells of the intestinal tract, bacteria, residues of digestive juices). Digestibility measured in this way is referred to as 'true digestibility', as distinct from the approximate measure 'apparent digestibility', which is simply the difference between intake and output.

digestion The breakdown of a complex compound into its constituent parts, achieved either chemically or enzymically. Most frequently refers to the digestion of food, enzymic hydrolysis of PROTEINS to AMINO ACIDS, STARCH to GLUCOSE, FATS to GLYCEROL and FATTY ACIDS.

See also GASTROINTESTINAL TRACT.

digestive juices The secretions of the GASTROINTESTINAL TRACT which are involved in the DIGESTION of foods: BILE, GASTRIC SECRETION, INTESTINAL JUICE, PANCREATIC JUICE, SALIVA.

digestive tract See GASTROINTESTINAL TRACT.

dihydrochalcones See NEOHESPERIDIN DIHYDROCHALCONE.

dihydrostreptomycin Poorly absorbed ANTIBIOTIC used in treatment of persistent bacterial DIARRHOEA and gastrointestinal infection.

dilatant COLLOIDAL SUSPENSION in which there is an increase in VISCOSITY with increasing shear stress.

See also PSEUDOPLASTIC; RHEOPEXIC; THIXOTROPIC.

dilatation of fats When fats melt from solids to liquid, at the same temperature, there is an increase in volume. Measurement of this increase, dilatometry, may be used to estimate the amount of solid fat present in a mixture at any given temperature. The precise measure is the difference between the volume of solid and liquid measured in millilitres per 25 g of fat.

dill The aromatic herb *Anethum graveolens* (parsley family). The dried ripe seeds are used in pickles, sauces, etc. The young leaves (dill weed) are used, fresh, dried or frozen.

dimethicone   Antifoaming agent added to ANTACIDS to reduce flatulence; used alone to treat gripe, colic and wind pain in infants. Also known as simethicone.

dim-sum (dim-sim)   Chinese; steamed dumplings and other delicacies.

dinitrofluorobenzene   See FLUORODINITROBENZENE.

dinitrophenol   Reacts with the amino group of AMINO ACIDS; used in separation of amino acids by thin-layer CHROMATOGRAPHY. Also a potent uncoupler of mitochondrial ELECTRON TRANSPORT and OXIDATIVE PHOSPHORYLATION; was formerly used as a slimming agent.

dinitrophenylhydrazine   Reacts with many reducing sugars to form dinitrophenylhydrazones that have characteristic absorption spectra and crystal shapes. Widely used for identification of sugars before the development of modern chromatographic techniques. Also used for colorimetric determination of dehydroascorbate and total VITAMIN C after oxidation to dehydro-ascorbate using Cu^{2+} salts.

dipeptidases   Enzymes (EC 3.4.14.x) in the intestinal mucosal brush border that hydrolyse dipeptides to their constituent amino acids.

dipeptide   A PEPTIDE consisting of two amino acids.

diphenoxylate   See ANTIDIARRHOEAL AGENTS; ANTIMOTILITY AGENTS.

diphenyl   Also known as biphenyl (E-230), one of two compounds (the other is orthophenylphenol, OPP, E-231) used for the treatment of fruit after harvesting, to prevent the growth of mould.

diphenylhydantoin   Anticonvulsant used in treatment of epilepsy; inhibits absorption of FOLIC ACID and can lead to folate deficiency and megaloblastic ANAEMIA.

diphosphopyridine nucleotide (DPN)   Obsolete name for nicotinamide adenine dinucleotide, NAD.

diphyllobothriasis   Intestinal infestation with the broad TAPEWORM *Diphyllobothrium latum* (also known as the fish tapeworm). Infection is from eating uncooked fish containing the larval stage. May cause VITAMIN B_{12} deficiency by impairing absorption.

dipsa   Foods that cause thirst.

dipsesis (dipsosis)   Extreme thirst, a craving for abnormal kinds of drinks.

dipsetic   Tending to produce thirst.

dipsogen   A thirst-provoking agent.

dipsomania   An imperative morbid craving for alcoholic drinks.

direct extract   See MEAT EXTRACT.

disaccharidases   Enzymes (EC 3.2.1.x) that hydrolyse DISACCHA-
RIDES to their constituent monosaccharides in the intestinal
mucosa: sucrase (also known as INVERTASE) acts on sucrose,
LACTASE on lactose and MALTASE on maltose.

disaccharide   Sugars composed of two monosaccharide units; the
nutritionally important disaccharides are SUCROSE, LACTOSE and
MALTOSE. See CARBOHYDRATE.

disaccharide intolerance   Impaired ability to digest lactose,
maltose or sucrose, due to lack of LACTASE, MALTASE or SUCRASE
in the small intestinal mucosa. The undigested sugars remain in
the intestinal contents, and are fermented by bacteria in the large
intestine, resulting in painful, explosive, watery DIARRHOEA. Treatment is by omitting the offending sugar from the diet.

   Lack of all three enzymes is generally caused by intestinal
infections, and the enzymes gradually recover after the infection
has been cured. Lack of just one of the enzymes, and hence intolerance of just one of the disaccharides, is normally an inherited
condition. Lactose intolerance due to loss of lactase is normal in
most ethnic groups after puberty.

displacement analysis   See RADIOIMMUNOASSAY.

distillers' dried solubles   See SPENT WASH.

DIT   See DIET-INDUCED THERMOGENESIS.

diuresis   Increased formation and excretion of urine; it occurs in
diseases such as DIABETES, and also in response to DIURETICS.

diuretics   Substances that increase the production and excretion
of urine. They may be either compounds that occur naturally in
foods (including CAFFEINE and ALCOHOL) or may be drugs used
medically to reduce the volume of body fluid (e.g. in the treatment of HYPERTENSION and OEDEMA).

diverticular disease   Diverticulosis is the presence of pouch-like
hernias (diverticula) through the muscle layer of the colon, associated with a low intake of DIETARY FIBRE and high intestinal pressure due to straining during defecation. Faecal matter can be
trapped in these diverticula, causing them to become inflamed,
causing pain and diarrhoea, the condition of diverticulitis.

   See also GASTROINTESTINAL TRACT.

djenkolic acid   A sulphur-containing amino acid found in the
djenkol bean, *Pithecolobium lobatum*, which grows in parts of
Sumatra. It is a derivative of CYSTEINE, and is metabolised but,
being relatively insoluble, unmetabolised djenkolic acid crystallises in the kidney tubules.

DNA   Deoxyribonucleic acid, the genetic material in the nuclei of
all cells. A polymer of deoxyribonucleotides, the PURINE bases
adenine and guanine, and the PYRIMIDINE bases thymidine and

cytidine, linked to deoxyribose phosphate. The sugar-phosphates form a double stranded helix, with the bases paired internally. See also NUCLEIC ACIDS.

dockage Name given to foreign material in wheat which can be removed readily by a simple cleaning procedure.

docosanoids Long chain polyunsaturated FATTY ACIDS with 22 carbon atoms.

docosahexaenoic acid A long chain polyunsaturated FATTY ACID (C22:6 ω3); see FISH OILS.

docusates See LAXATIVES.

dogfish A cartilaginous FISH, *Scilliorinus caniculum*, or *Squalis acanthias*, related to the sharks; sometimes called rock salmon or rock eel.

Composition/100 g: 644 kJ (154 kcal), protein 16.6 g, fat 9.7 g (20.8% saturated, 38.8% mono-, 40.2% polyunsaturated), cholesterol 76 mg, carbohydrate 0 g, Na 120 mg, K 290 mg, Ca 8 mg, Mg 21 mg, P 230 mg, Fe 0.9 mg, Cu 0.04 mg, Zn 0.4 mg, Se 55 μg, vitamin A 190 μg, D 9.1 μg, B_1 0.17 mg, B_2 0.29 mg, niacin 6 mg, B_6 0.37 mg, folate 3 μg, B_{12} 5 μg, pantothenate 0.8 mg. A 150 g serving is a source of vitamin B_1, pantothenate, Mg; good source of vitamin B_2, B_6; rich source of protein, vitamin A, D, niacin, B_{12}, Se.

dolomite Calcium magnesium carbonate.

Do-Maker process For continuous breadmaking. Ingredients are automatically fed into continuous dough mixer, the yeast suspension being added in a very active state.

domperidone DOPAMINE antagonist, stimulates gastric emptying and small intestinal transit; strengthens contraction of the oesophageal sphincter. Used in treatment of DYSPEPSIA and oesophageal reflux.

döner kebab See KEBAB.

dopa 3,4-Dihydroxyphenylalanine; a non-protein AMINO ACID, precursor of DOPAMINE, NORADRENALINE and ADRENALINE. M_r 197.2, pK_a 2.32, 8.72, 9.96, 11.79.

dopamine 3,4-Dihydroxyphenylethylamine; a neurotransmitter, and also precursor of NORADRENALINE and ADRENALINE.

double-labelled water Dual isotopically-labelled water, containing both deuterium (^{2}H) and ^{18}O (i.e. $^2H_2^{18}O$), used in studies of energy balance. ^{2}H is lost only as water, while ^{18}O is lost as both water and carbon dioxide; the difference in rate of loss of the two isotopes from body water permits estimation of total carbon dioxide production, and hence energy expenditure, over a period of 7–14 days.

See also CALORIMETRY; ISOTOPES.

dough cakes A general term to include crumpets, muffins and pikelets, all made from flour, water and milk. The batter is raised with yeast and baked on a hot plate or griddle (hence sometimes known as griddle cakes). Crumpets have sodium bicarbonate added to the batter; muffins are thick and well aerated, less tough than crumpets; pikelets are made from thinned crumpet batter.

Douglas bag An inflatable bag for collecting expired air to measure the consumption of oxygen and production of carbon dioxide, for the measurement of energy expenditure by indirect CALORIMETRY.

See also SPIROMETER.

Dowex An ION EXCHANGE RESIN.

DPN (diphosphopyridine nucleotide) Obsolete name for nicotinamide adenine dinucleotide, NAD.

dragée French; whole nuts with hard sugar or sugared chocolate coating. Silver dragées are coated with silver leaf.

dried solubles, distiller's See SPENT WASH.

dripping Unbleached and untreated fat from the adipose tissue or bones of sheep or oxen. Also the rendered fat that drips from meat as it is roasted.

Composition/100 g (beef dripping): 3729 kJ (891 kcal), protein 0 g, fat 99 g (58.2% saturated, 39% mono-, 2.6% polyunsaturated), cholesterol 94 mg, carbohydrate 0 g, Na 5 mg, K 4 mg, Ca 1 mg, P 13 mg, Fe 0.2 mg, I 5 μg, vitamin E 0.3 mg.

drisheen Irish; blood pudding, see BLACK PUDDING.

drop scones See SCONE, drop.

dropsy Popular name for OEDEMA.

drupe Botanical term for a fleshy fruit with a single stone enclosing the seed that does not split along defined lines to liberate the seed e.g. apricot, cherry, date, mango, olive, peach, plum.

DRV Dietary reference values, see REFERENCE INTAKES.

dry-blanch-dry process A method of drying fruit so as to retain the colour and flavour; it is faster than drying in the sun and preserves flavour and colour better than hot air drying. The material is dried to 50% water at about 82°C, blanched for a few minutes, then dried at 68°C over a period of 6–24 h to 15–20% water content.

dry frying Frying without the use of fat by using an antistick agent (silicone or a vegetable extract).

dry ice Solid carbon dioxide, used to refrigerate foodstuffs in transit and for carbonation of liquids. It sublimes from the solid to a gas (without liquefying) at −79°C.

drying oil Any highly unsaturated oil that absorbs oxygen and, when in thin films, polymerises to form a skin. Linseed and tung oil are examples of drying oils used in paints and in the manufacture of linoleum, etc. Nutritionally they are similar to edible oils, but toxic when polymerised.

See also IODINE VALUE.

du Bois formula   A formula for calculating BODY SURFACE AREA.

Dublin bay prawn   Scampi or Norway lobster; a shellfish, *Nephrops norvegicus*, see LOBSTER.

duck   Wild duck is mallard (*Anas platyrhynchos*), teal, small dabbling ducks of genus *Anas*.

Composition/100 g (roast meat with fat and skin): 1419 kJ (339 kcal), protein 19.6 g, fat 29 g (29.1% saturated, 57.9% mono-, 12.9% polyunsaturated), carbohydrate 0 g, Na 76 mg, K 210 mg, Ca 12 mg, Mg 16 mg, P 150 mg, Fe 2.7 mg, Cu 0.27 mg, Zn 1.8 mg, vitamin B_1 0.18 mg, niacin 8 mg, B_6 0.31 mg, B_{12} 2 μg. A 185 g serving is a good source of vitamin B_1, B_6, Zn; rich source of protein, niacin, vitamin B_{12}, Fe, Cu.

ductless glands   See ENDOCRINE GLANDS.

dulcin   A synthetic material (*p*-phenetylurea or *p*-phenetolcarbamide, discovered in 1883) which is 250 times as sweet as sugar but is not permitted in foods. Also called sucrol and valzin.

dulcitol   A six-carbon SUGAR ALCOHOL which occurs in some plants and is formed by the reduction of galactose; also known as melampyrin, dulcite or galacticol.

dulse   Edible purplish-brown seaweeds, *Rhodymenia palmata* and *Dilsea carnosa*, used in soups and jellies.

dUMP suppression test   Deoxyuridine suppression test, for FOLATE and VITAMIN B_{12} status. Preincubation of rapidly dividing cells with dUMP leads to a large intracellular pool of newly synthesised TMP (thymidine monophosphate), and hence little of the added [^{3}H]TMP is incorporated into DNA. In deficiency of either vitamin there is little endogenous synthesis of TMP and hence more incorporation of [^{3}H]TMP.

In folate deficiency addition of any form of folic acid will restore the suppression of incorporation of [^{3}H]TMP by dUMP, but vitamin B_{12} will have no effect. In vitamin B_{12} deficiency addition of vitamin B_{12} or any one-carbon folate derivative apart from methyl folate will be effective.

dun   Brown discoloration in salted fish caused by mould growth.

Dunaliella bardawil   A red marine alga discovered in 1980 in Israel, which is extremely rich in β-CAROTENE, containing 100 times more than most other natural sources.

dunst   Very fine SEMOLINA (starch from the endosperm of the wheat grain) approaching the fineness of flour. Also called break middlings (not to be confused with middlings, which is branny OFFAL).

duocrinin   Peptide hormone secreted by the duodenum; increases intestinal secretion and absorption.

duodenal ulcer   See ULCER.

duodenum   First part of the small intestine, between the stomach and the jejunum; the major site of DIGESTION. Pancreatic juice and bile are secreted into the duodenum. So called because it is about 12 finger breadths in length.

  See also GASTROINTESTINAL TRACT.

durian   Fruit of tree *Durio zibethinum*, grown in Malaysia and Indonesia. Each fruit weighs 2–3 kg and has a soft, cream-coloured pulp, with a smell considered disgusting by the uninitiated.

  Composition/100 g: 569 kJ (136 kcal), protein 2.4 g, fat 1.4 g, carbohydrate 28.4 g (23.2 g sugars, 5.2 g starch), dietary fibre 4 g, Na 1 mg, K 600 mg, Ca 14 mg, Mg 33 mg, P 52 mg, Fe 0.9 mg, vitamin A 1 µg (11 µg carotene), B_1 0.29 mg, B_2 0.29 mg, niacin 1.1 mg, C 41 mg. A 100 g serving is a source of vitamin B_2, Mg; good source of vitamin B_1; rich source of vitamin C.

durum wheat   A hard type of WHEAT of the species *Triticum durum* (most bread wheats are *T. vulgare*); mainly used for the production of semolina for preparation of PASTA.

Dutching   See COCOA, DUTCH.

Dutch oven   A semicircular metal shield which may be placed close to an open fire; fitted with shelves on which food is roasted. It may also be clamped to the fire bars.

D value   See DECIMAL REDUCTION TIME.

Dyox   Trade name for chlorine dioxide used to treat flour. See AGEING.

dysentery   Infection of the intestinal tract causing severe diarrhoea with blood and mucus. Amoebic dysentery is caused by *Entamoeba histolytica*, and occasionally other protozoans spread by contaminated food and water. Symptoms may develop many months after infection. Bacillary dysentery is caused by *Shigella* spp; symptoms develop 1–6 days after infection.

dysgeusia   Distortion of the sense of taste, a common side-effect of some drugs.

  See also GUSTIN; HYPOGEUSIA; PARAGEUSIA.

dyspepsia   Any pain or discomfort associated with eating; may be a symptom of gastritis, peptic ulcer, gall-bladder disease, etc; functional dyspepsia occurs when there is no obvious structural change in the intestinal tract. Treatment includes a BLAND DIET.

  See also INDIGESTION.

dysphagia   Difficulty in swallowing, commonly associated with disorders of the OESOPHAGUS. Inability to swallow is aphagia.

e   On food labels, before the weight or volume, to indicate that this has been notified to the regulatory authorities of the EU as a standard package size.

E   See E-NUMBERS and Table 6.

EAA index   Essential amino acid index, an index of PROTEIN QUALITY.

earth almond   See TIGER NUT.

earth nut   A very small variety of TRUFFLE, *Conopodium denudatum* also called pig nut and fairy potato. Also another name for the PEANUT.

eau de vie   Spirit distilled from fermented grape juice (sometimes other fruit juices); may be flavoured with fruits, etc.

See also MARC.

echoviruses   A group of RNA-containing viruses that infect the gastrointestinal tract and produce pathological changes in cells in culture, but not associated with any specific disease. Now usually classified as coxsackie viruses.

See also ENTEROVIRUSES; REOVIRUSES.

Eck fistula   See FISTULA.

EC numbers   Systematic classification of enzymes by the class, subclass, sub-subclass and individual reaction classified, shown as EC x.x.x.x. The classes are: (1) oxidoreductases, (2) transferases, (3) hydrolases, (4) lyases, (5) isomerases, (6) ligases (synthetases).

E. coli (*Escherichia coli*)   Group of bacteria including both harmless COMMENSALS in the human gut and strains that cause food poisoning by production of ENTEROTOXINS (TX 3.1.2.x, 3.1.3.x, 3.1.4.x, depending on the strain) after adhering to intestinal epithelial cells. For most pathogenic strains the infective dose is 10^5–10^7 organisms, onset 16–48 h, and duration 1–3 days.

Strain 0157:H7 (or VTEC) was first identified as a cause of food poisoning in the 1980s. It produces a toxin called verocytotoxin and is especially virulent; infective dose 10 organisms, onset 1–7 h and duration (if not fatal) of days or weeks.

ectomorph   Description given to a tall, thin person, possibly with underdeveloped muscles.

See also ENDOMORPH; MESOMORPH.

ecuelle   A device for obtaining peel oil from citrus fruit. It consists of a shallow funnel lined with spikes on which the fruit is rolled by hand. As the oil glands are pierced, the oil and cell sap collect in the bottom of the funnel.

eddo   See TARO.

edema See OEDEMA.

edetate See EDTA.

Edifas Trade name for CELLULOSE DERIVATIVES: Edifas A is methyl ethyl cellulose (E-465); Edifas B, sodium carboxymethylcellulose (E-466).

Edman reagent Phenylisothiocyanate (PIC); reacts with amino terminal amino acid of a protein; the basis of the Edman degradation used in sequencing proteins, and used in HPLC of amino acids for fluorimetric detection.

Edosol Trade name for a low-sodium milk substitute, containing 43 mg sodium/100 g, compared with dried milk at 400 mg.

EDTA Ethylene diamine tetra-acetic acid, a chelating agent that forms stable chelation complexes with metal ions. Also called versene, sequestrol and sequestrene. It can be used both to remove metal ions from a solution (or at least to remove them from activity) and also to add metal ions, for example in plant fertilisers (E-385).

eel A long thin fish, *Anguilla anguilla*; the conger eel is *Conger myriaster*. Eels live in rivers but go to sea to breed.

Composition/100 g (weighed with bones): 703 kJ (168 kcal), protein 16.6 g, fat 11.3 g (29.2% saturated, 54.5% mono-, 16.1% polyunsaturated), cholesterol 150 mg, carbohydrate 0 g, Na 89 mg, K 270 mg, Ca 19 mg, Mg 19 mg, P 310 mg, Fe 1.2 mg, Cu 0.07 mg, Zn 2.5 mg, Se 31 µg, I 80 µg, vitamin A 1200 µg, D 4.9 µg, E 4.1 mg, B_1 0.2 mg, B_2 0.35 mg, niacin 5.4 mg, B_6 0.25 mg, folate 12 µg, B_{12} 1 µg, pantothenate 0.1 mg. A 225 g serving is a source of folate, Mg, Fe, Cu; good source of vitamin B_6; rich source of protein, vitamin A, D, E, B_1, B_2, niacin, B_{12}, I, Se, Zn.

EFA Essential fatty acids, see FATTY ACIDS, ESSENTIAL.

egg Hens' eggs are sold by size in EU; large weigh 75 g or more, small 50–55 g (weighed with shell which is about 10% of the total weight). Duck eggs weigh around 85 g.

Composition/100 g: 615 kJ (147 kcal), protein 12.5 g, fat 10.8 g (34.4% saturated, 52.2% mono-, 13.3% polyunsaturated), cholesterol 385 mg, carbohydrate 0 g, Na 140 mg, K 130 mg, Ca 57 mg, Mg 12 mg, P 200 mg, Fe 1.9 mg, Cu 0.08 mg, Zn 1.3 mg, Se 11 µg, I 53 µg, vitamin A 190 µg, D 1.75 µg, E 1.1 mg, B_1 0.09 mg, B_2 0.47 mg, niacin 3.8 mg, B_6 0.12 mg, folate 50 µg, B_{12} 2.5 µg, pantothenate 1.8 mg, biotin 20 µg. A 70 g serving is a source of protein, vitamin A, B_2, niacin, folate, Se; good source of vitamin D, pantothenate, I; rich source of vitamin B_{12}.

egg plant See AUBERGINE.

egg proteins What is generally referred to as egg protein is a mixture of individual proteins, including ovalbumin, ovomucoid, ovoglobulin, conalbumin, vitellin and vitellenin. EGG-WHITE contains 11% protein, mostly ovalbumin; yolk contains 16% protein, mainly two phosphoproteins, vitellin and vitellenin.

eggs, Chinese (hundred years old) See CHINESE EGGS.

egg substitute Name formerly used for golden raising powder, a type of BAKING POWDER.

egg-white The white of an egg is in three layers: an outer layer of thin white, layer of thick white, richer in ovomucin, and inner layer of thin white surrounding the yolk. The ratio of thick to thin white varies, depending on the individual hen. A higher proportion of thick white is desirable for frying and poaching, since it helps the egg to coagulate into a small firm mass instead of spreading; thin white produces a larger volume of froth when beaten than does thick.

See also EGG PROTEINS.

egg-white injury BIOTIN deficiency caused by consumption of large quantities of uncooked egg-white.

EGRAC Erythrocyte GLUTATHIONE REDUCTASE activation coefficient.

EH See EQUILIBRIUM HUMIDITY.

eicosanoids Compounds formed in the body from C20 polyunsaturated FATTY ACIDS (eicosenoic acids), including the prostaglandins, prostacyclins, thromboxanes and leukotrienes, all of which act as local hormones, and are involved in wound healing, inflammation, platelet aggregation, and a variety of other functions.

eicosapentaenoic acid (EPA) A long-chain polyunsaturated FATTY ACID (C20:5 ω3), see FISH OILS.

eicosenoic acids Long-chain polyunsaturated FATTY ACIDS with 20 carbon atoms.

einkorn A type of WHEAT, the wild form of which, *Triticum boeoticum*, was probably one of the ancestors of all cultivated wheat. Still grown in some parts of southern Europe and Middle East, usually for animal feed. The name means 'one seed', from the single seed found in each spikelet.

eiswein WINE made from grapes that have frozen on the vine, picked and processed while still frozen, so that the juice is highly concentrated and very sweet. Similar Canadian wines are known as ice wine.

elastin Insoluble protein in CONNECTIVE TISSUE; the cause of tough meat, not changed by cooking.

electrofocusing See ISOELECTRIC FOCUSING.

electrolytes Salts that dissociate in solution and hence will carry an electric current; generally used to mean the inorganic ions in blood plasma and other body fluids, especially sodium, potassium, chloride, bicarbonate, and phosphate.

electronic heating   See MICROWAVE COOKING.

electron transport chain   A sequence of COENZYMES and CYTOCHROMES of differing redox potential. In the MITOCHONDRIA they carry electrons from the oxidation of metabolic fuels to (ultimately) the reduction of oxygen to water, and are obligatorily linked to OXIDATIVE PHOSPHORYLATION.

electrophoresis   Technique for separation of charged molecules (especially proteins and nucleic acids) by their migration in an electric field. The support medium may be a starch or polyacrylamide gel, paper or cellulose acetate.

electroporation   Use of high-voltage electric pulses at low voltage gradients to exchange genetic information between protoplast cells of microorganisms, plants or animals. At high voltage gradients (up to 30 kV/cm) used to sterilise (see STERILE) or pasteurise (see PASTEURISATION) food by permeabilisation of bacterial cell membranes.

electropure process   A method of pasteurising (see PASTEURISATION) milk by passing low-frequency, alternating current.

elemental diet   See FORMULA DIET.

elements, minor   See TRACE ELEMENTS.

ELISA (enzyme-linked immunosorbent assay)   Sensitive and specific analytical technique for determination of analytes present at very low concentrations in biological samples, in which either the tracer analyte or the antibody is bound to an enzyme; the product of the enzyme may be measured directly, or may be a catalyst or coenzyme for a second enzyme, giving considerable amplification, and hence permitting high sensitivity without the use of radioactive tracers.

   See also FLUORESCENCE IMMUNOASSAY; RADIOIMMUNOASSAY.

elixir   Alcoholic extract (tincture) of a naturally occurring substance; originally devised by medieval alchemists (the elixir of life), now used for a variety of medicines, liqueurs and BITTERS.

elute   To wash off or remove. Specifically applied to removal of adsorbed compounds in chromatography.

   See also ION-EXCHANGE RESINS.

elutriation   Technique for separating fine and coarse particles by suspending the mixture in water and decanting the upper layer while it still contains the finer particles.

elver   Young EEL, about 5 cm in length.

emaciation   Extreme thinness and wasting, caused by disease or undernutrition.

   See also CACHEXIA; MARASMUS; PROTEIN–ENERGY MALNUTRITION.

Embden groats   See GROATS.

emblic   Berry of the SE Asian malacca tree, *Emblica officinalis*, similar in appearance to the gooseberry. Also known as the

Indian gooseberry. An exceptionally rich source of vitamin C, 600 mg/100 g.

embolism Blockage of a blood vessel caused by a foreign object (embolus) such as a quantity of air or gas, a piece of tissue or tumour, a blood clot (thrombus) or fatty tissue derived from ATHEROMA, in the circulation.

embolus Blood clot that travels through the blood vessels.
See also THROMBUS.

emetic Substance that causes vomiting.

emmer A type of WHEAT known to have been used more than 8000 years ago. Wild emmer is *Triticum dicoccoides* and true emmer is *T. dicoccum*. Nowadays grown mainly for animal feed.

Emprote Trade name for a dried milk and cereal preparation consumed as a beverage, containing 33% protein.

emulsifying agents Substances that are soluble in both fat and water; enable fat to be uniformly dispersed in water as an EMULSION. STABILISERS maintain emulsions in a stable form. Emulsifying agents are also used in baking to aid the smooth incorporation of fat into the dough and to keep the crumb soft. Emulsifying agents used in foods include AGAR, ALBUMIN, ALGINATES, CASEIN, egg yolk, GLYCERYL MONOSTEARATE, GUMS, IRISH MOSS, LECITHIN, soaps. See Table 6.

emulsifying salts Sodium citrate, sodium phosphates and sodium tartrate, used in the manufacture of milk powder, evaporated milk, sterilised cream and processed cheese.

emulsin A mixture of enzymes (mainly β-glycosidase, EC 3.2.1.21) in bitter ALMOND which hydrolyse the glucoside AMYGDALIN to benzaldehyde, glucose and cyanide.

emulsion COLLOIDAL SUSPENSION of one liquid in another; the dispersed droplets are the internal phase and the dispersing liquid the external phase. Common emulsions in foods are either oil-in-water or water-in-oil.
See also EMULSIFYING AGENTS.

emulsoids See COLLOID, lyophilic.

en papillote French method of cooking in a closed container, a parchment paper or aluminium foil case. See also SOUS VIDE.

encopresis Faecal incontinence.

endergonic Used of chemical reactions that require an input of energy (usually as heat or light) such as the synthesis of complex molecules.

endive Curly serrated green leaves of *Cichorium endivia*. Called chicory in US and chicorée frisée in France.
Composition/100 g: 54 kJ (13 kcal), protein 1.8 g, fat 0.2 g, carbohydrate 1 g (1 g sugars), dietary fibre 2 g, nsp 2 g, Na 10 mg, K 380 mg, Ca 44 mg, Mg 10 mg, P 67 mg, Fe 2.8 mg, Cu 0.01 mg, Zn

0.2 mg, Se 1 μg, vitamin A 73 μg (440 μg carotene), B_1 0.06 mg, B_2 0.1 mg, niacin 0.6 mg, B_6 0.02 mg, folate 140 μg, pantothenate 0.9 mg, biotin 0.7 μg, C 12 mg. A 20 g serving is a source of folate. There is also broad-leaved Batavian endive which resembles lettuce.

See also CHICORY.

endocrine glands Those (ductless) glands that produce and secrete HORMONES, including the THYROID GLAND (secreting thyroxine and tri-iodothyronine), PANCREAS (INSULIN and GLU-CAGON), ADRENAL GLANDS (ADRENALINE, NORADRENALINE, GLUCO-CORTICOIDS, MINERALOCORTICOIDS), ovary and testes (sex steroids). Some endocrine glands respond directly to chemical changes in the bloodstream; others are controlled by hormones secreted by the pituitary gland, under control of the hypothalamus.

endomorph In relation to body build, means short and stocky. See ECTOMORPH; MESOMORPH.

endomysium See MUSCLE.

endopeptidases Enzymes that hydrolyse proteins (i.e. proteinases or peptidases), by cleaving PEPTIDE bonds inside protein molecules, as opposed to EXOPEPTIDASES, which remove amino acids from the end of the protein chain. The main endopeptidases in DIGESTION are chymotrypsin, elastase, pepsin and trypsin.

endosperm The inner part of cereal grains; in wheat it comprises about 83% of the grain. Mainly starch, and the source of SEMOLINA. Contains only about 10% of the vitamin B_1, 35% of the vitamin B_2, 40% of the niacin and 50% of the vitamin B_6 and pantothenic acid of the whole grain.

See also FLOUR, EXTRACTION RATE.

endothelium-derived relaxation factor See NITRIC OXIDE.

endotoxins Toxins produced by bacteria as an integral part of the cell, so cannot be separated by filtration; unlike EXOTOXINS, they do not usually stimulate antitoxin formation but the antibodies that they induce act directly on the bacteria. They are relatively stable to heat compared with exotoxins.

See also TX NUMBERS.

enema See NUTRIENT ENEMATA.

Energen rolls Trade name for a light BREAD roll of wheat flour plus added wheat GLUTEN.

energy The ability to do work. The SI unit of energy is the Joule, and nutritionally relevant amounts of energy are kilojoules (kJ, 1000 J) and megajoules (MJ, 1000000 J). The CALORIE is still widely used in nutrition; 1 cal = 4.186 J (approximated to 4.2).

While it is usual to speak of the calorie or joule content of a food it is more correct to refer to the energy content or yield.

The total chemical energy in a food, as released by complete combustion (in the bomb CALORIMETER) is gross energy. Allowing for the losses of unabsorbed food in the faeces gives digestible energy. Allowing for loss in the urine due to incomplete combustion in the body (e.g. urea from the incomplete combustion of proteins) gives metabolisable energy. Allowing for the loss due to DIET-INDUCED THERMOGENESIS gives net energy, i.e. the actual amount available for use in the body.

See also ENERGY CONVERSION FACTORS.

energy balance The difference between intake of energy from foods and ENERGY EXPENDITURE on BASAL METABOLISM and physical activity. Positive energy balance leads to increased body tissue, the normal process of growth. In adults positive energy balance leads to creation of body reserves of fat, resulting in overweight and OBESITY. Negative energy balance leads to utilisation of body reserves of fat and protein, resulting in wasting and undernutrition.

energy conversion factors Various factors are used to calculate the energy yields of foodstuffs:

The complete heats of combustion (gross energy) as determined by CALORIMETRY are: protein 23.9 kJ (5.7 kcal), fat 39.5 kJ (9.4 kcal); carbohydrate 17.2 kJ (4.1 kcal)/g.

The Rubner conversion factors for metabolic energy yield are: protein 17 kJ (4.1 kcal); fat 39 kJ (9.3 kcal); carbohydrate 17 kJ (4.1 kcal)/g.

The Atwater factors also allow for losses in digestion and incomplete oxidation of the nitrogen of proteins: protein 16.8 kJ (4 kcal); fat 37.8 kJ (9 kcal); carbohydrate 16.8 kJ (4 kcal)/g.

The following factors are generally used: carbohydrate 17 kJ (4 kcal); fat 38 kJ (9 kcal); carbohydrate (as monosaccharides) 17 kJ (4 kcal); alcohol 29 kJ (7 kcal); sugar alcohols 10 kJ (2.4 kcal); organic acids 13 kJ (3 kcal)/g.

energy expenditure The total energy cost of maintaining constant conditions in the body, i.e. homeostasis (BASAL METABOLIC RATE, BMR) plus the energy cost of physical activities. The average total energy expenditure in western countries is about 1.4 times BMR; a desirable level of physical activity is 1.7 times BMR.

energy requirements Energy requirements are calculated from estimated BASAL METABOLIC RATE and physical activity. Average energy requirements for adults are 8 MJ (1900 kcal)/day for women and 10 MJ (2400 kcal)/day for men.

energy-rich bonds An outdated and chemically incorrect concept in ENERGY metabolism, which suggested that the bond between ADP and phosphate in ATP, and between CREATINE and phosphate in creatine phosphate, which have a high chemical free energy of hydrolysis, somehow differs from 'ordinary' chemical bonds.

enfleurage A method of extracting essential oils from flowers by placing them on glass trays covered with purified LARD or other fat, which eventually becomes saturated with the oil.

enocianina Desugared grape extract used to colour fruit flavours. Prepared by acid extraction of the skins of black grapes; it is blue in neutral conditions and turns red in acid.

enrichment The addition of nutrients to foods. Although often used interchangeably, the term FORTIFICATION is used of legally imposed additions, and enrichment means the addition of nutrients beyond the levels originally present.

See also NUTRIFICATION; RESTORATION.

ensete See BANANA, FALSE.

Entamoeba Genus of protozoa, some of which are parasitic in the human gut. *Entamoeba coli* is harmless; *E. histolytica* causes amoebic DYSENTERY; *E. gingivalis* is found in spaces between the teeth and is associated with periodontal disease.

enteral nutrition Tube feeding with a liquid diet directly into the stomach or small intestine.

See also GASTROSTOMY FEEDING; NASOGASTRIC TUBE; NUTRIENT ENEMATA; PARENTERAL NUTRITION.

enteritis Inflammation of the mucosal lining of the small intestine, usually resulting from infection. Regional enteritis is CROHN'S DISEASE.

enterobiasis Infestation of the large intestine with PINWORM.

Enterococcus faecium See PROBIOTICS.

enterocolitis Inflammation of the mucosal lining of the small and large intestine, usually resulting from infection.

enterocrinin Peptide hormone secreted by the upper small intestine; increases intestinal secretion and absorption.

enterogastrone Peptide hormone secreted by the stomach and duodenum; decreases gastric secretion and motility. Its secretion is stimulated by fat; hence, fat in the diet inhibits gastric activity.

enteroglucagon Peptide hormone secreted by the ileum and colon; increases gut motility and mucosal growth.

enterohepatic circulation Excretion of metabolites in BILE, followed by reabsorption from the intestine, possibly after further metabolism by intestinal bacteria. Total flux through the gut may be several-fold higher than dietary intake or faecal excretion. Especially important with respect to the BILE SALTS, CHOLESTEROL, FOLIC ACID, VITAMIN B_{12} and STEROID hormones.

enterokinase Obsolete name for ENTEROPEPTIDASE.

enterolith Stone within the intestine, commonly builds up around a GALLSTONE or swallowed fruit stone.

entero-oxyntin Peptide hormone secreted by the upper small intestine; increases gastric secretion.

enteropathy Any disease or disorder of the intestinal tract.

enteropeptidase An enzyme (EC 3.4.21.9) secreted by the small intestinal mucosa which activates trypsinogen (from the pancreatic juice) to the active proteolytic enzyme TRYPSIN.
See also PROTEIN, digestion.

enterotoxin Substances more or less specifically toxic to the cells of the intestinal mucosa, normally produced by bacteria; they may be present in the food (e.g. BACILLUS CEREUS, CLOSTRIDIUM BOTULINUM, STAPHYLOCOCCUS AUREUS) or may be produced by the bacteria in the gut (e.g. CLOSTRIDIUM PERFRINGENS, VIBRIO CHOLERA, AEROMONAS spp, pathogenic E. COLI).
See also TX NUMBERS.

enteroviruses Viruses that multiply mainly in the intestinal tract, and commonly invade the central nervous system, including coxsackie virus and poliovirus.

entoleter A machine used to disinfest cereals and other foods. The material is fed to the centre of a high-speed rotating disc carrying studs so that it is thrown against the studs; the impact kills insects and destroys their eggs.

E-numbers Within the EU food additives may be listed on labels either by name or by their number in the EU list of permitted additives. See Table 6.

enzyme A PROTEIN that speeds up (catalyses) a metabolic reaction. Enzymes are specific for both the compounds acted on (the substrates) and the reactions carried out. Because of this, enzymes extracted from plant or animal sources, microorganisms or those produced by GENETIC MODIFICATION are widely used in the chemical, pharmaceutical and food industries (e.g. CHYMOSIN in cheese-making, MALTASE in beer production, synthesis of VITAMIN C and CITRIC ACID), as well as in washing powders.

Because they are proteins, enzymes are permanently inactivated by heat, strong acid or alkali and other conditions which cause DENATURATION of proteins.

Many enzymes contain non-protein components which are essential for their function. These are known as prosthetic groups, COENZYMES or cofactors and may be metal ions, metal ions in organic combination (e.g. haem in HAEMOGLOBIN and CYTOCHROMES) or a variety of organic compounds, many of which are derived from VITAMINS. The (inactive) protein without its prosthetic group is known as the apo-enzyme, and the active assembly of protein plus prosthetic group is the holo-enzyme.
See also EC NUMBERS; ENZYME ACTIVATION ASSAYS; TENDERISERS.

enzyme activation assays Used to assess the nutritional status of an individual with respect to VITAMINS B_1, B_2 and B_6. A sample of red blood cells is tested for activity of the relevant enzyme before and after adding extra vitamin-derived coenzyme; enhancement of the enzyme activity beyond a certain level serves as a biochemical index of deficiency of the vitamin in question. The enzymes involved are TRANSKETOLASE for vitamin B_1, GLUTATHIONE REDUCTASE for vitamin B_2 and either aspartate or alanine TRANSAMINASE for vitamin B_6.

enzyme electrodes An immobilised enzyme plus an electrochemical sensor, enclosed in a probe, used in food analysis and clinical chemistry, e.g. glucose oxidase (EC 1.1.3.4) produces hydrogen peroxide, which can be measured polarographically; lysine decarboxylase (EC 4.1.1.18) produces carbon dioxide which can be measured electrochemically.

enzyme, immobilised Enzyme bound physically to glass, plastic or other support, so permitting continuous flow processes, or recovery and re-utilisation of enzymes in batch processes.

enzyme induction Synthesis of new enzyme protein in response to some stimulus, normally a hormone, but sometimes a metabolic intermediate or other compound (e.g. a drug or food additive).

enzyme inhibition A number of compounds reduce the activity of enzymes; sometimes this is a part of normal metabolic regulation and integration (e.g. the responses to HORMONES), and sometimes it is the action of drugs. Some inhibitors are reversible, others act irreversibly on the enzymes, and therefore have a longer duration of action (the activity of the enzyme remains low until more has been synthesised).

enzyme precursors See ZYMOGENS.

enzyme repression Reduction in synthesis of enzyme protein in response to a stimulus such as a hormone or the presence of large amounts of the end-product of its activity.

EPA Eicosapentaenoic acid, a long-chain polyunsaturated fatty acid (C20:5 ω3). See FISH OILS.

epicarp See FLAVEDO.

epinephrine See ADRENALINE.

epiphysis The end of a long BONE; it develops separately from the shaft (DIAPHYSIS) and later undergoes fusion to form the complete bone. This fusion is impaired in RICKETS.

Epsom salts Magnesium sulphate, originally found in a mineral spring in Epsom, Surrey, UK; acts as a LAXATIVE because the OSMOTIC PRESSURE of the solution causes it to retain water in the intestine and so increase the bulk and moisture content of the faeces.

Equal   Trade name for ASPARTAME.

equilibrium humidity   The relative humidity of the atmosphere with which the substance under consideration is in equilibrium.

equilibrium, nitrogen   See NITROGEN BALANCE.

ercalciol   See VITAMIN D.

erepsin   Obsolete name for a mixture of enzymes contained in INTESTINAL JUICE, including aminopeptidases and dipeptidases.

ergocalciferol   See VITAMIN D.

ergosterol   A sterol isolated from yeast; when treated with ultraviolet light, it is converted to ercalciol (ergocalciferol, vitamin D_2). The main source of manufactured VITAMIN D.

ergot   A fungus that grows on grasses and cereal grains; the ergot of medical importance is *Claviceps purpurea*, which grows on rye. The consumption of infected rye is harmful, causing the disease known as St Anthony's Fire (ergotism), and can be fatal.

   The active principles in ergot are alkaloids (ergotinine, ergotoxine, ergotamine, ergometrine, etc), which yield lysergic acid (the active component) on hydrolysis. Its effect is to increase the tone and contraction of smooth muscle, particularly of the pregnant uterus. For this reason ergot has been used in obstetrics, but pure ergonovine maleate and ergotonine tartrate are preferable.

   Ergotism is poisoning due to ergot infection of rye which occurs from time to time among people eating rye bread. The last outbreak in the UK was in Manchester in 1925, when there were 200 cases. Symptoms appear when as little as 1% of ergot-infected rye is included in the flour.

eriodictin   A FLAVONOID (flavonone) found in citrus pith.

erucic acid   A mono-unsaturated FATTY ACID, *cis*-13-docosenoic acid (C22:1 ω9) found in RAPE seed (*Brassica napus*) and mustard seed (*B. junca* and *B. nigra*) oils; it may constitute 30–50% of the oil in some varieties. Causes fatty infiltration of heart muscle in experimental animals; low erucic acid varieties of rape seed have been developed for food use.

eructation   Belching, the act of bringing up air from the stomach, with a characteristic sound.

erythorbic acid   The D-isomer of ASCORBIC ACID, also called D-araboascorbic acid and *iso*-ascorbic acid; only slight VITAMIN C activity. Used in food processing as an antioxidant.

erythroamylose   Obsolete name for AMYLOPECTIN.

erythrocytes   See BLOOD CELLS, RED.

erythropoiesis   The formation and development of the red BLOOD CELLS in the bone marrow.

erythrosine BS   Red colour permitted in foods in most countries (E-127, Red number 3 in USA). Used in preserved cherries, sausages and meat and fish pastes; it is unstable to light and heat. Chemically the sodium or potassium salt of 2,4,5,7-tetraiodofluorescein.

esculin   See AESCULIN.

essential amino acid index   An index of PROTEIN QUALITY.

essential amino acid pattern   The quantities of essential AMINO ACIDS considered desirable in the diet.

essential amino acids   See AMINO ACIDS, essential.

essential fatty acids   See FATTY ACIDS, ESSENTIAL.

essential nutrients   Those nutrients that are required by the body and cannot be synthesised in the body in adequate amounts to meet requirements, so must be provided by the diet, includes the essential AMINO ACIDS and FATTY ACIDS, VITAMINS and MINERALS. Really a tautology, since by definition nutrients are essential dietary constituents.

essential oils   Volatile, aromatic or odoriferous oils found in plants and used for flavouring foods. Chemically distinct from the edible oils, since they are not glycerol esters.

See also TERPENES.

ester   Compound formed by condensation between an acid and an alcohol. FATS are esters of the alcohol glycerol and long-chain FATTY ACIDS. Many esters are used as synthetic FLAVOURS.

esterases   Enzymes (EC 3.1.x.x) that hydrolyse ESTERS to yield free acid and alcohol. Those that hydrolyse the ester linkages of fats are generally known as LIPASES, and those that hydrolyse PHOSPHOLIPIDS as phospholipases.

ester value   See SAPONIFICATION VALUE.

ethane   Hydrocarbon gas (C_2H_4) formed in small amounts by breakdown of oxidised linolenic acid and exhaled on the breath; used as an index of oxygen radical damage to tissue lipids, and indirectly as an index of ANTIOXIDANT status.

See also FATTY ACIDS; PENTANE.

ethanolamine   2-Amino-ethanol, one of the water-soluble bases of PHOSPHOLIPIDS. Used as softening agent for hides, as dispersing agent for agricultural chemicals and to peel fruits and vegetables.

ethene   See ETHYLENE.

ethionine   A toxic amino acid, the ethyl analogue of METHIONINE.

ethyl alcohol   See ALCOHOL.

ethyl carbamate   See URETHANE.

ethylene (ethene)   Hydrocarbon gas ($CH_2=CH_2$) produced by the oxidation of METHIONINE in CLIMACTERIC fruits as a hormone to speed ripening, the climacteric increase in respiration. This explains why some fruits ripen faster when stored in plastic bags. Used commercially in very small amounts (1 ppm) to speed fruit ripening after harvesting.

ethylene diamine tetra-acetic acid   See EDTA.

ethyl formate   Used as a fumigant against raisin moth, dried fruit beetle, fig moth, etc, and as a flavour; an ingredient of lemon, strawberry and artificial rum flavours.

ethylmethylcellulose   See CELLULOSE DERIVATIVES.

ethyl vanillin   See VANILLA.

euglobulin   The name given to that fraction of serum GLOBULIN which is precipitated by dialysis of blood serum against distilled water. The name implies that this fraction is a typical globulin by reason of its insolubility in water.

eukeratins   See KERATIN.

eutectic ice   The solid formed when a mixture of 76.7% water and 23.3% salt (by weight) is frozen. It melts at −21°C. It has about three times the refrigerant effect of solid carbon dioxide (DRY ICE), and is especially useful for icing fish on board trawlers.

eutrophia   Normal nutrition.

evaporation, flash   A short, rapid application of heat so that a small volume (about 1% of the total) is quickly distilled off, carrying with it the greater part of the volatile components. The flash distillate is collected separately from the later distillate and is added back to the concentrate to restore the flavour; applied to the concentration of products such as fruit juices.

evening primrose   *Oenothera biennis*, the oil from the seeds is a rich source of γ-LINOLENIC ACID, which may account for 8% of total FATTY ACIDS. Used as a dietary supplement and claimed to have beneficial effects in a number of conditions, although there is little evidence of efficacy.

exchange list   List of portions of foods in which energy yield, fat, carbohydrate and/or protein content are equivalent, so simplifying meal and diet planning for people with special needs.

exclusion diet   A limited diet excluding foods known possibly to cause food intolerance, to which foods are added in turn to test for intolerance (allergy). See ADVERSE REACTIONS TO FOODS.

exergonic   Chemical reactions that proceed with the output of energy, usually as heat (then sometimes known as exothermic reactions) or light. The reactions involved in the oxidation of foodstuffs are generally exergonic.

exon   A region of DNA within a gene that contains information coding for the protein that is retained during the post-transcriptional modification of mRNA.
See also INTRON.

exopeptidases   Proteolytic enzymes that hydrolyse the peptide bonds of the terminal amino acids of proteins or peptides, as opposed to ENDOPEPTIDASES, which cleave at sites in the middle of a peptide chain. There are two groups: aminopeptidases (EC

3.4.11.x) which remove the amino acid at the amino terminal of the protein, and carboxypeptidases (EC 3.4.16.x and 3.4.17.x), which remove the amino acid at the carboxyl terminal.

exophthalmus Protrusion of the eyeballs from the sockets, commonly associated with hyperthyroid GOITRE.

exotoxins Toxic substances produced by bacteria which diffuse out of the cells and stimulate the production of antibodies which specifically neutralise them (antitoxins). They are generally heat-labile and inactivated in about 1 h at 60°C. Exotoxins include those produced by the organisms responsible for BOTULISM, tetanus and diphtheria.

See also ENDOTOXINS; TX NUMBERS.

expansion rings In relation to cans, the concentric rings stamped into the ends of the can to allow bulging during heat processing without straining the seams unduly.

expeller cake The residue from oilseeds after most of the oil has been removed by pressing; a valuable source of protein for animal feeding.

extensograph (extensometer) An instrument for measuring the stretching strength of dough as an index of its baking quality.

extraction rate See FLOUR, EXTRACTION RATE.

extremophiles Microorganisms that can grow under extreme conditions of heat (THERMOPHILES and extreme thermophiles, some of which live in hot springs at 100°C), cold (PSYCHROPHILES), high concentrations of salt (HALOPHILES), high pressure or extremes of acid or alkali.

extrinsic factor See ANAEMIA, PERNICIOUS; VITAMIN B_{12}.

extrusion Process in which the raw materials are mixed, kneaded, sheared, shaped and extruded; essentially a screw press which forces the product through a restricted opening. When the food is also heated the process is termed extrusion cooking, a high-temperature short-time procedure.

exudative diathesis Vascular disease of VITAMIN E-deficient chicks, characterised by accumulation of greenish fluid under the skin of the breast and abdomen.

F

FAD See FLAVIN ADENINE DINUCLEOTIDE.

faeces Composed of undigested food residues, remains of digestive secretions that have not been reabsorbed, bacteria from the intestinal tract, cells, cell debris and mucus from the intestinal lining, substances excreted into the intestinal tract (mainly in the BILE). The average amount is about 100 g/day, but varies widely depending on the intake of DIETARY FIBRE.

faecolith Small hard mass of faeces, found especially in the vermiform APPENDIX.

faggot (1) Traditional British meatball made from pig OFFAL and meat.

(2) Bundle of herbs, BOUQUET GARNI.

fair maids Cornish name for PILCHARDS (thought to be a corruption of the Spanish *fumade* = smoked).

fairy potato See EARTH NUT.

famotidine See HISTAMINE RECEPTOR ANTAGONISTS.

FAO Food and Agriculture Organisation of the United Nations, founded in 1943; headquarters in Rome. Its goal is to achieve freedom from hunger worldwide. According to its constitution the specific objectives are 'raising the levels of nutrition and standards of living. . . . and securing improvements in the efficiency of production and distribution of all food and agricultural products.'

Farex Trade name for an infant cereal food.

farfals See PASTA.

farina General term for starch. More specifically in the UK refers to POTATO STARCH; in the USA is defined as the starch obtained from wheat other than DURUM WHEAT; starch from the latter is SEMOLINA. Farina dolce is Italian flour made from dried chestnuts.

farinaceous Starchy.

farinograph An instrument for measuring the physical properties of a dough.

farl Scottish; triangular oatmeal cake.

fascioliasis Infestation of the bile ducts and liver with the liver FLUKE *Fasciola hepatica*, commonly acquired by eating wild WATERCRESS on which the larval stage of the parasite is present.

fasciolopsiasis Infestation of the intestinal tract with the FLUKE *Fasciolopsis buski*, commonly acquired by eating uncooked water chestnuts contaminated with the larval stage of the parasite.

fast foods (fast service foods) General term used for a limited menu of foods that lend themselves to production line techniques; suppliers tend to specialise in products such as HAMBURGERS, PIZZAS, chicken or SANDWICHES.

fasting Going without food. The metabolic fasting state begins some 4 h after a meal, when the digestion and absorption of food are complete and body reserves of fat and GLYCOGEN begin to be mobilised. In more prolonged fasting the blood concentration of KETONE bodies rises, as they are exported from the liver for use by muscle and other tissues as a metabolic fuel.

fat (1) Chemically fats (or lipids) are substances that are insoluble in water but soluble in organic solvents such as ether, chloroform and benzene, and are actual or potential esters of FATTY ACIDS. The term includes TRIACYLGLYCEROLS (triglycerides), PHOSPHOLIPIDS, WAXES and STEROLS.

(2) In more general use the term 'fats' refers to the neutral fats which are mixtures of esters of fatty acids with GLYCEROL, triacylglycerols (or triglycerides).

fat, blood   Total blood fat in the fasting state is about 590 mg per 100 mL plasma: 150 mg neutral fats (TRIACYLGLYCEROLS), 160 mg (4 mmol) cholesterol, 200 mg phospholipids, mainly in the plasma LIPOPROTEINS. After a meal the total fat increases, as a result of the CHYLOMICRONS containing the recently absorbed dietary fat.

See also LIPIDS, PLASMA.

fat, brown   See BROWN ADIPOSE TISSUE.

fat-extenders   See SUPERGLYCINERATED FATS.

fat free   EU regulations restrict use of the term 'fat free' to foods that contain less than 0.15 g of fat/100 g; in USA low fat foods must state the percentage of fat; thus a product described as 95% fat free contains only 5 g of fat/100 g.

fat, high-ratio   See SUPERGLYCINERATED FATS.

fat, neutral   FATS that are chemically TRIACYLGLYCEROLS (triglycerides).

fat, non-saponifiable, saponifiable   See SAPONIFICATION.

fat replacers   Substances that provide a creamy, fat-like texture used to replace or partly replace the fat in a recipe food. Made from a variety of substances, e.g. Slendid is the trade name for a product derived from pectin, Olestra is sucrose polyester which is not absorbed by the body, Simplesse is a protein product, N-oil is made from tapioca.

fat, saturated   FATS containing only or mainly saturated FATTY ACIDS.

fat-soluble vitamins   VITAMINS A, D, E and K; they occur in food dissolved in the fats and are stored in the body to a greater extent than the water-soluble vitamins.

fat spread   A general term for fatty bread spreads (yellow fats), including BUTTER, MARGARINE and low-fat spreads. Reduced fat spreads contain not more than 60% fat, and low-fat spreads not more than 40%, compared with 80% fat in butter and margarine. Very low fat spreads contain less than 20% fat.

fatty acids   Organic ACIDS consisting of carbon chains with a terminal carboxyl group. The nutritionally important fatty acids have an even number of carbon atoms, commonly between 12 and 22. Saturated fatty acids are those in which there are only single bonds between adjacent carbon atoms. It is recommended that intake should not exceed about 10% of food energy intake, since they increase levels of blood CHOLESTEROL (a major risk factor in heart disease).

Unsaturated fatty acids have one or more carbon–carbon double bonds in the molecule. These double bonds can be reduced (saturated) with hydrogen, the process of hydrogenation, forming saturated fatty acids. Fatty acids with only one double bond are termed mono-unsaturated, OLEIC ACID is the main one found in fats and oils. Fatty acids with two or more double bonds are termed polyunsaturated fatty acids, often abbreviated to pufa.

Unsaturated fatty acids not only do not raise the levels of cholesterol in the blood but may be beneficial. In general fats from animal sources are high in saturated and relatively low in unsaturated fatty acids; vegetable and fish oils are generally higher in unsaturated and lower in saturated fatty acids.

In addition to their systematic and trivial names, fatty acids can be named by a shorthand giving the number of carbon atoms in the molecule (e.g. C18), then a colon and the number of double bonds (e.g. C18:2), followed by the position of the first double bond from the methyl end of the molecule as n- or ω (e.g. C18:2 n-6, or C18:2 ω6). See Table 7.

fatty acids, essential (EFA)   FATTY ACIDS that cannot be made in the body and are therefore dietary essentials; two polyunsaturated fatty acids: linoleic (C18:2 ω6) and α-linolenic (C18:3 ω3).

Several other fatty acids have some EFA activity in that they cure some, but not all, of the signs of (experimental) EFA deficiency. Arachidonic (C20:4 ω6), eicosapentaenoic (EPA C20:5 ω3) and docosahexaenoic (DHA C22:6 ω3) acids are physiologically important, although they are not dietary essentials since they can be formed from linoleic and α-linolenic acids.

Estimated average requirement for ω6 pufa is 1% of total energy intake (260 mg/MJ) and for ω3 pufa is 0.2% (50 mg/MJ), with a recommendation that total pufa intakes should not be more than 10–15% of total energy; a desirable intake, and the basis of REFERENCE INTAKES is 8–10% of energy intake, about 2–2.6 g/MJ.

fatty acids, free (FFA) or non-esterified (NEFA)   Fatty acids may be liberated from triacylglycerols (triglycerides) either by enzymic hydrolysis (when they are generally known as non-esterified fatty acids, NEFA, or unesterified fatty acids, UFA) or as a result of hydrolytic rancidity of the fat. Determination of NEFA is therefore an index of the quality of fats.

Free fatty acids circulate in the bloodstream, bound to albumin. They are released from ADIPOSE TISSUE, especially in the fasting state, as a fuel for muscle and other tissues. The normal concentration in plasma is between 0.5–2 μmol/L, increasing with fasting and exercise.

fatty acids, unesterified, non-esterified (NEFA)   See FATTY ACIDS, FREE.

fatty acids, volatile   Refers to acetic, propionic and butyric acids which, apart from their presence in some foods, are produced by bacteria in the human intestine and rumen of cattle from undigested starch and dietary fibre. To some extent they can be absorbed and used as a source of energy. Butyric acid formed in the colon may have some anticarcinogenic action.

fat, unsaturated   FATS containing a high proportion of unsaturated FATTY ACIDS.

fat, white   See ADIPOSE TISSUE.

fat, yellow   See FAT SPREAD.

favism   Acute haemolytic ANAEMIA induced in genetically sensitive people by eating broad beans, *Vicia faba*, or in response to various drugs, including especially antimalarials. The disease is due to a deficiency of the enzyme glucose-6-phosphate dehydrogenase (EC 1.1.1.19) in red BLOOD CELLS, which are then vulnerable to the toxins, vicine and convicine, in the beans. The condition affects some 100 million people worldwide, and is commonest in people of Mediterranean and Afro-Caribbean descent.

FDA   Food and Drug Administration; US government regulatory agency.

FD&C   USA, colours permitted for use in foods, drugs and cosmetics.

FDNB   See FLUORODINITROBENZENE.

fecula (fécule)   Foods that are almost solely starch; prepared from roots and stems by grating, e.g. TAPIOCA, SAGO and ARROWROOT; starchy powder from rice, potatoes, etc.

Fehling's reagent   Alkaline cupric tartrate solution used for detection and semi-quantitative determination of glucose and other reducing sugars.

   See also BENEDICT'S REAGENT, SOMOGYI–NELSON REAGENT.

feijoa beans   See BEANS, ADZUKI.

Feingold diet   Exclusion of foods containing synthetic colours, flavours and preservatives and limitation of intake of fruits and vegetables such as oranges, apricots, peaches, tomatoes and cucumbers; intended to treat hyperactive children. There is little evidence either that these foods are a cause of hyperactivity or that the exclusion diet is beneficial.

felafel   Middle Eastern; deep fried balls of CHICK PEA batter.

FEMA   US Flavor and Extract Manufacturers' Association.

fenfluramine An anorectic (appetite suppressant, see APPETITE CONTROL) drug with amphetamine-like actions used in the treatment of obesity. Only the D-isomer is active (dexfenfluramine).

fennel (1) Aromatic seeds and feathery green leaves of the perennial plant *Foeniculum vulgare*, used to flavour a variety of dishes.

(2) *Foeniculum dulce* (or *F. vulgare* var. *azoricum*). Annual plant, also called Florence fennel or finnochio; the swollen bases of the leaves are eaten as a vegetable, raw or cooked.

Composition/100 g: 46 kJ (11 kcal), protein 0.9 g, fat 0.2 g, carbohydrate 1.5 g (1.4 g sugars, 0.1 g starch), nsp 2.3 g, Na 96 mg, K 300 mg, Ca 20 mg, Mg 7 mg, P 21 mg, Fe 0.2 mg, Cu 0.01 mg, Zn 0.4 mg, vitamin A 10 µg (60 µg carotene), B_1 0.05 mg, B_2 0.01 mg, niacin 0.4 mg, B_6 0.08 mg, folate 26 µg, C 2 mg. A 100 g serving is a source of folate. The seeds are also used as flavouring .

fen-phen The combination of FENFLURAMINE and PHENTERMINE, formerly used as an appetite suppressant (APPETITE CONTROL) drug in the treatment of obesity; withdrawn in 1995 in response to reports of heart valve damage.

fenugreek *Trigonella feonumgraecum*, a leguminous plant eaten as a vegetable; the seeds are used for flavouring. Traditionally eaten by women in the Orient to help gain weight.

fermentation Anaerobic METABOLISM. Used generally of alcoholic fermentation of sugars, also production of acetic, lactic, and citric acids by microorganisms in pickling and manufacture of VINEGAR.

fermented milk See MILK, FERMENTED.

fermentograph An instrument for measuring the gas-producing power of a dough. The fermenting dough is contained in a balloon immersed in water and as gas is produced the balloon expands and rises in the water, the rise being measured continuously.

ferric ammonium citrate The form in which IRON is sometimes added to foods. Occurs as brown-red scales (16.5–18.5% iron) and as green scales (14.5–16% iron).

ferritin The main IRON storage protein in tissues; also found in serum, where the concentration reflects the total amount of storage iron in the body, and therefore permits assessment of iron status over the range from deficiency, through normal to overload. Although it provides the most sensitive index of iron depletion, its synthesis is also significantly reduced in response to trauma and infection.

See also ACUTE PHASE PROTEINS; TRANSFERRIN RECEPTOR.

ferrum redactum See IRON, REDUCED.

FFA Free fatty acids. See FATTY ACIDS, FREE.

fibre, crude The term given to indigestible part of foods, defined in the UK Fertiliser and Feedingstuffs Act of 1932 as the residue left after successive extraction under closely specified conditions with petroleum ether, 1.25% sulphuric acid and 1.25% sodium hydroxide, minus ash. No relationship to DIETARY FIBRE.

fibre, dietary See DIETARY FIBRE.

fibre, insoluble The part of DIETARY FIBRE (or NON-STARCH POLY-SACCHARIDE) that is not soluble in water, CELLULOSE, hemicelluloses and lignin. These increase the bulk of the intestinal contents.

fibre, soluble The plant GUMS and small oligosaccharides in DIETARY FIBRE that are soluble in water, forming viscous gels.

fibric acids A variety of analogues of clofibric acid (chlorophenoxy-isobutyrate), including bezafibrate, clofibrate (the ethyl ester), fenofibrate and gemfibrozil (which is not halogenated), used in treatment of HYPERLIPIDAEMIA. They lower VLDL and LDL, and raise HDL, by stimulation of lipoprotein LIPASE (EC3.1.1.34).

fibrin See FIBRINOGEN.

fibrinogen One of the proteins of the blood plasma responsible for COAGULATION. When PROTHROMBIN is activated to thrombin in response to injury, it hydrolyses fibrinogen to fibrin, which is deposited as strands that trap red cells and platelets, forming the clot.

fibronectin A protein found in blood plasma which has a very rapid rate of turnover, and can be used as an index of undernutrition.

fibrous proteins See ALBUMINOIDS.

ficin (ficain) Proteolytic enzyme (EC 3.4.22.3) from the FIG.

fiddleheads Canadian name for BRACKEN fronds.

field egg See AUBERGINE.

field mushroom *Agaricus campestris*, *A. vaporarius*, see MUSHROOMS.

fig The fruit of *Ficus carica*; eaten fresh or dried. Figs have mild laxative properties, e.g. syrup of figs is a medicinal preparation.

Composition/100 g (fresh): 179 kJ (43 kcal), protein 1.3 g, fat 0.3 g, carbohydrate 9.5 g (9.5 g sugars), dietary fibre 2.3 g, nsp 1.5 g, Na 3 mg, K 200 mg, Ca 38 mg, Mg 15 mg, P 15 mg, Fe 0.3 mg, Cu 0.06 mg, Zn 0.3 mg, vitamin A 25 μg (150 μg carotene), B_1 0.03 mg, B_2 0.03 mg, niacin 0.6 mg, B_6 0.08 mg, pantothenate 0.2 mg, C 2 mg. Serving 55 g.

fig, Adam's See PLANTAIN.

fig, berberry or Indian See PRICKLY PEAR.

FIGLU test For FOLIC ACID status. Measurement of urinary excretion of formiminoglutamate (FIGLU) after a test dose of 2–5 g of HISTIDINE. FIGLU formiminotransferase (EC 2.1.2.5) is a folate-dependent enzyme.

See also ANAEMIA, MEGALOBLASTIC.

filbert See HAZEL NUT.

filé powder   Dried powdered young leaves of the sassafras tree (*Sassafras albidum*); very aromatic, an ingredient of GUMBO.

filth test   Name given to a test originated in the USA for determining the contamination of a food with rodent hairs and insect fragments as an index of hygienic handling.

filtrate factor   Obsolete name for PANTOTHENIC ACID.

fines herbes   Mixture of chopped parsley, tarragon, chives, chervil, marjoram and sometimes watercress.

fingerware   Edible seaweed, *Laminaria digitata.*

fining agents   Substances used to clarify liquids by precipitation, e.g. EGG albumin, casein, bentonite, ISINGLASS, GELATINE, etc.

finnan haddock   Smoke-cured haddock (named after Findon in Scotland). See also ARBROATH SMOKIE.

finocchio   Variety of FENNEL with swollen leaf base; *Foeniculum vulgare* var *azoricum.*

fire point   The temperature at which a frying oil will sustain combustion; ranges between 340–360°C for different fats.
   See also FLASH POINT; SMOKE POINT.

fireless cooker   See HAYBOX COOKING.

firkin   A quarter of a barrel of beer, 9 Imperial gallons (40 L); also 56 lb (25.5 kg) of butter.

firming agents   Fresh fruits contain insoluble PECTINS as a gel around the fibrous tissues which keeps the fruit firm. Breakdown of cell structure allows conversion of pectin to pectic acid, with loss of firmness. The addition of calcium salts (chloride or carbonate) forms a calcium pectate gel which protects the fruit against softening; these are known as firming agents. Alum (aluminium potassium sulphate) is sometimes used to firm pickles.

fish, fatty   See FISH, OILY.

fish flour   See FISH PROTEIN CONCENTRATE.

fish ham   Japanese product made from a red fish such as tuna or marlin, pickled with salt and nitrite, mixed with whale meat and pork fat and stuffed into a large sausage-type casing.

fish meal   Surplus fish, waste from filleting (fish-house waste) and fish unsuitable for human consumption are dried and powdered. The resultant meal is a valuable source of protein for animal feedingstuff, or, after deodorisation, as human food since it contains about 70% protein of biological value up to 0.7. Meal made from white fish is termed white fish meal, distinct from the oily type which is sometimes of very poor quality and is then used as fertiliser.

fish oils   These contain long-chain polyunsaturated FATTY ACIDS which offer some protection against heart disease. The two main ones are eicosapentaenoic acid (EPA C20:5 ω3) and docosohexaenoic acid (DHA C22:6 ω3). Fish oil concentrates containing these fatty acids are sold as pharmaceutical preparations.

See also COD LIVER OIL; HALIBUT (liver oil); MENHADEN; Table 7.

fish, oily Anchovies, herring, mackerel, pilchard, salmon, sardine, trout, tuna, whitebait, containing about 15% fat (varying from 5–20% through the year) and containing 10–40 μg vitamin D per 100 g, as distinct from white fish, which contain 1–2% fat and only a trace of vitamin D.

See also HERRING.

fish paste A spread made from ground fish and cereal. In UK legally contains not less than 70% fish.

fish protein concentrate Deodorised, decolorised, defatted FISH MEAL, also known as fish flour.

fish solubles See STICKWATER.

fish, white Non-oily fish, i.e. 1–2% fat, e.g. cod, dogfish, haddock, halibut, plaice, saithe, skate, sole, whiting.

Average composition/100 g: 364 kJ (87 kcal), protein 18.1 g, fat 1.6 g, cholesterol 42.2 mg, carbohydrate 0 g, Na 85 mg, K 326 mg, Ca 31 mg, Mg 28 mg, P 218 mg, Fe 0.6 mg, Cu 0.03 mg, Zn 0.4 mg, Se 37 μg, I 80 μg, vitamin A 3 μg, E 0.4 mg, B_1 0.08 mg, B_2 0.12 mg, niacin 6.5 mg, B_6 0.4 mg, folate 8.9 μg, B_{12} 2.1 μg, pantothenate 0.4 mg, biotin 7.1 μg. A 120 g serving is a source of Mg; good source of vitamin B_6; rich source of protein, niacin, vitamin B_{12}, I, Se.

fistula An abnormal connection between two hollow organs, or between a hollow organ and the external environment; may occur as a result of infection, injury or surgery.

five-spice powder Chinese; a mixture of star ANISE, anise pepper, FENNEL, CLOVES and CINNAMON, and sometimes powdered dried orange peel.

flash 18 A method of canning foods (Swift & Co, USA) under pressure (126 kPa = 18 psi above atmospheric). The food is sterilised at 121 °C and then canned at that temperature, not requiring further heat. The process is claimed to give improved taste and texture compared with conventional canning, and the possibility of using large containers without overheating the food.

flash evaporation See EVAPORATION, FLASH.

flash pasteurisation See PASTEURISATION.

flash point With reference to frying oils, the temperature at which the decomposition products can be ignited, but will not support combustion; ranges between 290–330 °C.

See also FIRE POINT; SMOKE POINT.

flatfish FISH with a flattened shape, including dab, flounder, halibut, plaice, sole and turbot.

flatogens Substances that cause gas production, FLATULENCE, in the intestine, by providing fermentable substrate for intestinal bacteria. Those identified include small OLIGOSACCHARIDES such as raffinose, stachyose and verbascose in a variety of beans.

See also NON-STARCH POLYSACCHARIDES.

flat sours Bacteria such as *Bacillus stearothermophilus* render canned food sour by fermenting carbohydrates to lactic, formic and acetic acids, without gas production. This means that the ends of the can are not swelled out but remain flat. Economically they are the most important of the thermophilic spoilage agents (THERMOPHILES); some species can grow slowly at 25°C and thus spoil products after long storage periods.

flatulence (flatus) Production of gas in the intestine, hydrogen, carbon dioxide and methane. May be caused by a variety of foods which contain FLATOGENS.

flavanols, flavanones See FLAVONOIDS.

flavedo The coloured outer peel layer of citrus fruits, also called the epicarp or zest. It contains the oil sacs, and hence the aromatic oils, and numerous plastids which are green and contain chlorophyll in the unripe fruit, turning yellow or orange in the ripe fruit, when they contain carotene and xanthophyll.

flavin The group of compounds containing the iso-alloxazine ring structure, as in riboflavin (VITAMIN B₂); a general term for riboflavin derivatives.

flavin adenine dinucleotide (FAD) A COENZYME in oxidation reactions, derived from VITAMIN B₂, phosphate, ribose and adenine.

flavin mononucleotide (FMN) A COENZYME in oxidation reactions, chemically the phosphate of VITAMIN B₂ (riboflavin).

flavone See FLAVONOIDS.

flavonoids (bioflavonoids) Polyphenolic compounds widely distributed in plants where they are responsible for colour, taste and smell as well as attracting or repelling insects and microorganisms. Some 4000 have been identified, with a wide range of chemical properties. They occur as glycosides in which the sugar moiety is usually glucose or rhamnose.

At one time a mixture of flavonoids was shown to decrease capillary permeability and fragility in human beings and was named vitamin P, but later, 1950, when it was found that they are not dietary essentials, the name was dropped.

More recently there has been epidemiological evidence that flavonoids may have a rôle in protection against some forms of cancer from observations in population groups with a high intake of fruits and vegetables. Some are antioxidants and may help to prevent atherosclerosis; others have weak OESTROGEN activity (phyto-oestrogens).

Total dietary intake is around 1 g per day (650 mg when calculated as aglycones), a large part of which comes from tea, red wine, berries, and onions.

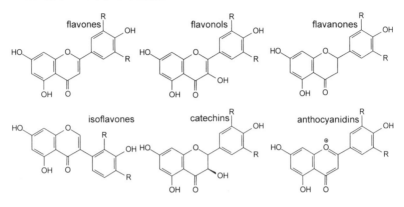

flavonols   See FLAVONOIDS.

flavoproteins   Enzymes that contain the vitamin RIBOFLAVIN, or a derivative such as flavin adenine dinucleotide or riboflavin phosphate, as the PROSTHETIC GROUP. Mainly involved in oxidation reactions in METABOLISM.

flavour   See TASTE; ORGANOLEPTIC.

flavour potentiator (enhancer)   A substance that enhances the flavours of other substances without itself imparting any characteristic flavour of its own, e.g. MONOSODIUM GLUTAMATE, RIBOTIDE, as well as small quantities of sugar, salt and vinegar.

flavour profile   A method of judging the flavour of foods by examination of a list of the separate factors into which the flavour can be analysed, the so-called character notes.

flavours, synthetic   Mostly mixtures of ESTERS, e.g. banana oil is ethyl butyrate and amyl acetate; apple oil is ethyl butyrate, ethyl valerianate, ethyl salicylate, amyl butyrate, glycerol, chloroform and alcohol; pineapple oil is ethyl and amyl butyrates, acetaldehyde, chloroform, glycerol, alcohol.

flea seed   See PSYLLIUM.

fleishig   Jewish term for dishes containing meat, which cannot be served with or before milk dishes.
      See also MILCHIG; PAREVE.

flint corn   See MAIZE.

flippers   See SWELLS.

Florence oil   Name given to high grade of OLIVE OIL.

floridean starch   A branched polysaccharide of glucose obtained from red algae (Florideae spp).

florigens   See PHYTOCHROMES.

flounder   Small flatfish, *Platichthys* spp, also called fluke.

Composition/100 g: 343 kJ (82 kcal), protein 16.4 g, fat 1.8 g, cholesterol 48 mg, carbohydrate 0 g, Na 92 mg, K 300 mg, Ca 27 mg, Mg 23 mg, P 190 mg, Fe 0.4 mg, Cu 0.03 mg, Zn 0.5 mg, Se 26 µg, I 25 µg, vitamin E 0.4 mg, B_1 0.14 mg, B_2 0.21 mg, niacin 6.5 mg, B_6 0.25 mg, folate 11 µg, B_{12} 1 µg. A 120 g serving is a source of vitamin B_1, B_2, B_6; good source of I; rich source of protein, niacin, vitamin B_{12}, Se.

flour   Most commonly refers to ground wheat, although also used for other cereals and applied to powdered dried matter such as FISH FLOUR, potato flour, etc.

See also BREAD; FLOUR, EXTRACTION RATE.

flour, ageing and bleaching   See AGEING.

flour, agglomerated   A dispersible form, easily wetted, produced by agglomerating the fine particles in steam; particles are greater than 100 µm in diameter, so the flour is dust-free.

flour enrichment   The addition of vitamins and minerals to flour, to contain not less than: (UK) vitamin B_1 0.24 mg, niacin 1.6 mg, iron 1.65 mg, calcium 120 mg/100 g; (USA) vitamin B_1 0.44–0.56 mg, vitamin B_2 0.2–0.33 mg, niacin 3.6–4.4 mg, iron 2.9–3.7 mg/100 g; calcium not specified.

flour, enzyme inactivated   Flour in which the enzyme α-AMYLASE has been inactivated by heat to prevent degradation when the flour is used as a thickening agent in gravies, soups, etc.

flour, extraction rate   The yield of flour obtained from wheat in the milling process. 100% extraction (or straight-run flour) is wholemeal flour containing all of the grain; lower extraction rates are the whiter flours from which progressively more of the BRAN and GERM (and thus B vitamins and iron) are excluded, down to a figure of 72% extraction, which is normal white flour. 'Patent' flours are of lower extraction rate, 30–50%, and so comprise mostly the ENDOSPERM of the grain.

See also BREAD.

flour, high-ratio   Flour of very fine, uniform particle size, treated with chlorine to reduce the GLUTEN strength. Used for making cakes, since it is possible to add up to 140 parts sugar to 100 parts of this flour, whereas only half this quantity of sugar can be incorporated into ordinary flour. See FLOUR STRENGTH.

flour improvers   See AGEING.

flour, national   See WHEATMEAL.

flour, patent   See FLOUR, EXTRACTION RATE.

flour, self-raising   Wheat flour to which BAKING POWDER has been added to produce carbon dioxide in the presence of water and heat; the dough is thus aerated without prolonged fermentation. Usually 'weaker' flours are used (see FLOUR STRENGTH). Legally, self-raising flour must contain not less than 0.4% available carbon dioxide.

flour strength A property of the flour proteins enabling the dough to retain gas during fermentation to give a 'bold' loaf. 'Strong' flour is higher in protein, has greater elasticity and resistance to extension, and greater ability to absorb water. A 'weak' flour gives a loaf that lacks volume.

See also EXTENSOMETER; FARINOGRAPH.

flour, wholemeal Flour made from the entire grain of wheat, i.e. 100% extraction rate.

fluid balance See WATER BALANCE.

fluid bed dryer A bed of solid particles is supported on a cushion of hot air jets (fluidised) and the material may be conveyed this way, while being dried. The method achieves intimate mixing without mechanical damage; applied to cereals, tableting granules, salt, coffee and dried vegetables.

fluke (1) Small flatfish, *Platichthys* spp, also called FLOUNDER.

(2) Parasitic flatworms of the order Trematoda.

flummery Old English pudding made by boiling down the water from soaked oatmeal until it becomes thick and gelatinous. Similar to FRUMENTY. Dutch flummery is made with gelatine or isinglass and egg yolk; Spanish flummery with cream, rice flour and cinnamon.

fluorescence The ability to absorb light at one wavelength and emit at another within 10–100 ns. See also FLUORIMETRY.

fluorescence immunoassay Sensitive and specific analytical technique for determination of analytes present at very low concentrations in biological samples; the ANTIBODY is labelled with a substrate that yields a fluorescent product, but in such a way that it does not act as a substrate for the enzyme when the antigen (analyte) is bound. Therefore only free antibody will yield the fluorescent product when the enzyme is added. Unlike RADIO-IMMUNOASSAY does not require separation of bound and free antigen.

See also ELISA.

fluoridation The addition of FLUORIDE to drinking water.

fluoride The ION of the element fluorine. Although it occurs in small amounts in plants and animals, and has effects on the formation of dental enamel and bones, it is not considered to be a dietary essential and no deficiency signs are known.

Drinking water containing about 1 part per million of fluoride protects teeth from decay, and in some areas fluoride is added to drinking water to achieve this level. Naturally, the fluoride content of water ranges between 0.05–14 ppm.

Water containing more than about 12 ppm fluoride can lead to chalky white patches on the surface of the teeth, known as mottled enamel. At higher levels there is strong brown mottling of the teeth and inappropriate deposition of fluoride in bones, fluorosis.

fluorimetry (fluorometry) Sensitive and relatively specific analytical technique dependent on emission of light more or less immediately (within 10–100 ns) after absorption of light by a compound in solution. Both the exciting and emitted wavelengths are characteristic of the analyte, and the intensity of fluorescence is proportional to the concentration of analyte present.

fluorodinitrobenzene (FDNB, dinitrofluorobenzene) Reacts with free amino groups; commonly used to determine free ε-amino groups of lysine (and hence AVAILABLE LYSINE) in proteins.

fluorosis Damage to teeth (brown mottling of the enamel) and bones caused by an excessive intake of FLUORIDE.

fluoxetine An antidepressant acting to stimulate serotoninergic activity (a SEROTONIN-specific reuptake inhibitor); also has anorectic activity, and is used in treatment of OBESITY and BULIMIA NERVOSA. Trade name Prozac.

FMN See FLAVIN MONONUCLEOTIDE.

foam COLLOIDAL SUSPENSION of gas bubbles in a liquid or semi-liquid phase. Most so-called aerosol foams (e.g. whipped cream) are correctly foams, since an aerosol is a colloidal suspension of liquid droplets in a gas phase.

foam cells Macrophages that have accumulated very large amounts of CHOLESTEROL as a result of uptake of (chemically modified) low density LIPOPROTEIN. They infiltrate the arterial wall and lead to the development of fatty streaks, and eventually ATHEROSCLEROSIS.

foam-mat drying A method of drying food. The liquid concentrate is whipped to a foam with the aid of a foaming agent, spread on a tray and dried in a stream of warm air. It reconstitutes very rapidly with water because of the fine structure of the foam.

foie gras (French, *fat liver*). The liver of goose or duck that has been force fed and fattened; may be cooked whole or used as the basis of PÂTÉ de foie gras, the most highly prized of the pâtés.

folacin, folate See FOLIC ACID.

folic acid A VITAMIN that functions as a carrier of one-carbon units in a variety of metabolic reactions. Essential for the synthesis of purines and pyrimidines (and so for NUCLEIC ACID synthesis and hence cell division); the principal deficiency disease is megaloblastic ANAEMIA, due to failure of the normal maturation of red BLOOD CELLS, with release into the circulation of immature precursors of red blood cells.

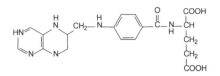

Occurs in foods as a variety of one-carbon substituted derivatives, and with a varying number of γ-glutamyl residues. Mixed food folate is about 50% as biologically active as synthetic tetrahydrofolic acid used in enrichment and supplements.

Supplements of 400 µg free folic acid/day begun before conception reduce the incidence of spina bifida and other neural tube defects in babies; it is unlikely that ordinary foods could provide this much folate, so supplements are advised.

See also DIETARY FOLATE EQUIVALENTS; dUMP SUPPRESSION TEST; FIGLU TEST; HOMOCYSTEINE; METHYLENETETRAHYDROFOLATE REDUCTASE.

folinic acid 5-Formyl FOLIC ACID, more stable to oxidation than folic acid itself, and commonly used in pharmaceutical preparations. The synthetic (racemic) compound is known as leucovorin.

fondant Minute sugar crystals in a saturated sugar syrup; used as the creamy filling in chocolates and biscuits and for decorating cakes. Prepared by boiling sugar solution with the addition of GLUCOSE syrup or an inverting agent (see INVERT SUGAR) and cooling rapidly while stirring.

fondue Swiss; cheese melted with wine and herbs, eaten by dipping small squares of bread into the hot mixture. Fondue bourguignonne is small cubes of marinated meat, cooked on a long fork in a vessel of hot oil at the table.

food Any solid or liquid material consumed by a living organism to supply ENERGY, build and replace tissue or participate in such reactions. Defined by the FAO/WHO CODEX ALIMENTARIUS Commission as a substance, whether processed, semiprocessed or raw, which is intended for human consumption and includes drink, chewing gum and any substance that has been used in the manufacture, preparation or treatment of food but does not include cosmetics, tobacco or substances used only as drugs.

food balance A national account of the annual production of food, changes in stocks, imports and exports, and distribution of food over various uses in the country. Permits estimation of *per capita* food availability, but not consumption.

foodborne disease Infectious or toxic disease caused by agents that enter the body through the consumption of food. The causative agents may be present in food as a result of infection of animals from which food is prepared or contamination at source or during manufacture, storage and preparation.

Three main categories: (1) diseases caused by microorganisms (including parasites) that invade and multiply in the body;

(2) diseases caused by toxins produced by microorganisms growing in the gastrointestinal tract;

(3) disease caused by the ingestion of food contaminated with poisonous chemicals or containing natural toxins or the toxins produced by microorganisms in the food.

See also FOOD POISONING.

food combining See HAY DIET.

food composition tables Tables of the chemical composition and energy and nutrient yield of foods, based on chemical analysis. Although the analyses are performed with great precision, they are, of necessity, only performed on a few samples of each type of food. There is considerable variation, especially in the content of vitamins and minerals, between different samples of the same food. Therefore, calculation of energy and nutrient intakes based on use of food composition tables, even when intake has been weighed, can only be considered to be accurate to within about ±10%, at best.

food intolerance See ADVERSE REACTIONS TO FOOD.

food phosphate factor Term applied to the resistance of bacteria to thermal destruction; defined as the ratio of the resistance to heat when present in a food to that when in phosphate buffer (at pH 6.98). The protective action of the ingredients of food renders the bacteria more resistant than buffer.

food poisoning May be due to:

(1) contamination with harmful bacteria or other microorganisms. The commonest bacterial contamination is due to AEROMONAS spp, BACILLUS CEREUS, CAMPYLOBACTER spp, CLOSTRIDIUM spp, E. COLI, LISTERIA spp, SALMONELLA spp, SHIGELLA spp, STAPHYLOCOCCUS AUREUS, YERSINIA ENTEROCOLITICA.

(2) toxic chemicals, either naturally present or the result of contamination;

(3) ADVERSE REACTIONS to certain proteins or other natural constituents of foods.

See also DYSENTERY; ENTEROTOXINS; TX NUMBERS.

food science The study of the basic chemical, physical, biochemical and biophysical properties of foods and their constituents, and of changes that these may undergo during handling, preservation, processing, storage, distribution and preparation for consumption. Hence food scientist.

172

food technology   The application of science and technology to the treatment, processing, preservation and distribution of foods. Hence food technologist.

food yeast   See YEAST.

forcemeat   A highly seasoned STUFFING made from chopped minced veal, pork or sausage meat mixed with onion and range of herbs (Fr *farce* = stuffing).

formiminoglutamic acid   See FIGLU TEST.

formula diet   Composed of simple substances that do not require digestion, are readily absorbed and leave a minimum residue in the intestine: glucose, amino acids or peptides, mono- and di-glycerides rather than starch, proteins and fats.

fortification   The deliberate addition of specific nutrients to foods in order to increase their content, sometimes to a higher level than normal, as a means of providing the population with an increased level of intake. Generally synonymous with enrichment, supplementation and restoration; in USA enrichment is used to mean the addition to foods of nutrients that they do not normally contain, while fortification is the restoration of nutrients lost in processing.

See also WINE, FORTIFIED.

four ale   BEER originally sold at four pence per quart. The four ale bar is the public bar.

fovantini   See PASTA.

FPLC (fast protein liquid chromatography)   Modification of HPLC for separation of proteins under denaturing conditions.

fractional test meal   A method of examining the secretion of gastric juices; the stomach contents are sampled at intervals after a test meal of gruel, and acidity (and sometimes also PEPSIN activity) measured.

frangipane (frangipani)   Originally a jasmine perfume which gave its name to an almond cream flavoured with the perfume. The term is used for a cake filling made from eggs, milk and flour with flavouring, and also for a pastry filled with an almond flavoured mixture.

frappé   (1) Iced, frozen or chilled.

(2) Egg-white and sugar syrup whipped until so aerated that the density reaches 5 lb per gallon (100 g in 200 mL).

freedom food   UK, animals maintained under relatively extensive conditions (but not FREE RANGE), with high standard of animal welfare monitored by the Royal Society for the Prevention of Cruelty to Animals.

free from   For a food label or advertising to bear a claim that it is free from fat, saturates, cholesterol, sodium or alcohol it must contain no more than a specified (low) amount. The precise levels at which such claims are permitted differ from one country to another. In USA the food so described must contain only a trivial or physiologically insignificant amount of the specified nutrient.

free radical   A highly reactive molecular species with an unpaired electron.

See also ANTIOXIDANT.

free range   Applied to laying hens kept at no more than 1000 birds to the hectare with free access to open air and grass during daylight.

freeze concentration   Concentration of a liquid by freezing out pure ice, leaving a more concentrated solution; it requires less input of energy, and causes less loss of flavour, than concentration by evaporation. Used especially in the concentration of fruit juices, VINEGAR and BEER.

See also APPLE JACK.

freeze drying   Also known as lyophilisation. A method of drying in which the material is frozen and subjected to high vacuum. The ice sublimes off as water vapour without melting. Materials dried in this way are damaged little, if at all. Freeze-dried food is very porous, since it occupies the same volume as the original and so rehydrates rapidly. There is less loss of flavour and texture than with most other methods of drying. Controlled heat may be applied to the process without melting the frozen material, this is accelerated freeze drying.

freezerburn   A change in the texture of frozen meat, fish and poultry during storage due to sublimation of the ice.

freezer temperatures   For long-term storage of frozen foods (up to 2–3 months), domestic freezers run at −18°C (0°F); in UK this is a three star (***) rated deep freeze. A freezing compartment of a refrigerator (for short-term storage of frozen foods) is between −11°C (12°F), two star (**) rated, for storage up to four weeks and −4°C (25°F), one star (*) rated, for storage up to a week.

See also DATE MARKING.

A three star (***) deep freeze with a snowflake symbol is one that is suitable for freezing foods, as opposed to storing ready-frozen food; it has a higher cooling capacity than a simple storage cabinet.

frenching   Breaking up the fibres of meat by cutting, usually diagonally or in a criss-cross pattern.

fresh   For food labelling and advertising purposes, the US Food and Drug Administration has defined fresh to mean a food that is raw, has never been frozen or heated and contains no preservatives. (IRRADIATION at low levels is permitted.) 'Fresh frozen' and 'frozen fresh' may be used for foods that are quickly frozen while still fresh, and BLANCHING before freezing is permitted.

frigi-canning A process of preserving food by controlled heating sufficient to destroy the vegetative form of microorganisms (and possibly to damage spores sufficiently to prevent germination) followed by sealing aseptically and storing at a low temperature but above freezing point.

frijole bean *Phaseolus acutifolius*, also known as Mexican haricot bean, tepary or pinto. Able to withstand drought.

frijoles A Mexican dish based on boiled fava or lima (butter) beans which have been left to cool, then fried. Also known as refried beans.

fromage frais (fromage blanc) French 'fresh cheese', soft, unripened cheese, 80% water, made from skim milk or semi-skim milk and may include added cream.

Composition/100 g: 470–550 kJ (110–130 kcal), protein 6.8 g, fat 5.8–7.1 g (65.4% saturated, 30.9% mono-, 3.6% polyunsaturated), cholesterol 21 mg; very low fat varieties 242 kJ (58 kcal), protein 7.7 g, fat 0.2 g (50% saturated, 50% mono-, 0% polyunsaturated), cholesterol 1 mg; carbohydrate 5.7–13.8 g (5.7–13.8 g sugars), Na 35 mg, K 110 mg, Ca 86 mg, Mg 8 mg, P 110 mg, Fe 0.1 mg, Cu 0.02 mg, Zn 0.4 mg, Se 2 μg, vitamin A 82 μg, D 0.04 μg, B_1 0.02 mg, B_2 0.35 mg, niacin 1.7 mg, B_6 0.04 mg, folate 15 μg, B_{12} 1.4 μg. A 45 g serving (one tablespoon) is a source of vitamin B_2; rich source of vitamin B_{12}.

fructosan A general name for polysaccharides of FRUCTOSE, such as INULIN. Not digested, and hence a part of DIETARY FIBRE or NON-STARCH POLYSACCHARIDES.

fructose Also known as fruit sugar or laevulose. A six-carbon monosaccharide SUGAR (hexose) with a keto group on carbon-2. Found as the free sugar in fruits and honey, and as a constituent of the DISACCHARIDE SUCROSE. 1.7 times sweeter than sucrose.

See also CARBOHYDRATES; INVERT SUGAR.

fructose syrups Glucose SYRUP made by hydrolysis of starch and then half the glucose converted into fructose, similar to invert syrup produced from sucrose but cheaper. Also known as iso-syrups, high fructose syrups (HFS), high fructose corn syrups (HFCS).

See also GLUCOSE ISOMERASE.

fruitarian A person who eats only fruits, nuts and seeds; an extreme form of VEGETARIAN.

frumenty An old English pudding made from whole wheat

stewed in water for 24 h until the grains have burst and set in a thick jelly, then boiled with milk. Similar to FLUMMERY.

frying Cooking foods with oil at temperatures well above the boiling point of water. Deep frying, in which a food is completely covered with oil, reaches a temperature around 185°C. Nutrient losses are less than in roasting, about 10–20% thiamin, 10–15% riboflavin and nicotinic acid from meat; about 20% thiamin from fish.

fudge CARAMEL in which crystallisation of the sugar (graining) is deliberately induced by the addition of FONDANT (saturated SYRUP containing sugar crystals).

fuga The Japanese puffer fish, *Fuga* spp, responsible for TETRODONTIN POISONING.

fuller's earth An adsorbent clay, calcium montmorillonite, or bentonite; adsorbs both by physical means and by ion exchange. Used to bleach oils, clarify liquids and absorb grease.

fumeol Refined smoke with the bitter principles removed; used for preparing 'liquid' smokes for dipping foods such as fish to give them a smoked flavour.

See also SMOKING.

fumonisin Carcinogenic MYCOTOXIN from *Fusarium* spp growing on cereals; inhibits synthesis of ceramides by inhibition of sphingosine *N*-acetyltransferase (EC 2.3.1.24).

functional foods Foods eaten for specified health purposes, because of their (rich) content of one or more nutrients or non-nutrient substances which may confer health benefits.

fungal protein See MYCOPROTEIN.

fungi Subdivision of Thallophyta, plants without differentiation into root, stem and leaf; cannot photosynthesise, all are parasites or saprophytes. Microfungi are MOULDS, as opposed to larger fungi, which are mushrooms and toadstools. YEASTS are sometimes classed with fungi.

Species of moulds such as *Penicillium*, *Aspergillus*, etc are important causes of food spoilage in the presence of oxygen and relatively high humidity. Those that produce toxins (MYCOTOXINS) are especially problematical.

On the other hand species of *Penicillium* such as *P. cambertii* and *P. rocquefortii* are desirable and essential in the ripening of certain CHEESES.

A number of larger fungi (MUSHROOMS) are cultivated, and other wild species are harvested for their delicate flavour. The mycelium of smaller fungi (including *Graphium*, *Fusarium* and *Rhizopus* species) are grown commercially on waste carbohydrate as a rich source of protein (MYCOPROTEIN) for food manufacture.

furcellaran Danish agar; an anionic, sulphated polysaccharide extracted from the red alga, *Furcellaria fastigiata*, structurally similar to CARRAGEENAN; used as a gelling agent.

fusel oil Alcoholic fermentation produces about 95% alcohol and 5% fusel oil, a mixture of organic acids, higher alcohols (propyl, butyl and amyl), aldehydes and esters, known collectively as CONGENERS. Present in low concentration in wines and beer, and high concentration in pot-still spirit. On maturation of the liquor fusel oil changes and imparts the special flavour to the spirit. Many of the symptoms of HANGOVER can be attributed to fusel oil in alcoholic beverages.

fussol Monofluoroacetamide, a systemic insecticide for treating fruit.

F value A unit of measurement used to compare relative sterilising effects of different procedures (total time–temperature combination); equal to 1 min at 121.1°C.

G

gaffelbitar Semi-preserved HERRING in which microbial growth is checked by the addition of 10–12% salt and sometimes BENZOIC ACID.

galacticol See DULCITOL.

Galactomin Trade name for preparation free from lactose and galactose, for people suffering from lactose intolerance.

galacto-oligosaccharides Small oligosaccharides consisting of glucosyl-(galactose)$_{2-5}$, formed from LACTOSE by galactosyl transfer catalysed by LACTASE (EC 3.2.1.23). Considered to be a PREBIOTIC.

galactorrhoea Abnormal secretion of milk, due to excessive secretion of PROLACTIN.

galactosaemia Congenital lack of UDP-glucose galactosyltransferase (EC 2.7.7.12), or more rarely galactokinase (EC 2.7.1.6) leading to elevated blood concentration of GALACTOSE, and hence non-enzymic GLYCATION of proteins, and the development of cataract and neurological damage; subjects suffer mental retardation, growth failure, vomiting and jaundice, with enlargement of liver and spleen. Treatment is by severe restriction of LACTOSE intake, since this is the only significant source of galactose.

galactose A six-carbon monosaccharide (hexose), differing from GLUCOSE in orientation of the hydroxyl group on carbon-4. About one third as sweet as sucrose. The main dietary source is the disaccharide LACTOSE in milk, important in formation of the galactolipids (cerebrosides) of nerve tissue.

See also CARBOHYDRATES; GALACTOSAEMIA.

β-galactosidase Enzyme (EC 3.2.1.23) that hydrolyses β-galactans in NON-STARCH POLYSACCHARIDES; responsible for loss of firmness during ripening and storage of fruits.

galenicals Crude drugs; infusions, decoctions and tinctures prepared from medicinal plants.

gallates Salts and esters of gallic acid, found in many plants. Used in making dyes and inks, and medicinally as an astringent. Propyl, octyl and dodecyl gallates are legally permitted antioxidants in foods (E-310–312).

gall bladder The gland in the liver that stores the BILE before secretion into the small intestine. See GALLSTONES; GASTROINTESTINAL TRACT.

gallon A unit of volume. The Imperial gallon is 4.546 litres, and the US gallon is 3.7853 litres; therefore 1 Imperial gallon = 1.2 US gallons.

gallstones (cholelithiasis) Crystals of cholesterol, bile salts and calcium salts, formed in the bile duct of the GALL BLADDER when the bile becomes supersaturated.

game Non-domesticated (i.e. wild) animals and birds shot for sport and eaten. RABBIT and PIGEON may be shot at any time, but other game species, such as GROUSE, HARE, PARTRIDGE, PHEASANT, QUAIL, deer (VENISON) and wild DUCK, may not be shot during the closed season, to protect breeding stocks. Game birds are generally raised on farms to provide sport, rather than being hunted in the wild, and increasingly game species are farmed and killed in conventional ways to provide food. Traditionally, game is hung for several days to soften the meat, when it develops a strong flavour.

gammon See BACON.

gangliosides Glycolipids, structurally similar to cerebrosides, but with a charged polar oligosaccharide head region.

garam masala A mixture of aromatic spices widely used in Indian cooking; contains powdered black pepper, cumin, cinnamon, cloves, mace, cardamom seeds and sometimes also coriander and/or bay leaf.

garbanzo See CHICKPEA.

gari Fermented CASSAVA meal.

garlic The bulb of *Allium sativum* with a pungent odour when crushed, widely used to flavour foods. There is some evidence that garlic has a beneficial effect in lowering blood CHOLESTEROL.

Composition/100 g: 410 kJ (98 kcal), protein 7.9 g, fat 0.6 g, carbohydrate 16.3 g (1.6 g sugars, 14.7 g starch), nsp 4.1 g, Na 4 mg, K 620 mg, Ca 19 mg, Mg 25 mg, P 170 mg, Fe 1.9 mg, Cu 0.06 mg, Zn 1 mg, Se 2 μg, I 3 μg, vitamin B_1 0.13 mg, B_2 0.03 mg, niacin 2.2 mg, B_6 0.38 mg, folate 5 μg, C 17 mg. Serving 12 g.

garlic mustard   A common wild plant of hedgerows and woodland (*Alliaria petiolata*), the leaves have a garlic-like flavour and can be used in salads or cooked as a vegetable .

gas storage, controlled (modified)   Storage of fruits, vegetables and prepacked red meat in a controlled atmosphere in which a proportion of the oxygen is replaced by carbon dioxide, sometimes with the addition of other gases.

gastrectomy   Surgical removal of part or all of the stomach.

gastric inhibitory peptide   Peptide HORMONE secreted by the mucosa of the duodenum and jejunum in response to absorbed fat and carbohydrate; stimulates the pancreas to secrete INSULIN. Also known as glucose-dependent insulinotropic polypeptide.

gastric secretion   Gastric juice contains the enzymes CHYMOSIN (EC 3.4.23.4), lipase (EC 3.1.1.3), pepsinogen (the inactive precursor of PEPSIN, EC 3.4.23.1), INTRINSIC FACTOR, mucin and hydrochloric acid.

The acid is secreted by the parietal (oxyntic) cells at a strength of 0.16 mol/L (0.5–0.6% acid); the same cells also secrete intrinsic factor, and failure of acid secretion (ACHLORHYDRIA) is associated with pernicious ANAEMIA due to failure of VITAMIN B_{12} absorption.

Pepsinogen is secreted by the chief cells of the gastric mucosa, and is activated to pepsin by either gastric acid or the action of existing pepsin; it is a proteolytic enzyme (see PROTEOLYSIS).

See also ANAEMIA, PERNICIOUS; PROTON PUMP.

gastric ulcer   See ULCER.

gastrin   Peptide hormone secreted by G-cells of the antrum of the stomach; stimulates PARIETAL CELLS to secrete acid.

gastroenteritis   Inflammation of the mucosal lining of the stomach (gastritis) and/or small or large intestine, normally resulting from infection, or, in the case of gastritis, from excessive alcohol consumption.

gastroenterology   The study and treatment of diseases of the GASTROINTESTINAL TRACT.

gastrointestinal tract   A term for the whole of the digestive tract, from the mouth to the anus. Average length 4.5 m (15 feet).

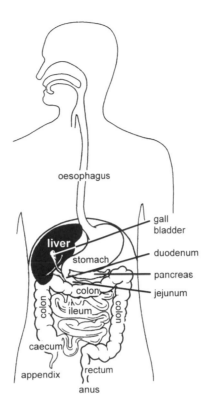

oesophagus

gall bladder

liver

stomach

duodenum

pancreas

jejunum

colon

ileum

colon

colon

caecum

rectum

appendix

anus

gastrolith Stone in the stomach, usually builds up around a BEZOAR.

gastroplasty Surgical alteration of the shape of the stomach without removing any part. Has been used to reduce the physical capacity of the stomach as a treatment for severe OBESITY.

gastrostomy feeding Feeding a liquid diet directly into the stomach through a tube that has been surgically introduced through the abdominal wall.

See also ENTERAL NUTRITION; NASOGASTRIC TUBE.

gavage The process of feeding liquids by stomach tube. Also feeding an excessive amount (hyperalimentation).

gean Scottish name for the fruit of *Prunus avium*; also known as wild cherry, sweet cherry and mazzard.

gefillte fish (gefilte, gefüllte) German for stuffed fish; of Russian or Polish origin, where it is commonly referred to as Jewish fish. The whole fish is served and the filleted portion chopped and stuffed back between the skin and the backbone. More frequently today, the fish is simply chopped and made into balls, which are either fried or boiled. In the UK has been legally referred to as 'fish cutlets in fish sauce' instead of a fish cake.

gel   COLLOIDAL SUSPENSION consisting of a continuous phase (commonly water) and a dispersed phase (the gelling agent); the water molecules are held in a three-dimensional network of the gelling agent. Examples include plant GUMS, GELATINE, PECTIN.

gelatine   A soluble protein prepared from COLLAGEN or bones by boiling with water: used for sugar confectionery, in canned meats, for table jellies and in pharmaceutical capsules. Gelatine from fish (especially the swim bladder) is ISINGLASS. As a protein it is of poor nutritive value, since it lacks TRYPTOPHAN. Chinese gelatine is AGAR.

gelatine sugar   Obsolete name for GLYCINE.

gelatinisation   Formation of a water-retentive gel by expansion of starch granules when heated in moist conditions.
See also STALING.

gellan gum   A POLYSACCHARIDE produced by fermentation of the bacterium, *Pseudomonas elodea*, used in some foods.

gelometer   See BLOOM GELOMETER.

gemfibrizol   See FIBRIC ACID.

generic descriptor   The name used to cover the different chemical forms of a VITAMIN, compounds that have the same vitamin activity.

genetic diseases   Also known as inborn errors of metabolism. Diseases due to a single defective gene, with a characteristic pattern of inheritance in families. Many affect the ability to metabolise individual AMINO ACIDS or CARBOHYDRATES and can be treated by dietary restriction.
See also AMINO ACID DISORDERS; DISACCHARIDE INTOLERANCE.

genetic modification   A change in the genes in a living organism, as occurs in nature, and which has been used for many years in selective breeding, or, more quickly and specifically, in the laboratory (genetic engineering).
See also SUBSTANTIAL EQUIVALENCE.

gentiobiose   A disaccharide consisting of two molecules of glucose joined β-1,6.

Gentleman's relish   Trade name for a paste of anchovies, butter, cereal, salt and spices developed in the UK in the nineteenth century; also called patum peperium.

geophagia   Eating of dirt or soil. See also PICA.

Gerber test   For fat (CREAM) in milk. The milk is mixed with sulphuric acid (or detergent) and amyl alcohol; the protein and carbohydrate are dissolved, and the fat separates out. The reaction is carried out in a Gerber bottle with a thin graduated neck, in which the fat collects for measurement after centrifugation.

germ, wheat The embryo or sprouting portion of the wheat berry, comprising about 2.5% of the seed. Contains 64% of the vitamin B_1, 26% of the vitamin B_2, 21% of the vitamin B_6 and most of the fat of the wheat grain. It is discarded, with the bran, when the grain is milled to white FLOUR. See FLOUR, EXTRACTION RATE.

ghee (ghrt) Clarified BUTTER fat; may also be made from vegetable oils.

Composition/100g: 3759 kJ (898 kcal), protein 0g, fat 99.8g (70.5% saturated, 25.7% mono-, 3.6% polyunsaturated), cholesterol 280mg, carbohydrate 0g, Na 2mg, K 3mg, Fe 0.2mg, vitamin A 758μg (500μg carotene), D 1.9μg, E 3.3mg. A 100g serving is a rich source of vitamins A, D, E.

gherkin Young green CUCUMBER of a small variety (*Cucumis anguira*), used mainly for pickling.

ghrt See GHEE.

giardiasis Intestinal inflammation and DIARRHOEA caused by infection with the protozoan parasite *Giardia lamblia*.

giberellins Plant growth substances derived from giberellic acid, originally found in the fungus *Gibberella fujikori* growing on rice. About 30 giberellins are known; they cause stem extension and allow mutant dwarf forms of plants to revert to normal size, induce flower formation and break bud dormancy. Used in horticulture to control flowering and fruit maturation, also to induce α-AMYLASE in malting (see MALT) of barley.

giblets The edible part of the entrails of a bird; gizzard, liver, heart and neck.

gigot French; leg of lamb or mutton. In Ireland gigot chops are neck chops used for stewing.

gill Obsolete British measure of liquid, 5 or 10 fl oz ($^1/_4$ or $^1/_2$ pint), varying regionally.

gin Alcoholic drink made by distilling fermented starch or other carbohydrate, flavoured mainly with juniper berries together with coriander seeds, angelica, cinnamon, orange and lemon peel. Distillate is diluted to 40% ALCOHOL by volume, 925 kJ (220 kcal) / 100 mL. Name derived from French *genièvre* (juniper); originally known as geneva, schiedam or hollands, since it is Dutch in origin.

There are two types of English gin: Plymouth gin with a fuller flavour and London gin. Dutch and German gins are more strongly flavoured than English or American; steinhäger and schinkenhäger are distilled from a mash of wheat, barley and juniper berries; wacholder is made from neutral spirit flavoured with juniper. Dutch gin may be *jonge* (young) or *oude* (aged, matured).

gingelly (gingili)   See SESAME.

ginger   The rhizome of *Zingiber officinale*, used as a spice. Preserved ginger is made from young fleshy rhizomes boiled with sugar and either packed in syrup or crystallised.

ginger paralysis   See JAMAICA GINGER PARALYSIS.

gingivitis   Inflammation, swelling and bleeding of the gums; may be due to SCURVY, but most commonly the result of poor oral hygiene.

GIP   See GASTRIC INHIBITORY PEPTIDE.

gipping (of fish)   Partial evisceration to remove intestines but not pyloric caeca which contain enzymes responsible for the characteristic flavour of HERRING when it is subsequently salted.

Glamorgan sausage   Welsh; dish based on Caerphilly cheese, breadcrumbs and egg, fried in sausage shape.

Glasgow magistrate   See RED HERRINGS.

gliadin   A PROLAMIN, one of the proteins that make up wheat GLUTEN. Allergy to, or intolerance of, gliadin is COELIAC DISEASE.

globins   PROTEINS that are rich in the AMINO ACID HISTIDINE (and hence basic), relatively deficient in ISOLEUCINE and contain average amounts of ARGININE and TRYPTOPHAN. Often found as the protein part of conjugated proteins such as haemoglobin.

globulins   Class of PROTEINS that are heat-coagulated and soluble in dilute solutions of salts; they differ from ALBUMINS in being relatively insoluble in water. They occur in blood (serum globulins), milk (lactoglobulins) and some plants, e.g. edestin from hemp seed and amandin from almonds.

glossitis   Inflammation of the tongue; may be one of the signs of RIBOFLAVIN deficiency.

glucagon   Peptide HORMONE secreted by the α-islet cells of the PANCREAS. Elevates blood glucose by increasing the breakdown of liver GLYCOGEN and stimulating GLUCONEOGENESIS; also stimulates hormone-sensitive LIPASE (EC 3.1.1.x) in adipose tissue, leading to release of fatty acids.

glucagon-like peptide   Peptide hormone secreted by the terminal ileum; increases secretion of INSULIN and decreases that of GLUCAGON.

glucans   Soluble undigested polysaccharide of glucose; found particularly in oats, barley and rye.
    See also FIBRE, SOLUBLE; NON-STARCH POLYSACCHARIDES.

glucaric acid   Alternative name for saccharic acid, the dicarboxylic acid derived from glucose.

glucide (gluside)   Name occasionally used for SACCHARIN.

glucitol Obsolete name for sorbitol, one of the SUGAR ALCOHOLS or GLYCITOLS.

glucoamylase See AMYLASE; DEBRANCHING ENZYME.

glucocorticoids The STEROID HORMONES secreted by the adrenal cortex (see ADRENAL GLANDS) which regulate carbohydrate metabolism. See CORTICOSTEROIDS.

glucokinase An isoenzyme of HEXOKINASE (EC 2.7.1.1), with a high K_m, found only in liver and β-islet cells of the pancreas. A rare form of DIABETES mellitus (maturity onset diabetes of the young) is due to a genetic defect in glucokinase.

glucomannan A polysaccharide consisting of glucose and mannose.

gluconeogenesis The synthesis of glucose from non-carbohydrate precursors, such as lactate, pyruvate, glycerol, and glucogenic AMINO ACIDS.

gluconic acid The acid formed by oxidation of the hydroxyl group on carbon-1 of glucose to a carboxylic acid group. Also termed dextronic acid, maltonic acid and glycogenic acid.

glucono-δ-lactone GLUCONIC ACID lactone; liberates acid slowly, and used in chemically leavened (aerated) BREAD to form carbon dioxide from bicarbonate.

glucosaccharic acid See SACCHARIC ACID.

glucosamine The amino derivative of GLUCOSE, a constituent of a variety of complex POLYSACCHARIDES.

glucosan A general term for polysaccharides of GLUCOSE, such as STARCH, CELLULOSE and GLYCOGEN.

glucose A six-carbon monosaccharide sugar (hexose), with the chemical formula $C_6H_{12}O_6$, occurring free in plant and animal tissues and formed by the hydrolysis of STARCH and GLYCOGEN. Also known as dextrose, grape sugar and blood sugar.

The circulating carbohydrate in blood is glucose; normal concentration is between 4.5–5.5 mmol/L (80–100 mg/100 mL). In the fed state glucose is used for the synthesis of GLYCOGEN in liver and muscle, as well as for synthesis of fats; in the fasting state glycogen is hydrolysed as a source of glucose to maintain the blood concentration. Used in the manufacture of confectionery, since its mixture with FRUCTOSE prevents sucrose from crystallising (see boiled sweets); it is 74% as sweet as sucrose.

See also CARBOHYDRATES; DEXTROSE.

glucose, confectioners' Glucose SYRUPS known as glucose in confectionery making (GLUCOSE is referred to as dextrose).

glucose isomerase Bacterial enzyme (EC 5.3.1.5) that catalyses isomerisation of glucose to fructose. Used in the production of FRUCTOSE syrups. Main commercial source is *Streptomyces* spp.

glucose metabolism   Series of reactions in which glucose is oxidised to carbon dioxide and water as a metabolic fuel (i.e. to provide energy). The overall reaction is: $C_6H_{12}O_6 + 6O_2 \rightarrow 6CO_2 + 6H_2O$, yielding 16.4 kJ (3.9 kcal)/g, or 2.88 MJ (686 kcal)/mol.

The first series of reactions does not require oxygen and is referred to as (anaerobic) glycolysis or glucose fermentation, yielding two molecules of the three-carbon compound pyruvic acid. Under anaerobic conditions this can be reduced to LACTIC ACID. Pyruvic acid is normally oxidised to acetyl CoA, which is then oxidised to carbon dioxide and water via the citric acid or Krebs cycle. Both glycolysis and the citric acid cycle are linked to the formation of ATP from ADP and phosphate, as a metabolically usable energy source.

An alternative to part of glycolysis, the pentose phosphate pathway or hexose monophosphate shunt, is important in formation of reduced NADPH for FATTY ACID synthesis.

glucose oxidase   Enzyme (EC 1.1.3.4) that oxidises glucose to gluconic acid, with the formation of hydrogen peroxide. Used for specific quantitative determination of glucose, including urine and blood glucose, and to remove traces of glucose from foodstuffs (e.g. from dried egg to prevent the MAILLARD REACTION during storage). Also used to remove traces of oxygen from products such as beer, wine, fruit juices and mayonnaise to prevent oxidative rancidity. Originally isolated from *Penicillium notatum* and called notatin; main commercial source is *Aspergillus niger*.

glucose-6-phosphate dehydrogenase deficiency   See FAVISM.

glucose syrups   See SYRUP; DEXTROSE EQUIVALENT VALUE.

glucose tolerance   The ability of the body to deal with a relatively large dose of glucose is used as a test for DIABETES mellitus. The fasting subject ingests 50 or 75 g of glucose and the concentration of blood glucose is measured at intervals. In normal subjects the fasting sugar concentration is between 4.5–5.5 mmol/L, and rises to about 7.5 mmol/L, returning to the starting level within $1–1\frac{1}{2}$ h. In diabetes, it rises considerably higher and takes longer to return to the baseline value. The graph of the results forms a glucose tolerance curve.

glucose tolerance factor (GTF)   Organic chelate of CHROMIUM, M_r around 1500, variously reported to contain NICOTINIC ACID, GLUTATHIONE and other amino acid derivatives. Potentiates the action of INSULIN, but has no activity in the absence of insulin. Acts by increasing the protein kinase activity of the insulin receptor when insulin is bound.

glucosides   See GLYCOSIDES.

glucosinolates   Substances occurring widely in *Brassica* spp (e.g.

Brussels sprouts, cabbage, watercress, radishes); broken down by the enzyme myrosinase (thioglucosidase, EC 3.2.3.1) to yield, among other products, the mustard oils which are responsible for the pungent flavour (especially in mustard and horseradish).

Several of the glucosinolates interfere with the metabolism of IODINE by the thyroid gland (thyroid hormones), and hence are GOITROGENS; chemically they are thioesters. There is evidence that the various glucosinolates in vegetables may have useful anti-cancer activity, since they increase the rate at which a variety of potentially toxic and carcinogenic compounds are conjugated and excreted.

See also PHASE II METABOLISM.

glucostatic mechanism   A theory that appetite depends on the difference between arterial and venous concentrations of glucose; when the difference falls, the hunger centres in the hypothalamus are stimulated.

glucosuria   (Also glycosuria); appearance of GLUCOSE in the urine, as in DIABETES and after the administration of drugs that lower the renal threshold.

glucuronic acid   The acid derived from glucose by the oxidation of the hydroxyl group on carbon-6. Many substances, including hormones and potentially toxic ingested substances, are excreted as conjugates with glucuronic acid, known as glucuronides. It is present in various complex polysaccharides.

glucuronides   A variety of compounds are metabolised by conjugation with GLUCURONIC ACID to yield water-soluble derivatives for excretion from the body.

glutamic acid   A non-essential AMINO ACID; abbr Glu (E), M_r 147.1, pK_a 2.10, 4.07, 9.47, CODONS GAPu. Acidic since it has two carboxylic acid groups; the amide is GLUTAMINE.

See also MONOSODIUM GLUTAMATE.

glutamine   A non-essential amino acid, abbr Gln (Q), M_r 146.1, pK_a 2.17, 9.13, CODONS CAPu. The amide of GLUTAMIC ACID.

glutathione   A tripeptide, γ-glutamyl-cysteinyl-glycine (GSH). Important in protection against oxidative damage, since it can be oxidised to the disulphide compound (GSSG), which can then be reduced back to active glutathione. Also important in PHASE II METABOLISM of foreign compounds, yielding mercapturic acids as a result of S-conjugation, and transport of amino acids into cells.

glutathione peroxidase   SELENIUM-containing enzyme (EC 1.11.1.9) that protects tissues from oxidative damage by removing peroxides resulting from free radical action, linked to oxidation of GLUTATHIONE; part of the body's ANTIOXIDANT protection. Low activity in red blood cells indicates selenium deficiency, but not useful as an index of marginal status.

glutathione reductase Enzyme (EC 1.6.4.2) that catalyses the reduction of oxidised GLUTATHIONE (GSSG) to glutathione (GSH), and hence an important antioxidant system. Activation of this enzyme *in vitro* by added cofactor (flavin adenine dinucleotide, derived from vitamin B_2) provides a means of assessing vitamin B_2 nutritional status, sometimes known as the erythrocyte glutathione reductase activation coefficient (EGRAC) test. An activation coefficient above 1.7 indicates deficiency.

See also ENZYME ACTIVATION ASSAYS.

glutelins Proteins insoluble in water and neutral salt solutions but soluble in dilute acids and alkalis, e.g. wheat glutenin.

gluten The protein complex in wheat, and to a lesser extent rye, which gives dough the viscid property that holds gas when it rises. None in oats, barley, maize. It is a mixture of two proteins, gliadin and glutelin. Allergy to, or intolerance of, the gliadin fraction of gluten is COELIAC DISEASE (gluten-sensitive enteropathy). In the undamaged state with extensible properties it is termed vital gluten; when overheated, these properties are lost and the product is termed devitalised gluten, used for protein enrichment of foods.

gluten-free foods Formulated without any wheat or rye protein (although the starch may be used) for people suffering from COELIAC DISEASE.

gluten-sensitive enteropathy See COELIAC DISEASE.

glutose A six-carbon sugar (hexose) with a keto group on carbon-3; not metabolised and non-fermentable.

glycaemic index The increase in blood glucose after a test dose of a carbohydrate, relative to that in response to an equivalent amount of glucose. A measure of the rate and extent of small intestinal digestion of the carbohydrate.

glycation Any non-enzymic reaction between glucose and amino groups in proteins, resulting in formation of a glycoprotein. Glycation of collagen, crystallin and other proteins is probably the basis of many of the adverse effects of poor glycaemic control in diabetes.

See also GLYCOSYLATION; HAEMOGLOBIN, GLYCATED; MAILLARD REACTION.

glycerides Esters of GLYCEROL with FATTY ACIDS. See TRIACYL-GLYCEROL; SUPERGLYCERINATED FATS.

glycerol (glycerine) 1,2,3-Propane triol (CH_2OH-$CHOH$-CH_2OH), a trihydric alcohol. Simple or neutral FATS are esters of glycerol with three molecules of FATTY ACID, i.e. triacylglycerols, sometimes known as triglycerides. Glycerol is a clear, colourless, odourless, viscous liquid, sweet to taste; it is made from fats by alkaline hydrolysis (saponification). Used as a solvent for flavours, as a humectant to keep foods moist, and in cake batters to improve texture and slow staling.

glycerose Glyceraldehyde, a three-carbon sugar (CHO—CHOH—CH$_2$OH) derived from GLYCEROL.

glyceryl lactostearate Or lactostearin. Formed by glycerolysis of hydrogenated soya bean oil followed by esterification with lactic acid, resulting in a mixture of mono- and diacylglycerols and their lactic mono-esters. Used as an emulsifier in shortenings (E-472b).

glyceryl monostearate See SUPERGLYCERINATED FATS.

glycine A non-essential AMINO ACID, abbr Gly (G), M_r 75.1, pK_a 2.35, 9.78, CODONS CGNu. It has a sweet taste (70% of the sweetness of sucrose) and is sometimes used mixed with SACCHARIN as a sweetener. Known at one time as collagen sugar.

glycinin Globulin protein in soya bean.

glycitols See SUGAR ALCOHOLS. Glycitol was used at one time as an alternative name for SORBITOL.

glycochenodeoxycholic acid The GLYCINE conjugate of CHENO-DEOXYCHOLIC ACID, one of the BILE acids.

glycocholic acid The GLYCINE conjugate of CHOLIC ACID, one of the BILE acids.

glycogen The storage carbohydrate in the liver and muscles, a branched polymer of GLUCOSE units, with the same structure as AMYLOPECTIN, and sometimes referred to as animal starch. In an adult there are about 250 g of glycogen in the muscles and 100 g in the liver in the fed state. Since glycogen is rapidly broken down to glucose after an animal is killed, meat and animal liver do not contain glycogen; the only dietary sources are oysters and other shellfish that are eaten virtually alive and contain about 5% glycogen.

glycogenesis The synthesis of glycogen from glucose in liver and muscle after a meal, stimulated by the hormone INSULIN.

glycogenic acid See GLUCONIC ACID.

glycogenolysis The breakdown of GLYCOGEN to GLUCOSE for use as a metabolic fuel and to maintain the normal blood glucose in the fasting state. Stimulated by the hormone GLUCAGON.

glycogen storage diseases A group of rare GENETIC DISEASES caused by a defect of one or another of the various enzymes involved in glycogen synthesis and mobilisation, characterised by excessive accumulation of GLYCOGEN in liver and/or muscle and, in some forms, profound fasting HYPOGLYCAEMIA. Treatment is by feeding small frequent meals, rich in carbohydrate.

glycolysis The first sequence of reactions in GLUCOSE metabolism, leading to the formation of two molecules of pyruvic acid from each glucose molecule.

glycoproteins Also known as proteoglycans; polysaccharides covalently bound to a protein, commonly via *N*- or *O*-acylglucosamine linkage to the hydroxyl group of SERINE or THREONINE.

See also MUCOPOLYSACCHARIDES; MUCOPROTEINS.

glycosides Compounds of a sugar attached to another molecule; called glucosides when glucose is the sugar.

glycosuria See GLUCOSURIA.

glycosylation Chemical reaction leading to the substitution of one or more glycosyl groups into a compound; GLYCATION is a general term for any reaction leading to incorporation of glucose into a protein.

glycyrrhizin Triterpenoid glycoside extracted from LIQUORICE root *Glycyrrhiza glabra*; 50–100 times as sweet as sucrose but with liquorice flavour. Used to flavour tobacco and pharmaceutical preparations, and as a foaming agent in some non-alcoholic beverages.

GMP See GOOD MANUFACTURING PRACTICE.

GMS Glyceryl monostearate, see SUPERGLYCERINATED FATS.

goblet cell Secretory cell in the intestinal mucosa which secretes the major constituents of MUCUS.

goitre Enlargement of the thyroid gland, seen as a swelling in the neck, most commonly due to deficiency of IODINE in the diet or to the presence of GOITROGENS in foods. In such cases there is commonly underproduction of the THYROID HORMONES, i.e. hypothyroid goitre. Euthyroid goitre is a condition in which the enlargement of the thyroid gland is sufficient to compensate for a deficiency of iodine and permit normal production of thyroid hormones. In infancy iodine deficiency can also lead to severe mental retardation, goitrous cretinism. Supplementation with iodide often prevents the condition, hence the use of iodised SALT.

Rarely, goitre may be due to other causes, including excessive stimulation of the thyroid gland. In this case there is overproduction of the thyroid hormones, hyperthyroid goitre.

goitrogens Compounds in foods (especially *Brassica* spp, groundnuts, cassava and soya bean) that inhibit either synthesis of THYROID HORMONES (GLUCOSINOLATES) or uptake of iodide into the thyroid gland (thiocyanates), and hence can cause GOITRE, especially when the dietary intake of iodine is marginal.

golden berry See CAPE GOOSEBERRY.

golden syrup Light coloured SYRUP made by evaporation of cane sugar juice.

See also TREACLE; SUGAR.

Gomez classification One of the earliest systems for classifying PROTEIN–ENERGY MALNUTRITION in children, based on percentage of expected weight for age: over 90% is normal, 76–90% is mild (first degree), 61–75% is moderate (second degree) and less than 60% is severe (third degree) malnutrition.

good manufacturing practice (GMP)   Part of a food and drink control operation aimed at ensuring that products are consistently manufactured to a quality appropriate to their intended use (detailed in *Good Manufacturing Practice – A Guide to Responsible Management*, Institute of Food Science and Technology, 1987).

goose   Domesticated water-fowl, *Anser anser*.

Composition/100 g (roast meat only): 1335 kJ (319 kcal), protein 29.3 g, fat 22.4 g, carbohydrate 0 g, Na 80 mg, K 320 mg, Ca 10 mg, Mg 23 mg, P 270 mg, Fe 303 mg, Cu 0.15 mg, Zn 2.6 mg, vitamin B_1 0.12 mg, B_2 0.51 mg, niacin 10.1 mg, B_6 0.42 mg, folate 12 μg, B_{12} 1.9 μg, pantothenate 1.4 mg, biotin 3 μg. A 150 g serving is a source of vitamin B_1, Mg; good source of Cu, Zn; rich source of protein, vitamin B_2, niacin, B_6, B_{12}, pantothenate, Fe.

gooseberry   Berry of the shrub, *Ribes grossularia*. The British National Fruit Collection contains 155 varieties.

Composition/100 g: 80–170 kJ (20–40 kcal), protein 0.7–1.1 g, fat 0.3–0.4 g, carbohydrate 3–9 g (3–9 g sugars), dietary fibre 3 g, nsp 2.4 g, Na 2 mg, K 210 mg, Ca 28 mg, Mg 7 mg, P 34 mg, Fe 0.3 mg, Cu 0.06 mg, Zn 0.1 mg, vitamin A 18 μg (110 μg carotene), E 0.4 mg, B_1 0.03 mg, B_2 0.03 mg, niacin 0.5 mg, B_6 0.02 mg, folate 8 μg, pantothenate 0.3 mg, biotin 0.5 μg, C 14 mg. A 140 g serving is a source of Cu; rich source of vitamin C.

gooseberry, Indian   See EMBLIC.

gossypol   Yellow toxic pigment found in some varieties of cottonseed. When included in chicken feed, it causes discoloration of the yolk, but has not been found to be toxic to human beings, and has been investigated as a possible male contraceptive agent. Chemically a dialdehyde, it reacts with the ε-amino group of lysine, thus reducing AVAILABLE LYSINE and PROTEIN QUALITY.

gossypose   See RAFFINOSE.

goujon   Small deep fried pieces of FISH. The name is derived from gudgeon, a small freshwater fish. Now also used for small pieces of chicken breast.

gourds   Vegetables of the family Cucurbitaceae, including calabash or bottle gourd (*Lagenaria vulgaris*), ash gourd (*Benincasa hispida*), snake gourd (*Trichosanthes anguina*), cucumber (*Cucumis sativus*), vegetable marrow (*Cucurbita pepo*), pumpkin (*Cucurbita moschata*), squash (*Cucurbita maxima*), coocha or chayote (*Sechium edule*), cantaloup melon (*Cucumis melo*), water melon (*Citrullus vulgaris*).

All contain more than 90% water and have little food value

apart from vitamin C at 10 mg/100 g. In addition, yellow pumpkin contains 900 µg carotene/100 g. Melons are sometimes grown for their seeds, which contain 20–40% oil and 20% protein.

gout Painful disease caused by accumulation of crystals of URIC ACID in the synovial fluid of joints; may be due to excessive synthesis and metabolism of PURINES, which are metabolised to uric acid, or to impaired excretion of uric acid. Traditionally associated with a rich diet, although there is little evidence for dietary factors in causing the condition. May be exacerbated by alcohol.

G proteins Guanine nucleotide binding proteins. Part of the transmembrane signalling mechanism in response to hormones, etc, that bind to cell surface receptors, leading to activation of enzymes that form intracellular SECOND MESSENGERS.

Graham bread Wholewheat bread in which the bran is very finely ground. Graham cakes are made from wholemeal flour and milk. The name is that of a miller of wholemeal flour who advocated its use in the USA (*Treatise on Bread and Bread Making*, 1837). See also ALLINSON BREAD.

graining Crystallisation of refined sugar when boiled. Prevented by adding glucose or cream of tartar as SUGAR DOCTORS.

grains of paradise See PEPPER, MELEGUETA.

Gram-negative, Gram-positive A method of classifying bacteria depending on whether or not they retain crystal-violet dye (Gram stain). Named after the Danish botanist HCJ Gram (1858–1938).

grams, Indian Various small dried peas (LEGUMES), e.g. green gram (*Phaseolus aureus*), black gram (*Phaseolus mungo*), red gram (*Cajanus indicus*), Bengal gram or CHICK PEA (*Cicer aretinum*).

granadilla See PASSION FRUIT.

grape Fruit of a large number of varieties of *Vitis vinifera*. One of the oldest cultivated plants; three main groups: dessert grapes, WINE grapes and varieties that are used for drying to produce raisins, currants and sultanas. Of the many varieties of grape that are grown for wine making, nine are considered classic varieties: cabernet sauvignon, chardonnay, chenin blanc, merlot, pinot noir, riesling, sauvignon blanc, sémillon, syrah.

Composition/100 g: 238 kJ (57 kcal), protein 0.4 g, fat 0.1 g, carbohydrate 14.6 g (14.6 g sugars), dietary fibre 0.8 g, nsp 0.7 g, Na 2 mg, K 200 mg, Ca 12 mg, Mg 7 mg, P 17 mg, Fe 0.3 mg, Cu 0.11 mg, Zn 0.1 mg, Se 1 µg, I 1 µg, vitamin A 2 µg (16 µg carotene), B_1 0.05 mg, B_2 0.01 mg, niacin 0.2 mg, B_6 0.09 mg, folate 2 µg, pantothenate 0.1 mg, biotin 0.3 µg, C 3 mg. A 100 g serving is a source of Cu.

grapefruit Fruit of *Citrus paradisi*; thought to have arisen as sport of the POMELO or shaddock (*Citrus grandis*), a coarser CITRUS fruit, or as a hybrid between pomelo and sweet orange. The pith contains NARINGIN, which is very bitter. Name said to have arisen because the fruit is borne on the tree in clusters (like grapes).

Composition/100 g: 83 kJ (20 kcal), protein 0.5 g, fat 0.1 g, carbohydrate 4.6 g (4.6 g sugars), dietary fibre 1.1 g, nsp 0.9 g, Na 2 mg, K 140 mg, Ca 16 mg, Mg 6 mg, P 14 mg, Fe 0.1 mg, Cu 0.01 mg, Se 1 µg, vitamin A 1 µg (11 µg carotene), E 0.1 mg, B_1 0.03 mg, B_2 0.01 mg, niacin 0.3 mg, B_6 0.02 mg, folate 18 µg, pantothenate 0.2 mg, biotin 0.7 µg, C 24 mg. A 170 g serving ($^1/_2$ fruit) is a source of folate; rich source of vitamin C.

grape sugar See GLUCOSE.

grappa See MARC.

GRAS (Generally regarded as safe) Designation given to food additives when further evidence is required before the substance can be classified more precisely (US usage).

grass tetany MAGNESIUM deficiency in cattle.

gratin (1) A fireproof dish.

(2) Also gratiné, French term for the thin brown crust formed on top of foods that have been covered with butter and breadcrumbs, then heated under the grill or in the oven. Au gratin when cheese is also used.

grattons (gratterons) French; crispy remains of melted fat tissue of poultry or pork. German equivalent is gribbens.

gravadlax (gravlaks, gravlax) Scandinavian; pickled or marinated raw salmon.

Graves' disease See THYROTOXICOSIS.

gray (Gy) The SI unit for ionising radiation (= 100 rad). The gray is equivalent to 1 J/kg.

great millet See SORGHUM.

green butter See VEGETABLE BUTTERS.

greengage Green variety of PLUM introduced into England in the early eighteenth century by Sir William Gage.

Composition/100 g: 159 kJ (38 kcal), protein 0.7 g, fat 0.1 g, carbohydrate 9.2 g (9.2 g sugars), dietary fibre 2.2 g, nsp 2 g, Na 1 mg, K 290 mg, Ca 16 mg, Mg 8 mg, P 22 mg, Fe 0.4 mg, Cu 0.08 mg, Zn 0.1 mg, vitamin A 15 µg (90 µg carotene), E 0.7 mg, B_1 0.05 mg, B_2 0.04 mg, niacin 0.7 mg, B_6 0.05 mg, folate 3 µg, pantothenate 0.2 mg, C 5 mg. Serving 80 g.

green S Food COLOUR, also known as Wool green S and Brilliant acid green BS, E-142.

gribbens (greben, gribbenes) See GRATTONS.

griddle Also girdle; iron plate used for baking scones, etc on top of stove.

grilse Young SALMON that has returned to freshwater after one year in the sea.

griskin CHINE of pork, also used for a thin piece of loin.

grissini Italian 'finger rolls' or stick bread 15–45 cm (6–18 in) long, and normally crisp and dry.

grist Cereal for grinding.

gristle The CONNECTIVE TISSUE of the meat, consisting mainly of the insoluble proteins COLLAGEN and elastin. Usually inedible and accounts for the toughness of some cuts of meat. Prolonged slow cooking converts collagen to GELATINE, but has no effect on elastin.

grits, corn See HOMINY.

groats Oats from which the husk has been entirely removed; when crushed, Embden groats result. Used to make gruel and porridge.

grog British naval drink; sugared rum mixed with hot water. Named after Admiral Vernon (early eighteenth century) nicknamed 'Old Grog' because of his grosgrain (heavy corded silk) coat.

groundnut See PEANUT.

ground tomato See CAPE GOOSEBERRY.

grouse GAME bird, *Lagopus lagopus*. Shooting period in UK August 12–December 10; eaten fresh or after being hung for 2–4 days to develop flavour. The whole bird weighs about 700 g.

Composition/100 g: 477 kJ (114 kcal), protein 20.6 g, fat 3.5 g (24.2% saturated, 12.1% mono-, 63.6% polyunsaturated), carbohydrate 0 g, Na 63 mg, K 310 mg, Ca 20 mg, Mg 27 mg, P 220 mg, Fe 5 mg, Cu 0.05 mg, Zn 0.7 mg, vitamin B_1 0.1 mg, B_2 0.41 mg, niacin 7.5 mg, B_6 0.33 mg, folate 19 µg, B_{12} 0.5 µg. A 350 g serving (weighed with bone) is a source of Zn; good source of vitamin B_1, Cu; rich source of protein, vitamin B_2, niacin, B_6, folate, B_{12}, Mg, Fe.

gruel Thin porridge made from oatmeal, barley or other cereal.

GTF See GLUCOSE TOLERANCE FACTOR.

guanine One of the PURINES.

guarana Dried paste from the seeds of a climbing shrub, *Paullina cupana*, native of the Amazon region. It contains caffeine and related compounds; used in UK as an ingredient of drinks, chewing gum, a powder to be sprinkled on food and capsules and tablets.

guar gum Cyamopsis gum; from the cluster bean, *Cyamopsis tetragonoloba*. Member of Leguminosae, used in India as livestock feed. The GUM is a water-soluble galactomannan; used in 'slimming' preparations, since it is not digested by digestive enzymes, and experimentally in the treatment of DIABETES, since it slows the absorption of glucose after a meal.

guava   Fruit of the central and south American tropical shrub *Psidium guajava*.

Composition/100 g: 100 kJ (24 kcal), protein 0.7 g, fat 0.5 g, carbohydrate 4.5 g (4.4 g sugars, 0.1 g starch), dietary fibre 4.2 g, nsp 3.3 g, Na 5 mg, K 210 mg, Ca 12 mg, Mg 11 mg, P 23 mg, Fe 0.4 mg, Cu 0.09 mg, Zn 0.2 mg, vitamin A 65 µg (390 µg carotene), B_1 0.04 mg, B_2 0.04 mg, niacin 1 mg, B_6 0.13 mg, pantothenate 0.1 mg, C 210 mg. A 100 g serving is a source of Cu; rich source of vitamin C.

guinea corn   See SORGHUM.

guinea fowl   Game bird, now farmed, *Numida meleagris*, not seasonal. Nutritionally similar to CHICKEN.

guinea pepper   See PEPPER, MELEGUETA.

gum   Carbohydrate polymers that can disperse in water to form a viscous mucilaginous mass. Used in food processing to stabilise emulsions, as a thickening agent and in sugar confectionery. Most (apart from dextrans) are not digested and have no food value, although they contribute to the intake of NON-STARCH POLYSACCHARIDES.

Exudate gums: karaya (sterculia) from *Sterculia arens*, partially acetylated high-molecular-weight heteropolymers of rhamnose, galactose and galacturonic acid; tragacanth from *Astralagus* spp a neutral arabinogalactan; ghatti from *Anageissus latifolia*.

Seed gums: guar from *Cyamopsis tetragonolobus*; locust bean is *Ceratonia siliqua*; psyllium *Plantago* spp esp *P. ovata*; quince seed *Cydonia vulgaris* and *C. oblongata*.

Dextran gums: α-D-glucose polymers produced by *Leuconostoc mesenteroides*. Xanthan gum produced by *Xanthomonas campestris*.

gum arabic (gum acacia)   Exudate from the stems of several species of acacia; the best product comes from *Acacia senegal*. Used as thickening agent, as stabiliser, often in combination with other gums, in gum drops and soft jelly gums and to prevent crystallisation in sugar confectionery.

gumbo   (1) American (Creole); soup or stew made from okra, onions, celery and pepper, flavoured with filé powder (powdered dried SASSAFRAS leaves), and containing chicken, meat, fish or shellfish.

(2) OKRA.

gum, British   Partly hydrolysed starch, DEXTRIN.

gum, chewing   See CHEWING GUM.

gum drops (fruit gums)   SUGAR CONFECTIONERY based on SUCROSE and GLUCOSE with GUM ARABIC (hard gums) or a mixture of GELATINE and gum arabic (soft gums).

gum tragacanth   Obtained from the trees of *Astralagus* spp, used as a stabiliser.

gur Mixture of sugar crystals and syrup, brown and toffee-like, made by evaporation of juice of sugar cane; also called jaggery.

gustin ZINC-containing protein associated with taste acuity.
See also HYPOGEUSIA; DYSGEUSIA.

gut See GASTROINTESTINAL TRACT.

Guthrie test Test for a number of GENETIC DISEASES (especially PHENYLKETONURIA) based on measuring the concentrations of AMINO ACIDS in a small sample of blood taken by pricking the heel of the child a few days after birth, by biological assay using mutated bacteria for which the amino acid is a growth factor. Now largely superseded by chromatographic methods.

gut sweetbread See PANCREAS.

GYE Guinness yeast extract, see YEAST EXTRACT.

gyle ALCOHOL solution formed in the first stage of VINEGAR production, 6–9% alcohol. Subsequent fermentation with *Acetobacter* spp converts the alcohol to ACETIC ACID.

H

hachis Minced or chopped mixture of meat and herbs.

haddock White FISH, *Melanogrammus aeglefinus*.
Composition/100 g: 339 kJ (81 kcal), protein 19 g, fat 0.6 g, cholesterol 36 mg, carbohydrate 0 g, Na 67 mg, K 360 mg, Ca 14 mg, Mg 24 mg, P 200 mg, Fe 0.1 mg, Cu 0.03 mg, Zn 0.4 mg, Se 27 μg, I 250 μg, vitamin E 0.4 mg, B_1 0.04 mg, B_2 0.07 mg, niacin 8 mg, B_6 0.39 mg, folate 9 μg, B_{12} 1 μg, pantothenate 0.3 mg, biotin 2 μg. A 120 g serving is a good source of vitamin B_6; rich source of protein, niacin, vitamin B_{12}, I, Se.

haem (heme) The iron-containing PORPHYRIN which, in combination with the protein globin, forms HAEMOGLOBIN and MYOGLOBIN. It is also part of a wide variety of other proteins, collectively known as haem proteins, including the CYTOCHROMES.
See also PROTOPORPHYRIN.

haemagglutinins (hemagglutinins) See LECTINS.

haematemesis (hematemesis) Vomiting bright red blood, due to bleeding in the upper GASTROINTESTINAL TRACT.

haematin (hematin) Formed by the oxidation of HAEM; the iron is oxidised from the ferrous (Fe^{2+}) to the ferric (Fe^{3+}) state.

haematinic (hematinic) General term for those nutrients, including iron, folic acid, vitamin B_{12}, required for the formation and development of blood cells in bone marrow (the process of haematopoiesis), deficiency of which may result in ANAEMIA.

haematocrit (hematocrit) Packed volume of red blood cells, expressed as fraction of the total volume of blood; determined by centrifugation in calibrated capillary tube (haematocrit tube), as an index of ANAEMIA, and especially microcytic and MEGALOBLASTIC ANAEMIAS. Not a sensitive index of IRON status, because it only falls after HAEMOGLOBIN synthesis has been impaired.

haemin (hemin) The hydrochloride of HAEMATIN, derived from HAEMOGLOBIN. The crystals are readily recognisable under the microscope and used as a test for blood.

haemochromatosis IRON overload due to GENETIC DISEASE. Increased intestinal absorption of iron leading to deposition in parenchymal cells, and hence causing damage especially to liver, pancreas, heart and pituitary. The biochemical defect has not been identified, but it is closely linked to the HLA-A gene, so that HLA (human leucocyte-associated antigen) genotyping permits detection of asymptomatic subjects.

haemoglobin (hemoglobin) The HAEM-containing protein in red blood cells, is responsible for the transport of oxygen and carbon dioxide in the bloodstream.

See also ANAEMIA; IRON.

haemoglobin, glycated Also known as glycosylated haemoglobin or haemoglobin A_{1c}. The result of non-enzymic reaction between GLUCOSE and ε-amino groups of LYSINE. Measurement of glycated haemoglobin is used as an index of glycaemic control in DIABETES mellitus over the preceding 2–3 months; normally 3–6% of haemoglobin is glycated, but when there has been prolonged HYPERGLYCAEMIA as much as 20% may be glycated.

See also GLYCATION; MAILLARD REACTION.

haemoglobinometer (hemoglobinometer) Instrument to measure the amount of haemoglobin in blood by colorimetry.

haemolysis (hemolysis) Destruction of red blood cells by lysis of the cell membrane; may occur in a variety of pathological conditions, as a result of incorrectly matched blood transfusion or in VITAMIN E deficiency.

See also ANAEMIA, HAEMOLYTIC; FAVISM.

haemorrhagic (hemorrhagic) disease of the newborn Excessive bleeding due to VITAMIN K deficiency; in most countries infants are given vitamin K by injection shortly after birth to prevent this rare but serious (potentially fatal) condition.

haemorrhoids (hemorrhoids) Or piles, varicosity in the lower rectum or anus due to congestion of the veins; caused or exacerbated by a low-fibre diet and consequent straining to defecate.

See also DIETARY FIBRE.

haemosiderin (hemosiderin) See IRON STORAGE.

Hagberg test Measure of α-AMYLASE (EC 3.2.1.1) activity of flour based on the change in viscosity of flour paste.

haggis Traditional Scottish dish made from sheep's heart, liver and lungs cooked and chopped with suet, onions, oatmeal and seasoning, stuffed into a sheep's stomach. Said to have been originated by the Romans when campaigning in Scotland; when breaking camp in an emergency, the food was wrapped in the sheep's stomach. A similar Norman-French dish was afronchemoyle.

Composition/100 g: 1297 kJ (310 kcal), protein 10.7 g, fat 21.7 g (47.7% saturated, 43.3% mono-, 8.8% polyunsaturated), cholesterol 91 mg, carbohydrate 19.2 g (19.2 g starch), Na 770 mg, K 170 mg, Ca 29 mg, Mg 36 mg, P 160 mg, Fe 4.8 mg, Cu 0.44 mg, Zn 1.9 mg, vitamin A 1800 µg, D 0.1 µg, E 0.4 mg, B_1 0.16 mg, B_2 0.35 mg, niacin 3.5 mg, B_6 0.07 mg, folate 8 µg, B_{12} 2 µg, pantothenate 0.5 mg, biotin 12 µg. A 150 g serving is a source of vitamin B_1, biotin, pantothenate, Mg, Zn; good source of niacin; rich source of protein, vitamin A, B_2, B_{12}, Fe, Cu.

hair analysis Measurement of various minerals, including CHROMIUM, SELENIUM and ZINC in hair has been proposed as an index of status, but interpretation of the results is confounded by adsorption of minerals onto the hair from shampoo, etc.

hake A white FISH, *Merluccius bilinearis*.

halal Food conforming to the Islamic (Muslim) dietary laws. Meat from permitted animals (in general grazing animals with cloven hooves, and thus excluding pig meat) and birds (excluding birds of prey). The animals are killed under religious supervision by cutting the throat to allow removal of all blood from the carcass, without prior stunning. Food that is not halal is haram.

haldi See TURMERIC.

half-life (1) The time taken for half of the PROTEIN or tissue in question to be replaced. Proteins are continuously being degraded and replaced even in the mature adult, and the half-life is used as a quantitative measure of this dynamic equilibrium. The values of half-life of different proteins range from a few minutes or hours for enzymes which control the rate of metabolic pathways, to almost a year for structural proteins such as collagen. The average half-life of human liver and serum proteins is 10 days, and of the total body protein is 80 days.

(2) Of radioactive ISOTOPES, the time in which half of the original material undergoes radioactive decay.

halibut A white FISH, *Hippoglossus* spp.

Composition/100 g: 431 kJ (103 kcal), protein 21.5 g, fat 1.9 g, cholesterol 35 mg, carbohydrate 0 g, Na 60 mg, K 410 mg, Ca 29 mg, Mg 25 mg, P 200 mg, Fe 0.5 mg, Cu 0.04 mg, Zn 0.4 mg, I 40 µg, vitamin E 0.9 mg, B_1 0.07 mg, B_2 0.07 mg, niacin 9.8 mg, B_6 0.38 mg, folate 9 µg, B_{12} 1 µg, pantothenate 0.3 mg, biotin 3 µg. A

120 g serving is a source of vitamin E, Mg; good source of vitamin B_6; rich source of protein, niacin, vitamin B_{12}, I.

Halibut liver oil is one of the richest natural sources of vitamins A and D, containing 50 mg vitamin A and 80 µg vitamin D per gram.

halophiles (halophilic bacteria) Able to grow at up to 25% salt. The growth of colonic bacteria is inhibited at 8–9% salt, *Clostridia* at 7–10%, food poisoning staphylococci at 15–20% and *Penicillium* at 20%. Film-forming YEASTS can grow in 24% salt.

Halphen test For the presence of cottonseed oil in other oils and fats.

halvah (halva, halwa, halawa, chalva) (1) A sweetmeat composed of an aerated mixture of glucose, sugar and crushed sesame seeds; because of the seeds, the sweet contains 25% fat.

(2) Indian desserts of various types, made from carrot, pumpkin or banana, sweetened and flavoured.

halverine Name sometimes given to low-fat spreads with less than the statutory amount of fat in a MARGARINE.

ham The whole hind leg of the pig, removed from the carcass and cured individually; sometimes the process is secret. Hams cured or smoked in different ways have different flavours. Green ham has been cured but not smoked.

See also BACON.

hamburger Or Hamburg steak, also known as beefburger. A flat cake made from ground (minced) BEEF, seasoned with salt, pepper and herbs, and bound with egg and flour. Commercial beefburgers are usually 80–100% meat, but must by law (in UK) contain 52% lean meat, of which 80% must be beef. Cereal, cereal fibre or bean fibre may be added as filler or 'meat extender'.

Hammarsten's casein See CASEIN.

hammer mill Continuous process mill in which material is powdered by impact from a set of hammers.

hand of pork The foreleg of PORK; usually salted and boiled.

hangover Headache and feeling of malaise resulting from excessive consumption of ALCOHOLIC BEVERAGES. The severity differs with different beverages and is not due to the toxic effects of alcohol alone, but to the presence of higher alcohols and esters (collectively known as CONGENERS or FUSEL oil), the substances that give different beverages their distinctive flavours.

Hansa can An all-aluminium can (developed in Germany) with easily opened ends.

haram Food forbidden by Islamic law. See HALAL.

hardening of oils   See HYDROGENATION.

hardness of water   See WATER, HARDNESS.

hare   Game animal, similar to RABBIT but larger; caught wild but not farmed commercially. *Lepus europaeus* is the common hare; some 20 *Lepus* spp occur in Europe.

Hartnup disease   Rare genetic defect of tryptophan transport, leading to development of PELLAGRA.

Harvard standard   Tables of height and weight for age used as reference values for the assessment of growth and nutritional status in children, based on data collected in the USA. Now largely replaced by the NCHS (US National Center for Health Statistics) standards.

hash   Dish of cooked meat reheated in highly flavoured sauce. In USA canned CORNED BEEF is known as corned beef hash.

haslet (harslet)   Old English country dish made from pig's offal (heart, liver, lungs and sweetbreads) cooked in small pieces with seasoning and flour. Also known as pig's fry.

hasty pudding   English, sixteenth century; made from flour, milk, butter and spices, which since they were usually readily available, could be quickly made into the pudding for unexpected visitors. Made in the USA with maize (corn) flour instead of wheat flour.

Hausa groundnut   LEGUME grown in West Africa, *Kerslingiella geocarpa*; 20% protein, 60% fat.

haybox cooking   The food is cooked for only a short time, then placed in a well-lagged container, the haybox, where it remains hot for many hours, so cooking continues without further use of fuel. Also known as the fireless cooker.

Hay diet   A system of eating based on the concept that carbohydrates and proteins should not be eaten at the same meal, for which there is no scientific basis, originally proposed by William Hay in 1936. It ignores the fact that almost all carbohydrate-rich foods also contain significant amounts of protein. In any case, in the absence of adequate carbohydrate, protein is oxidised as a metabolic fuel and therefore not available for tissue building. Also called combining diet or food combining.

haze   Term in brewing to indicate cloudiness of BEER. Chill haze appears at 0°C and disappears at 20°C; permanent haze remains at 20°C but there is no fundamental difference. Caused by GUMS derived from the barley, leucoanthocyanins and tannins from the malt and hops, and glucose, pentoses and amino acids.

See also CHILLPROOFING.

hazel nut   Fruit of the tree *Corylus avellana*; cultivated varieties include Barcelona nut, cob nut and filbert (*C. maxima*).

Composition/100 g (shelled): 2720 kJ (650 kcal), protein 14.1 g, fat 63.5 g (7.7% saturated, 82.5% mono-, 9.7% polyunsaturated), carbohydrate 6 g (4 g sugars, 2 g starch), dietary fibre 8.9 g, nsp 6.5 g, Na 6 mg, K 730 mg, Ca 140 mg, Mg 160 mg, P 300 mg, Fe 3.2 mg, Cu 1.23 mg, Zn 2.1 mg, I 17 µg, vitamin E 25 mg, B_1 0.43 mg, B_2 0.16 mg, niacin 5.1 mg, B_6 0.59 mg, folate 72 µg, pantothenate 1.5 mg, biotin 76 µg. A 10 g serving (ten nuts) is a source of Cu; good source of vitamin E.

HDL High-density lipoprotein, see LIPOPROTEINS, PLASMA.

headcheese Mock BRAWN.

health foods Substances whose consumption is advocated by various reform movements, including vegetable foods, whole grain cereals, food processed without chemical additives, food grown on organic compost, 'magic' foods (bees' royal jelly, LECITHIN, seaweed, etc) and pills and potions. Numerous health claims are made but rarely is there any evidence to support these claims.

healthy US legislation permits a claim of 'healthy' for a food that is LOW IN fat and saturated fat, and contains no more than 480 mg of sodium and 60 mg of cholesterol per serving.

heartburn A burning sensation in the chest usually caused by reflux (regurgitation) of acid digestive juices from the stomach, into the oesophagus. A common form of INDIGESTION, treated by ANTACIDS.

heart sugar See INOSITOL.

heat exchanger Equipment for heating or cooling liquids rapidly by providing a large surface area and turbulence for the rapid and efficient transfer of heat. Used for continuous PASTEURISATION and subsequent cooling.

heat of combustion ENERGY released by complete combustion, as for example, in the BOMB CALORIMETER. See ENERGY CONVERSION FACTORS.

heat pump System of producing heat or cold by compression or expansion of air, also known as Joule cycle or air cycle. Modern systems can produce temperatures as low as –80°C or as high as +200°C and are being introduced as an environmentally friendly method of refrigeration, replacing fluorocarbon and chlorofluorocarbon refrigerants.

hedonic scale Term used in tasting panels where the judges indicate the extent of their like or dislike for the food.

heel-prick test See GUTHRIE TEST.

Helicobacter pylori Bacterium commonly infecting the gastric mucosa. Believed to be the underlying cause of ULCERS, and implicated in the development of gastric cancer. Formerly classified as *CAMPYLOBACTER*.

helminths Various parasitic worms, including FLUKES, TAPEWORMS and nematodes.

hemicelluloses Complex CARBOHYDRATES included as DIETARY FIBRE, composed of polyuronic acids combined with xylose, glucose, mannose and arabinose. Found together with cellulose and lignin in plant cell walls; most GUMS and mucilages are hemicelluloses.

hemoglobin American spelling of HAEMOGLOBIN; similarly, hematin = haematin, heme = haem, hemosiderin = haemosiderin.

heparin Complex carbohydrate (glycosaminoglycan) from mast cells in liver, lung, muscle, heart and blood which prevents blood coagulation by activating antithrombin III, and so inhibiting the conversion of prothrombin to thrombin. *In vivo* cleared rapidly from the bloodstream, but *in vitro* 10 mg prevents the coagulation of 100 mL of blood.

hepatic encephalopathy Impairment of brain function, leading to coma, as a result of liver disease.

hepatitis Inflammatory liver disease, characterised by jaundice, abdominal pain and anorexia. May be due to bacterial or viral infection, alcohol abuse or various toxins. Treatment is usually conservative, with a very low fat diet (secretion of BILE is impaired) and complete abstinence from alcohol. Even after recovery, people may continue to be carriers of the virus, especially for hepatitis B and C, which are transmitted through blood and other body fluids. Liver cancer and cirrhosis are more common among people who have suffered from hepatitis B or C.

hepatoflavin Name given to a substance isolated from liver, later shown to be RIBOFLAVIN.

hepatolenticular degeneration See WILSON'S DISEASE.

hepatomegaly Enlargement of the liver as a result of congestion (e.g. in heart failure), inflammation or fatty infiltration (as in KWASHIORKOR).

herbs Soft-stemmed aromatic plants used fresh or dried to flavour and garnish dishes, and sometimes for medicinal effects. Not clearly distinguished from SPICES, except that herbs are usually the leaves or the whole of the plant while spices are only part of the plant, commonly the seeds, or sometimes the roots or rhizomes.

herb tea See TISANE.

Hermesetas Trade name for SACCHARIN.

herring Oily FISH, *Clupea harengus*; young herrings are sild. Sprat is *Clupea sprattus*; young are brislings. Pilchard is *Clupea pilchardus*; young are sardines. Kippers, bloaters and red herrings are salted and smoked herrings; bucklings are hot-smoked herrings. GAFFELBITAR are preserved herring.

Composition/100 g: 795 kJ (190 kcal), protein 17.8 g, fat 13.2 g (28.6% saturated, 47.8% mono-, 23.4% polyunsaturated), cholesterol 50 mg, carbohydrate 0 g, Na 120 mg, K 320 mg, Ca 60 mg, Mg 32 mg, P 230 mg, Fe 1.2 mg, Cu 0.14 mg, Zn 0.9 mg, Se 35 μg, I 29 μg, vitamin A 44 μg, D 19 μg, E 0.8 mg, B_1 0.01 mg, B_2 0.26 mg, niacin 7.4 mg, B_6 0.44 mg, folate 9 μg, B_{12} 13 μg, pantothenate 0.8 mg, biotin 7 μg. A 120 g serving is a source of vitamin B_2, pantothenate, Mg, Fe; good source of vitamin B_6, Cu, I; rich source of protein, vitamin D, niacin, B_{12}, Se.

hesperidin A FLAVONOID found in the pith of unripe citrus fruits; chemically a complex of glucose and rhamnose with the flavonone hesperin. At one time called VITAMIN P, since it affects the fragility of the capillary walls, although there is no evidence that it is a dietary essential.

Hess test A test for capillary fragility in SCURVY. A slight pressure is applied to the arm for 5 min and a shower of petechiae (small blood spots) appear on the skin below the area of application.

heterofermentative Fermentation by microorganisms producing several products.

heterophysiasis Intestinal infestation with the parasitic FLUKE *Heterophyes heterophyes* after consumption of raw fish containing the larval stage.

heterosides See HOLOSIDES.

heterotrophes See AUTOTROPHES.

hexamethylene tetramine Preservative (fungicide), E-239. Also known as hexamine.

hexamic acid Cyclohexyl sulphamic acid, the free acid of CYCLAMATE.

hexamine See HEXAMETHYLENE TETRAMINE.

hexosans POLYSACCHARIDES of HEXOSE sugars, including STARCH, GLYCOGEN, CELLULOSE and hemicellulose.

hexose monophosphate shunt The pentose phosphate pathway of GLUCOSE metabolism.

hexoses Six-carbon (monosaccharide) SUGARS such as GLUCOSE or FRUCTOSE.

hexuronic acid The acid derived from a hexose SUGAR by oxidation of the hydroxyl group on carbon-6. Originally proposed as a name for ASCORBIC ACID. The hexuronic acid derived from glucose is glucuronic acid.

HFCS High-fructose corn syrup. See FRUCTOSE SYRUPS.

HF heating High-frequency heating. See MICROWAVE HEATING.

hiatus hernia Protrusion of a part of the stomach upwards through the diaphragm. The condition occurs in about 40% of the population, most people suffering no ill effects; in a small number of people there is reflux of stomach contents into the oesophagus, causing HEARTBURN.

See also GASTROINTESTINAL TRACT.

hickory nut   North American walnut, *Carya* spp; the best known is the PECAN NUT.

high-density lipoproteins (HDL)   One of the classes of plasma LIPIDS.

high-frequency heating   See MICROWAVE HEATING.

high-fructose corn syrup   See FRUCTOSE SYRUPS.

high in   EU legislation states that for a food label or advertising to bear a claim that it is 'high in' a nutrient it must contain 50% more of the claimed nutrient than a similar product for which no claim is made. Claims may also be made for foods containing more than 12 g of protein, 6 g of dietary fibre or more than 30% of the labelling reference amount of a vitamin or mineral/100 g (see Table 2).

US legislation permits a claim of 'high in' for foods containing more than 20% of the daily value for a particular nutrient in a serving. For a claim that a food is 'higher in' a nutrient it must contain at least 25% more of the claimed nutrient than a similar food for which no claim is made.

high performance (high pressure) liquid chromatography, HPLC   An extremely sensitive analytical technique, typically able to separate and measure nanogram or smaller amounts of compounds in 10–100 μL samples.

high-ratio fats, shortenings   See SUPERGLYCERINATED FATS.

high-ratio flour   See FLOUR, HIGH-RATIO.

high-temperature short-time treatment (HTST)   Sterilisation by heat for times ranging from a few seconds to minutes; usually applied to flow sterilisation, in which the process time is less than about 1 min; based on the fact that at higher temperatures bacteria are destroyed more rapidly than damage occurs to nutrients and texture.

hindle wakes   Old English (fourteenth century) method of cooking chicken, stuffed with fruit and spices, including prunes. Possibly a corruption of *hen de la wake* (feast).

Hirschsprung's disease   Congenital failure of development of the nerve network of the lower colon or rectum, so that it neither expands nor conducts the contents of the bowel, which therefore accumulate in, and distend, the upper colon.

Hi-soy   Trade name for full-fat SOYA FLOUR.

histamine   The amine formed by decarboxylation of the amino acid HISTIDINE, found in cheese, beer, chocolate, sauerkraut and wine. Excessive release of histamine from mast cells is responsible for many of the symptoms of allergic reactions. Stimulates secretion of gastric acid, and administration of histamine is used as test for ACHLORHYDRIA.

histamine receptor antagonists Inhibitors of the histamine H_2 receptor, including cimetidine, ranitidine, famotidine and nisatidine, are used in treatment of gastric ULCERS; they act to reduce secretion of gastric acid in response to hormone or nerve stimulation.

histidinaemia GENETIC DISEASE due to a lack of histidase (EC 4.3.1.3), leading to impaired metabolism of the AMINO ACID HISTIDINE. If untreated leads to mental retardation and nervous system abnormalities. Treatment is by feeding a diet very low in histidine.

histidine An essential AMINO ACID, abbr His (H), M_r 155.2, pK_a 1.80, 6.04 (imidazole), 9.76, CODONS CAPy.

histidine load test See FIGLU TEST.

histones Proteins rich in arginine and lysine, soluble in water but not dilute ammonia. They occur mainly in the cell nucleus and are concerned with the regulation of DNA.

HMG CoA reductase Hydroxymethylglutaryl CoA reductase (EC 1.1.1.34), the first and rate-limiting enzyme of CHOLESTEROL synthesis. The STATINS are a family of HMG CoA reductase inhibitors used to treat HYPERCHOLESTEROLAEMIA.

HMT See HEXAMETHYLENE TETRAMINE.

hock (1) Generic term for white wines from the Rhine region of Germany, known in USA as Rhine wines; bottled in brown glass, to distinguish from Moselle wines (in green glass).

(2) The knuckle of PORK; also used in USA for foreleg pork shank.

hogget One year old sheep. See LAMB.

hogshead A traditional UK measure of volume or size of barrel: for beer or cider contains 54 gallons (243 L); for wine contains $52^1/_2$ gallons (236 L).

holocellulose Mixture of CELLULOSE and hemicellulose in wood, the fibrous residue that remains after the extractives, the lignin, and the ash-forming elements, have been removed.

holoenzyme An enzyme protein together with its COENZYME or PROSTHETIC GROUP.

See also ENZYME ACTIVATION TESTS.

holosides Complexes of sugars that yield only sugars on hydrolysis. As distinct from heterosides which yield other substances as well as sugars on hydrolysis, e.g. tannins, anthocyanins, nucleosides.

hominy Prepared MAIZE kernels. Lye hominy, pericarp and germ removed by soaking in caustic soda. Pearled hominy, degermed hulled maize. Corn grits are ground hominy.

homocysteine An amino acid formed as an intermediate in the metabolism of METHIONINE; demethylated methionine; M_r 117.2, pK_a 2.22, 8.87, 10.86 (-SH). Does not occur in foods to any significant extent, and is not generally considered to be of nutritional importance. High blood homocysteine (possibly a result of poor FOLIC ACID, VITAMIN B$_6$ and B$_{12}$ status) has been implicated in the development of ATHEROSCLEROSIS and heart disease, associated with a genetic polymorphism in METHYLENE TETRAHYDROFOLATE REDUCTASE, EC 1.7.99.5).

homocystinuria A GENETIC DISEASE caused by lack of cystathionine synthetase (EC 4.2.1.22), leading to impaired conversion of the AMINO ACID methionine to cysteine, characterised by excretion of HOMOCYSTEINE and its derivatives. May result in mental retardation and early death from ATHEROSCLEROSIS and coronary thrombosis if untreated, as well as fractures of bones and dislocation of the lens of the eye. Treatment (which must be continued throughout life) is either by feeding a diet low in methionine and supplemented with cysteine or, in some cases, by administration of high intakes of VITAMIN B$_6$ (about 100–500 times the normal requirement).

homofermentative Fermentation by microorganisms producing a single product.

homogenisation Emulsions usually consist of a suspension of globules of varying size. Homogenisation reduces these globules to a smaller and more uniform size. In homogenised milk the smaller globules adsorb more of the protein, which acts as a stabiliser, and the cream does not rise to the top.

homogeniser, ultrasonic See ULTRASONIC HOMOGENISER.

homopantothenic acid See HOPANTHATE.

honey Syrupy liquid made by bees (the honey bee is *Apis mellifera*) from the nectar of flowers (which is essentially sucrose). The flavour and colour depend on the flowers from which the nectar was obtained and the composition varies with the source. If the ratio of fructose : glucose is high, there is a tendency for the honey to crystallise. Comb honey is stored by bees in cells of freshly built broodless combs and sold in the comb; drained honey is drained from decapped combs.

Composition/100 g: 1205 kJ (288 kcal), protein 0.4 g, fat 0 g, carbohydrate 76.4 g (76.4 g sugars), Na 11 mg, K 51 mg, Ca 5 mg, Mg 2 mg, P 17 mg, Fe 0.4 mg, Cu 0.05 mg, Zn 0.9 mg, Se 1 µg, vitamin B$_2$ 0.05 mg, niacin 0.2 mg. Serving 20 g.

honeydew honey During periods of prolonged drought, bees may supplement their nectar supplies with honeydew, the sweet fluid excreted on leaves by leaf-sucking insects. The resultant honey is dark, with an unpleasant taste.

honeyware See BADDERLOCKS.

hookworm   Intestinal parasitic nematodes (*Ancyclostoma duode-nale* and *Necator americanus*); infestation causes severe damage to the intestinal wall, leading to blood loss, and is a common cause of IRON deficiency and ANAEMIA.

hopanthate   Homopantothenic acid (pantoyl-γ-aminobutyric acid); a homologue of PANTOTHENIC ACID reported to enhance cholinergic function in the central nervous system, and used to improve cognitive function in ALZHEIMER'S DISEASE.

hops   Perennial climbing plant, *Humulus lupulus*; the dried female flowers contain bitter aromatic acids (HUMULONES and isohumulones) and ESSENTIAL OILS, and are added to beer both to preserve it and enhance the flavour. The tender shoots are eaten as a vegetable in some countries.

hordein   A protein in barley; one of the PROLAMINS.

hordenin   Alkaloid found in germinated barley, sorghum and millet which can cause HYPERTENSION and respiratory inhibition.

Horlick's   Trade name for a preparation of malted milk, for consumption as a beverage when added to milk.

hormones   Compounds produced in the body in ENDOCRINE GLANDS, and released into the bloodstream, where they act as chemical messengers to affect other tissues and organs.

hormones, human   Originally the hormones extracted from human tissues, used therapeutically, now applied to proteins such as INSULIN and growth hormone produced in microorganisms into which the human gene has been introduced, and correctly known as recombinant human hormones.

hormones, sex   Male hormones, or androgens, include testosterone, dihydrotestosterone and androsterone; female hormones, or OESTROGENS, include oestradiol, oestrone and progesterone. Chemically, all are STEROIDS, derived from CHOLESTEROL. The synthetic female hormones stilboestrol and hexoestrol have similar biological activities to the oestrogens, but are quite different chemically. Apart from clinical use the oestrogens have been used for chemical caponisation (see CAPON) of cockerels and to enhance the growth rate of cattle.

horseradish   The root of *Armoracia lapathifolia*. Pungency is caused by volatile oils. Used as a condiment, usually as a creamed sauce or grated and mixed with beetroot.

Hortvet freezing test   Test for the adulteration of milk with water by measuring the freezing point; milk normally freezes between −0.53 and −0.55°C; if diluted with water it will freeze above −0.53°C.

hot break   Coagulation and precipitation of high molecular weight proteins during the boiling of WORT for BEER production. Also known as trub.

Hot Springs Conference   International Conference held in 1943 at which the Food and Agriculture Organisation (FAO) of the United Nations originated.

Hovis Trade name for a mixture of brown flour and wheat germ; from Latin *hominis vis*, strength of man; originally, in the 1880s, called Smith's Old Patent Germ Bread.

Composition/100g: 887kJ (212kcal), protein 9.5g, fat 2g, carbohydrate 41.5g (1.8g sugars, 39.7g starch), dietary fibre 5.1g, nsp 3.3g, Na 600mg, K 200mg, Ca 120mg, Mg 56mg, P 190mg, Fe 3.7mg, Cu 0.24mg, Zn 2.1mg, I 22µg, vitamin B_1 0.8mg, B_2 0.09mg, niacin 6.1mg, B_6 0.11mg, folate 39µg, pantothenate 0.3mg, biotin 2µg. A 120g serving (four slices) is a source of Ca, I, Zn; good source of protein, folate, Mg; rich source of vitamin B_1, niacin, Fe, Cu.

Howard mould count Standardised microscope technique for measuring mould contamination.

howtowdie Scottish; boiled chicken with poached egg and spinach.

HPLC See HIGH PERFORMANCE (OR PRESSURE) LIQUID CHROMATOGRAPHY.

5HT See 5-HYDROXYTRYPTAMINE.

HTST See HIGH-TEMPERATURE SHORT-TIME TREATMENT.

huckleberry Wild north American berry, the fruit of *Gaylussacia baccata* and other species, named after the French chemist Gay-Lussac (1778–1850).

Composition/100g: 125kJ (30kcal), protein 0.6g, fat 0.2g, carbohydrate 6.9g (6.9g sugars), dietary fibre 2.5g, nsp 1.8g, Na 3mg, K 88mg, Ca 12mg, Mg 5mg, P 14mg, Fe 0.5mg, Cu 0.08mg, Zn 0.2mg, vitamin A 5µg (30µg carotene), B_1 0.03mg, B_2 0.03mg, niacin 0.5mg, B_6 0.05mg, folate 6µg, pantothenate 0.3mg, biotin 1.1µg, C 17mg. A 110g serving is a source of Cu; rich source of vitamin C.

huff paste Northern British name for pastry made from suet, flour and water, used to enclose meat, fish or poultry while baking.

hull See HUSK.

humble pie See UMBLES.

humectants Substances such as GLYCEROL, SORBITOL, INVERT SUGAR, HONEY which prevent loss of moisture from foods, especially flour confectionery, which would make them unappetising; also prevent sugar crystallising and prevent growth of ice crystals in frozen foods. Also used in other products such as tobacco, inks, glues, etc.

humidity The moistness of air. Weight of water per unit weight of air is absolute or specific humidity. Saturation humidity is the absolute humidity of air that is saturated with water vapour at a given temperature. Relative humidity is the degree of saturation:

the ratio of water vapour pressure in the atmosphere to water vapour pressure that would be exerted by pure water at the same temperature.

hummus Middle Eastern hors d'œuvre; a purée of CHICKPEAS and TAHINI with garlic, oil and lemon juice.

Composition/100 g: 782 kJ (187 kcal), protein 7.6 g, fat 12.6 g, carbohydrate 11.6 g (1.9 g sugars, 9.3 g starch), dietary fibre 3.2 g, nsp 2.4 g, Na 670 mg, K 190 mg, Ca 41 mg, Mg 62 mg, P 160 mg, Fe 1.9 mg, Cu 0.3 mg, Zn 1.4 mg, vitamin B_1 0.16 mg, B_2 0.05 mg, niacin 2.1 mg, C 1 mg. A 60 g serving is a source of Mg; good source of Cu.

humulones Bitter aromatic acids (humulone, cohumulone and adhumulone) in HOPS, used to flavour and preserve BEER. Converted to isohumulones during boiling of the WORT. Also known as α-acids, to distinguish them from the lupulones (β-acids).

Hursting mill Horizontal stone grinders formerly used for grain milling.

husk (or hull) The outer woody cellulose covering of seeds and grains. In wheat it is loosely attached and removed during threshing; in rice it is firmly attached. High in fibre content and of limited use as animal feed.

hyaluronidase Enzyme that catalyses random cleavage of 1,4 links between N-acetylglucosamine and glucuronic acid (EC 3.2.1.35) or 1,3 links between glucuronic acid and N-acetylglucosamine (EC 3.2.1.36) in hyaluronic acid. Injected under the skin of poultry before slaughter to enhance tenderness and flavour.

See also TENDERISERS.

hydrocooling Vegetables are washed in cold water, then subjected to vacuum while still wet. The evaporation of the water chills the vegetables for transport. The term is also applied to vegetables washed in ice-water without the vacuum treatment.

hydrogen Formed in small amounts by intestinal bacterial fermentation; measurement of exhaled hydrogen on the breath provides a sensitive way of diagnosing DISACCHARIDE intolerance.

hydrogenation Conversion of liquid oils to semi-hard fats by the addition of hydrogen across carbon–carbon double bonds; used for margarines and shortenings intended for bakery products. See FATTY ACIDS, unsaturated.

hydrogen peroxide Antimicrobial agent; can be used at 0.1% to preserve milk (Buddeised milk), but destroys vitamin C, methionine and tryptophan. Not permitted in the UK. Formula H_2O_2, readily loses active oxygen, the effective sterilising agent, forming water.

hydrogen swells See SWELLS.

hydrolyse   To split a complex compound into its constituent parts by the action of water, either enzymically or catalysed by the addition of acid or alkali. Hence hydrolysis.

hydroponics   The practice of growing plants without soil in a solution of inorganic salts.

hydrostatic steriliser   Continuous steriliser in which the process is carried out under sufficient depth of water to maintain the required pressure. Used for continuous sterilisation of canned foods on a large scale.

hydrotalcite   Aluminium magnesium carbonate/hydroxide hydrate used as an ANTACID.

hydroxocobalamin   See VITAMIN B_{12}.

hydroxyapatite   Calcium orthophosphate hydroxide, the main mineral of bones, $Ca_{10}(PO_4)_6(OH)_2$.

hydroxybenzoic acid esters   See PARABENS.

hydroxycholecalciferol   See VITAMIN D.

hydroxylysine   Amino acid found only in CONNECTIVE TISSUE proteins (collagen and elastin); incorporated into the protein as LYSINE and then hydroxylated in a vitamin C-dependent reaction; abbr Hyl, M_r 162.2, pK_a 2.13, 8.62, 9.67.

hydroxyproline   Amino acid mainly in CONNECTIVE TISSUE proteins (collagen and elastin); incorporated into the protein as PROLINE and then hydroxylated in a vitamin C-dependent reaction; abbr Hyp, M_r 131.1, pK_a 1.82, 9.66. Peptides of hydroxyproline are excreted in the urine and the output is increased when collagen turnover is high, as in rapid growth or resorption of tissue. Excretion is significantly lower than normal in children whose growth is impaired by protein–energy malnutrition.

hydroxyproline index   The ratio of urinary hydroxyproline: creatinine/kg body weight; low in malnourished children.

5-hydroxytryptamine (5HT)   Also called serotonin. A neurotransmitter amine synthesised from the AMINO ACID TRYPTOPHAN, also formed in blood platelets; it acts as a vasoconstrictor. Found in PLANTAINS and some other foods, but metabolised in the intestinal mucosa.

hygroscopic   Readily absorbing water, as when table salt becomes damp. Materials such as calcium chloride and silica gel absorb water very readily and are used as drying agents.

hyoscine   See ATROPINE.

hyperalimentation   Provision of unusually large amounts of energy, either intravenously (PARENTERAL NUTRITION) or by NASO-GASTRIC TUBE or GASTROSTOSTOMY TUBE (ENTERAL NUTRITION).

hyperammonaemia   High blood ammonia concentration (normal < 80 μmol/L), especially after protein intake, leading to coma, convulsions and possibly death. May be due to a variety of

GENETIC DISEASES affecting amino acid metabolism, or liver failure. Treatment is normally by severe restriction of protein intake.

See also AMINO ACID DISORDERS.

hypercalcaemia Elevated plasma calcium believed to be due to hypersensitivity of some children to VITAMIN D toxicity. There is excessive absorption of calcium, with loss of appetite, vomiting, constipation, flabby muscles and calcinosis, deposition of calcium in the tissues. It can be fatal in infants.

hyperchlorhydria Excess secretion of hydrochloric acid in the stomach due to secretion of a greater volume of gastric juice (GASTRIC SECRETION) rather than to a higher concentration.

hypercholesterolaemia Abnormally high concentrations of CHOLESTEROL in the blood; normal total plasma cholesterol is below 5.2 mmol/L; above 6.5 mmol/L is considered abnormal and indicative of the need for intervention. Generally considered to be a sign of high risk for ATHEROSCLEROSIS and ISCHAEMIC HEART DISEASE. Treatment is by restriction of fat (especially saturated fat, see FAT, SATURATED) and cholesterol intake and a high intake of non-starch polysaccharides, which increase the excretion of cholesterol and its metabolites (the BILE SALTS) in the faeces.

In severe cases, ION-EXCHANGE RESINS may be fed, to increase further the excretion of bile salts, and drugs (HMG COA REDUCTASE inhibitors) may be given to inhibit the synthesis of cholesterol in the body. Familial hypercholesterolaemia is a GENETIC DISEASE in which affected individuals have extremely high blood concentrations of cholesterol, frequently dying from ischaemic heart disease in early adulthood; treatment is as for other forms of hypercholesterolaemia, but more rigorous.

See also LIPIDS, PLASMA.

hyperfiltration (reverse osmosis) See OSMOSIS, REVERSE.

hyperglycaemia High blood glucose (normal is 3.5–5.5 mmol/L), caused by a failure of the normal hormonal mechanisms of blood glucose control.

See also DIABETES (mellitus); GLUCOSE TOLERANCE.

hyperkinetic syndrome (hyperkinesis) Mental disorder of children, characterised by excessive activity and impaired attention and learning ability. Has been attributed to ADVERSE REACTIONS TO FOOD additives, but there is little evidence.

hyperlipidaemia (hyperlipoproteinaemia) A variety of conditions in which there are increased concentrations of LIPIDS in plasma, PHOSPHOLIPIDS, TRIGLYCERIDES, free and esterified CHOLESTEROL or free FATTY ACIDS.

See also HYPERCHOLESTEROLAEMIA; LIPIDS, PLASMA.

hyperoxaluria GENETIC DISEASE leading to excessive formation of OXALIC ACID, which causes the formation of kidney stones. Treatment includes a diet low in those fruits and vegetables that are sources of oxalic acid and in some cases supplements of VITAMIN B$_6$ some 50–100 times greater than reference intakes.

hypersalivation Excessive flow of SALIVA.

hypertension High BLOOD PRESSURE; a risk factor for ischaemic disease, stroke and kidney disease. May be due to increased sensitivity to SALT (correctly sensitivity to SODIUM), and treated by restriction of salt intake, together with drugs; increased intake of fruits and vegetables (as a safe source of potassium) is recommended.

See also SALT-FREE DIET.

hyperthyroidism See THYROTOXICOSIS.

hypertonic A solution more concentrated than the body fluids; see ISOTONIC.

hypervitaminosis Overdosage with vitamins, leading to toxic effects. A problem with high levels of intake of VITAMINS A, D, B$_6$ and NIACIN, normally at levels of intake from supplements considerably higher than might be obtained from foods, although hypervitaminosis A and D may result from (enriched) foods.

See also HYPERCALCAEMIA; REFERENCE INTAKES; UL.

hypocalcaemia Low blood CALCIUM, leading to tetany (uncontrollable twitching of muscles) if severe; may be due to underactivity of the parathyroid gland, kidney failure or VITAMIN D deficiency.

hypochlorhydria Partial deficiency of hydrochloric acid secretion in the gastric juice (GASTRIC SECRETION).

See also ACHLORHYDRIA; ANAEMIA, PERNICIOUS.

hypogeusia Diminished sense of taste. An early sign of marginal zinc deficiency, and potentially useful as an index of zinc status.

See also DYSGEUSIA; GUSTIN; PARAGEUSIA.

hypoglycaemia Abnormally low blood glucose; (normal is 3.5–5.5 mmol/L); may result in loss of consciousness, hypoglycaemic coma.

hypoglycaemic agents Two groups of compounds are used as oral hypoglycaemic agents for treatment of non-insulin-dependent DIABETES mellitus: the sulphonylureas (chlorpropamide, glibenclamide, glicazide, glimepiride, glipizide, gliquidone, tolazamide, tolbutamide) act to enhance secretion of INSULIN; buformin, metformin and phenformin are biguanides that act to decrease GLUCONEOGENESIS and increase peripheral utilisation of glucose.

hypokalaemia Abnormally low plasma potassium (Latin name *kalium*).

hypoproteinaemia Abnormally low total plasma protein concentration.

hyposite Little used word, from Greek, for low-energy food.

hypothermia Low body temperature (normal is around 37°C). Occurs among elderly people far more readily than in younger adults, often with fatal results. Also used in connection with deliberate reduction of body temperature to 28°C to permit heart and brain surgery.

hypothyroidism Underactivity of the thyroid gland, leading to reduced secretion of THYROID HORMONES and a reduction in BASAL METABOLIC RATE. Commonly associated with GOITRE due to IODINE deficiency. In hypothyroid adults there is a characteristic moon-faced appearance, lethargy and dull mental apathy. In infants, hypothyroidism can lead to severe mental retardation, CRETINISM. See also THYROTOXICOSIS.

hypotonic A solution more dilute than the body fluids, see ISOTONIC.

hypovitaminosis VITAMIN deficiency.

hypoxanthine A PURINE, an intermediate in the metabolism of ADENINE and GUANINE to URIC ACID.

hyssop Pungent aromatic herb, *Hyssopus officinalis*, used in salads, soups and in making liqueurs.

I

iatrogenic A condition caused by medical intervention or drug treatment; iatrogenic nutrient deficiency is caused by drug–nutrient interactions.

Iberian moss See CARRAGEENAN.

ice-cream A frozen confection made from fat, milk solids and sugar. Some European countries permit the use of non-milk fat and term the product ice-cream, while if milk fat is used, it is termed dairy ice-cream. According to UK regulations, contains not less than 5% fat and 7% other milk solids; according to US regulations, 10% milk fat and 20% other milk solids. Stabilisers such as carboxymethylcellulose, GUMS and alginates are included, and emulsifiers such as polysorbate and monoglycerides. Mono- and diglycerides bind the looser globules of water and are added in 'non-drip' ice-cream.

Composition/100 g (dairy ice-cream): 812 kJ (194 kcal), protein 3.6 g, fat 9.8 g (70.3% saturated, 26.3% mono-, 3.2% polyunsaturated), cholesterol 31 mg, carbohydrate 24.4 g (22.1 g sugars), Na 69 mg, K 160 mg, Ca 130 mg, Mg 13 mg, P 110 mg, Fe 0.1 mg, Cu 0.02 mg, Zn 0.3 mg, vitamin A 147 µg (195 µg carotene),

D 0.12 µg, E 0.2 mg, B_1 0.04 mg, B_2 0.25 mg, niacin 0.9 mg, B_6 0.08 mg, folate 7 µg, B_{12} 0.4 µg, pantothenate 0.4 mg, biotin 2.5 µg, C 1 mg. A 60 g serving is a source of vitamin A; good source of vitamin B_{12}.

Composition/100 g (non-dairy): 745 kJ (178 kcal), protein 3.2 g, fat 8.7 g (52.3% saturated, 38% mono-, 9.5% polyunsaturated), cholesterol 7 mg, carbohydrate 23.1 g (19.2 g sugars), Na 76 mg, K 170 mg, Ca 120 mg, Mg 13 mg, P 100 mg, Fe 0.1 mg, Zn 0.3 mg, vitamin A 2 µg (6 µg carotene), E 0.8 mg, B_1 0.04 mg, B_2 0.24 mg, niacin 0.8 mg, B_6 0.07 mg, folate 8 µg, B_{12} 0.5 µg, pantothenate 0.4 mg, biotin 3 µg, C 1 mg. A 60 g serving is a rich source of vitamin B_{12}.

ice, eutectic   See EUTECTIC ICE.

Iceland moss   A lichen, *Cetraria islandica*, that can be boiled to make a jelly.

ichthyosarcotoxins   Toxins in fish.

IDDM   Insulin-dependent DIABETES mellitus.

idiopathic   A condition of unknown origin or cause.

idiosyncrasy   Unusual and unexpected sensitivity or reaction to a drug or food.

IDL   Intermediate-density lipoprotein, see LIPOPROTEINS, PLASMA.

idli   SE Asian; small cakes made from a mixture of cooked rice and black gram, fermented with the aid of mould.

IHD   Ischaemic heart disease.

ileitis   Inflammation of the ILEUM.

ileocolitis   Inflammation of the ILEUM and COLON.

ileostomy   Surgical formation of an opening of the ileum on the abdominal wall, performed to treat severe ulcerative COLITIS; see GASTROINTESTINAL TRACT.

ileotomy   Surgical removal of (part of) the ILEUM.

ileum   Last portion of the small intestine, between the jejunum and the colon (large intestine), see GASTROINTESTINAL TRACT.

ileus   Obstruction of the intestines, see GASTROINTESTINAL TRACT.

immune system   Series of defence mechanisms of the body. There are two major parts: humoral, mediated through antibodies secreted into the circulation (IMMUNOGLOBULINS); and cell-mediated. Lymphocytes produce antibodies against, and bind to, the antigens of foreign cells, leading to death of the invading organisms; other white blood cells are phagocytic and engulf the invading organisms.

immunoglobulins   Specific antibodies produced in the blood in response to foreign proteins or other ANTIGENS. Five classes, IgA, IgE, IgG, IgM and IgI; present in circulating blood as a result of previous exposure to the antigens, and also present in breast milk to confer passive immunity.

IMP (1) INTEGRATING MOTOR PNEUMOTACHOGRAPH.

(2) Inosine monophosphate, one of the PURINE nucleotides.

improvers, flour See AGEING.

inanition Exhaustion and wasting due to complete lack or non-assimilation of food; a state of starvation.

inborn errors of metabolism See GENETIC DISEASE.

Incaparina A number of protein-rich dietary supplements developed by the Institute of Nutrition of Central America and Panama (INCAP), based on cottonseed flour, or soya and vegetables, with various nutrient supplements, containing 27.5% protein.

incidence rate Measure of morbidity based on the number of new episodes of a disease arising in a population over a given period of time.

See also PREVALENCE RATE.

index of nutritional quality (INQ) An attempt to provide an overall figure for the nutrient content of a food or diet. The ratio of the amount of the nutrient/1000 kcal: the REFERENCE INTAKE/1000 kcal.

Indian corn See MAIZE.

Indian fig See PRICKLY PEAR.

Indian rice grass Perennial, growing wild in the USA, *Oryzopsis hymenoides*; tolerant to drought. The seeds resemble MILLET, small, round, dark in colour, covered with white hairs. Traditionally used by native Americans for flour, now almost exclusively for forage.

indigestion Discomfort and distension of the stomach after a meal, also known as dyspepsia, including HEARTBURN. Persistent indigestion may be a symptom of a digestive disorder such as HIATUS HERNIA or peptic ULCER.

indigo carmine Blue food colour (E-132), derivative of indigotin, which comes from tropical leguminous plants *Indigofera* spp.

induction Of enzymes; an increase in the total amount of the enzyme protein in a cell as a result of increased TRANSCRIPTION of DNA, leading to an increased amount of mRNA.

See also REPRESSION.

induction period The lag period during which a fat or oil shows stability to oxidation because of its content of ANTIOXIDANTS, natural or added, which are oxidised preferentially. After this there is a sudden and large consumption of oxygen and the fat becomes rancid.

INFOODS International Network of Food Data Systems, created to develop standards and guidelines for collection of food composition data, and standardised terminology and nomenclature.

infuse (infusion) To extract the flavour from herbs, spices, etc, by steeping them in a liquid, usually by pouring on boiling liquid, covering and leaving to stand without further cooking, as in making tea.

inorganic   Materials of MINERAL, as distinct from animal or vegetable, origin. Apart from carbonates and cyanides, inorganic chemicals are those that contain no carbon.

inositol   A carbohydrate derivative which is an essential nutrient for microorganisms and many animals and sometimes classified as a vitamin, although there is no evidence that it is a dietary essential for human beings. Deficiency causes alopecia in mice and 'spectacle eye' (denudation around the eye) in rats. Obsolete names inosite and meat sugar.

Chemically hexahydrocyclohexane $(CHOH)_6$; there are nine isomers, but only one, *meso-* or *myo*-inositol, is of physiological importance. It is a constituent of many PHOSPHOLIPIDS (phosphatidyl inositols) involved in membrane structure and as part of the signalling mechanism for HORMONES which act at the cell surface. The insecticide gammexane is hexachlorocyclohexane, and appears to function by competing with inositol. Inositol hexaphosphate is PHYTIC ACID.

INQ   See INDEX OF NUTRITIONAL QUALITY.

instant foods   Dried foods that reconstitute rapidly when water is added, e.g. tea, coffee, milk, soups, precooked cereal products, potatoes, etc. The dried powders may be agglomerated to control particle size and improve solubility. 'Instant puddings' are formulated with pregelatinised starch and disperse rapidly in cold milk.

insulin   Peptide HORMONE secreted by the β-islet cells of the PANCREAS; controls CARBOHYDRATE METABOLISM. DIABETES mellitus is the result of inadequate supply of insulin or failure of its function. Since insulin is a protein it would be digested if taken by mouth so must be injected. Originally the hormone was prepared from beef or pork pancreas, but these differ slightly in structure from human insulin, and lead to antibody formation after prolonged use. Most insulin for therapeutic use is now human insulin, the product of biosynthesis from the human insulin gene.

See also DIABETES (mellitus); GLUCOSE TOLERANCE.

insulin-like growth factors   See SOMATOMEDINS.

integrating motor pneumotachograph (IMP)   Apparatus for measuring ENERGY EXPENDITURE indirectly from oxygen consumption. It meters the expired air and removes a proportion for analysis.

See also SPIROMETER.

intense sweeteners   See SWEETENERS, NON-NUTRITIVE.

interesterification   Exchange of FATTY ACIDS between TRIACYL-GLYCEROLS in order to modify the properties of the fat; may be achieved by heat treatment or using fungal LIPASE.

interferon A family of proteins that are secreted by macrophages (IFN-α), fibroblasts (IFN-β) and lymphocytes (IFN-γ) in response to viral, bacterial or LECTIN stimulation. They have potent antiviral activity, acting by inhibiting TRANSLATION of viral RNA, and inhibit proliferation of cancer cells.

interleukins A family of CYTOKINES that act as signalling molecules between leukocytes.

intermediate moisture foods These are semimoist with about 25% (15–50%) moisture but with some of the water bound (and so unavailable to MICROORGANISMS) by the addition of glycerol, sorbitol, salt or certain organic acids, so preventing the growth of microorganisms.

international units (iu) Used as a measure of comparative potency of natural substances, such as vitamins, before they were obtained in a sufficiently pure form to measure by weight. Still sometimes used (3.33 iu VITAMIN A = 1 µg; 40 iu VITAMIN D = 1 µg; 1 iu VITAMIN E = 1 mg).

intervention study Comparison of an outcome (e.g. morbidity or mortality) between two groups of people deliberately subjected to different dietary or drug regimes.

intestinal flora Bacteria and other microorganisms that are normally present in the GASTROINTESTINAL TRACT.

intestinal juice Also called succus entericus. Digestive juice secreted by the intestinal glands lining the small intestine. It contains a variety of enzymes, including ENTEROPEPTIDASE, the enzyme that converts trypsinogen to active TRYPSIN, AMINOPEPTIDASE, nucleases and nucleotidases.

See also GASTROINTESTINAL TRACT.

intestine The GASTROINTESTINAL TRACT; the small intestine (duodenum, jejunum and ileum) where the greater part of digestion and absorption take place, and the large intestine where water is absorbed.

intolerance (to foods) See ADVERSE REACTIONS TO FOODS.

intravenous nutrition See PARENTERAL NUTRITION.

intrinsic factor A protein secreted in the gastric juice by the parietal (oxyntic) cells of the gastric mucosa; essential for the absorption of VITAMIN B_{12}; impaired secretion results in pernicious ANAEMIA.

See also ACHLORHYDRIA; dUMP SUPPRESSION TEST; SCHILLING TEST.

intron A region of DNA within a gene that does not contain information coding for the protein and is spliced out during the post-transcriptional modification of mRNA.

See also EXON.

intussusception Telescoping or invagination of one part of the bowel into another.

inulin   Soluble but undigested polymer of FRUCTOSE found in root vegetables, especially Jerusalem ARTICHOKE. Included with NON-STARCH POLYSACCHARIDES (DIETARY FIBRE). Also called dahlin and alant starch. Filtered at the glomerulus and not reabsorbed. Used clinically to measure glomerular filtration rate and kidney function.

inversion   Applied to SUCROSE, means its hydrolysis to glucose and fructose (INVERT SUGAR).

invertase   Also known as sucrase or saccharase; either of two enzymes, glucohydrolase (EC 3.2.1.20) or fructohydrolase (EC 3.2.1.26), with differing specificity, that hydrolyse SUCROSE to yield glucose and fructose. Used in the manufacture of INVERT SUGAR and in chocolate confectionery to hydrolyse crystalline sucrose to a liquid syrup. The bifunctional sucrase–isomaltase of the intestinal mucosa is glucohydrolase.

invert sugar   The mixture of glucose and fructose produced by hydrolysis of sucrose, 1.3 times sweeter than sucrose. So called because the OPTICAL ACTIVITY is reversed in the process. It is important in the manufacture of sugar confectionery, and especially boiled sweets, since the presence of 10–15% invert sugar prevents the crystallisation of sucrose.

in vitro   Literally 'in glass'; used to indicate an observation made experimentally in the test tube, as distinct from the natural living conditions, *in vivo*.

in vivo   In the living state, as distinct from *in vitro*.

iodine   An essential mineral, a TRACE ELEMENT; the reference intake is about 140 µg per day. Iodine is required for synthesis of the THYROID HORMONES, which are iodotyrosine derivatives. A prolonged deficiency of iodine in the diet leads to GOITRE. It is plentifully supplied by sea foods and by vegetables grown in soil containing iodide. In areas where the soil is deficient in iodide, locally grown vegetables are iodine deficient, and hence goitre occurs in defined geographical regions, especially inland upland areas over limestone soil. Where deficiency is a problem, salt may be iodised (IODISED SALT) to increase iodide intake.

iodine number (iodine value)   Measurement of the degree of unsaturation of fatty acids by iodination of the carbon–carbon double bonds. The Wijs method uses iodine chloride, Hanus iodine bromide, and Rosenmund–Kuhnhenn a pyridine sulphate/bromine reagent.

iodine, protein-bound   See THYROGLOBULIN.

iodised oil   Oil intended for administration either by injection or orally in regions of severe IODINE deficiency; prepared by treating vegetable oils with iodine which adds across double bonds. Oils used include poppyseed (relatively scarce), peanut and rape seed oils; injections provide protection for 2–4 years, oral administration about 1 year.

iodised salt In areas of mild IODINE deficiency, salt is often enriched with iodate of levels of 10–25 mg iodate/kg; in areas of moderate deficiency to levels of 25–40 mg/kg. Where there is severe deficiency, IODISED OIL is used. In some areas all salt is enriched, in others it is optional. In some countries by law bread is made with iodised salt.

iodopsin See RHODOPSIN.

ion An atom or molecule that has lost or gained one or more electrons, and thus has an electric charge. Positively charged ions are known as cations, because they migrate towards the cathode (negative pole) in solution, while negatively charged ions migrate towards the positive pole (anode) and hence are known as anions.

ion-exchange resin An organic compound that will adsorb ions under some conditions and release them under other conditions. The best-known example is in water softening, where calcium ions are removed from the water by binding to the resin, displacing sodium ions. The resin is then regenerated by washing with a concentrated solution of salt, when the sodium ions displace the calcium ions. Ion-exchange resins are used for purification of chemicals, metal recovery, a variety of analytical techniques and treatment of HYPERCHOLESTEROLAEMIA.

ionisation The process whereby the positive and negative IONS of a salt or other compound separate when dissolved in water. The degree of ionisation of an ACID or ALKALI determines its strength (see pH).

ionising radiation See IRRADIATION.

IQB (individual quick blanch) Steam BLANCHING method in which all particles receive the same heat treatment, unlike conventional steam blanching where particles at the periphery of the bed are overheated when those in the centre are adequately treated.

Irish moss A red seaweed, *Chondrus crispus*; source of the polysaccharide CARRAGEENAN.

iron An essential MINERAL. The average adult has 4–5 g of iron, of which 60–70% is present in the blood as haem in the circulating HAEMOGLOBIN, and the remainder present in MYOGLOBIN in muscles, a variety of enzymes and tissue stores. Iron is stored in the liver as ferritin, in other tissues as haemosiderin, and as the blood transport protein transferrin.

Iron balance: losses in faeces 0.3–0.5 mg per day, in sweat and skin cells 0.5 mg, traces in hair and urine, total loss 0.5–1.5 mg per day. Blood loss leads to a considerable loss of iron. The average diet contains 10–15 mg, of which 0.5–1.5 mg is absorbed. The haem iron of meat and fish is considerably better absorbed than the inorganic iron of vegetable foods. Absorption of iron is enhanced by VITAMIN C taken at the same time as iron-containing foods, and reduced by phosphate, calcium and PHYTIC ACID.

See also ANAEMIA; FERRITIN; HAEMOCHROMATOSIS; IRON STORAGE; TRANSFERRIN.

iron ammonium citrate   See FERRIC AMMONIUM CITRATE.

iron binding capacity, total   See TRANSFERRIN.

iron, reduced   Metallic iron in finely divided form, produced by reduction of iron oxide. The form in which iron is sometimes added to foods, such as bread. Also known by its Latin name *ferrum redactum*.

iron storage   Ferritin is the iron storage protein in the intestinal mucosa, liver, spleen and bone marrow. It is a ferric hydroxide–phosphate–protein complex containing 23% iron. Haemosiderin is a long-term reserve (storage form) of iron in tissues; colloidal iron hydroxide combined with protein and phosphate, probably formed by agglomeration of FERRITIN, the short-term storage form. Abnormally high levels of haemosiderin occur in SIDEROSIS.

irradiation   IONISING RADIATION (X-rays or γ-rays) kills microorganisms and insects, so used for sterilisation of foods; also inhibits sprouting of potatoes.

See also MICROWAVE COOKING; ULTRAVIOLET RADIATION.

irritable bowel syndrome   Also known as spastic colon or mucous colitis. Abnormally increased motility of the large and small intestines, leading to pain and alternating diarrhoea and constipation; often precipitated by emotional stress.

ischaemic heart disease   Or coronary heart disease. Group of syndromes arising from failure of the coronary arteries to supply sufficient blood to heart muscles; associated with ATHEROSCLEROSIS of coronary arteries.

isinglass   GELATINE prepared from the swim bladder of fish (especially sturgeon). Used commercially to clear wine and beer, and sometimes in jellies and ice cream. Japanese isinglass is AGAR.

islets of Langerhans   The ENDOCRINE parts of the PANCREAS; GLUCAGON is secreted by the α-cells and INSULIN by the β-cells of the islets.

isoamylase   See DEBRANCHING ENZYMES.

isoascorbic acid   See ERYTHORBIC ACID.

isodesmosine   See DESMOSINE.

isoelectric focusing (electrofocusing)   A technique for separating proteins etc, by ELECTROPHORESIS on a support medium that provides a pH gradient, so that each comes to rest at a position determined by its isoelectric point (the pH at which it has no net charge).

isoenzymes   Enzymes that have the same catalytic activity, but different structures, properties and/or tissue distribution.

isoflavones   See FLAVONOIDS.

isohumulones   See HUMULONES.

isoleucine   An essential AMINO ACID, abbr Ile (I), M_r 131.2, pK_a 2.32, 9.76, CODONS AUA, AUPu. Rarely limiting in food. It is one of the branched-chain amino acids, together with leucine and valine.

isomalt   A bulk SWEETENER, about half as sweet as sucrose, consisting of a mixture of two disaccharide POLYOLS, glucosorbitol and glucomannitol. About 50% metabolised, yielding 9 kJ (2.4 kcal)/gram. Thought to be less laxative than SORBITOL or MANNITOL, and does not encourage tooth decay, so is used in TOOTH-FRIENDLY SWEETS.

isomaltose   A disaccharide of glucose linked α-1,6 (MALTOSE is linked α-1,4); not fermentable. Also known as brachyose.

Isomerose   Trade name of high-fructose corn syrup (see FRUCTOSE SYRUPS): 70–72% solids, 42% fructose, 55% glucose, 3% polysaccharides.

isomers   Molecules containing the same atoms but differently arranged, so that the chemical and biochemical properties differ.

(1) In positional isomers the functional groups are on different carbon atoms; e.g. leucine and isoleucine, citric and isocitric acids.

(2) D- and L-isomerism refers to the spatial arrangement of four different chemical groups on the same carbon atom (stereoisomerism or optical isomerism). *R*- and *S*-isomerism is the same, but determined by a set of systematic chemical rules. See D-, L- AND DL-.

(3) *Cis*- and *trans*-isomerism refers to the arrangement of groups adjacent to a carbon–carbon double bond; in the *cis*-isomer the groups are on the same side of the double bond, while on the *trans*-isomer they are on opposite sides.

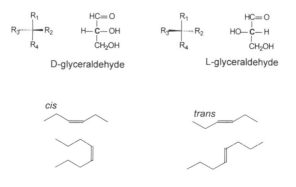

D-glyceraldehyde   L-glyceraldehyde

cis   *trans*

isoniazid Isonicotinic acid hydrazide, used in the treatment of tuberculosis. Separately from its antimycobacterial action, forms an inactive adduct with pyridoxal, leading to depletion of VITAMIN B_6, and secondary PELLAGRA as a result of impaired synthesis of NIACIN from TRYPTOPHAN.

isosyrups See FRUCTOSE SYRUPS.

isotonic Solutions with the same OSMOTIC PRESSURE (concentration of solids); often refers to a solution with the same osmotic pressure as body fluids. Hypertonic and hypotonic refer to solutions that are respectively more and less concentrated.

isotopes Forms of elements with the same chemical properties, differing in atomic mass because of differing numbers of neutrons in the atomic nucleus. Thus, hydrogen has three isotopes, of atomic masses 1, 2 and 3, generally written as ^1H (the most abundant isotope of hydrogen), ^2H (deuterium) and ^3H (tritium). The incorporation of isotopes into compounds (labelled compounds or tracers) permits the metabolic fates of those compounds in the body to be followed easily.

Stable isotopes can be detected only by their different atomic mass. Since they emit no radiation, they are considered completely safe for use in labelled compounds given to human beings. Examples of stable isotopes commonly used in nutrition research include ^2H, ^{13}C, ^{15}N and ^{18}O.

Unstable isotopes decay to stable elements, emitting radiation in the process. This may be α-particles, β-radiation (electrons), γ-radiation or X-rays, depending on the particular isotope. Radioactive isotopes can readily be detected by the radiation emitted. The time taken for half the radioactive isotope to decay is the HALF-LIFE of the isotope, and can vary from a fraction of a second, through several days to years (e.g. the half-life of ^3H is 12.5 years, that of ^{14}C is 5200 years).

isotretinoin 13-*Cis* retinoic acid, a RETINOID used in the treatment of severe acne.

isozymes See ISOENZYMES.

ispaghula A bulk-forming LAXATIVE.

itai-itai disease See CADMIUM.

iu See INTERNATIONAL UNITS.

J

jaggery (1) Coarse dark sugar made from the sap of the coconut palm.

(2) Raw sugar cane juice, used in India as sweetening agent, also known as gur.

jaguar gum See GUAR GUM.

jak fruit (jack fruit)   Large fruit, up to 30 kg, from tropical tree *Artocarpus* spp, related to BREADFRUIT. Both pulp and seeds are eaten.

jake paralysis   See JAMAICA GINGER PARALYSIS.

jam   A conserve of fruit boiled to a pulp with sugar; sets to a PECTIN jelly on cooling (known in USA as jelly). Standard jam, with certain exceptions, contains a minimum of 35 g of fruit per 100 g; extra jam, with certain exceptions, contains 45 g.

Composition/100 g: 1092 kJ (261 kcal), protein 0.6 g, fat 0 g, carbohydrate 69 g (69 g sugars), dietary fibre 1 g, Na 16 mg, K 110 mg, Ca 24 mg, Mg 10 mg, P 18 mg, Fe 1.5 mg, Cu 0.23 mg, Zn 0.2 mg, I 7 μg, vitamin C 10 mg. Serving 15 g.

Reduced sugar jam: composition/100 g: 502 kJ (120 kcal), protein 0.5 g, fat 0 g, carbohydrate 32 g (32 g sugars), Na 17 mg, K 230 mg, Ca 20 mg, Mg 7 mg, P 15 mg, Fe 0.4 mg, vitamin C 25 mg. Serving 15 g.

Jamaica ginger paralysis   Polyneuritis caused by poisoning from an extract of Jamaica ginger ('jake') due to triorthocresyl phosphate.

Jamaican pepper   See ALLSPICE.

Japanese isinglass   See AGAR.

jasmine tea   A perfumed or scented tea made by adding petals of jasmine flowers to Chinese tea.

jejuno–ileostomy   Surgical procedure in which the terminal JEJUNUM or proximal ILEUM is removed or by-passed. Was formerly used as a treatment for severe OBESITY.

jejunostomy feeding   See ENTERAL NUTRITION.

jejunum   Part of the small intestine, between the duodenum and the ileum; see GASTROINTESTINAL TRACT.

jelly   (1) Clear JAM made from strained fruit juice by boiling with sugar. Also used in this sense in N America to mean any jam.

(2) Table jelly is a dessert made from GELATINE, sweetened and flavoured; known in N America as jello.

(3) Savoury gelatine jelly made from calf's foot or gelatinous stock; see ASPIC.

jerked beef, jerky   See CHARQUI.

Job's tears   See ADLAY.

jodbasedow   See THYROTOXICOSIS.

jojoba oil   Liquid wax of long-chain FATTY ACIDS (eicosenoic and docosenoic (erucic) acids) esterified with long-chain alcohols (eicosanol and docosanol) from seeds of the shrub *Simmondsia chinensis*. Of interest in cosmetics as a replacement for sperm whale oil but also has food applications, e.g. coating agent for dried fruits.

jonathan   Calcined, ground oat chaff used in nineteenth century as adulterant for maize and other cereals.

Joule   The SI (Système Internationale) unit of ENERGY; used to express energy content of foods and energy expenditure of man and animals. Gradually adopted as a replacement for the CALORIE from about 1970; 4.2 kilojoules (kJ) is equivalent to 1 kilocalorie (kcal).

Joule cycle   See HEAT PUMP.

jowar   Indian name for SORGHUM (*Sorghum vulgare*), also known as great millet, kaffir corn, guinea corn.

jujube   (1) Sweet made from gum and sugar.

(2) Chinese date, Indian plum, fruit of the shrub *Zisiphus mauritania* or *Z. jujuba*, important fruit crop in India; the fruit is reddish-brown up to 2 cm in diameter with a single stone.

Composition/100 g: 364 kJ (87 kcal), protein 1.5 g, fat 0.3 g, carbohydrate 19.7 g (19.7 g sugars), Na 4 mg, K 240 mg, Ca 30 mg, Mg 10 mg, P 22 mg, Fe 0.6 mg, Cu 0.07 mg, Zn 0.1 mg, vitamin A 4 µg (24 µg carotene), B_1 0.03 mg, B_2 0.03 mg, niacin 1 mg, B_6 0.08 mg, C 57 mg. A 30 g serving is a good source of vitamin C.

juniper   The ripened berries of the bush *Juniperis communis*, used as a flavouring in GIN.

junket   Dessert made from milk by treating with RENNET to curdle the protein.

K

kaffir beer   African BEER brewed from millet.

kaffir corn   See SORGHUM.

kaffir manna corn   See MILLET.

kaki   See PERSIMMON.

kale   Scottish name for any type of cabbage; in England means specifically open-headed varieties of cabbage with curly leaves, also known as curly kale or borecole. Distinct from sea kale or SWISS CHARD.

Composition/100 g: 100 kJ (24 kcal), protein 2.4 g, fat 1.1 g (22.2% saturated, 11.1% mono-, 66.6% polyunsaturated), carbohydrate 1 g (0.9 g sugars, 0.1 g starch), dietary fibre 2.6 g, nsp 2.8 g, Na 100 mg, K 160 mg, Ca 150 mg, Mg 8 mg, P 39 mg, Fe 2 mg, Cu 0.02 mg, Zn 0.2 mg, Se 2 µg, vitamin A 562 µg (3375 µg carotene), E 1.3 mg, B_1 0.02 mg, B_2 0.06 mg, niacin 1.3 mg, B_6 0.13 mg, folate 86 µg, pantothenate 0.1 mg, biotin 0.4 µg, C 71 mg. A 95 g serving is a source of vitamin E, Ca, Fe; rich source of vitamin A, folate, C.

kaolin   Adsorbent clay used to treat diarrhoea and vomiting.

karaya gum   Obtained from E Indian tree *Sterculia arens.* Used as stabiliser, e.g. in frozen water ices; also used in combination with other stabilisers; sometimes used as laxative. Also called sterculia gum (E-416).

Karl Fischer method   For determination of the moisture content of dehydrated foods. Water is extracted from the sample into anhydrous methanol, then titrated against the Karl Fischer reagent (sulphur dioxide, pyridine and iodine in anhydrous methanol) with electrometric determination of the end-point.

Karo Syrup   Trade name for a dextromaltose preparation made from maize starch, used as carbohydrate modifier in milk preparations for infant feeding. Consists of a mixture of dextrin, maltose, glucose and sucrose.

kasha   See BUCKWHEAT.

Kashin–Beck syndrome   Osteo-articular disorder that is endemic in regions of China where there is severe SELENIUM deficiency, and responds to selenium supplementation.
See also KESHAN DISEASE.

katadyn process   See MATZKA PROCESS; OLIGODYNAMIC.

katemfe   An intensely sweet African fruit, *Thaumatococcus daniellii,* called katemfe in Sierra Leone and miraculous fruit of Sudan (not the same as MIRACLE BERRY). The active principle is the protein THAUMATIN.

kathepsins   See CATHEPSINS.

kb   Kilobase, a measure of the size of DNA and RNA by the number of bases in the sequence under consideration.

kcal   Abbreviation for kilocalorie (1000 CALORIES), sometimes shown as Cal.

kebab   Turkish for roast meat. Shishkebab is small pieces of mutton rubbed with salt, pepper, etc and roasted on a skewer (*shish* in Turkish) sometimes interspaced with vegetables. Shashlik is a Georgian version. Döner kebab is a Turkish speciality consisting of marinated mutton or lamb packed into a cylindrical mass and grilled on a vertical rotating spit (*showarma* in Arabic).

kedgeree   Indian; dish of rice and pulses. Modified to Victorian breakfast dish of flaked fish with egg and rice.

kefir   See MILK, FERMENTED.

kelp   Large brown seaweeds, *Laminaria* spp. Occasionally used as food or food ingredient but mostly the ash is used as a source of alkali and iodine. Sometimes claimed as a HEALTH FOOD with unspecified properties.

Kelvin   SI unit of absolute temperature; $°K = °C - 273.15$.

kephalins   Or cephalins; PHOSPHOLIPIDS containing ethanolamine, hence PHOSPHATIDYLETHANOLAMINES. Found especially in brain and nerve tissue.

Kepler extract of malt Trade name for one of the earliest of the MALT EXTRACTS, intended as a dietary supplement to aid digestion, since it was rich in DIASTASE compared with ordinary malt extracts.

keratin The insoluble protein of hair, horn, hoof, feathers and nails. Not hydrolysed by digestive enzymes, and therefore nutritionally useless. Used as fertiliser, since it is slowly broken down by soil bacteria. Steamed feather meal is used to some extent as a supplement for ruminants.

keratinisation Process by which epithelial cells become horny due to deposition of KERATIN; may occur excessively and inappropriately in VITAMIN A deficiency.

keratomalacia Progressive softening and ulceration of the cornea, due to VITAMIN A deficiency. Blindness is usually inevitable unless the deficiency is corrected at an early stage.

kesari dhal A legume, *Lathyris sativus*.
See also LATHYRISM.

Keshan disease Cardiomyopathy that is endemic in regions of China where there is severe SELENIUM deficiency, and responds to selenium supplementation, although other factors, including COXSACKIE VIRUS and the MYCOTOXIN MONILIFORMIN, may also be involved.
See also KASHIN–BECK SYNDROME.

Kesp Trade name for a texture vegetable protein product made by a spinning process.

ketchup (catsup or catchup) From the Chinese koechap or kitsiap, originally meaning brine of pickled fish. Now used for spicy sauce or condiment made with juice of fruit or vegetables, vinegar and spices.

ketoacidosis The result of synthesis of KETONE bodies so far in excess of the capacity for their metabolism that the blood level rises sufficiently to affect pH. May occur in patients with insulin-dependent DIABETES mellitus, but rare in those with non-insulin-dependent diabetes.

ketogenic amino acids See AMINO ACIDS, KETOGENIC.

ketogenic diet A diet poor in carbohydrate (20–30 g) and rich in fat; causes accumulation of KETONE bodies in tissue; formerly used in the treatment of epilepsy.

ketonaemia High concentrations of KETONE bodies in the blood.

ketone bodies Acetone, acetoacetate and β-hydroxybutyric acid (not chemically a KETONE) synthesised in liver from acetyl CoA (the product of β-oxidation of fatty acids), especially in the fasting state, and exported for use by other tissues as a metabolic fuel. When production exceeds the rate of utilisation the plasma concentration may rise high enough to cause significant ketoacidosis (especially in uncontrolled insulin-dependent DIABETES mellitus), and significant amounts may be excreted in the urine (ketonuria).

ketones Chemical compounds containing a carbonyl group (C=O), with two alkyl groups attached to the same carbon; the simplest ketone is ACETONE (dimethylketone, $(CH_3)_2$-C=O).

ketonic rancidity Moulds of *Penicillium* and *Aspergillus* spp attack fats containing short-chain fatty acids and produce KETONES with a characteristic odour and taste, so-called ketonic rancidity. Fats such as butter, coconut and palm kernel are most susceptible.

Ketonil Trade name for protein-rich food low in PHENYLALANINE for feeding patients with PHENYLKETONURIA.

ketonuria Excretion of KETONE bodies in the urine.

ketosis High concentrations of KETONE bodies in the blood.

khushkhash See ORANGE, BITTER.

kibble To grind or chop coarsely.

kid Young goat (*Capra aegragus*) usually under three months old; similar to LAMB, but with a stronger flavour.

kidney Usually from lamb, ox, pig.

Composition/100 g (average): 370 kJ (88 kcal), protein 16.2 g, fat 2.7 g (50% saturated, 35% mono-, 15% polyunsaturated), cholesterol 400 mg, carbohydrate 0 g, Na 200 mg, K 260 mg, Ca 9 mg, Mg 17 mg, P 250 mg, Fe 6 mg, Cu 0.55 mg, Zn 2.3 mg, Se 150 μg, I 7 μg, vitamin A 120 μg, E 0.4 mg, B_1 0.3933 mg, B_2 1.9 mg, niacin 10.8 mg, B_6 0.29 mg, folate 50 μg, B_{12} 33 μg, pantothenate 3.5 mg, biotin 31 μg, C 10 mg. A 110 g serving is a source of vitamin A, B_6, C, Zn; good source of folate, biotin; rich source of protein, vitamin B_1, B_2, niacin, B_{12}, pantothenate, Fe, Cu, Se.

kieves Irish name for MASH TUNS.

kilderkin Cask for beer (18 gallons = 80.1 L) and ale (16 gallons = 71.2 L).

Kiliani reaction Colorimetric reaction for CHOLESTEROL; the development of a purple colour on reaction with ferric chloride.

kimchi Korean; dish based on fermented cabbage with garlic, red peppers and pimientos, often with the addition of fish and other foods.

kipper HERRING that has been lightly salted and smoked, invented by John Woodger, a fish curer of Seahouses, Northumberland, 1843.

Composition/100 g: 673 kJ (161 kcal), protein 12.7 g, fat 12.2 g (18% saturated, 57.6% mono-, 24.3% polyunsaturated), cholesterol 44 mg, carbohydrate 0 g, Na 590 mg, K 240 mg, Ca 38 mg, Mg 20 mg, P 160 mg, Fe 1.1 mg, Cu 0.09 mg, Zn 0.7 mg, Se 23 μg, I 40 μg, vitamin A 24 μg, D 5.9 μg, E 0.2 mg, B_2 0.17 mg, niacin

5.2 mg, B_6 0.16 mg, folate 3 µg, B_{12} 7 µg, pantothenate 0.3 mg, biotin 3 µg. A 130 g serving is a source of vitamin B_2, B_6, Fe, Cu; rich source of protein, vitamin D, niacin, B_{12}, I, Se.

kiwano The horned melon, a New Zealand fruit with a spiky yellow skin and green flesh.

kiwi Fruit of *Actinidia sinensis*, originally native of China and also known as Chinese gooseberry.

Composition/100 g: 175 kJ (42 kcal), protein 1 g, fat 0.4 g, carbohydrate 9.1 g (8.9 g sugars, 0.3 g starch), nsp 1.6 g, Na 3 mg, K 250 mg, Ca 21 mg, Mg 13 mg, P 27 mg, Fe 0.3 mg, Cu 0.11 mg, Zn 0.1 mg, vitamin A 5 µg (32 µg carotene), B_1 0.01 mg, B_2 0.03 mg, niacin 0.6 mg, B_6 0.13 mg, C 51 mg. A 60 g serving is a rich source of vitamin C.

Kjeldahl determination Widely used method of determining total nitrogen in a substance by digesting with sulphuric acid and a catalyst first described in 1883; the nitrogen is reduced to ammonia which is then measured. In foodstuffs most of the nitrogen is PROTEIN, and the term crude protein is the total 'Kjeldahl nitrogen' multiplied by factor 6.25 (since most proteins contain 16% nitrogen).

See also NITROGEN CONVERSION FACTOR.

Klim Trade name for dried milk.

klipfish Salted and dried cod, mainly produced in Norway, also known as bacalao or bacalau. The fish is boned, stored in salt for a month, washed and dried slowly.

See also STOCKFISH.

K_m The Michaelis constant of an enzyme. A measure of the affinity of the enzyme for its substrate, equal to the concentration of substrate at which the enzyme achieves half its maximum rate of activity.

kneading To work dough by stretching and folding until it achieves the required consistency.

knee height Distance from the heel to the anterior surface of the thigh, proximal to the patella. Highly correlated with stature, and used to estimate height in people with severe spinal curvature or those who are unable to stand.

kohlrabi Swollen stem of *Brassica oleracea gongylodes* (turnip-rooted cabbage, kale turnip); green and purple varieties.

Composition/100 g: 75 kJ (18 kcal), protein 1.2 g, fat 0.2 g, carbohydrate 3.1 g (3 g sugars, 0.1 g starch), nsp 1.9 g, Na 110 mg, K 240 mg, Ca 21 mg, Mg 6 mg, P 30 mg, Fe 0.2 mg, Cu 0.01 mg, Zn 0.1 mg, I 1 µg, vitamin B_1 0.08 mg, B_2 0.01 mg, niacin 0.4 mg, B_6 0.11 mg, folate 47 µg, pantothenate 0.1 mg, C 27 mg. A 25 g serving is a source of vitamin C.

koilonychia   Development of (brittle) concave fingernails, commonly associated with IRON deficiency ANAEMIA.

koji   See MISO.

kokoh   In the Zen macrobiotic diet this is a mixture of ground seeds and cereals fed to young infants; it is deficient in a number of nutrients and can result in growth retardation unless supplemented.

konjac   GUM derived from tubers of *Amorphophallus konjac*; eaten in Japan as a firm jelly.

Korsakoff's psychosis   Failure of recent memory, although events from the past are recalled, with CONFABULATION; associated with VITAMIN B₁ deficiency, especially in alcoholics.

See also WERNICKE'S ENCEPHALOPATHY.

kosher   The selection and preparation of foods in accordance with traditional Jewish ritual and dietary laws. Foods that are not kosher are traife. The only kosher flesh foods are from animals that chew the cud and have cloven hooves, such as cattle, sheep, goats and deer; the hindquarters must not be eaten. The only fish permitted are those with fins and scales; birds of prey and scavengers are not kosher. Moreover, the animals must be slaughtered according to ritual before the meat can be considered kosher. From Hebrew *kosher* = right (Deuteronomy, Ch. 14).

See also HALAL; FLEISHIG; MILCHIG; PAREVE.

koumiss   See MILK, FERMENTED.

Krebs' cycle   Or citric acid cycle, a central pathway for the METABOLISM of fats, carbohydrates and amino acids. Named for Sir Hans Krebs (1900–81), who first described the pathway.

krill   Term that refers to many species of planktonic crustaceans but mostly the shrimp *Euphausia superba*. This is the main food of whales, and some penguins and other seabirds; occurs in shoals in the Antarctic, containing up to 12 kg/m³. Collected in limited quantities for use as human food.

kryptoxanthin   See CRYPTOXANTHIN.

kuban   See MILK, FERMENTED.

kumiss   See MILK, FERMENTED.

kumquat   A CITRUS fruit of the genus *Fortunella*; widely distributed in S China and now cultivated elsewhere; resembles other citrus fruits, but very small, ovoid shape, with acid pulp, and sweet, edible skin.

Composition/100 g: 179 kJ (43 kcal), protein 0.9 g, fat 0.5 g, carbohydrate 9.3 g (9.3 g sugars), nsp 3.8 g, Na 6 mg, K 180 mg, Ca 25 mg, Mg 13 mg, P 49 mg, Fe 0.6 mg, Cu 0.11 mg, Zn 0.1 mg, vitamin A 29 µg (175 µg carotene), B₁ 0.07 mg, B₂ 0.07 mg, niacin 0.6 mg, C 39 mg. A 30 g serving (four fruits) is a source of vitamin C.

kuru Or trembling disease; progressive degeneration of central nervous system cells, associated with cannibalism in Papua-New Guinea, and believed to be caused by a PRION. More or less eradicated since ritual cannibalism was abolished.

kwashiorkor See PROTEIN–ENERGY MALNUTRITION.

kyphosis Excessive outward curvature of the spine, causing hunching of the back. May result from collapse of the vertebrae in OSTEOPOROSIS.

L

l- See D-, L- and DL-

laccase See PHENOL OXIDASES.

lacquer With reference to canned foods (see CANNING), a layer of gum and gum resin coated onto the tinplate and hardened with heat. The layer of lacquer protects the tin lining from attack by acid fruit juices.

lactalbumin One of the proteins of milk. Not precipitated from acid solution as is CASEIN; hence, during cheese-making the whey contains lactalbumin and lactoglobulin. They are precipitated by heat and a whey CHEESE can be made in this way.

lactase The enzyme (β-galactosidase, EC 3.2.1.23) that hydrolyses LACTOSE to glucose and galactose; normally present in the brush border of the intestinal mucosal cells; deficiency of lactase is alactasia, leading to lactose intolerance. Fungal lactase is used to produce lactose-free MILK for people suffering from ALACTASIA.
  See also DISACCHARIDE INTOLERANCE.

lactic acid The acid produced by the anaerobic metabolism of glucose. Originally discovered in sour milk, it is responsible for the flavour of fermented MILK and for the precipitation of the CASEIN curd in cottage CHEESE. Also produced by fermentation in silage, PICKLING, SAUERKRAUT, cocoa, tobacco; its value here is in suppressing the growth of unwanted organisms.
  It is formed in mammalian muscle under conditions of maximum exertion (see GLUCOSE METABOLISM) and by metabolism of glycogen in meat immediately after death of the animal. Lactic acid in muscle was at one time known as sarcolactic acid.
  Used as an acidulant (as well as citric and tartaric acids) in sugar confectionery, soft drinks, pickles and sauces. (E-270; salts of lactic acid are E-325–327.)

lactic acid, buffered A mixture of LACTIC ACID and sodium lactate used in sugar confectionery to provide an acid taste without INVERSION of the sugar, which occurs at lower pH.

lactitol SUGAR ALCOHOL derived from LACTULOSE. Not digested by digestive enzymes but fermented by intestinal bacteria to short chain fatty acids, some of which are absorbed; it yields about 8 kJ (2 kcal)/g and hence has a potential use as a low-calorie bulk sweetener; also retards crystallisation and improves moisture retention in foods (E-966). Because of bacterial fermentation in the colon, it is also used as an osmotic LAXATIVE. Also known as lactit, lactositol, lactobiosit.

Lactobacillus Genus of bacteria capable of growth in acidic medium, and producing LACTIC ACID by fermentation of carbohydrates. Responsible for souring of MILK, and production of flavour in YOGHOURT and other fermented milk products.

See also PROBIOTICS.

***Lactobacillus casei* factor** See FOLIC ACID.

lactobiose See LACTOSE.

lactobiosit See LACTITOL.

lactochrome Obsolete name for riboflavin (VITAMIN B₂).

lactoferrin Iron–protein complex in human milk (only a trace cow's milk) only partly saturated with iron; has a rôle inhibiting the growth of *E. coli* and other potentially pathogenic organisms.

lactoflavin Obsolete name for RIBOFLAVIN, so named because it was isolated from milk.

See VITAMIN B₂.

lactogen A drug or other substance that increases the production and secretion of milk. Lactogenic hormone is PROLACTIN.

lactoglobulin See LACTALBUMIN.

lactometer Floating device used to measure the specific gravity of milk (1.027–1.035).

Lac-tone Trade name; protein-rich baby food (26% protein) made in India from peanut flour, skim milk powder, wheat flour and barley flour with added vitamins and calcium.

lacto-ovo-vegetarian One whose diet excludes animal foods (i.e. flesh) but permits milk and eggs.

lactose Milk sugar, the CARBOHYDRATE of milk; a DISACCHARIDE, β-1,4-glucosyl-galactose. Used pharmaceutically as a tablet filler and as a medium for growth of microorganisms. The fermentation of lactose to LACTIC ACID by bacteria is responsible for the souring of milk. Ordinary lactose is α-lactose, which is 16% as sweet as sucrose; if crystallised above 93°C, it is converted to the β-form which is more soluble and sweeter.

See also DISACCHARIDE INTOLERANCE.

lacto-serum See WHEY.

lactositol See LACTITOL.

lactostearin See GLYCERYL LACTOSTEARATE.

lactosucrose A trisaccharide (galactosyl-glucosyl-fructose) formed from sucrose and lactose by fructosyl transfer catalysed by INVERTASE (EC 3.2.1.6). Considered to be a PREBIOTIC.

lactulose   A DISACCHARIDE, β-1,4-fructosyl-galactose, which does not occur naturally but is formed in heated or stored milk by isomerisation of LACTOSE. About half as sweet as sucrose. Not hydrolysed by human digestive enzymes but fermented by intestinal bacteria to form LACTIC ACID and pyruvic acid. Thought to promote the growth of *Lactobacillus bifidus* and so added to some infant formulae. Because of bacterial fermentation in the colon it is an osmotic LAXATIVE.

See also LACTITOL.

ladies' fingers   See OKRA; also a short kind of banana.

laetrile   See AMYGDALIN.

laevorotatory   See OPTICAL ACTIVITY.

laevulose   See FRUCTOSE.

lamb   Meat from sheep (*Ovis aries*) younger than 12–14 months. Composition/100 g: 535–1054 kJ (128–252 kcal), protein 17–29 g, fat 8–16 g (52.7% saturated, 41.6% mono-, 5.5% polyunsaturated), cholesterol 50–110 mg, carbohydrate 0 g, Na 87 mg, K 267.5 mg, Ca 8 mg, Mg 21 mg, P 172.5 mg, Fe 1.85 mg, Cu 0.2175 mg, Zn 4.85 mg, Se 1 μg, I 4.5 μg, vitamin E 0.1 mg, B_1 0.0925 mg, B_2 0.2625 mg, niacin 9.5 mg, B_6 0.1925 mg, folate 3.5 μg, B_{12} 1.75 μg, pantothenate 0.625 mg, biotin 1.75 μg. A 90 g serving is a source of vitamin B_2, Fe; good source of Cu, Zn; rich source of protein, niacin, vitamin B_{12}.

lamb's lettuce   Or corn salad, hardy annual plant, *Valerianella locusta* or *V. olitoria* used in salads in winter and early spring.

lamb's wool   Old English drink made by pouring hot ale over pulped roasted apples and adding sugar and spices.

lamprey (lampern)   Cartilaginous fish resembling eel; sea lamprey is *Petromyzon marinus*, river lamprey or lampern is *Lampetra fluviatilis*.

langouste   SHELLFISH, *Palinurus vulgaris*; see LOBSTER.

lanolin   The fat from wool. Consists of a mixture of cholesterol oleate, palmitate and stearate, and not useful as food; used in various cosmetics.

lansoprazole   See PROTON PUMP.

larch gum   A POLYSACCHARIDE of galactose and arabinose (ratio of 1:6), found in the aqueous extract of the Western larch tree (*Larix occidentalis*); a potential substitute for GUM ARABIC, since it is readily dispersed in water.

lard   Originally rendered fat from pig carcass (sheep and cattle also used). The best quality is from the fat surrounding the kidneys; neutral lard is the highest quality, prepared by agitating the minced fat with water at a temperature below 50°C; kidney fat provides No. 1 quality; back fat provides No. 2 quality. Leaf lard is made from the residue of kidney and back fat after the preparation of neutral lard by heating with water above 100°C in an autoclave. Prime steam lard is fat from any part of the carcass, rendered in the autoclave. Lard used to be stored in pig's bladder, hence the expression 'bladder of lard' for a grossly obese person.

lard compounds Blends of animal fats, such as oleostearin or PREMIER JUS, with vegetable oils, to produce products similar to lard in consistency and texture.

See also LARD SUBSTITUTES.

lardine See MARGARINE.

lard substitutes Vegetable shortenings made from mixtures of partially hardened vegetable fats with the consistency of LARD.

See also LARD COMPOUNDS.

lardy cake West of England; made from bread dough, lard, sugar and dried fruit.

lasagne Wide ribbons of PASTA; lasagne verdi is flavoured with spinach. Narrow ribbons are lasagnette.

latent heat Heat absorbed or released when a substance changes phase. This property is used in refrigeration, e.g. latent heat of solid carbon dioxide when changing into a gas is 352 kJ per kg at −78°C; liquid nitrogen 358 kJ per kg at −196°C.

lathyrism The effect of consuming *Lathyrus* spp peas (chickling vetch, flat-podded vetch, Spanish vetchling, Indian vetch), which contain the neurotoxin oxalyl-diaminopropionic acid. Although growing *Lathyrus* spp has been banned in many countries, lathyrism continues to be a public health problem in India since kesari dhal, *Lathyrus sativa*, is a hardy crop that survives adverse conditions and can become a large part of the diet in times of drought.

See also ODORATISM.

lauric acid A medium-chain length saturated FATTY ACID (C12:0) in butter, coconut oil and palm oil.

lauter tun Vertical cylindrical tank for extracting and clarifying WORT and separating it from spent grain in malting and brewing.

laver Edible seaweed, *Porphyra* spp. Laver bread is made by boiling in salted water and mincing to a gelatinous mass. It is made into a cake with oatmeal or fried. Locally known in S Wales as bara lawr.

lax Scandinavian name for salmon.

See also GRAVADLAX; LOX.

laxarinic acid See MALTOL.

laxative Compounds used to treat CONSTIPATION. Bulk-forming laxatives include various preparations of non-starch polysaccharide.

Stimulant or contact laxatives include senna and cascara

(*Rhamnus purshianus, Frangula purshiana*) in which the active ingredients are anthroquinones, aloe vera extract, bisacodyl (a diphenylmethene derivative), phenolphthalein and sodium picosulphate.

Osmotic laxatives include magnesium salts and LACTULOSE.

Emollient laxatives (faecal softeners) include liquid paraffin and docusates (which act as detergents to permit penetration of water into the faecal mass).

A number of drugs are used to increase intestinal motility.

LD$_{50}$ An index of acute toxicity (lethal dose 50%); the amount of the substance that kills 50% of the test population of experimental animals when administered as a single dose.

LDL Low-density lipoprotein, see LIPOPROTEINS, PLASMA.

lead A mineral of no nutritional interest, since it is not known to have any function in the body. It is toxic and its effects are cumulative. May be present in food from traces naturally present in the soil, as contamination of vegetables grown near main roads, which absorb volatile lead compounds from car exhausts, from shellfish that have absorbed it from seawater, from lead glazes on cooking vessels and in drinking water where lead pipes are used. Traces are excreted in the urine.

lean body mass Measure of body composition excluding adipose tissue, i.e. cells, extracellular fluid and skeleton.

Lean Cuisine Trade name for a range of frozen meals prepared to a specified energy content.

leathers, fruit Fruit purées dried in air in thin layers, 4–5 mm thick, then built up into thicker preparations.

leaven YEAST, or a piece of dough kept to ferment the next batch.

leben See MILK, FERMENTED.

lecithin Chemically lecithin is phosphatidyl choline; a PHOSPHOLIPID containing CHOLINE. Commercial lecithin, prepared from soya bean, peanut and maize, is a mixture of phospholipids in which phosphatidyl choline predominates.

Used in food processing as an EMULSIFIER, e.g. in salad dressing, processed cheese and chocolate, and as an antispattering agent in frying oils. Is plentiful in the diet and not a dietary essential.

lecithinase Any of a number of PHOSPHOLIPASES that hydrolyse LECITHIN.

lectin One of a series of proteins found especially in LEGUME seeds that are both mitogenic, stimulating cell division, and act to agglutinate cells (especially red blood cells, hence the old names haemagglutinin and phytoagglutinin). Lectins may be a cause of serious non-bacterial food poisoning, after consumption of raw or undercooked beans of some varieties of *Phaseolus vul-*

garis (red kidney beans) causing vomiting and diarrhoea within 2 h, and severe damage to the intestinal mucosa; they are denatured, and hence inactivated, only by boiling for about 10 min.

leek *Allium ampeloprasum*; a member of the onion family which has been known as a food for over 4000 years. The lower part is usually blanched by planting in trenches or earthing up, and eaten along with the upper long green leaves.

Composition/100 g: 87 kJ (21 kcal), protein 1.2 g, fat 0.7 g, carbohydrate 2.6 g (2 g sugars, 0.2 g starch), dietary fibre 2.4 g, nsp 1.7 g, Na 6 mg, K 150 mg, Ca 20 mg, Mg 2 mg, P 32 mg, Fe 0.7 mg, Cu 0.02 mg, Zn 0.2 mg, Se 1 μg, vitamin A 95 μg (575 μg carotene), E 0.8 mg, B_1 0.02 mg, B_2 0.02 mg, niacin 0.6 mg, B_6 0.1 mg, folate 40 μg, biotin 1 μg, C 7 mg. A 160 g serving is a source of vitamin A, E, C; rich source of folate.

leghaemoglobin Haem-containing protein in the root nodules of leguminous plants that binds O_2 for transport within the root, and so permits the growth of obligate anaerobic nitrogen-fixing microorganisms, *Rhizobium* spp.

See also NITROGENASE.

legumes Food seeds of members of the leguminosae family. Consumed in the immature green state in the pod or as the dried mature seed (grain legumes and pulses) after boiling; 100 g cooked portion contains approximately 50 g of the dried product.

Include ground nut, *Arachis hypogea* and soya bean, *Glycine max* and African yam bean *Sphenostylis stenocarpa*, grown for their edible tubers as well as seeds.

Phaseolus vulgaris Navy, Boston, pinto, string, snapbean (USA); haricot, kidney and when unripe, French, wax bean (UK); flageolet (yellow variety).

P. coccineus (*P. multiflora*) runner, scarlet runner, multiflora bean.

P. acutifolius (var. *latifolius*) tepary, rice haricot bean, Texan bean (USA).

P. lunatus (*lumensis, inamoensus*) Lima bean (USA), butter, Madagascar butter, Rangoon, Burma, Sieva bean.

Cajanus cajan (*C. indicus*) pigeon, Angola, non-eye pea, Congo bean or pea, red gram, yellow dhal.

Vigna umbellata (*P. calcaratus*) rice bean, red bean (also used for adzuki bean). *Vigna mango* (*P. mungo*) urd bean, black gram, mash. *V.* or *P. angularis* adzuki bean.

Vigna unguiculata (or *V. sesquipedalis* or *sinensis*, systematics confused) cow pea, black-eyed bean or pea, China pea, cowgram, catjang, southern pea. *Vigna unguiculata sesquipedalis* (L) asparagus bean, pea bean, yard-long bean.

V. aconitifolia (*P. aconitifolia*) moth, mat bean, Turkish gram.

V. radiata (*P. aureus*, *P. radiatus*) mung bean, green or golden gram. *Lablab purpureus* (*Dolichos lablab*) bonavista, dolichos, Egyptian kidney, Indian butter, lablab, tonga, hyacinth bean.

Canavalia ensiformis jack, overlook, sword bean. *Lens culinaris* (*esculenta*) lentil, red dhal, masur dhal, split pea.

Pisum sativa garden, green pea. *Pisum aevense* field pea. *Voandzeia subterranea* bambar(r)a groundnut, earth pea, ground bean, Kaffir pea, Madagascar groundnut.

Cicer aretinum chick pea, Bengal gram.

Cyamopsis tetragonoloba cluster bean. *Lathyrus sativus* grass, lathyrus, chickling pea, Indian vetch, khesari dhal. *Macrotyloma uniflorum* (*Dolichos uniflorus*) horse gram, horse grain, kulthi bean, Madras gram. *Macuna pruriens* velvet bean. *Psophocarpus tetragonolobus* winged bean, asparagus bean or pea, four-cornered, Goa, Manila, Mauritius bean. *Vicia faba* broad bean, faba, field, horse, pigeon, trick, windsor bean.

legumin Globulin protein in legumes.

lemon Sour fruit of *Citrus limon*.

Composition/100 g: 79 kJ (19 kcal), protein 1 g, fat 0.3 g, carbohydrate 3.2 g (3.2 g sugars), dietary fibre 4.7 g, Na 5 mg, K 150 mg, Ca 85 mg, Mg 12 mg, P 18 mg, Fe 0.5 mg, Cu 0.26 mg, Zn 0.1 mg, Se 1 μg, vitamin A 3 μg (18 μg carotene), B_1 0.05 mg, B_2 0.04 mg, niacin 0.3 mg, B_6 0.11 mg, pantothenate 0.2 mg, biotin 0.5 μg, C 58 mg. An 80 g serving is a good source of Cu; rich source of vitamin C.

lemon grass Lemon-scented grasses (*Cymbopogon* spp), native to SE Asia, widely used in Thai, Indonesian and Malay cooking.

lentils LEGUMES; dried seeds of many varieties of *Lens esculenta*, they may be green, yellow or orange-red.

Composition/100 g (boiled, green): 439 kJ (105 kcal), protein 8.8 g, fat 0.7 g, carbohydrate 16.9 g (0.4 g sugars, 15.9 g starch), nsp 3.8 g, Na 3 mg, K 310 mg, Ca 22 mg, Mg 34 mg, P 130 mg, Fe 3.5 mg, Cu 0.33 mg, Zn 1.4 mg, Se 40 μg, vitamin B_1 0.14 mg, B_2 0.08 mg, niacin 1.8 mg, B_6 0.28 mg, folate 30 μg. A 120 g serving is a source of vitamin B_1, niacin, B_6, folate, Mg, Zn; good source of protein; rich source of Fe, Cu, Se.

Composition/100 g (boiled, red): 418 kJ (100 kcal), protein 7.6 g, fat 0.4 g, carbohydrate 17.5 g (0.8 g sugars, 16.2 g starch), dietary fibre 3.3 g, nsp 1.9 g, Na 12 mg, K 220 mg, Ca 16 mg, Mg 26 mg, P 100 mg, Fe 2.4 mg, Cu 0.19 mg, Zn 1 mg, Se 2 μg, vitamin A 3 μg (20 μg carotene), B_1 0.11 mg, B_2 0.04 mg, niacin 1.4 mg, B_6 0.11 mg, folate 5 μg, pantothenate 0.3 mg. A 120 g serving is a source of protein, Mg; good source of Fe, Cu.

leptin A peptide hormone synthesised in adipose tissue which acts to regulate appetite. Its crystal structure suggests that it is a member of the CYTOKINE family. The *ob* gene (defective in the *ob/ob* genetically obese mouse) codes for leptin; the *db* gene (defective in the *db/db* genetically obese diabetic mice) codes for the hypothalamic leptin receptor.

lettuce Leaves of the plant *Lactuca sativa*; many varieties are grown commercially.

Composition/100 g: 58 kJ (14 kcal), protein 0.8 g, fat 0.5 g, carbohydrate 1.7 g (1.7 g sugars), dietary fibre 1.3 g, nsp 0.9 g, Na 3 mg, K 220 mg, Ca 28 mg, Mg 6 mg, P 28 mg, Fe 0.7 mg, Cu 0.01 mg, Zn 0.2 mg, Se 1 μg, I 2 μg, vitamin A 59 μg (355 μg carotene), E 0.6 mg, B_1 0.12 mg, B_2 0.02 mg, niacin 0.5 mg, B_6 0.04 mg, folate 55 μg, pantothenate 0.2 mg, biotin 0.7 μg, C 5 mg. Serving 20 g.

leucine An essential AMINO ACID; rarely limiting in foods; abbr Leu (L), M_r 131.2, pK_a 2.33, 9.74, CODONS UUPu, CUNu. Chemically, amino-isocaproic acid.

leucocytes White blood cells, normally 5000–9000/mL; includes polymorphonuclear neutrophils, lymphocytes, monocytes, polymorphonuclear eosinophils and polymorphonuclear basophils. A 'white cell count' determines the total; a differential cell count estimates the numbers of each type. Fever, haemorrhage and violent exercise cause an increase (leucocytosis); starvation and debilitating conditions a decrease (leucopenia).

leucocytosis Increase in the number of LEUCOCYTES in the blood.

leucopenia Decrease in the number of LEUCOCYTES in the blood.

leucosin One of the water-soluble proteins of wheat flour.

leucovorin See FOLINIC ACID.

levans Polymers of FRUCTOSE (the principal one is INULIN) that occur in tubers and some grasses.

levitin One of the proteins of egg yolk; about 20% of the total, the remainder being vitellin. Rich in sulphur, accounting for half of the sulphur in the yolk.

Lieberkühn, crypts of Glands lining the small intestine which secrete the intestinal juice.

Liebermann–Burchard reaction Colorimetric reaction for CHOLESTEROL; the development of a blue colour on reaction with acetic anhydride and sulphuric acid.

light (or lite) As applied to foods usually indicates:

(1) a lower content of fat compared with the standard product (e.g. BREADSPREADS, sausages).

(2) Sodium chloride substitutes lower in SODIUM (see SALT, LIGHT).

(3) Low-alcohol BEER or WINE.

US legislation restricts the term light to modified foods that contain one-third less energy or half the fat of a reference unmodified food, or that the sodium content of a low-fat, low-calorie food has been reduced by half.

See also FAT FREE; FREE FROM; LOW IN; REDUCED.

lights Butchers' term for the lungs of an animal.

lignin (lignocellulose) A polymer of aromatic alcohols, in plant cell walls; included in measurement of DIETARY FIBRE, but not of NON-STARCH POLYSACCHARIDE.

limb fat area Cross-sectional area of arm or leg fat, calculated from SKINFOLD THICKNESS and limb circumference, as an index of total body fat.

See also ANTHROPOMETRY.

lime The fruit of *Citrus aurantifolia*, cultivated almost solely in the tropics, since it is not as hardy as other CITRUS fruits. Used to prevent scurvy in the British Navy (replacing, at the time, lemon juice) and so giving rise to the nickname of 'Limeys' for British sailors and for British people in general.

Composition/100 g: 25 kJ (6 kcal), protein 0.5 g, fat 0.2 g, carbohydrate 0.6 g (0.6 g sugars), Na 1 mg, K 96 mg, Ca 17 mg, Mg 8 mg, P 13 mg, Fe 0.3 mg, Cu 0.04 mg, Zn 0.1 mg, vitamin A 1 µg (9 µg carotene), B_1 0.02 mg, B_2 0.01 mg, niacin 0.2 mg, B_6 0.06 mg, folate 6 µg, pantothenate 0.2 mg, C 34 mg. A 60 g serving is a rich source of vitamin C.

limit dextrin See DEXTRINS.

Limmisax Trade name for SACCHARIN.

Limmits Trade name for a 'slimming' preparation composed of wholemeal biscuits with a methyl cellulose mixture as filling, containing some vitamins and minerals; intended as a meal replacement.

limonin The bitter principle in the albedo of the Valencia orange. Isolimonin in the navel orange. Both are present as a non-bitter precursor which is liberated into the juice during extraction and is slowly hydrolysed, making the juice bitter.

limosis Abnormal hunger or excessive desire for food.

linamarin Cyanogenic (CYANOGENIC GLYCOSIDES) GLUCOSIDE found in CASSAVA (manioc) which may be a cause of neuropathies in areas where cassava is major food; the cyanide is removed in traditional processing by grating and exposing to air.

linguini See PASTA.

linoleic acid An essential polyunsaturated FATTY ACID (C18:2 ω6), predominant in most edible vegetable oils.

α-linolenic acid An essential polyunsaturated FATTY ACID (C18:3 ω3).

γ-linolenic acid A non-essential polyunsaturated FATTY ACID (C18:3 ω6) which has some pharmacological actions. Found in oils from the seeds of evening primrose, borage and blackcurrant.

linseed oil Vegetable oil from the seeds of flax, *Linum usitatissimum*; rich in LINOLEIC ACID.

liothyronine Alternative name for the THYROID HORMONE tri-iodothyronine (T3).

lipaemia Increase in blood lipids, as occurs normally after a meal.

lipase Enzyme (EC 3.1.1.x) that hydrolyses triacylglycerols to free fatty acids and 2-mono-acylglycerol. Lipase secreted by the tongue and in gastric and pancreatic juice is EC 3.1.1.3; lipases are also present in many seeds and grains. Final hydrolysis to yield glycerol is catalysed by acylglycerol lipase (EC 3.1.1.23).

Most lipases have low specificity and will hydrolyse any triacylglycerol. Sometimes responsible for the development of (hydrolytic) RANCIDITY in stored foods, and the development of flavour in cheese.

See also ACID NUMBER; INTERESTERIFICATION.

Hormone-sensitive lipase in ADIPOSE TISSUE is activated by hormones such as GLUCAGON and ADRENALINE, which are secreted when there is a need for the release of free fatty acids as a metabolic fuel.

Lipoprotein lipase (EC 3.1.1.34, also known as clearing factor lipase) in muscle and adipose tissue is responsible for the uptake of free fatty acids from triacylglycerols in LIPOPROTEINS.

lipectomy Surgical removal of subcutaneous fat.

lipidema Condition in which fat deposits accumulate in the lower extremities, from hips to ankles, with tenderness of the affected parts.

lipids (Also sometimes lipides, lipins.) A general term for fats and oils (chemically TRIACYLGLYCEROLS), WAXES, PHOSPHOLIPIDS, steroids and terpenes. Their common property is insolubility in water and solubility in hydrocarbons, chloroform and alcohols. Fats are solid at room temperature, while oils are liquids.

Non-saponifiable lipids are not hydrolysed by treatment with sodium or potassium hydroxide and therefore cannot be extracted into an aqueous medium: CHOLESTEROL and other sterols, SQUALENE, CAROTENOIDS and VITAMINS A, D, E and K. The saponifiable lipids are triacylglycerols (and mono- and diacylglycerols) and phospholipids, which can be extracted into an aqueous medium after alkaline hydrolysis (saponification).

lipids, plasma See LIPOPROTEINS, PLASMA.

lipochromes Plant pigments soluble in lipids and organic solvents, e.g. chlorophyll, carotenoids.

lipodystrophy Abnormality in the metabolism or deposition of fats; abnormal pattern of subcutaneous fat deposits.

lipofuscin A group of pigments that accumulate in several body tissues, particularly the myocardium, during life and are consequently associated with the ageing process.

lipoic acid 1,2-Dithiolane-3-valeric acid (6,8-thioctic acid), co-enzyme in the oxidative decarboxylation of pyruvate, α-ketoglutarate and branched-chain keto-acids. Not a dietary essential.

lipolysis Hydrolysis of triacylglycerols to mono- and diacylglycerols, glycerol and free fatty acids, catalysed by LIPASE.

lipolytic rancidity Spoilage of foods as a result of HYDROLYSIS (see HYDROLYSE) of fats to free fatty acids on storage (by the action of LIPASE, either bacterial lipase or the enzyme naturally present in the food). Since the enzyme is inactivated by heat, occurs only in uncooked foods.

See also ACID NUMBER.

lipoprotein [a] (Lp[a]) Complex of low-density lipoprotein in which an additional protein, apo-a, is bound to apo-protein B-100 by a disulphide bridge. It is genetically determined and there is a strong association between Lp[a] and coronary artery disease.

lipoproteins, plasma Lipids, encased in protein, in the blood plasma.

Chylomicrons are assembled in the intestinal mucosa, and contain the products of digestion of dietary fat. They are absorbed into the lymphatic circulation, and enter the bloodstream at the thoracic duct. Triacylglycerol is hydrolysed by lipoprotein LIPASE in adipose tissue and muscle, and the chylomicron remnants are cleared by the liver.

Very low-density lipoproteins are secreted by the liver, containing mainly newly synthesised triacylglycerol and cholesterol; hydrolysis by lipoprotein LIPASE in muscle and adipose tissue yields progressively intermediate density and then low-density lipoprotein (LDL). LDL is normally cleared by the liver, but oxidative damage may prevent uptake by the liver, when macrophages scavenge LDL, leading to the formation of foam cells and the development of atherosclerotic plaque.

High-density lipoprotein is secreted by the liver as the apo-protein, and accumulates cholesterol from tissues, which is normally transferred to LDL for clearance by the liver.

liposis See ADIPOSIS.

liposuction Procedure for removal of subcutaneous adipose tissue in obese people using a tube inserted through the skin at different locations.

lipovitellenin A lipoprotein complex in egg comprising about one-sixth of the solids of the yolk.

lipoxygenase Enzyme (EC 1.13.11.12) that catalyses the oxidation of polyunsaturated FATTY ACIDS to *trans*-hydroperoxides (an intermediate step in PROSTAGLANDIN synthesis); in plant oils may be important in the development of oxidative RANCIDITY. Lipoxygenase from soya or fava bean flour is used in breadmaking to improve mixing tolerance and dough stability; it also bleaches carotenoids and other lipid pigments in the flour.

liquefied herring HERRING reduced to liquid state by enzyme action at slightly acid pH; used as protein concentrate for animal feed.

liqueurs Distilled, flavoured and sweetened alcoholic liquors, 20–40% alcohol by volume.

liquid oleo See PREMIER JUS.

liquid paraffin See MEDICINAL PARAFFIN.

liquorice Used in confectionery and to flavour medicines; liquorice root and extract are obtained from the plant *Glycyrrhiza glabra*; stick liquorice is the crude evaporated extract of the root. The plant has been grown in the Pontefract district of Yorkshire since the sixteenth century; hence the name Pontefract cakes for the sugar confection of liquorice.

See also GLYCYRRHIZIN.

Listeria A genus of bacteria commonly found in soil of which the commonest is *Listeria monocytogenes*. They can cause FOOD POISONING (listeriosis). *Listeria* spp are especially found in unwashed vegetables and some soft cheeses; they resist cold and the presence of salt and can multiply in a refrigerator. Symptoms of listeriosis are flu-like, with high fever and dizziness. Pregnant women, babies and the elderly are especially at risk. *L. monocytogenes* causes systemic infection; minimum infective dose not known; onset within days, duration weeks.

litchi See LYCHEE.

lite See LIGHT.

lithium Metal not known to have any physiological function, although it occurs in food and water; lithium salts are used in the treatment of manic-depressive illness.

lithocholic acid One of the secondary BILE SALTS, formed by intestinal bacterial metabolism of CHENODEOXYCHOLIC ACID.

liver Usually from calf, pig, ox, lamb, chicken, duck or goose.

Composition/100 g: 565–750 kJ (135–180 kcal), protein 19–21 g, fat 6.3–10.3 g (37–46% saturated, 23–38% mono-, 24–30% polyunsaturated), cholesterol 260–430 mg, carbohydrate 0.6–2.2 g (2.2 g starch), Na 76–93 mg, K 290–330 mg, Ca 6–8 mg, Mg 19–21 mg, P 320–370 mg, Fe 7–21 mg, Cu 0.5–11 mg, Zn 3.4–7.8 mg, Sc 28 µg, I 13 µg, vitamin A 11 000–30 000 µg (1540 µg carotene), D 0.2–1.1 µg, E 0.2–0.5 mg, B_1 0.21–0.36 mg, B_2 2.7–3.3 mg, niacin 14–19 mg, B_6 0.4–0.8 mg, folate 110–590 µg, B_{12} 25–110 µg, pantothenate 6–8 mg, biotin 25–210 µg, C 10–23 mg. A 100 g serving is a good source of vitamin D, B_1; rich source of protein, vitamin A, B_2, niacin, B_6, folate, B_{12}, biotin, pantothenate, C, Fe, Cu, Se, Zn.

The vitamin A content of liver is high enough for it to pose a possible hazard to unborn children, and pregnant women have been advised not to eat liver. See VITAMIN A TOXICITY.

Fish liver is a particularly rich source of vitamins A and D, and fish liver oils (especially cod and halibut) are used as sources of these vitamins as nutritional supplements.

livetin A water-soluble protein fraction of egg yolk.

lobster Crustacean, *Homarus vulgaris*.

Composition/100 g: 175 kJ (42 kcal), protein 7.9 g, fat 1.2 g, cholesterol 43 mg, carbohydrate 0 g, Na 120 mg, K 93 mg, Ca 22 mg, Mg 12 mg, P 100 mg, Fe 0.3 mg, Cu 0.65 mg, Zn 0.6 mg, vitamin E 0.5 mg, B_1 0.03 mg, B_2 0.02 mg, niacin 2 mg, folate 6 µg, pantothenate 0.6 mg, biotin 2 µg. A 250 g serving ($^1/_4$ dressed lobster) a source of vitamin E, Mg, Zn; good source of niacin, pantothenate; rich source of protein, Cu.

lobster, rock or spiny See CRAWFISH.

Locasol Trade name for a low-calcium milk substitute.

locksoy Chinese fine-drawn rice macaroni.

locoweed *Astralagus* and *Oxytropus* spp common in arid areas of western USA. Toxic to cattle, causing locoism: neurological damage, abortion and birth defects. Apparently caused by an alkaloid, swainsonine, which is also found in mouldy hay.

locust bean (1) CAROB seed. (2) African locust bean, *Parkia* spp.

Loeb membrane. Thin layer of membrane used in reverse OSMOSIS, supported on thicker layer of porous support material.

Lofenalac Trade name for food low in PHENYLALANINE for treatment of PHENYLKETONURIA.

loganberry Cross between European raspberry and Californian blackberry, *Rubus ursinus* var *loganobaccus*, named after LH Logan.

Composition/100 g: 71 kJ (17 kcal), protein 1.1 g, fat 0 g, carbohydrate 3.4 g (3.4 g sugars), dietary fibre 5.6 g, nsp 2.5 g, Na 3 mg, K 260 mg, Ca 35 mg, Mg 25 mg, P 24 mg, Fe 1.4 mg, Cu 0.14 mg, Zn 0.3 mg, vitamin A 1 µg (6 µg carotene), E 0.5 mg, B_1 0.03 mg, B_2 0.05 mg, niacin 0.7 mg, B_6 0.06 mg, folate 33 µg, pantothenate 0.2 mg, biotin 1.9 µg, C 35 mg. An 80 g serving is a source of folate, Cu; rich source of vitamin C.

logarithmic phase The most rapid period of bacterial growth, when the numbers increase in geometric progression. Under ideal conditions bacteria can double in number every 20 min.

Lonalac Trade name for a milk preparation free from SODIUM.

London broil American name for steak, broiled or grilled and sliced thinly against the grain.

loonzein Rice from which the husk has been removed; also known as brown rice, hulled rice and cargo rice.

loperamide See ANTIDIARRHOEAL AGENTS; ANTIMOTILITY AGENTS.

loquat The small pear-shaped fruit of *Eriobotyra japonica*, a member of the apple family, also known as Japanese medlar or plum.

Composition/100 g: 117 kJ (28 kcal), protein 0.7 g, fat 0.2 g, carbohydrate 6.3 g (6.3 g sugars), Na 1 mg, K 220 mg, Ca 20 mg, Mg 10 mg, P 22 mg, Fe 0.4 mg, Cu 0.04 mg, Zn 0.2 mg, vitamin A 85 μg (515 μg carotene), B_1 0.02 mg, B_2 0.03 mg, niacin 0.2 mg, C 3 mg. A 100 g serving is a source of vitamin A.

lotus The sacred lotus of India and China, *Nelumbium nuciferum*, a water plant whose rhizomes and seeds are eaten.

lovage Herb of the carrot family, *Ligusticum scoticum*, with a strong musky scent of celery. The stems can be candied like ANGELICA or used as a vegetable, and the leaves and stems are used in soup. The seeds can also be used as a seasoning, with a flavour like dill or fennel seed.

lovastatin See STATINS.

love apple Old name for TOMATO.

low birth weight Infants born weighing significantly less than normal (2.5–4.5 kg) are considered to be premature; their chances of survival and normal development are considerably improved if they are fed special formula preparations to meet their needs, rather than being breast fed or fed normal infant formula.

low in EU legislation states that for a food label or advertising to bear a claim that it is low in fat, saturates, cholesterol, sodium or alcohol, it must provide less than half of the amount of the specified nutrient of a reference product for which no claim is made. US legislation sets precise levels at which claims may be made.

Lowry reaction Sensitive technique for colorimetric determination of protein using the Folin–Cioucalteau tungstate, molybdate, phosphate reagent, which reacts with tyrosine in proteins. Sensitivity 1 ng/mL, maximum absorbance 660 nm.

lox American (originally Yiddish) name for smoked salmon; See also LAX.

lozenges Shapes stamped out of mixture of icing sugar, glucose syrup and gum arabic or gelatine with flavourings, then hardened at 32–43°C.

LRNI Lower reference nutrient intake; see REFERENCE INTAKES.

LSM Trade name (USA) for a low-sodium milk containing 50 mg/L; ordinary milk contains 500 mg/L.

lucerne See ALFALFA.

Luff–Schoorl method For determination of starch and sugars. Sugars are extracted using ethanol, then starch is hydrolysed using hydrochloric acid and the resultant glucose is extracted after neutralisation. Sugars are determined in the extracts after oxidation using copper reagent, linked to the reduction of potassium iodide to iodine, and titration of iodine with sodium thiosulphate.

lumichrome Product of ultraviolet irradiation of riboflavin (VITAMIN B$_2$) in neutral solution; some is formed *in vivo* on exposure to sunlight and is excreted in the urine. May also arise as a result of intestinal bacterial metabolism of riboflavin. Formed in milk on exposure to sunlight.

See also LUMIFLAVIN; SUNLIGHT FLAVOUR.

lumiflavin Product of ultraviolet irradiation of riboflavin (VITAMIN B$_2$) in alkaline solution; soluble in chloroform, and provides the basis of a fluorimetric assay for the vitamin.

See also LUMICHROME.

lumpfish Large sea fish, *Cylopterus lumpus*, the eggs of which are salted, pressed and coloured, as Danish or German CAVIARE.

luncheon meat Precooked, canned meat, usually pork.

lupeose See STACHYOSE.

lupins Legumes of *Lupinus* spp. The ordinary garden lupin contains toxic quinolizidine alkaloids and tastes bitter; varieties selected for animal feed and grain crop, low in alkaloids are known as sweet lupins; rich in protein and fat.

lupulones Aromatic acids in HOPS. See HUMULONES.

lutein (or luteol) Alternative names for XANTHOPHYLL.

luteotrophin (luteotrophic hormone) See PROLACTIN.

luxus konsumption See DIET-INDUCED THERMOGENESIS.

Lycasin Trade name for hydrogenated glucose syrup, a bulk SWEETENER.

lychee (litchi) The fruit of *Litchi chinensis*, native of China; the size of a small plum, with a hard case and translucent white jelly-like sweet flesh surrounding the seed.

Composition/100 g: 150 kJ (36 kcal), protein 0.5 g, fat 0.1 g, carbohydrate 8.9 g (8.9 g sugars), dietary fibre 0.9 g, nsp 0.4 g, Na 1 mg, K 99 mg, Ca 4 mg, Mg 6 mg, P 19 mg, Fe 0.3 mg, Cu 0.09 mg, Zn 0.2 mg, vitamin B$_1$ 0.02 mg, B$_2$ 0.04 mg, niacin 0.3 mg, C 28 mg. A 95 g serving (four fruits) is a source of Cu; rich source of vitamin C.

lycopene A CAROTENOID, not VITAMIN A active, found especially in TOMATOES. It does not have a characteristic ionone ring, both rings are open. Epidemiological evidence suggests that it may be associated with lower incidence of cardiovascular disease and cancer of the prostate and gastrointestinal tract. Sometimes used as a food colour (E-160d).

lye-peeling A method of removing skins from vegetables by immersion in hot caustic soda solution (lye) followed by tumbling in a wash to remove the skin and chemicals.

lymph The fluid between blood and the tissues; the medium in which oxygen and nutrients are conveyed from the blood to the tissues, and waste products back to the blood. Similar to BLOOD PLASMA in composition. Dietary fat is absorbed into the lacteals (lymphatic vessels of the intestinal villi) as chylomicrons which are formed in the intestinal mucosa, and enters the bloodstream at the thoracic duct. After a fatty meal the lymph is rich in emulsified fat and is called chyle.

lymphatics Vessels through which the LYMPH flows, draining from the tissues and entering the bloodstream at the thoracic duct.

lymphocytes See LEUCOCYTES.

lymphokine See CYTOKINE.

lyophilisation See FREEZE DRYING.

lysergic acid The toxin of ERGOT.

lysine An essential AMINO ACID, abbr Lys (K), M_r 146.2, pK_a 2.16, 9.18, 10.79, CODONS AAPu. Of nutritional importance, since it is the limiting AMINO ACID in many cereals.

lysinoalanine An amino acid formed when proteins are heated or treated with alkali by reaction between ε-amino group of lysine and dehydroalanine formed from cysteine or serine. Present in many foods at about 1000 ppm. Although high doses cause kidney tubule lesions (nephrocytomegaly) in rats, it is not considered hazardous to health.

lysozyme An enzyme (EC 3.2.1.17) that hydrolyses some high molecular weight carbohydrates of bacterial cell walls, and so lyses bacteria. Widely distributed (e.g. in tears); egg-white is especially rich.

lyxoflavin An analogue of RIBOFLAVIN isolated from human heart muscle, containing the sugar lyxose; its function is unknown.

lyxulose See XYLULOSE.

M

MA Modified atmosphere. See GAS STORAGE, CONTROLLED.

maatjes Dutch; cured HERRING made only from young female herrings.

macadamia nut Or Queensland nuts, fruit of *Macadamia ternifolia*.

Composition/100 g: 3131 kJ (748 kcal), protein 7.9 g, fat 77.6 g

(15.2% saturated, 82.6% mono-, 2.1% polyunsaturated), carbohydrate 4.8 g (4 g sugars, 0.8 g starch), nsp 5.3 g, K 300 mg, Ca 47 mg, Mg 100 mg, P 200 mg, Fe 1.6 mg, Cu 0.43 mg, Zn 1.1 mg, Se 7 μg, vitamin E 1.5 mg, B_1 0.28 mg, B_2 0.06 mg, niacin 3.3 mg, B_6 0.28 mg, pantothenate 0.6 mg, biotin 6 μg. Serving 10 g (six nuts).

macaroni, maccaroncelli   See PASTA.

macassar gum   See AGAR.

mace   See NUTMEG.

macedoine   Mixture of fruits or vegetables, diced, or cut into small even-shaped pieces.

macerases   A group of enzymes (usually extracted from the mould *Aspergillus*) used to break down PECTIN in fruits to facilitate maximum extraction of the juice.

mackerel   An oily FISH, *Scomber scombrus*.
Composition/100 g: 920 kJ (220 kcal), protein 18.7 g, fat 16.1 g (22.7% saturated, 54.4% mono-, 22.7% polyunsaturated), cholesterol 54 mg, carbohydrate 0 g, Na 63 mg, K 290 mg, Ca 11 mg, Mg 24 mg, P 200 mg, Fe 0.8 mg, Cu 0.08 mg, Zn 0.6 mg, Se 30 μg, I 140 μg, vitamin A 45 μg, D 5 μg, E 0.4 mg, B_1 0.14 mg, B_2 0.29 mg, niacin 12.1 mg, B_6 0.41 mg, B_{12} 8 μg, pantothenate 0.8 mg, biotin 5 μg. A 160 g serving is a source of vitamin B_1, Mg, Cu; good source of vitamin B_2, pantothenate; rich source of protein, vitamin D, niacin, B_6, B_{12}, I, Se.

macon   'BACON' made from mutton.

maconochie   A canned meat stew much used in the first World War; made by Maconochie Brothers.

macrobiotic diet   A system of eating associated with Zen Buddhism; consists of several stages finally reaching Diet 7 which is restricted to cereals. Cases of severe malnutrition have been reported on this diet. Based loosely on the Buddhist concept of *yin* and *yang* whereby foods (and indeed everything in life) are predominantly one or the other and must be balanced.

macrocytes   Large immature precursors of red BLOOD CELLS found in the circulation in PERNICIOUS ANAEMIA and in FOLIC ACID deficiency, due to impairment of the normal maturation of red cells; hence macrocytic ANAEMIA.

macrogols   Polyethylene glycols used as osmotic LAXATIVES.

mad cow disease   Bovine spongiform encephalopathy, see BSE.

Madeira nuts   See WALNUTS.

Madeira wines   Fortified wines from the island of Madeira: sercial (dry); verdelho (semi-dry); bual (semi-sweet); malmsey (sweet).

magma   Mixture of sugar syrup and sugar crystals produced during sugar refining.

magnesium   An essential mineral; present in all human tissues, especially bone. Involved in the metabolism of ATP. Present in chlorophyll and so in all green plant foods, and therefore generally plentiful in the diet. Deficiency in human beings leads to disturbances of muscle and nervous system; in cattle, grass tetany. Magnesium-deficient plants are yellow (chlorosed).

Magnesium salts (especially the sulphate) are used as osmotic LAXATIVES because they are poorly absorbed from the small intestine; magnesium carbonate and hydroxide are used as ANTACIDS and LAXATIVES; magnesium hydroxide is milk of magnesia, magnesium sulphate is Epsom salts (also used as a laxative) and magnesium trisilicate is used in the treatment of peptic ULCERS.

magnum Double size wine BOTTLE, 1.5 L.

mahleb Spice prepared from black cherry kernels, Syrian in origin, widely used in Greek baked goods.

maids of honour Small tartlets filled with almond-flavoured custard; said to have originated in the court of Henry VIII, where they were made by Ann Boleyn when she was lady-in-waiting to Catherine of Aragon.

Maillard reaction Non-enzymic reaction between LYSINE in proteins and reducing sugars leading to a brown colour. A similar reaction occurs in the GLYCATION of proteins in DIABETES mellitus.

The first step in the reaction is the formation of a Schiff base (aldimine) between the aldehyde group of the sugar and the ε-amino group of lysine, followed by isomerisation (Amadori rearrangement). May also occur with other amino acids at the amino terminal of a protein.

It takes place on heating or prolonged storage and is one of the deteriorative processes that take place in stored foods. It is accompanied by a loss in nutritive value, since the amino acid that reacts with the sugar is not available.

See also AVAILABILITY; AVAILABLE LYSINE.

maître d'hôtel (1) Simply prepared dishes garnished with butter creamed with parsley and lemon juice (maître d'hôtel butter); literally *in the style of the chief steward*.

(2) Especially in USA, the head waiter.

maize Grain of *Zea mays*, also called Indian corn and (in US) simply corn. Staple food in many countries, made into TORTILLAS in Latin America, POLENTA in Italy, and flaked as corn flakes breakfast cereal; various preparations in the southern states of the USA are known as hominy, samp and cerealine.

Two varieties of major commercial importance are flint corn (*Zea mays indurata*), which is very hard, and dent corn (*Z. mays dentata*); there is also sweet corn *Z. mays saccharata*, and a variety that expands on heating (*Zea mays everta*, see POPCORN).

The starch prepared from *Z. mays dentata* is termed cornflour;

the ground maize is termed maize meal. There is a white variety; the usual yellow colour is partly due to cryptoxanthin (a vitamin A precursor). Because of its low content of the amino acid TRYP-TOPHAN (and available NIACIN), diets based largely on maize are associated with the development of PELLAGRA.

Composition/100 g (sweetcorn): 276 kJ (66 kcal), protein 2.5 g, fat 1.4 g, carbohydrate 11.6 g (1.4 g sugars, 10 g starch), dietary fibre 2.5 g, nsp 1.3 g, Na 1 mg, K 140 mg, Ca 2 mg, Mg 20 mg, P 48 mg, Fe 0.3 mg, Cu 0.02 mg, Zn 0.2 mg, vitamin A 11 µg (71 µg carotene), E 0.5 mg, B_1 0.11 mg, B_2 0.03 mg, niacin 1.5 mg, B_6 0.09 mg, folate 20 µg, pantothenate 0.4 mg, C 4 mg. A 210 g serving (one cob) is a source of protein, vitamin E, B_1, niacin, pan-tothenate, C, Mg; a good source of folate.

maize, flaked Partly gelatinised maize used for animal feed. The grain is cracked to small pieces, moistened, cooked and flaked between rollers.

maize flour Highly refined and very finely ground maize meal from which all bran and germ have been removed.

maize oil See CORN OIL.

maize rice Finely cut MAIZE with bran and germ partly removed, also called mealie rice.

maize starch, waxy STARCH obtained from hybrids of MAIZE con-sisting wholly or largely (99%) of AMYLOPECTIN, compared with ordinary maize starch with 26% AMYLOSE and 74% amylopectin. The paste is semi-translucent, cohesive and does not form a gel.

malabsorption syndrome Defect of absorption of one or more nutrients; signs include diarrhoea, STEATORRHOEA, abdominal dis-tension, weight loss and specific signs of nutrient deficiency.

malacia Abnormal softening of tissue or organ. See KERATOMA-LACIA; OSTEOMALACIA.

malai Indian; cream prepared by boiling milk, leaving it to cool and then skimming off the clotted cream.

malic acid Dicarboxylic acid ($COOH-CHOH-CH_2-COOH$), a metabolic intermediate occurring in many fruits, particularly in apples, tomatoes and plums. Used as a food additive to increase acidity (E-296).

mallorising PASTEURISATION at high temperatures (up to 130°C).

malmsey See MADEIRA WINES.

malnutrition Disturbance of form or function arising from deficiency or excess of one or more nutrients.

See also CACHEXIA; OBESITY; PROTEIN–ENERGY MALNUTRITION; VITAMIN TOXICITY (various).

malolactic fermentation The conversion of the malic acid in grape juice (and other fruit juices) into lactic acid, especially in red wines and CIDER as they mellow and become less acidic.

malpighia See CHERRY, WEST INDIAN.

malt, malt extract Mixture of starch breakdown products containing mainly MALTOSE (malt sugar), prepared from barley or wheat. The grain is allowed to sprout, when the enzyme diastase (AMYLASE) develops and HYDROLYSES the starch to maltose. The mixture is then extracted with hot water, and this malt extract contains a solution of starch breakdown products together with diastase. Malt extract may be the concentrated solution or evaporated to dryness.

maltase Enzyme (EC 3.2.1.20) that hydrolyses MALTOSE.

malt flour Germinated barley or wheat, in dried form. As well as dextrins, glucose, proteins and salts derived from the cereal, it is rich in diastase and is added to wheat flour of low DIASTATIC ACTIVITY for breadmaking; used as an ingredient of malt loaf.

malt sugar See MALTOSE.

Malthus TR Malthus (1766–1835), author of an essay in 1798 postulating that any temporary or local improvement in living conditions will increase population faster than the food supply, and that disasters such as war and pestilence, which check population growth, are inescapable features of human society.

maltin, maltodextrin See DEXTROSE EQUIVALENT VALUE.

maltitol A SUGAR ALCOHOL produced by hydrogenation of maltose. Slowly hydrolysed in the digestive tract to GLUCOSE and SORBITOL and fairly completely utilised, providing 16 kJ (4 kcal)/g; sweeter than maltose, and 90% as sweet as sucrose (E-965).

maltobiose See MALTOSE.

maltol Also called laxarinic acid, palatone, veltol; chemically 3-hydroxy 2-methyl-γ-pyrone. Found in the bark of young larch trees, pine needles, chicory and roasted malt; synthesised for use as a fragrant, caramel-like flavour for addition to foods; imparts a 'freshly baked' flavour to bread and cakes.

maltonic acid See GLUCONIC ACID.

maltose Malt sugar, or maltobiose, a DISACCHARIDE, α-1,4-glucosyl-glucose. Hydrolysed by MALTASE. Does not occur in foods (unless specifically added as MALT) but formed during the acid or enzymic hydrolysis of starch. 33% as sweet as sucrose.

maltose figure See DIASTATIC ACTIVITY.

maltose intolerance See DISACCHARIDE INTOLERANCE.

mandarin Loose-skinned CITRUS fruit, *Citrus reticulata* or *C. nobilio*. Varieties include satsumas and tangerines (although all three names are used indiscriminately) with various hybrids including tangelo, tangor, temple, clementine.

manganese An essential trace mineral which functions as the PROSTHETIC GROUP in a number of enzymes. Dietary deficiency has not been reported in man; in experimental animals manganese deficiency leads to impaired synthesis of MUCOPOLYSACCHARIDES. Requirements are not known; intakes greater than 1.4 mg/day are considered SAFE AND ADEQUATE.

mangelwurzel, mangoldwurzel   A root vegetable used as cattle feed, *Beta vulgaris rapa*; a cross between red and white BEETROOT.

mange tout   See PEA, MANGE TOUT.

mango   A fruit, originally of Indo-Burmese origin and now grown widely throughout the tropics, *Mangifera indica*. The fruit is ovoid, with orange-coloured sweet aromatic flesh surrounding a central stone.

Composition/100 g: 163 kJ (39 kcal), protein 0.5 g, fat 0.1 g, carbohydrate 9.6 g (9.4 g sugars, 0.2 g starch), dietary fibre 2 g, nsp 1.8 g, Na 1 mg, K 120 mg, Ca 8 mg, Mg 9 mg, P 11 mg, Fe 0.5 mg, Cu 0.08 mg, Zn 0.1 mg, vitamin A 204 µg (1225 µg carotene), E 0.7 mg, B_1 0.03 mg, B_2 0.03 mg, niacin 0.4 mg, B_6 0.09 mg, pantothenate 0.1 mg, C 25 mg. A 110 g serving ($^1/_2$ fruit) is a source of Cu; good source of vitamin A; rich source of vitamin C.

mangosteen   Fruit of *Garcinea mangostana*, the size of an orange with thick purple rind and sweet white pulp in segments.

Composition/100 g: 305 kJ (73 kcal), protein 0.6 g, fat 0.5 g, carbohydrate 16.4 g (16.1 g sugars, 0.3 g starch), dietary fibre 1.3 g, Na 1 mg, K 130 mg, Ca 14 mg, P 14 mg, Fe 0.3 mg, vitamin B_1 0.05 mg, B_2 0.01 mg, niacin 0.4 mg, C 3 mg.

manihot starch   See CASSAVA.

manioc   See CASSAVA.

manna   Dried exudate from the manna-ash tamarisk tree (*Fraxinus ornus*). Abundant in Sicily and used as a mild laxative for children; it consists of 40–60% MANNITOL, 10–16% mannotetrose, 6–16% mannotriose, plus glucose, mucilage and fraxin. This is thought to be the food eaten by the children of Israel in the wilderness. Manna sugar or mannite is MANNITOL.

manna bread   A cake-like product made from crushed, sprouted wheat without yeast; said to be a recipe of the Essenes who lived by the Dead Sea around the beginning of the Christian era.

mannitol   Mannite or manna sugar, a six-carbon SUGAR ALCOHOL found in beets, pumpkin, mushrooms, onions; 50–60% as sweet as sucrose. Extracted commercially from seaweed (*Laminaria* spp) or by reduction of MANNOSE (E-421).

mannosans   POLYSACCHARIDES containing MANNOSE.

mannose   A six-carbon (hexose) sugar found in small amounts in legumes, MANNA and some gums. Also called seminose and carubinose.

mannotetrose   See STACHYOSE.

manothermosonication   Method of sterilisation using mild heat treatment combined with ultrasonication and moderately raised pressure.

Manucol Trade name for sodium ALGINATE.

maple syrup Sap of the north American sugar maple tree, *Acer saccharum*. Evaporated either to syrup (63% sucrose, 1.5% invert sugar) or to dry sugar for use in confectionery.

maple syrup urine disease A rare GENETIC DISEASE affecting catabolism of the branched-chain AMINO ACIDS LEUCINE, ISOLEUCINE and VALINE, due to deficiency of branched-chain keto-acid dehydrogenase (EC 1.2.4.4), leading to accumulation of high concentrations of these amino acids and their keto-acids in plasma and urine. The keto-acids give the urine a characteristic smell like that of maple syrup. If untreated leads to severe mental retardation and death in infancy.

marasmic kwashiorkor The most severe form of PROTEIN–ENERGY MALNUTRITION in children, with weight for height less than 60% of that expected and the oedema and other signs of KWASHIORKOR.

marasmus See PROTEIN–ENERGY MALNUTRITION.

marc French; spirit distilled from the fermented residue of grape skins, stalks and seeds after the grapes have been pressed for wine making. The same as grappa (Italian), bagaciera (Portugal) and aguardiente (Spain). Often a harsh raw spirit, drunk young, although some are matured and smooth.

margarine (butterine, lardine, oleomargarine) Emulsion of about 80% vegetable, animal and/or marine fats and 20% water, originally made as a substitute for butter. Usually contains emulsifiers, antispattering agents, colours, vitamins A and D (sometimes E) and preservatives.

Composition/100 g: 3097 kJ (740 kcal), protein 0.2 g, fat 81.6 g, cholesterol 7 mg, carbohydrate 1 g (1 g sugars), Na 800 mg, K 5 mg, Ca 4 mg, Mg 1 mg, P 12 mg, Fe 0.3 mg, Cu 0.04 mg, I 27 μg, vitamin A 900 μg (750 μg carotene), D 7.94 μg. A 15 g serving is a source of vitamin A; good source of vitamin D.

Ordinary margarines contain roughly equal proportions of saturated (see SATURATES), mono-unsaturated and poly-unsaturated fatty acids; special soft varieties are rich in POLY-UNSATURATES. Low-fat spreads are made with 20–60% fat and correspondingly higher contents of air and water and less energy.

Kosher and vegetarian margarines are made only from vegetable fats, because ordinary margarine can include animal fats. It is fortified with carotene (which is derived from vegetable sources) as the source of vitamin A, instead of retinol (which may be obtained from non-kosher sources).

marinade   Mixture of oil with wine, lemon juice or vinegar and herbs in which meat or fish is soaked before cooking, both to give flavour and to make it more tender. Hence to marinate.

marine biotoxins   Toxins in shellfish and marine fish, either produced naturally or accumulated by the fish from their diet (includes CIGUATERA and PARALYTIC SHELLFISH POISONING).

marine oils   See FISH OILS.

marjoram   Dried leaves of a number of aromatic plants of different species, used as seasoning. The most widely accepted marjoram herbs are the perennial bush *Origanum majorana* and the annual sweet marjoram *Majorana hortensis*. Spanish wild marjoram is *Thymus mastichina*.

Composition/100 g: 276 kJ (66 kcal), protein 2.2 g, fat 2 g, carbohydrate 9.7 g, Na 3 mg, K 330 mg, Ca 310 mg, Mg 53 mg, P 39 mg, Zn 0.9 mg, vitamin A 135 μg (810 μg carotene), B_1 0.07 mg, C 45 mg. Serving 5 g.

marmalade   Defined by EU Directive as JAM made from citrus peel; what was known as ginger marmalade is now known as ginger preserve. The name comes from the Portuguese *marmalada*, the quince, which was used to make preserves. Used in French and German to mean jam or preserve in general.

Composition/100 g: 1092 kJ (261 kcal), protein 0.1 g, fat 0 g, carbohydrate 69.5 g (69.5 g sugars), dietary fibre 0.6 g, nsp 0.6 g, Na 18 mg, K 44 mg, Ca 35 mg, Mg 4 mg, P 13 mg, Fe 0.6 mg, Cu 0.12 mg, Zn 0.2 mg, Se 1 μg, I 7 μg, vitamin A 8 μg (50 μg carotene), folate 5 μg, C 10 mg. Serving 15 g.

marmite   (1) The original form of pressure cooker used by Papin in 1681; it was an iron pot with a sealing lid.

(2) Cookery term for a stock, or the pot in which stock is prepared.

Marmite   Trade name for YEAST EXTRACT flavoured with vegetable extract.

marron glacé   Chestnuts preserved in syrup; semi-crystallised.

marrow   (1) Bone marrow; tissue within internal cavities of bones. Red marrow is the site of formation of red BLOOD CELLS. In infants almost all of the marrow is red, and is gradually replaced by fat (yellow marrow) in the limb bones.

(2) Varieties of the gourd *Cucurbita pepo*.

See also COURGETTE; SQUASHES; PUMPKIN.

Composition/100 g: 37 kJ (9 kcal), protein 0.4 g, fat 0.2 g, carbohydrate 1.6 g (1.4 g sugars, 0.2 g starch), dietary fibre 1 g, nsp 0.6 g, Na 1 mg, K 110 mg, Ca 14 mg, Mg 7 mg, P 18 mg, Fe 0.1 mg, Cu 0.01 mg, Zn 0.2 mg, vitamin A 18 μg (110 μg carotene), B_1 0.08 mg, niacin 0.3 mg, B_6 0.01 mg, folate 15 μg, pantothenate 0.1 mg, biotin 0.4 μg, C 3 mg. Serving 65 g.

marshmallow   Soft sweetmeat made from an aerated mixture of gelatine or egg albumin with sugar or starch syrup. NOUGAT is harder, containing less water, and usually incorporating dried fruit and nuts. Originally using the root of the marshmallow plant (*Althaea officinalis*), which contains a mucilaginous substance as well as starch and sugar.

Marumillon 50   Trade name for mixture of the sweet glycosides extracted from stevia leaves.
See also STEVIOSIDE; REBAUDIOSIDE.

marzipan   See ALMOND PASTE.

mascarpone   Italian; soft cream CHEESE from the Lombardy region.

mashing   In the brewing of BEER, the process in which the malted barley is heated with water, to extract the soluble sugars and to continue enzymic reactions started during malting.

mash tun   Vessel used for MASHING.

maslin, mashum   (1) Old term still used in Scotland, for mixed crop of beans and oats used as cattle food.
(2) In Yorkshire and N England, a mixed crop of 2–3 parts of wheat and 1 part of rye, used for making bread.

Mason jar   Screw-topped glass jar for home bottling; patented 1858.

massecuite   The mixture of sugar crystals and syrup (mother liquor) obtained during the crystallisation stage of sugar refining.

mast   See MILK, FERMENTED.

mastic (mastic gum)   Resin from the evergreen shrub *Pistacia lenticus* and related species, with a flavour similar to liquorice, used in Greek and Balkan cookery.

mastication   Chewing, grinding and tearing food with the teeth while it becomes mixed with saliva.

matai   Chinese water chestnut, see CHESTNUT.

maté   Also yerba maté, or Paraguay or Brazilian tea. Infusion of the dried leaves of *Ilex paraguayensis*.

matoké   Steamed green BANANA or PLANTAIN.

matrix Gla protein   See OSTEOCALCIN.

matsutake   Edible wild fungus, widely collected in Japan and exported canned or dried, *Tricholoma matsutake*, see MUSHROOMS.

Matzka process   A low-temperature sterilisation process used for fruit juices by adding silver salts; in the presence of silver ions the pasteurisation temperature is only 8–11°C. The KATADYN PROCESS employs silver ions alone.
See also OLIGODYNAMIC.

matzo, motza (matzoth is the plural)   Unleavened bread or Passover bread made as thin, flat, round or square water biscuits, and, according to the injunction in Exodus, eaten by Jews during the eight days of Passover in place of leavened bread.

Composition/100 g: 1607 kJ (384 kcal), protein 10.5 g, fat 1.9 g, carbohydrate 86.6 g (4.2 g sugars, 82.4 g starch), dietary fibre 3.5 g, nsp 3 g, Na 17 mg, K 150 mg, Ca 32 mg, Mg 20 mg, P 100 mg, Fe 1.5 mg, Cu 0.16 mg, Zn 0.7 mg, vitamin B_1 0.11 mg, B_2 0.03 mg, niacin 3.1 mg, B_6 0.06 mg. Serving 23 g (one large square).

maw   Fourth stomach of the ruminant.

mawseed   See POPPYSEED.

MaxEPA   Trade name for a standardised mixture of long-chain marine FATTY ACIDS, eicosapentaenoic (EPA, C20:5 ω3) and docosohexaenoic (DHA, C22:6 ω3) acids.

mayonnaise   See SALAD DRESSING.

maysin   Coagulable globulin protein of maize.

mazindol   Anorectic (appetite suppressing, see APPETITE CONTROL) drug used in the treatment of OBESITY.

mazun   See MILK, FERMENTED.

mazzard   See GEAN.

mcv   See MEAN CELL VOLUME.

mead   A traditional wine made by fermentation of honey, sometimes flavoured with herbs and spices. One of the most ancient of alcoholic drinks.

mealie pudding   See SKIRLIE.

mealie rice   See MAIZE RICE.

mealie(s)   See MAIZE.

mean cell volume (mcv)   Average size of red BLOOD CELLS, determined using an electronic counter, or calculated from the HAEMATOCRIT and red cell count/L of blood. Low values occur with severe iron deficiency (microcytic ANAEMIA) and high values in FOLIC ACID and VITAMIN B_{12} deficiency (megaloblastic anaemia).

meat   Generally refers to the muscle tissue of animal or bird, other parts being termed OFFAL. Legally defined in UK as all that is found between the skin and bone of the animal.

meat bar   Dehydrated cooked meat and fat; a modern form of PEMMICAN; 50% protein and 40% fat; provides 560 kcal (2350 kJ)/100 g.

meat conditioning   After an animal has been slaughtered, muscle glycogen breaks down and is metabolised to lactic acid, which tends to improve the texture and keeping qualities of the meat. Meat that has been left until these changes have occurred is 'conditioned'.

See also DFD MEAT; RIGOR MORTIS.

meat, curing   Pickling with the aid of sodium chloride (SALT), sodium nitrate (saltpetre) and some sodium nitrite, which permits the growth of only salt-tolerant bacteria and inhibits the growth of *Clostridium botulinum*. The nitrite is the effective preserving agent and the nitrate is converted into nitrite during the process. The red colour of cured meat is due to the formation of nitrosomyoglobin from MYOGLOBIN.

meat extender   Vegetable proteins added to meat products to replace part of the meat.

meat extract   The water-soluble part of meat that is mainly responsible for its flavour. Commercially is made during the manufacture of CORNED BEEF; chopped meat is immersed in boiling water, when the water-soluble extractives are partially leached out and concentrated. Rich in the B vitamins (particularly vitamins B_1, B_{12} and niacin), meat bases and potassium, and a potent stimulator of gastric secretion.

meat factor   Factor used to calculate the fat-free meat content of sausages and similar meat products from a NITROGEN estimation.

meat, reformed   An artefact having the appearance of a cut slice or portion of meat, formed by 'tumbling' chopped meat, with or without the addition of finely comminuted meat, the soluble proteins of which bind the small pieces together.

meat speciation   Identification of species of animal from which the meat originated.

meat sugar   Obsolete name for INOSITOL.

medicinal paraffin   Liquid paraffin, a mineral oil of no nutritive value since it is not affected by digestive enzymes and passes through the intestine unchanged. Used as a LAXATIVE because of its lubricant properties.

medlar   The fruit of *Mespilus germanica*. Can be eaten fresh from tree in Mediterranean areas but in colder climates, as Great Britain, does not become palatable until it is half rotten (bletted).
  Composition/100 g: 175 kJ (42 kcal), protein 0.5 g, fat 0 g, carbohydrate 10.6 g (10.6 g sugars), dietary fibre 9.2 g, Na 6 mg, K 250 mg, Ca 30 mg, Mg 11 mg, P 28 mg, Fe 0.5 mg, Cu 0.17 mg, vitamin niacin 0.1 mg, C 2 mg. A 60 g serving is a source of Cu.

medlar, Japanese   See LOQUAT.

Meeh formula   See BODY SURFACE AREA.

megaloblast   Abnormal form of any of the cells that are precursors of red BLOOD CELLS; they occur in bone MARROW in ANAEMIA due to deficiency of FOLIC ACID or VITAMIN B_{12}.

megavitamin therapy   Treatment of diseases with very high doses of vitamins, several hundred-fold higher than REFERENCE INTAKES. Little or no evidence of efficacy; VITAMINS A, D, B_6 and NIACIN are known to be toxic at high levels of intake.

mejing   See MONOSODIUM GLUTAMATE.

melaena   Tarry black faeces due to partly digested blood as a result of bleeding into the gut.

melalgia, nutritional   See BURNING FOOT SYNDROME.

melampyrin   See DULCITOL.

melangeur   Mixing vessel consisting of rollers riding on a rotating horizontal bed. Used to mix substances of pasty consistency (hence melangeuring).

melba   Peach poached in vanilla syrup, set in vanilla ice-cream with a purée of raspberries. Created by Escoffier, 1892, in honour of Dame Nellie Melba.

melegueta pepper   See PEPPER, MELEGUETA.

melezitose   Trisaccharide, glucosyl-glucosyl-fructose, hydrolysed to glucose plus the disaccharide turanose (α-1,3-glucosyl-fructose).

melibiose   *DISACCHARIDE, α-1,6-galactosyl-glucose.

melitose, melitriose   See RAFFINOSE.

mellorine   US term for ICE-CREAM made from non-butter fat.

melon   GOURDS, sweet fruit of *Cucumis melo*.

Composition/100 g (depending on variety): 54–79 kJ (13–19 kcal), protein 0.4 g, fat 0.1 g, carbohydrate 2.8–4.3 g (2.8–4.3 g sugars), dietary fibre 0.6 g, nsp 0.7 g, Na 5–21 mg, K 100–140 mg, Ca 6–13 mg, Mg 7–8 mg, Fe 0.1–0.2 mg, I 3 µg, vitamin A 5–110 µg (31–660 µg carotene), E 0.1 mg, B_1 0.03 mg, B_2 0.01 mg, niacin 0.4 mg, B_6 0.07 mg, folate 3 µg, pantothenate 0.1 mg, C 6–17 mg. A 230 g serving is a rich source of vitamin C, and may be a good source of vitamin A.

Melon seeds, Composition/100 g: 2440 kJ (583 kcal), protein 28.5 g, fat 47.7 g (25.8% saturated, 17.8% mono-, 56.3% polyun-saturated), carbohydrate 9.9 g, Na 99 mg, K 650 mg, Ca 71 mg, Mg 510 mg, P 690 mg, Fe 7.6 mg, Cu 2.39 mg, Zn 4 mg, vitamin B_1 0.17 mg, B_2 0.15 mg, niacin 11.8 mg, folate 58 µg. A 15 g serving is a good source of Mg; rich source of Cu.

See also WATERMELON.

melting point   The temperature at which a compound melts to a liquid. Often characteristic of a particular chemical and used as a means of identification. Particularly valuable as an index of purity, since impurities lower the melting point.

melts   See SPLEEN.

membrane, semipermeable (selectively permeable)   One that allows the passage of small molecules but not large ones; e.g. pig's bladder is permeable to water but not salt; collodion is perme-able to salt but not protein molecules.

See also DIALYSIS; OSMOSIS; ULTRAFILTRATION.

menadione, menadiol   Synthetic vitamin K analogue (vitamin K_3, sometimes known as menaquinone-0). Formerly used in pro-phylaxis of HAEMORRHAGIC DISEASE OF THE NEWBORN, but its use has declined since it was shown to support redox cycling reactions and may be associated with later development of cancers.

menaquinones Bacterial metabolites with VITAMIN K activity; vitamin K_2.

menarche The initiation of menstruation in adolescent girls, normally occurring between the ages of 11–15. The age at menarche has become younger in western countries, possibly associated with a better general standard of nutrition, and is later in less developed countries.

menhaden Oily FISH, *Brevoortia patronus, B. tyrannus*, from Gulf of Mexico and Atlantic seaboard of USA, a rich source of FISH oils.

Menke's syndrome A GENETIC DISEASE involving failure of the intestinal copper transport mechanism, resulting in functional copper deficiency. Because of the effects on hair colour and structure, sometimes known as Menke's kinky or steely hair syndrome.

mescal See TEQUILA.

mesocarp See ALBEDO.

meso-inositol See INOSITOL.

mesomorph Description given to a well-covered individual with well-developed muscles.

See also ECTOMORPH; ENDOMORPH.

mesophiles Pathogenic microorganisms that grow best at temperatures between 25–40°C; usually will not grow below 5°C.

metabolic equivalent (MET) Unit of measurement of heat production by the body; 1 MET = 50 kcal/hour/m^2 body surface area.

metabolic rate Rate of utilisation of ENERGY. See BASAL METABOLIC RATE.

metabolic water Produced in the body by the oxidation of foods. 100 g of fat produces 107.1 g, 100 g of starch produces 55.1 g and 100 g of protein produces 41.3 g of water.

See also WATER BALANCE.

metabolic weight ENERGY EXPENDITURE and BASAL METABOLIC RATE depend on the amount of metabolically active tissue in the body, not the total body weight; body weight to the power of 0.75 is generally used to calculate the weight of active tissue.

metabolism The processes of interconversion of chemical compounds in the body. Anabolism is the process of forming larger and more complex compounds, commonly linked to the utilisation of metabolic energy. Catabolism is the process of breaking down larger molecules to smaller ones, commonly oxidation reactions linked to release of energy.

metalloproteins Proteins containing a metal. For example,

HAEMOGLOBIN, CYTOCHROMES, peroxidase, ferritin and siderophilin all contain iron; many enzymes contain copper, manganese or zinc as a prosthetic group.

metallothionein A small protein (M_r 6.8k, 61 amino acids) that binds zinc, copper and cadmium. Important in both absorption and metabolism of essential metal ions, and also sequestration and hence detoxication of metals such as cadmium. Plasma concentration may be a useful index of zinc status.

metaphysis Growing portion of a long BONE, between the EPIPHYSES and the shaft (DIAPHYSIS).

metaproteins Products of the action of dilute acid or alkali on proteins; they are no longer soluble at their ISOELECTRIC points but will dissolve in weak acid or alkali.

metformin See HYPOGLYCAEMIC AGENTS.

methaemoglobin Oxidised HAEMOGLOBIN (unlike oxyhaemoglobin in which oxygen is reversibly bound without oxidising the iron); cannot transport oxygen. Present in small quantities in normal blood, increased after certain drugs and after smoking, and in babies after consumption of food or water containing moderately high levels of nitrates. Rarely occurs as a GENETIC DISEASE, methaemoglobinaemia.

methaglen (metheglin) A traditional British wine made from honey (and thus a form of MEAD) to which herbs are added before fermentation. Originally for medicinal purposes.

methanogens Archebacteria found in RUMEN flora that produce methane (and hydrogen) as a metabolic end-product.

methanol (methyl alcohol, wood alcohol) The first member of the alcohol series, chemically CH_3-OH. It is a highly toxic substance and leads to mental disturbance, blindness and death when consumed over a period. See ALCOHOL, DENATURED.

methionine An essential AMINO ACID, abbr Met (M), M_r 149.2, pK_a 2.13, 9.28, codon AUG. One of the three containing sulphur; cystine and CYSTEINE are the other two. Cystine and cysteine are not essential, but can only be made from methionine, and therefore the requirement for methionine is lower if there is an adequate intake of cyst(e)ine. For this reason the sulphur amino acids are considered together.

methionine load test For VITAMIN B_6 status, measurement of urinary excretion of HOMOCYSTEINE after a test dose of 3g of METHIONINE; the enzyme cystathionine synthetase (EC 4.2.1.22) is pyridoxal phosphate-dependent.

methionine sulphoximine Formed by reaction between nitrogen trichloride (AGENE) and the amino acid METHIONINE when flour is treated with agene as a bleaching agent. Causes running fits in dogs, and although it has never been shown to be toxic to man, the use of agene as a FLOUR IMPROVER was abandoned in UK in 1955.

Methocel   Trade name for methyl CELLULOSE.

méthode champenoise   Sparkling WINES made by a second fermentation in the bottle, as for CHAMPAGNE, but outside the Champagne region of north-eastern France.

Methofas   Trade name for methyl hydroxypropyl CELLULOSE.

methotrexate   4-Amino-10-methyl folic acid, a FOLIC ACID antagonist used in cancer chemotherapy; inhibits dihydrofolate reductase (EC 1.5.1.3).

methylated spirits   See ALCOHOL, DENATURED.

methyl cellulose   See CELLULOSE.

methylene blue dye-reduction test   When the dye methylene blue is added to milk, the bacteria present take up oxygen and change the colour of the dye; methylene blue loses its colour. A similar test uses resazurin, which changes from blue-purple to pink.

The speed of the change indicates the bacterial content. Pasteurised milk (see PASTEURISATION) must not reduce dye in 30 min.

methylene tetrahydrofolate reductase   Enzyme (EC 1.7.99.5) involved in FOLIC ACID metabolism. A thermolabile variant occurs in 10–20% of the population leading to high blood levels of HOMOCYSTEINE, associated with ATHEROSCLEROSIS, THROMBOSIS and possibly NEURAL TUBE DEFECT.

methyl folate trap   Hypothesis to explain the occurrence of megaloblastic ANAEMIA and functional FOLIC ACID deficiency in VITAMIN B_{12} deficiency. Folic acid is transported between tissues as methyl folate, which can only be utilised by the vitamin B_{12}-dependent enzyme methionine synthetase (EC 2.1.1.13), so in vitamin B_{12} deficiency there is accumulation of folate as methyl folate, which cannot be utilised.

3-methyl-histidine   Derivative of the amino acid, HISTIDINE, found almost exclusively in the contractile proteins of muscle (myosin and actin). Useful among other purposes as an index of lean meat content of prepared foods, because it is not present in collagen or other added materials. Formed in protein after synthesis, and not reutilised when protein is catabolised. Urinary excretion has been proposed as an index of muscle protein turnover, but smaller pools of methyl histidine in non-muscle tissues turn over faster than muscle, and confound the interpretation of results.

methylmalonic acid   Methylmalonyl CoA is an intermediate in the metabolism of VALINE, ISOLEUCINE and the side-chain of CHOLESTEROL, as well as (rare) odd-carbon FATTY ACIDS. It is normally metabolised by a VITAMIN B_{12}-dependent enzyme, methylmalonyl CoA mutase (EC 5.4.99.2); in deficiency the activity of this enzyme is impaired and methylmalonic acid is excreted in the urine, especially after a test dose of valine or isoleucine. Methylmalonic aciduria also occurs as a GENETIC DISEASE due to deficiency of methylmalonyl CoA mutase.

N^1-methyl nicotinamide Major urinary metabolite of NIACIN, and measured as an index of niacin status. Some methyl nicotinamide is oxidised to methyl pyridone carboxamide, and measurement of the ratio of the two metabolites is a more sensitive index of status.

methyl pyridone carboxamide See N^1-METHYL NICOTINAMIDE.

metmyoglobin Brown oxidation product of MYOGLOBIN in meat when the iron has been oxidised to Fe^{3+}. Storage of pre-packed meat under low oxygen conditions slows the rate of oxidation. See also GAS STORAGE, CONTROLLED; NITROSOMYOGLOBIN.

metronidazole Drug used to treat intestinal (and other) infections, including AMOEBIASIS and GIARDIASIS.

Meulengracht diet For peptic ulcer patients; sieved foods such as meat, chicken, vegetables, at two-hourly intervals. Differs from the SIPPY DIET in being much richer in protein. The intention is to neutralise the acid in the stomach by the buffering effect of the protein.

meunière, à la Fish dredged with flour, fried in butter and served with this butter and chopped parsley; (literally *in the style of the miller's wife*).

micelle Droplet of dietary lipid, emulsified by non-esterified FATTY ACIDS, mono-acylglycerol and BILE SALTS, small enough to be absorbed into intestinal mucosal cells.

micro-aerophiles Microorganisms that grow best at oxygen concentrations well below atmospheric, but not ANAEROBIC (see AEROBIC). Lead to spoilage of foodstuffs unless all oxygen is excluded.

microbiological assay Biological method of measuring compounds such as vitamins and amino acids, using microorganisms. The principle is that the organism is inoculated into a medium containing all the growth factors needed except the one under examination; the rate of growth is then proportional to the amount of this nutrient added in the test substance.

microcapsules See MICROENCAPSULATION.

microcytosis Presence of abnormally small red BLOOD CELLS (microcytes) in the circulation; occurs in IRON deficiency ANAEMIA and other anaemias associated with impairment of HAEMOGLOBIN synthesis.

microencapsulation Preparation of small particles of solids, or droplets of liquids, inside thin coatings (e.g. beeswax, starch, gelatine or polyacrylic acid). The microcapsules range from 1–100 nm in size. Used to prepare liquids as free-flowing powders or compressed solids, to separate reactive materials, reduce toxicity, protect against oxidation and control the rate of release; used for enzymes, flavours, nutrients, etc.

microfiltration Filtration under pressure through a membrane of small pore size (0.1–10 μm; larger pores than for ULTRAFILTRATION). Used for clarification of beverages and to sterilise liquids by filtering out bacteria.

micronisation Extremely rapid heating with infrared radiation produced by heating propane on a ceramic tile or with nichrome wire elements. Suggested as an alternative to steam heating or toasting since the shorter heating time is less damaging to the foodstuff.

micronutrients VITAMINS and MINERALS, which are needed in very small amounts (μg or mg per day), as distinct from fats, carbohydrates and proteins which are macronutrients, needed in considerably greater amounts.

microorganisms Bacteria, yeasts and moulds; can cause food spoilage, and disease (pathogens); used to process and preserve food by FERMENTATION and have been used as foodstuffs (single cell protein and mycoprotein).

See also FOOD POISONING.

microvilli Hair-like projections (~5 μm long) from the surface of epithelial cells, e.g. in the GASTROINTESTINAL TRACT. When microvilli form a dense covering on the surface of a cell, this is the brush border.

microwave cooking Rapid heating by passing high-frequency electromagnetic waves (commonly 2450 MHz, sometimes 896 MHz in Europe and 915 MHz in USA) from a magnetron through the food or liquid to be heated. The process is based on the negatively charged oxygen atom and the positively charged hydrogen atoms in water which form an electric dipole. The application of a rapidly oscillating electric field causes the dipoles to reorient with each change in the field direction, dissipating the energy as heat. The ratio of the capacitance of the food to the capacitance of air is the dielectric constant and depends on the number of dipoles, temperature and the changes induced by the electric fields.

middlings See WHEATFEED.

mid-upper-arm circumference (MUAC) A rapid way of assessing nutritional status, especially applicable to children.

See also ANTHROPOMETRY; QUAC STICK.

milchig Jewish term for dishes containing milk or milk products, which cannot be served with or after meat dishes.

See also FLEISHIG, PAREVE.

milfoil   A common wild plant (*Achillea millefolium*, or yarrow) with finely divided leaves which can be used in salads or chopped to replace chervil or parsley as a garnish.

milk   The secretion of the mammary gland of animals including cow, buffalo, goat, ass, mare, ewe, camel and human beings. Cow's milk:

Composition /100 g (full cream): 276 kJ (66 kcal), protein 3.2 g, fat 3.9 g (66.6% saturated, 30.5% mono-, 2.7% polyunsaturated), cholesterol 14 mg, carbohydrate 4.8 g (4.8 g sugars);

Channel Island milk: 326 kJ (78 kcal), protein 3.6 g, fat 5.1 g (70.2% saturated, 27.6% mono-, 2.1% polyunsaturated), cholesterol 16 mg carbohydrate 4.8 g (4.8 g sugars);

semiskimmed milk: 192 kJ (46 kcal), protein 3.3 g, fat 1.6 g (66.6% saturated, 33.3% mono-, 0% polyunsaturated), cholesterol 7 mg, carbohydrate 5 g (5 g sugars);

skimmed: 138 kJ (33 kcal), protein 3.3 g, fat 0.1 g (100% saturated, 0% mono-, 0% polyunsaturated), cholesterol 2 mg, carbohydrate 5 g (5 g sugars);

Na 55 mg, K 140 mg, Ca 115 mg, Mg 11 mg, P 92 mg, Fe 0.1 mg, Zn 0.4 mg, Se 1 μg, I 15 μg, vitamin A 55 μg (21 μg carotene), D 0.03 μg, E 0.1 mg, B_1 0.03 mg, B_2 0.17 mg, niacin 0.8 mg, B_6 0.06 mg, folate 6 μg, B_{12} 0.4 μg, pantothenate 0.4 mg, biotin 1.9 μg, C 1 mg. A 585 mL serving (one pint) is a source of vitamin B_1, B_6, folate, Se, Zn; good source of Mg; rich source of protein, vitamin A (full cream and Channel Island only), B_2, B_{12}, pantothenate; Ca, I.

milk, accredited   Term not used after October 1954. Referred to milk untreated by heat, from cows examined at specified intervals for freedom from disease.

milk, acidophilus   A preparation similar to cultured BUTTERMILK but soured by *Lactobacillus* spp instead of acid-producing streptococci.

milk alkali syndrome   Weakness and lethargy caused by prolonged adherence to a diet rich in milk, more than about 1 L (2 pints daily) and alkalis.

milk baby   Infant with iron deficiency ANAEMIA caused by excessive ingestion of milk and delayed or inadequate addition of iron-rich foods to the diet.

milk, citrated   Milk to which sodium citrate has been added to combine with the calcium and inhibit the curdling of CASEINOGEN which would normally occur in the stomach. Claimed, with little evidence, to be of value in feeding infants and invalids.

milk, dye-reduction test   See METHYLENE BLUE DYE-REDUCTION TEST.

milk, evaporated, condensed   Full fat, skimmed or partly skimmed milk, sweetened or unsweetened, that has been concentrated by partial evaporation; fat and total solids for each type defined by law.

milk fat test See GERBER TEST.

milk, fermented In various countries, milk is fermented with a mixture of bacteria (and sometimes yeasts) when the lactose is converted to lactic acid and in some cases to alcohol. The acidity (and alcohol) prevent the growth of potentially hazardous microorganisms, and the fermentation thus acts to preserve the milk for a time.

Include busa (Turkestan), cieddu (Italy), dadhi (India), kefir (Balkans), kumiss (Steppes), laban zabadi (Egypt), mazun (Armenia), taette (N Europe), skyr (Iceland), masl (Iran), crowdies (Scotland), kuban and YOGHURT.

See also PROBIOTIC.

milk, filled Milk from which the natural fat has been removed and replaced with fat from another source. The reason may be economic, if the butter-fat can be replaced by a cheaper one, or more recently, to replace a fat rich in saturated FATTY ACIDS with a vegetable oil with a lower content of saturates.

milk, freezing-point test A test for the adulteration of milk with water. Milk normally freezes between -0.53 and $-0.56°C$; when it has been diluted the freezing point rises nearer to that of water. A freezing point above $-0.53°C$ is indicative of adulteration.

milk, homogenised Mechanical treatment breaks up and redistributes the fat globules throughout the milk to prevent the cream rising to the surface.

milk, humanised Cow's milk that has had its composition modified to resemble human milk, for infant feeding. The main change is a reduction in protein content, often achieved by dilution with carbohydrate and restoration of the fat content.

milk, human mature

Composition/100 g: 288 kJ (69 kcal), protein 1.3 g, fat 4.1 g (46.1% saturated, 41% mono-, 12.8% polyunsaturated), cholesterol 16 mg, carbohydrate 7.2 g (7.2 g sugars), Na 15 mg, K 58 mg, Ca 34 mg, Mg 3 mg, P 15 mg, Fe 0.07 mg, Cu 0.04 mg, Zn 0.3 mg, Se 1 μg, I 7 μg, vitamin A 62 μg (24 μg carotene), D 0.04 μg, E 0.34 mg, B_1 0.02 mg, B_2 0.03 mg, niacin 0.69 mg, B_6 0.01 mg, folate 5 μg, B_{12} 0.01 μg, pantothenate 0.25 mg, biotin 0.7 μg, C 4 mg.

milk, irradiated Milk that has been subjected to uv light, when the 7-dehydrocholesterol naturally present is partly converted into VITAMIN D.

milk, lactose-hydrolysed Milk in which the LACTOSE has been hydrolysed to glucose and galactose by treatment with the enzyme LACTASE, intended for infants who are lactose intolerant.

Lactose-free milk may also be prepared by physical removal of lactose by ULTRAFILTRATION.

See also DISACCHARIDE INTOLERANCE.

milk, long (ropy) A Scandinavian soured milk which is viscous because of 'ropiness' caused by bacteria. See ROPE.

milk, malted A preparation of milk and the liquid separated from a mash of barley malt and wheat flour, evaporated to dryness.

Milkman's syndrome Form of OSTEOMALACIA with characteristic X-ray appearance of the bones; named after the American radiologist L A Milkman.

milk, methylene blue test See METHYLENE BLUE DYE-REDUCTION TEST.

milk of magnesia Magnesium hydroxide solution used as an ANTACID and LAXATIVE.

milk, pasteurised See PASTEURISATION.

milk, ropy See MILK, LONG; ROPE.

milk stone Deposit of calcium and magnesium phosphates, protein, etc, produced when milk is heated to temperatures above 60°C.

milk, toned Dried skim milk added to a high-fat milk such as buffalo milk, to reduce the fat content but maintain the total solids.

milk, tuberculin tested (TT) Applied to milk from a herd that has been attested free from tuberculosis.

milk, UHT (or long-life) Milk sterilised for a very short time (2 s) at ultra-high temperature (137°C).

milk, witches' See WITCHES' MILK.

millerator Wheat-cleaning machine consisting of two sieves, the upper one retaining particles larger than wheat, the lower one rejecting particles smaller than wheat.

miller's offal See WHEATFEED.

millet Cereal of a number of species of Gramineae (grass family) smaller than wheat and rice and high in fibre content. Common millet (*Panicum* and *Setaria* spp) also known as China, Italian, Indian, French hog, proso, panicled and broom corn millet, foxtail millet (*Setaria italica*); grows very rapidly, 2–2¹/₂ months from sowing to harvest. Protein 10%, fat 2.5%, carbohydrate 73%. Red, finger, South India millet, coracan or ragi is *Eleusine coracana*. Protein 6%, fat 1.5%, carbohydrate 75%.

Bulrush millet, pearl millet, bajoa or Kaffir manna corn is *Pennisetum typhoideum* or *P. americanum*; the staple food in poor parts of India. Protein 11%, fat 5%, carbohydrate 69%.

Other species are hungry rice (*Digitaria exilis*), jajeo millet (*Acroceras amplectens*), Kodo or haraka millet (*Paspalum scrobiculatum*), teff (*Eragrostis tefor, E abyssinica*).

See also SORGHUM.

milling The term usually refers to the conversion of cereal grain into its derivative, e.g. wheat into flour, brown rice to white rice. Flour milling involves two types of rollers:

(1) break rolls are corrugated and exert shear pressure and forces which break up the wheat grain and permit sieving into fractions containing varying proportions of GERM, BRAN and ENDOSPERM;

(2) reducing rolls that are smooth and subdivide the endosperm to fine particles.

See also FLOUR, EXTRACTION RATE.

mills Various types of equipment, including a number of mills, are used to reduce the size of fibrous foods to smaller pieces or to pulp and dry foods to powders. See HAMMER MILL; QUERNS; ROLLER MILL.

milt (melt) Soft ROE (testes) of male fish. Also SPLEEN of animals.

miltone A toned MILK developed in India in which peanut protein is added to buffalo or cow's milk to extend supplies.

Minafen Trade name for food low in PHENYLALANINE for treatment of PHENYLKETONURIA.

Minamata disease Poisoning by organic mercurial compounds, named after Minamata Bay in Japan, where fish contained high levels of organic mercurials during 1953–1956, as a result of mercury-rich industrial waste entering the river estuary.

minarine Name sometimes given to low-fat spreads with less than the statutory amount of fat in a MARGARINE.

mince (1) To chop or cut into small pieces with a knife or, more commonly, in a mincing machine or electric mixer.

(2) Meat which is finely divided by chopping or passing through a mincing machine; known as ground meat in USA.

mincemeat A traditional product made from apple, sugar, vine fruits and citrus peel with suet, spices and acetic acid, coloured with caramel. Preserved by the sugar content and acid. Also called fruit mince. Originally a meat product; in USA a spiced mixture of chopped meat, apples and raisins.

Composition/100g: 1146kJ (274kcal), protein 0.6g, fat 4.3g (58.5% saturated, 39% mono-, 2.4% polyunsaturated), cholesterol 4mg, carbohydrate 62.1g (62.1g sugars), dietary fibre 3g, nsp 1.3g, Na 140mg, K 190mg, Ca 30mg, Mg 10mg, P 17mg, Fe 1.5mg, Cu 0.2mg, Zn 0.2mg, vitamin A 1µg (9µg carotene), B_1 0.04mg, B_2 0.02mg, niacin 0.5mg, B_6 0.1mg, folate 8µg. Serving 25g.

mineola A CITRUS fruit.

mineralocorticoids A general term for the STEROID hormones secreted by the adrenal cortex (ADRENAL GLANDS) which control the excretion of salt and water.

See also WATER BALANCE.

mineral salts The inorganic salts, including sodium, potassium, calcium, chloride, phosphate, sulphate, etc. So-called because they are (or originally were) obtained by mining.

minerals, trace Those MINERAL SALTS present in the body, and required in the diet, in small amounts (parts per million): COPPER, CHROMIUM, IODINE, MANGANESE, SELENIUM; although required in larger amounts, ZINC and IRON are sometimes included with the trace minerals.

minerals, ultratrace Those MINERAL SALTS present in the body, and required in the diet, in extremely small amounts (parts per thousand million or less); known to be dietary essentials, although rarely if ever a cause for concern since the amounts required are small and they are widely distributed in foods and water, e.g. COBALT, MOLYBDENUM, SILICON, TIN, VANADIUM.

mineral water Natural, untreated, spring waters, some of which are naturally carbonated, may be slightly alkaline or salty. Numerous health claims have been made for the benefits arising from the traces of a large number of minerals found in solution. They are normally named after the town nearest the source. Examples are Evian, Malvern, Apollinaris, Vichy, Vittel, Perrier. Sparkling mineral water may either contain the gases naturally present at the source or may be artificially carbonated (SODA WATER, Seltzer water or club soda). Carbonated beverages are sometimes called minerals.

miners' cramp Cramp due to loss of SALT from the body caused by excessive sweating. Occurs in tropical climates and with severe exercise; mining often combines the two. Prevented by consuming salt, e.g. salt tablets in the tropics and for athletes.

minimum lethal dose (MLD) Smallest amount of a toxic compound that has been recorded as causing death.
See also LD$_{50}$; NO ADVERSE EFFECT LEVEL.

mint Aromatic herbs, *Mentha* spp, including spearmint, *M. spicata*; peppermint, *M. piperita*, garden mint is *M. spicata*. Oil of peppermint is distilled from stem and leaves of *M. piperita*, and used both pharmaceutically and as a flavour.
Composition/100 g: 179 kJ (43 kcal), protein 3.8 g, fat 0.7 g, carbohydrate 5.3 g, Na 15 mg, K 260 mg, Ca 210 mg, P 75 mg, Fe 9.5 mg, vitamin A 123 µg (740 µg carotene), E 5 mg, B$_1$ 0.12 mg, B$_2$ 0.33 mg, niacin 1.1 mg, folate 110 µg, C 31 mg. Serving 5 g.

miracle berry The fruit of the west African bush *Richardella dulcifica* (*Synsepalum dulcificum*). It contains a taste-modifying glycoprotein (miraculin) that causes sour foods to taste sweet, hence the name.

miraculin The taste-modifying glycoprotein of the MIRACLE BERRY.

miso   A Japanese sauce, prepared from autoclaved soya beans mixed with cooked rice and partly fermented with *Aspergillus oryzae* and *A. sojae* to form koji. Salt is added to stop further mould growth, bacterial fermentation continues with the addition of *Lactobacillus* (1–2 months).

mistelles   French; partially fermented grape juice.

mitochondrion (mitochondria)   The subcellular organelles in all cells apart from red blood cells in which the major oxidative reactions of METABOLISM occur, linked to the formation of ATP from ADP.

mitogen   Any compound that acts to stimulate cell division (mitosis).

mixed function oxidases   A group of enzymes (EC 1.14.x.x) that catalyse oxidation of two substrates simultaneously, using molecular oxygen as the donor. Most hydroxylases and the CYTOCHROMES P450 are mixed-function oxidases.

mixiria   Process of preserving meat and fish by roasting in their own fat and preserving in jars covered with a layer of fat.

mixograph   American instrument for measuring the physical properties of a dough, similar in principle to the FARINOGRAPH.

MLD   See minimum lethal dose.

mocca   Mixture of coffee and cocoa used in bakery and confectionery products.

mocha   (1) Variety of arabica coffee.
(2) Flavoured with coffee.
(3) In USA a combination of coffee and chocolate flavouring. See also MOCCA.

mock turtle soup   Gelatinous soup made from calf's head, beef, bacon and veal; similar to turtle soup, but without the TURTLE; mock turtle is a calf's head dressed to resemble a turtle.

modified atmosphere   See GAS STORAGE, CONTROLLED.

MODY   Maturity onset diabetes of the young. See GLUCOKINASE.

molality   Concentration of a solution expressed as mol of solute per kg of solvent.

molarity   Concentration of a solution expressed as mol of solute per litre of solution.

molasses   The residue left after repeated crystallisation of sugar; it will not crystallise. Contains 67% sucrose, together with glucose and fructose and (if from beet) raffinose and small quantities of dextrans; 1100 kJ (260 kcal), >500 mg iron/100 g, with traces of other minerals.

molluscs   Marine bivalve shellfish with soft unsegmented body, most are enclosed in a hard shell and include ABALONE, CLAMS, COCKLES, MUSSELS, OYSTERS, SCALLOPS, WHELKS, WINKLES.

molybdenum   A dietary essential mineral, required for a number of enzymes in which it forms the functional part of the coenzyme MOLYBDOPTERIN. Deficiency is unknown, and there are no estimates of requirements. Average intakes are between 50–400 µg/day, and are considered to be SAFE AND ADEQUATE.

molybdopterin A pterin derivative with MOLYBDENUM chelated by two sulphydryl groups; not a dietary essential but synthesised in the body. The coenzyme of molybdenum-dependent enzymes, including XANTHINE (EC 1.1.3.22), sulphite (EC 1.8.3.1), aldehyde (EC 1.2.3.1) and pyridoxal (EC 1.1.3.12) oxidases.

monellin The active sweet principle, a protein, from the serendipity berry, *Dioscoreophyllum cumminsii*. 1500–2000 times as sweet as sucrose.

monethanolamine See ETHANOLAMINE.

Monilia Obsolete name for genus of fungi now known as CANDIDA.

moniliformin MYCOTOXIN formed by *Fusarium moniliforme*, *F. oxysporum*, *F. anthopilum* and *F. graminearum*, growing especially on maize. Toxic to experimental animals and associated with KESHAN DISEASE in areas of China where SELENIUM intake is extremely low.

monkey nut See PEANUT.

monkfish White FISH, *Lophius piscatorius*.
Composition /100 g: 276 kJ (66 kcal), protein 15.7 g, fat 0.4 g, cholesterol 14 mg, carbohydrate 0 g, Na 18 mg, K 300 mg, Ca 8 mg, Mg 21 mg, P 330 mg, Fe 0.3 mg, Cu 0.01 mg, Zn 0.5 mg, vitamin B_1 0.03 mg, B_2 0.06 mg, niacin 2.9 mg. A 70 g serving is a source of niacin; good source of protein.

monoacylglycerol, monoglyceride See SUPERGLYCERINATED FATS.

monocalcium phosphate See CALCIUM ACID PHOSPHATE.

monoglycerides See SUPERGLYCERINATED FATS.

monokine See CYTOKINE.

monophagia Desire for one type of food.

monophenol oxidase See PHENOL OXIDASES.

monosaccharides Group name of the simplest sugars, including those composed of three carbon atoms (trioses), four (tetroses), five (pentoses), six (hexoses) and seven (heptoses). Formerly known as monoses or monosaccharoses. See CARBOHYDRATES.

monosaccharose (monose) Obsolete names for MONOSACCHA-RIDES.

monosodium glutamate (MSG) The sodium salt of GLUTAMIC ACID, used to enhance flavour of savoury dishes and often added to canned meat and soups. Originally called Aginomoto.
See also FLAVOUR POTENTIATORS; UMAMI.

mono-unsaturates Commonly used term for mono-unsaturated FATTY ACIDS.

monstera   Fruit of the Swiss cheese plant, *Monstera deliciosa*, also known as fruit salad fruit (Australia), and delicious fruit.

montmorillonite   See FULLER'S EARTH.

mooli   Long, white oriental variety of RADISH, *Raphanus sativa*. Composition/100 g: 62 kJ (15 kcal), protein 0.8 g, fat 0.1 g, carbohydrate 2.9 g (2.9 g sugars), dietary fibre 1.5 g, Na 27 mg, K 220 mg, Ca 30 mg, Mg 15 mg, P 25 mg, Fe 0.4 mg, Zn 0.3 mg, vitamin B_1 0.03 mg, B_2 0.02 mg, niacin 0.6 mg, B_6 0.07 mg, folate 38 μg, pantothenate 0.2 mg, C 24 mg. A 30 g serving is a source of vitamin C.

morbidity   The state of being diseased. Morbidity rate is the number of cases of a disease/million of the population. See also INCIDENCE RATE; PREVALENCE RATE.

morel   Edible fungus *Morchella esculenta*, much prized for its delicate flavour; see MUSHROOMS.

Moreton Bay bug   Or Bay lobster, a variety of sand lobster found in Australia.

morphine   See ANTIMOTILITY AGENTS.

mortality   The incidence of death in a population in a given period of time.

mortoban   See PHYLLO PASTRY.

moss, Irish   See CARRAGEENAN.

motilin   Peptide hormone secreted by the stomach and upper small intestine; increases intestinal motility.

mottled teeth   See FLUORIDE; FLUOROSIS.

motza   See MATZO.

mould bran   A fungal AMYLASE preparation produced by growing mould on moist wheat bran.

mould inhibitors   Scc ANTIMYCOTICS.

moulds   FUNGI characterised by their branched filamentous structure (mycelium), including MUSHROOMS and smaller fungi. They can cause food spoilage very rapidly, e.g. white *Mucor*, grey-green *Penicillium*, black *Aspergillus*. Many also produce MYCOTOXINS.

Used for large-scale manufacture of citric acid (*Aspergillus niger*), ripening of cheeses (*Penicillium* spp) and as source of enzymes for industrial use. A number of foods are fermented with moulds, e.g. IDLI, MISO and TEMPEH. The mycelium of *Fusarium* spp is used as MYCOPROTEIN. Most of the ANTIBIOTICS are mould products.

mowrah fat   See VEGETABLE BUTTERS.

MPD   Modified POLYDEXTROSE.

M_r   Relative molecular mass, sometimes also known as molecular weight.

mRNA   Messenger RNA, synthesised in the nucleus as a copy of one strand of a region of DNA containing the information for the synthesis of one or more proteins.

See also TRANSCRIPTION; TRANSLATION.

MSG See MONOSODIUM GLUTAMATE.

MUAC See MID-UPPER-ARM CIRCUMFERENCE.

mucilages Soluble but undigested polymers of the sugars arabinose and xylose found in some seeds and seaweeds; used as thickening and stabilising agents in food processing by virtue of their water-holding and viscous properties.

See also GUM.

mucin A GLYCOPROTEIN, the main protein of MUCUS secreted by goblet cells of mucous epithelium as protection; it is resistant to hydrolysis by digestive enzymes. Especially rich in CYSTEINE and THREONINE; some 60% of the dietary requirement for threonine is accounted for by losses in intestinal mucus.

mucopolysaccharides GLYCOPROTEINS with a short polypeptide chain covalently linked to a long linear polysaccharide; commonly found in connective tissue.

mucoproteins GLYCOPROTEINS consisting of acidic MUCOPOLYSACCHARIDES covalently linked to specific proteins; sticky and slippery, found for example in saliva and mucous membrane secretions.

mucosa Moist tissue lining, e.g. the mouth (buccal mucosa), stomach (gastric mucosa), intestines and respiratory tract.

mucous colitis See IRRITABLE BOWEL SYNDROME.

mucus Viscous fluid secreted by mucous membranes, in the GASTRO-INTESTINAL TRACT acts both to lubricate the intestinal wall and also to prevent digestion of intestinal mucosal cells. Main constituent is MUCIN.

muesli Breakfast cereal; a mixture of raw cereal flakes (oats, wheat, rye, barley and millet) together with dried fruit, apple flakes, nuts, sugar, bran and wheatgerm. Originated in Switzerland in late nineteenth century.

mulberry Dark purple-red fruit of the tree *Morus nigra*, slightly sweet and acid, similar shape and size to a raspberry or loganberry. There is also a white mulberry, *M. alba*. Of little commercial importance as a fruit; the leaves of the mulberry are the only food plant of the silkworm.

Composition/100 g: 150 kJ (36 kcal), protein 1.3 g, fat 0 g, carbohydrate 8.1 g (8.1 g sugars), dietary fibre 1.5 g, Na 2 mg, K 260 mg, Ca 36 mg, Mg 15 mg, P 48 mg, Fe 1.6 mg, Cu 0.06 mg, Zn 0.2 mg, vitamin A 2 µg (14 µg carotene), B_1 0.03 mg, B_2 0.05 mg, niacin 0.9 mg, B_6 0.06 mg, folate 33 µg, pantothenate 0.2 mg, biotin 1.9 µg, C 19 mg. An 80 g serving is a source of folate; good source of vitamin C.

mulled ale   Beer that has been spiced and heated, traditionally by plunging a red-hot poker into the liquid.

mulled wine   Wine mixed with fruit juice, sweetened and flavoured with spices (especially cinnamon, cloves and ginger), served hot.

mulligatawny   Anglo-Indian; CURRY-flavoured soup made with meat or chicken stock.

multiple sclerosis   A slowly progressive disease involving nerve degeneration; it may take many years to develop to the stage of paralysis, and the disease is subject to random periods of spontaneous remission. There is some evidence that supplements of polyunsaturated FATTY ACIDS slow the progression of the disease.

muscatels   Made by drying the large seed-containing grapes grown almost exclusively around Malaga (Spain). They are partially dried in the sun and drying is completed indoors; they are left on the stalk and pressed flat for sale. Muscatel is a sweet wine made from the grapes.

muscle   The contractile unit of skeletal muscle is the cylindrical fibre, composed of many myofibrils. Chemically, muscle consists of four main proteins, actin, myosin, tropomyosin and troponin, as well as structural proteins such as COLLAGEN and ELASTIN. Contraction is achieved by formation of a complex between actin and myosin. The muscle fibre is surrounded by a thin membrane, the sarcolemma; within the muscle fibre, surrounding the myofibrils, is the sarcoplasm. Individual fibres are separated by a thin network of CONNECTIVE TISSUE, the endomysium, and the muscle as a whole is enclosed in the epimysium.

muscovado sugar   See SUGAR.

mushrooms   Various edible FUNGI (botanically both mushrooms and toadstools); correctly the fruiting bodies of the fungi. Altogether some 300 species are sold, fresh or dried, in markets around the world; most of these are gathered wild rather than cultivated. The common cultivated mushroom, including flat, cup and button mushrooms is *Agaricus bisporus*, as is the chestnut or Paris mushroom.

Composition/100 g: 54 kJ (13 kcal), protein 1.8 g, fat 0.5 g, carbohydrate 0.4 g (0.2 g sugars, 0.2 g starch), dietary fibre 2.3 g, nsp 1.1 g, Na 5 mg, K 320 mg, Ca 6 mg, Mg 9 mg, P 80 mg, Fe 0.6 mg, Cu 0.72 mg, Zn 0.4 mg, Se 9 μg, I 3 μg, vitamin E 0.1 mg, B_1 0.09 mg, B_2 0.31 mg, niacin 3.5 mg, B_6 0.18 mg, folate 44 μg, pantothenate 2 mg, biotin 12 μg, C 1 mg. A 45 g serving is a source of pantothenate, Se; rich source of Cu.

Other cultivated mushrooms include: shiitake or Black Forest mushroom; oyster mushroom; Chinese straw mushroom.

Some wild species are especially prized, including field mushroom; horse mushroom; parasol mushroom; beefsteak fungus; blewits; wood blewits; cèpe or boletus; chanterelle; matsutake; puffballs; morels; truffles, wood ears or Chinese black fungus; yellow mushroom. Many other wild fungi are also edible, but many are also poisonous.

mussels Various marine bivalve molluscs, *Mytilus edulis, M. californianus.*

Composition/100 g: 108 kJ (26 kcal), protein 5.2 g, fat 0.6 g, cholesterol 12 mg, carbohydrate 0 g, Na 63 mg, K 28 mg, Ca 59 mg, Mg 8 mg, P 99 mg, Fe 2.3 mg, Cu 0.16 mg, Zn 0.6 mg, Se 9 µg, I 23 µg, vitamin B_2 0.08 mg, niacin 1.7 mg, B_6 0.01 mg, B_{12} 4.4 µg, pantothenate 0.1 mg, biotin 2 µg. A 130 g serving (weighed with shell) is a source of protein, niacin, I; good source of Fe, Cu, Se; rich source of vitamin B_{12}.

mustard Powdered seeds of black or brown mustard (*Brassica nigra* or *B. juncea*) or white or yellow (*Sinapsis alba*) or a mixture. English mustard contains not more than 10% wheat flour and turmeric (still referred to in parts of England as Durham mustard, after Mrs Clements of Durham). French mustard: Dijon made from dehusked seeds (and therefore light coloured) or black or brown seeds with salt, spices and white wine or unripe grape juice. Bordeaux (usually called French mustard) black and brown seeds mixed with sugar, vinegar and herbs. Meaux mustard is grainy and made with mixed seeds. American mustard is mild and sweet made with white seeds, sugar, vinegar and turmeric.

mustard and cress Salad herb mixture of leaves of mustard (*Brassica alba*) and garden cress (*Lepidium sativum*). Often mustard is replaced with rape (*Brassica napus* var *oleifera*), a different strain from that used for RAPE seed oil, it has a larger leaf and grows faster than mustard.

mustard oil Used as cooking fat in Bengal and Bihar. The seeds are often contaminated with seeds of *Argemone mexicana*, which contains the toxic ALKALOID, argemone; contaminated mustard oil is the cause of epidemic DROPSY.

mutachrome A yellow CAROTENOID pigment in orange peel which has vitamin A activity. Also known as citroxanthin.

mutagen Any compound that can modify DNA, causing a mutation in bacteria. Many mutagens are also CARCINOGENS, and early screening of compounds for safety involves testing for mutagenicity (the AMES TEST).

mutton Meat from fully grown sheep, *Ovis aries* (LAMB is from animals under 1 year old).

mycelium   Mass of fine branching threads that make up the feed-ing and growing (vegetative) part of a FUNGUS that produces a MUSHROOM or toadstool as a fruiting body.

mycoprotein   Name given to mould MYCELIUM prepared as food-stuff. *Fusarium* and *Neurospora* spp grown on carbohydrate have been used.

mycose   See TREHALOSE.

mycotoxins   Compounds produced by FUNGI that may accumulate to harmful levels in foods without any adverse effect on the flavour or appearance of the food; many are acutely or chroni-cally toxic or carcinogenic. The most important are: AFLATOXINS (produced by *Aspergillus* spp), ochratoxins (*Aspergillus* and *Penicillium* spp), monoliformin (*Fusarium* spp), PATULIN (*Asper-gillus* and *Penicillium* spp) and ergot alkaloids formed by *Clavi-ceps purpurea* growing on rye.

myenteron   Muscle layers of the intestine, a layer of circular muscles inside a layer of longitudinal muscles, responsible for PERISTALSIS.

myocardial infarction   Damage to heart muscle due to failure of the blood supply to the muscle (ischaemia).

myofibril   See MUSCLE.

myoglobin   HAEM-containing oxygen binding protein in muscle. Responsible for the red colour of fresh meat, oxidised to brown METMYOGLOBIN as meat ages, or on cooking. When meat is cured (see CURING) with nitrite, the myoglobin is converted to the bright red NITROSOMYOGLOBIN.

myo-inositol   See INOSITOL.

myosin   The major protein of MUSCLE, about 40% of the total. A globulin, insoluble in water but soluble in salt solution.

myristic acid   A saturated FATTY ACID with 14 carbon atoms (C14:0).

myrosinase   The enzyme (thioglycosidase, EC 3.2.3.1) in MUSTARD seed and HORSERADISH that hydrolyses myrosin or sinigrin to glucose and allyl isothiocyanate, the pungent principle.

Mysore flour   A blend of 75% tapioca flour and 25% peanut flour, used as a partial substitute for cereals in large-scale feeding trials in Madras State, India.

myxoedema   Severe hypothyroidism (underactivity of the thyroid gland, see THYROID HORMONES) in the adult; the name is derived from puffiness of hands and face due to thickening of skin. Signs include coarsening of the skin, intolerance of cold, weight gain and dull mental apathy, as well as reduced BASAL METABOLIC RATE.

myxoxanthin   CAROTENOID pigment in algae with VITAMIN A activity.

N

naartje   Afrikaans; a small tangerine; see CITRUS fruit.

NAD, NADP   Nicotinamide adenine dinucleotide and nicotinamide adenine dinucleotide phosphate, the coenzymes derived
from NIACIN. Involved as hydrogen acceptors in a wide variety of
oxidation and reduction reactions.

NAEL   See NO ADVERSE EFFECT LEVEL.

nalidixic acid   Quinolone antibiotic used to treat intestinal (and
urinary tract) infections.

nan   Indian flat bread, an egg dough prepared with white flour and
leavened with sodium bicarbonate, normally baked in a tandoor
(see TANDOORI).

naphthoquinone   The chemical ring structure of VITAMIN K; the
various chemical forms of vitamin K can be referred to as substituted naphthoquinones.

naringenin   See NARINGIN.

naringin   A GLYCOSIDE (trihydroxyflavonone rhamnoglucoside)
found in grapefruit, especially in the immature fruit. Extremely
bitter: dilutions of 1 part in 10 000 parts of water can be detected.
Sometimes found in canned grapefruit segments as tiny, white
beads. Hydrolysed to the aglycone, trihydroxyflavonone (naringenin), which is not bitter.

nasogastric tube   Fine plastic tube inserted through the nose and
thence into the stomach for ENTERAL NUTRITION.

nasturtium   Both the leaves and seeds of *Tropaeolum officinalis*
can be eaten; they have a hot flavour. The seeds can be pickled
as a substitute for CAPERS, and the flowers can be used to decorate salads.

national flour   See WHEATMEAL.

natriuretic   Any compound that promotes excretion of sodium
salts in the urine; most DIURETICS are natriuretics.

natto   Japanese; soya bean fermented using *Bacillus natto*.

natural foods   A term widely used but with little meaning and
sometimes misleading since all foods come from natural sources.
No legal definition seems possible but guidelines suggest the
term should be applied only to single foods that have been subjected only to mild processing, i.e. largely by physical methods
such as heating, concentrating, freezing, etc, but not chemically
or 'severely' processed.

natural water   See MINERAL WATER.

nature-identical   Term applied to food additives that are synthesised in the laboratory and are identical to those that occur in
nature.

N balance (equilibrium)   See NITROGEN BALANCE.

NCHS standards Tables of height and weight for age used as reference values for the assessment of growth and nutritional status of children, based on data collected by the US National Center for Health Statistics. The most comprehensive such set of data, and used in most countries of the world.

N conversion factor See NITROGEN CONVERSION FACTOR.

NDGA See NORDIHYDROGUAIARETIC ACID.

NDpCal See NET DIETARY PROTEIN–ENERGY RATIO.

neat's foot Ox or calf's foot used for making soups and jellies. Now called cow heels. Neat's foot oil is obtained from the knuckle bones of cattle; used in leather working and for canning sardines.

Necator Genus of HOOKWORMS that are parasitic in the small intestine; the human parasite is *N americanus*.

nectarine Smooth-skinned peach (*Prunus persica* var. *nectarina*). Composition/100 g: 167 kJ (40 kcal), protein 1.4 g, fat 0.1 g, carbohydrate 9 g (9 g sugars), dietary fibre 2.2 g, nsp 1.2 g, Na 1 mg, K 150 mg, Ca 6 mg, Mg 9 mg, P 20 mg, Fe 0.4 mg, Cu 0.05 mg, Zn 0.1 mg, Se 1 µg, I 3 µg, vitamin A 8 µg (52 µg carotene), B_1 0.02 mg, B_2 0.04 mg, niacin 0.8 mg, B_6 0.03 mg, pantothenate 0.1 mg, biotin 0.2 µg, C 33 mg. A 150 g serving is a rich source of vitamin C.

Neeld–Pearson method See CARR–PRICE REACTION.

neep Scottish name for root vegetables; now used for TURNIP (and sometimes for SWEDE in England).

NEFA Non-esterified FATTY ACIDS.

negus Drink made from port or sherry with spices, sugar and hot water.

NEL See NO EFFECT LEVEL.

nematode Any one of a large group of unsegmented worms; most are free-living, but some, including HOOKWORMS and pinworms, are intestinal parasites.

neohesperidin dihydrochalcone (NEO-DHC) A non-nutritive SWEETENER, 1000 times as sweet as sucrose; formed by hydrogenation of the naturally occurring FLAVONOID neohesperidin.

neomycin Broad spectrum aminoglycoside ANTIBIOTIC isolated from *Streptomyces fradii* that is poorly absorbed from the GASTROINTESTINAL TRACT and is used to treat persistent intestinal bacterial infections.

neonate Literally new-born, used to describe infants in the first four weeks of life.

nephrocalcinosis Presence of calcium deposits in the kidneys, may result from VITAMIN D toxicity.

neroli oil Prepared from blossoms of the bitter orange by steam distillation. Yellowish oil with intense odour of orange blossom.

net dietary protein calories See NET DIETARY PROTEIN–ENERGY RATIO.

net dietary protein–energy ratio (NDpE) A way of expressing the protein content of a diet or food taking into account both the amount of protein (relative to total energy intake) and the PROTEIN QUALITY. It is protein energy multiplied by net protein utilisation divided by total energy. If energy is expressed in kcal and the result expressed as a percentage, this is net dietary protein calories percent, NDpCal%.

See also NET PROTEIN VALUE.

net protein ratio (NPR), net protein utilisation (NPU) Measures of PROTEIN QUALITY.

net protein value A way of expressing the amount and quality of the protein in a food; the product of NET PROTEIN UTILISATION and protein content percent.

See also NET DIETARY PROTEIN–ENERGY RATIO; PROTEIN QUALITY.

neural tube defect Congenital malformations of the spinal cord caused by failure of the closure of the neural tube in early embryonic development (before day 28 of gestation). Supplements of FOLIC ACID (400μg/day) begun before conception reduce the risk.

neuritis Inflammatory disease of peripheral nerves.

See also NEUROPATHY.

neuropathy Any disease of peripheral nerves, usually causing weakness and numbness.

See also NEURITIS.

neuropeptide Y A peptide neurotransmitter believed to be important in the control of appetite and feeding behaviour, especially in response to LEPTIN.

neutron activation analysis The nuclei of a number of elements will capture a neutron on exposure to a neutron beam, leading to the formation of unstable (radioactive) ISOTOPES which can then be measured by the radiation emitted as they decay. Used for determination of whole body CALCIUM, chlorine and nitrogen.

new cocoyam See TANNIA.

New Zealand process Drying process applied to meat. It is immersed in hot oil under vacuum when it dries to 3% moisture in about 4h. The fat is removed from the dry meat in a hydro-extractor.

NFE See NITROGEN-FREE EXTRACT.

niacin A VITAMIN; one of the B complex without a numerical designation. Sometimes (incorrectly) referred to as vitamin B_3, and formerly vitamin PP (pellagra preventative). Deficiency leads to PELLAGRA, photosensitive dermatitis resembling severe sunburn, a depressive psychosis and intestinal disorders; fatal if untreated.

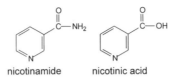

nicotinamide   nicotinic acid

Niacin is the GENERIC DESCRIPTOR for two compounds in foods which have the biological activity of the vitamin: nicotinic acid (pyridine carboxylic acid) and nicotinamide (the amide of nicotinic acid). In the USA niacin is sometimes used specifically to mean nicotinic acid, and niacinamide for nicotinamide.

The metabolic function of niacin is in the COENZYMES NAD (nicotinamide adenine dinucleotide) and NADP (nicotinamide adenine dinucleotide phosphate), which act as intermediate HYDROGEN carriers in a wide variety of oxidation and reduction reactions. In cereals niacin is largely present as NIACYTIN, which is not biologically AVAILABLE (see AVAILABILITY); therefore the preformed niacin content of cereals is generally ignored when calculating intakes.

niacinamide   American name for NICOTINAMIDE.

niacin equivalents   Nicotinamide can also be formed in the body from the amino acid TRYPTOPHAN; on average 60 mg dietary tryptophan is equivalent to 1 mg preformed niacin. The total niacin content of foods is generally expressed as mg niacin equivalents; the sum of preformed niacin plus one-sixtieth of the tryptophan.
  See also NIACYTIN.

niacinogens   Name given to protein–niacin complexes found in cereals; see also NIACYTIN.

niacin toxicity   High doses of nicotinic acid have been used to treat HYPERCHOLESTEROLAEMIA; they can cause an acute flushing reaction, with vasodilatation and severe itching (nicotinamide does not have this effect, but is not useful for treatment of hypercholesterolaemia). Intakes of niacin above 500 mg/day (the reference intake is 17 mg/day) can cause liver damage over a period of months; the risk is greater with sustained release preparations of niacin.

niacytin   The main form of NIACIN in cereals. Nicotinic acid esterified as nicotinoyl-glucose in oligosaccharides and non-starch polysaccharides; susceptible to alkaline hydrolysis and partially susceptible to acid hydrolysis in the stomach. However, because of variable availability, it is conventional to exclude the niacin content of cereals from calculations of intake.

nib   See CHOCOLATE.

niceritol   Penta-erythritol tetranicotinate, a derivative of NIACIN used in gram doses to reduce plasma CHOLESTEROL levels.

nickel   An ultratrace MINERAL; known to be essential to experimental animals, although its function is not known. There is no information on requirements. Metallic nickel is used as a catalyst in the HYDROGENATION of fats.

nicotinamide (niacinamide)   One of the vitamers of NIACIN.

nicotinamide adenine dinucleotide (phosphate)   See NAD.

nicotinate, sodium   Sodium salt of nicotinic acid; has been used, among other purposes, to preserve the red colour in fresh and processed meats.

Nigerian berry   See SERENDIPITY BERRY.

nigerseed   *Guizotia abyssinica*, or nug; grown in India and Ethiopia as food crop.

night blindness   Nyctalopia. Inability to see in dim light as a result of VITAMIN A deficiency.
See also DARK ADAPTATION; VISION.

nim leaf   Sweet nim, an aromatic Indian herb with an aroma resembling that of TRUFFLES.

ninhydrin test   For proteins and amino acids (actually for the amino group). Pink, purple or blue colour is developed on heating the amino acid or peptide with ninhydrin (triketohydrindene hydrate).

nisatidine   See histamine receptor antagonists.

nisin   ANTIBIOTIC isolated from lactic *Streptococcus* group N; inhibits some but not all *Clostridia*; not used medically. The only antibiotic permitted in UK to preserve specified foods. It is naturally present in cheese, being produced by a number of strains of cheese starter organisms. Useful to prolong storage life of cheese, milk, cream, soups, canned fruits and vegetables, canned fish and milk puddings. It also lowers the resistance of many thermophilic bacteria (see THERMOPHILES) to heat and so permits a reduction in the time and/or temperature of heating when processing canned vegetables.

nitrates   The inorganic form of nitrogen used by plants; found in soils and included in inorganic fertiliser. Nitrate is a natural constituent of crops in amounts sometimes depending on the content in the soil. Also found in drinking water as a result of excessive use of fertilisers. Health problems can arise because within a day or two of harvesting some crop nitrates are converted into NITRITES which can react with the HAEMOGLOBIN (especially foetal haemoglobin) to form METHAEMOGLOBIN which cannot transport oxygen. An upper limit of 45–50 mg nitrate/L drinking water has been recommended for infants. Also used, together with nitrite, for CURING meat products.
See also NITROSAMINES.

nitric oxide (NO)   Synthesised in most mammalian cells by the action of nitric oxide synthetase (EC 1.14.13.39) on ARGININE. It causes vasodilatation and inhibits platelet aggregation; it also has anticoagulant and fibrinolytic action, acting by cell surface receptors and intracellular guanylate cyclase (EC 4.6.1.2), leading to increased formation of cyclic GMP. Before it was identified, NO was known as the endothelium-derived relaxation factor.

nitrites Found in many plant foods, since they are rapidly formed by the reduction of naturally occurring NITRATE. Nitrite is the essential agent in preserving meat by pickling, since it inhibits the growth of *Clostridia*; it also combines with the MYOGLOBIN of meat to form the characteristic red NITROSOMYOGLOBIN.

See also NITROSAMINES.

nitrogen A gas comprising about 80% of the atmosphere; in nutrition the term 'nitrogen' is used to refer to ammonium salts and nitrates as plant fertilisers, proteins and amino acids as animal nutrients, and urea and ammonium salts as excretory products.

nitrogenase The enzyme (EC 1.18.6.1 or 1.19.6.1) in nitrogen-fixing microorganisms that catalyses the reduction of N_2 to ammonia. Irreversibly inactivated by oxygen.

See also LEGHAEMOGLOBIN.

nitrogen balance (N balance) The difference between the dietary intake of nitrogen (mainly protein) and its excretion (as urea and other waste products). Healthy adults excrete the same amount as is ingested, and so are in nitrogen equilibrium. During growth and tissue repair (convalescence) the body is in positive N balance, i.e. ingestion is greater than loss and there is an increase in the total body pool of nitrogen (protein). In fevers, fasting and wasting diseases the loss is greater than the intake and the individual is in negative balance; there is a net loss of nitrogen from the body.

nitrogen conversion factor Factor by which total nitrogen content of a material (measured chemically) is multiplied to determine the PROTEIN; depends on the amino acid composition of the protein of the food. Wheat and most cereals 5.8, rice 5.95, soya 5.7, most legumes and nuts 5.3, milk 6.38, other foods 6.25. Errors arise if part of the nitrogen is present as non-protein nitrogen. In mixtures of proteins, as in dishes and diets, the factor of 6.25 is used. Crude protein is defined as N × 6.25.

See also KJELDAHL DETERMINATION.

nitrogen equilibrium See NITROGEN BALANCE.

nitrogen-free extract (NFE) In the analysis of foods and animal feedingstuffs, the fraction that contains the sugars and starches plus small amounts of other materials.

nitrogen, metabolic Nitrogen in the faeces derived from internal or endogenous sources, as distinct from nitrogen-containing dietary sources (exogenous nitrogen). This nitrogen consists of unabsorbed digestive juices, the shed lining of the gastrointestinal tract and bacteria from the intestine, and continues to be excreted in a protein-free diet.

nitrogen trichloride   See AGENE.

nitro-keg   BEER conditioned in kegs under nitrogen, to give a smoother, creamier beverage than traditional conditioning under carbon dioxide.

nitrosamines   *N*-Nitroso derivatives of AMINES. Found in trace amounts in mushrooms, fermented fish meal and smoked fish, and in pickled foods, where they are formed by reaction between NITRITE and amines. They cause cancer in experimental animals, but it is not known whether the small amounts in foods affect human beings, especially since they have also been found in human gastric juice, possibly formed by reaction between amines and nitrites or nitrates from the diet.

nitrosomyoglobin   The red colour of cured meat, formed by the reaction of NITRITE with MYOGLOBIN. Fades in light to yellow-brown metmyoglobin.

nitrous oxide N_2O, a gas used as a propellant in pressurised containers, e.g. to eject cream or salad dressing from containers.

NO   See NITRIC OXIDE.

no adverse effect level (NAEL)   Highest dose or intake of a compound at which no adverse effect can be detected.

See also LD_{50}; MINIMUM LETHAL DOSE.

noble rot   White grapes affected by the fungus *Botrytis cinerea*. It spoils the grapes if they are damaged by rain, but if they are ripe and healthy, and the weather is sunny, it causes them to shrivel and concentrates the sugar, so that top quality sweet wines can be made.

See also WINE CLASSIFICATION, Germany.

No Effect Level (NEL)   With respect to food additives, the maximum dose of an additive that has no detectable adverse effects.

See also ACCEPTABLE DAILY INTAKE.

noggin   Traditional measure of volume of liquor = $^1/_4$ pint (140 mL); also known as a quartern.

N-oil   See FAT REPLACERS.

non-essential amino acids   Those AMINO ACIDS that can be synthesised in the body and therefore are not dietary essentials.

non-esterified fatty acids (NEFA)   See FATTY ACIDS, FREE.

non-nutritive sweeteners   See SWEETENERS, INTENSE.

non-saponifiable fats   See SAPONIFICATION.

non-starch polysaccharides (nsp) Those POLYSACCHARIDES (complex carbohydrates) found in foods other than STARCHES. They
are the major part of DIETARY FIBRE and can be measured more
precisely than total dietary fibre; include CELLULOSE, PECTINS,
GLUCANS, GUMS, MUCILAGES, INULIN, and CHITIN (and exclude
lignin). The nsp in wheat, maize and rice are mainly insoluble and
have a laxative effect, while those in oats, barley, rye and beans
are mainly soluble and have a blood cholesterol-lowering effect.
In vegetables the proportions of soluble to insoluble are roughly
equal but vary in fruits.

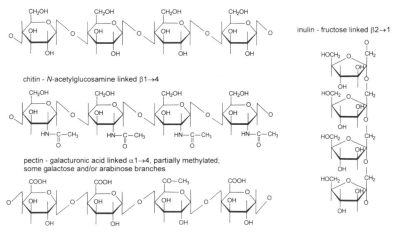

noodles Type of PASTA made with flour and water, or with added
egg, the flour being made from various grains such as rice, wheat,
buckwheat and mung bean starch. Made into a vast range of
shapes and sizes.

nor- Chemical prefix to the name of a compound indicating:
(1) one methyl (CH_3) group has been replaced by hydrogen
(e.g. NORADRENALINE can be considered to be a demethylated
derivative of adrenaline).
(2) An analogue of a compound containing one fewer methylene (CH_2) groups than the parent compound.
(3) An isomer with an unbranched side-chain (e.g. norleucine,
norvaline).

noradrenaline Hormone secreted by the adrenal medulla
together with ADRENALINE; also a neurotransmitter. Physiological effects similar to those of adrenaline. Also known as norepinephrine.

norconidendrin See CONIDENDRIN.

nordihydroguaiaretic acid (NDGA) Extracted from the creosote bush, *Larrea divaricata* (*Covillea tridentata*); used as an antioxidant for fats.

norepinephrine See NORADRENALINE.

nori Edible seaweed, *Porphyra umbilicalis.*

norite Activated charcoal used to decolorise solutions.

norleucine 2-Aminohexanoic acid, a non-physiological AMINO ACID, a straight-chain isomer of LEUCINE, commonly used as an internal standard in amino acid analysis.

northern blot See BLOTTING.

notatin See GLUCOSE OXIDASE.

nougat Sweetmeat made from a mixture of gelatine or egg albumin with sugar and starch syrup, and the whole thoroughly aerated. Originated in Montelimar in southern France.

Novadelox Trade name for benzoyl peroxide used for treating (AGEING) flour.

novain Old name for CARNITINE.

novel foods Foods and food ingredients consisting of, or containing, chemical substances not hitherto used for human consumption to a significant extent in the locality in question (including microorganisms, fungi or algae and substances isolated from them and organisms obtained using genetic modification techniques). A food or ingredient to which has been applied a process not currently used for food manufacture or which has not been previously marketed and which gives rise to changes that affect its nutritional value or safety.

See also SUBSTANTIAL EQUIVALENCE.

NPR Net protein ratio, a measure of PROTEIN QUALITY.

NPU Net protein utilisation, a measure of PROTEIN QUALITY.

NPV Net protein value, a measure of PROTEIN QUALITY.

NSP See NON-STARCH POLYSACCHARIDES.

nubbing Term used in the canning industry for 'topping and tailing' of gooseberries.

nucellar layer Of wheat, the layer of cells that surrounds the endosperm and protects it from the entry of moisture.

nucleic acids Polymers of PURINE and PYRIMIDINE sugar phosphates; two main classes: ribonucleic acid (RNA) and deoxyribonucleic acid (DNA). Collectively the purines and pyrimidines are called bases. DNA is a double-stranded polymer (the so-called 'double helix') containing the five-carbon sugar deoxyribose. RNA is a single-stranded polymer containing the sugar ribose.

Not nutritionally important, since dietary nucleic acids are hydrolysed to their bases, ribose and phosphate in the intestinal tract; purines and pyrimidines can readily be synthesised in the body, and are not dietary essentials.

nucleoproteins The complex of proteins and NUCLEIC ACIDS found in the cell nucleus.

nucleosides Compounds of PURINE or PYRIMIDINE bases with a sugar, most commonly ribose. For example, ADENINE plus ribose forms adenosine. With the addition of phosphate a NUCLEOTIDE is formed.

nucleotides Compounds of PURINE or PYRIMIDINE base with a sugar phosphate; the monomer units of DNA and RNA. Natural constituents of human milk, often used to supplement infant formulae.

nug See NIGERSEED.

nuoc mam Vietnamese, Cambodian; fermented fish sauce. The fish is digested by autolytic enzymes in the presence of salt added to inhibit bacterial growth.

nutmeg Dried ripe seed of *Myristica fragrans*; mace is the seed coat (arillus). Both mace and nutmeg are used as flavourings in meat products and bakery goods.

nutraceuticals Term for compounds in foods that are not nutrients but have (potential) beneficial effects.

See also FUNCTIONAL FOODS.

Nutrasweet Trade name for ASPARTAME.

nutrient density A way of expressing the nutrient content of a food or diet relative to the energy yield (i.e. per 1000 kcal or per MJ) rather than per unit weight.

nutrient enemata Rectal feeding can be carried out with nutrient solutions as the colon can absorb 1–2 L of solution per day; maximum daily amount of glucose that can be given is 75 g (equivalent to 1260 kJ, 300 kcal), and 1 g of nitrogen, in the form of hydrolysed protein (equivalent to 6 g of protein).

See also ENTERAL NUTRITION; PARENTERAL NUTRITION.

nutrients Essential dietary factors such as VITAMINS, MINERALS, AMINO ACIDS and FATTY ACIDS. Metabolic fuels (sources of energy) are not termed nutrients so that a commonly used phrase is 'energy and nutrients'.

nutrification The addition of nutrients to foods at such a level as to make a major contribution to the diet.

nutrition The process by which living organisms take in and use food for the maintenance of life, growth, the functioning of organs and tissues and the production of energy; the branch of science that involves these processes.

See also ENTERAL NUTRITION; NUTRIENT ENEMATA; PARENTERAL NUTRITION.

nutritional claim Any representation that states, suggests or

implies that a food has particular nutrition-related health properties. The extent of such claims on food labelling (see NUTRI-
TIONAL LABELLING) and advertising are controlled by law in most
countries.

nutritional disorder Any morbid process or functional abnormality of the body due to the consumption of a diet not conforming to physiological requirements, or to failure in absorption
or utilisation of the food after ingestion.

nutritional labelling Any information appearing on labelling or
packaging of foods relating to energy and nutrients in the
food. The information which must or may be given, and the
format in which it must appear, is governed by law in most
countries.

nutritional recommendations Recommendations comprising
nutrient goals, food goals and dietary guidelines. In addition to
REFERENCE INTAKES of nutrients, key recommendations in developed countries are reduction of total FAT intake to 30% of energy
intake, with a more severe restriction of saturated fats (see FAT,
SATURATED) (to 10% of energy intake); increase of CARBOHYDRATE
intake to 55% of energy intake (with a reduction of sugars to
10% of energy intake); increased intake of NON-STARCH POLYSAC-
CHARIDES and reduced intake of SALT.

nutritional status assessment For adults, general adequacy of
nutrition is assessed by measuring weight and height; the result
is commonly expressed as the BODY MASS INDEX, the ratio of
weight (kg)/height^2 (m). Body fat may also be estimated, by measuring SKINFOLD THICKNESS, and muscle diameter is also measured. For children, weight and height for age are compared with
standard data for adequately nourished children. The increase
in the circumference of the head and the development of
bones may also be measured. Status with respect to individual
vitamins and minerals is normally determined by laboratory
tests, either measuring the blood and urine concentrations of the
nutrients and their metabolites, or by testing for specific metabolic responses.

See also ANTHROPOMETRY; ENZYME ACTIVATION TESTS.

nutritionist According to the United States Department of
Labor's *Dictionary of Occupational Titles*, one who applies the
science of nutrition to the promotion of health and control of
disease; instructs auxiliary medical personnel; participates in
surveys. Not legally defined in UK, but there is a Register of
Accredited Nutritionists maintained by the Nutrition Society.

See also DIETITIAN.

nutrition policy (or planning) A set of concerted actions, based
on a governmental mandate, intended to ensure good health of

the population through informed access to safe, healthy and adequate food.

nutrition surveillance Monitoring the state of health, nutrition, eating behaviour and nutrition knowledge of a given population for the purpose of planning and evaluating NUTRITION POLICY. Especially in developing countries, monitoring may include factors that may be potential causes of nutritional emergencies, in order to give early warning of such emergencies.

nutritive ratio In animal feeding; a measure of the value of a feeding ration for growth (or milk production) compared with its fattening value. It is the sum of the digestible carbohydrate, protein and $2.3 \times$ fat, divided by digestible protein. (Energy yield of fat is 2.3 times that of carbohydrate and protein.) Ratio 4–5 for growth, 7–8 for fattening.

nutritive value index In animal feeding; intake of digestible energy expressed as energy digestibility multiplied by voluntary intake of dry matter of a particular feed, divided by METABOLIC WEIGHT (weight to the power of 0.75), compared with standard feed.

nutro-biscuit Indian; biscuit baked from a mixture of 60% wheat flour and 40% peanut flour, contains 16–17% protein.

nutro-macaroni Indian; mixture of 80 parts wheat flour, 20 parts defatted peanut meal (total 19% protein).

nuts Hard-shelled fruit of a wide variety of trees, e.g. ALMONDS, BRAZIL, CASHEW, PEANUT, WALNUT, all have high fat content, 45–60%; high protein content, 15–20%; 15–20% carbohydrate. The CHESTNUT is an exception, with 3% fat and 3% protein, being largely carbohydrate, 37%. A number of nuts are grown specially for their oils; see OILSEED.

nyctalopia See NIGHT BLINDNESS.

nystagmus Paralysis of the eye muscles; occurs e.g. in the WERNICKE–KORSAKOFF SYNDROME due to VITAMIN B_1 deficiency.

O

oats Grain from *Avena* spp, esp *A. sativa*, *A. steritis* and *A. strigosa*. Oatmeal, ground oats; oatflour, ground and bran removed; groats, husked oats; Embden groats, crushed groats; Scotch oats, groats cut into granules of various sizes; Sussex ground oats, very finely ground oats; rolled oats, crushed by rollers and partially precooked.

obesity Excessive accumulation of body fat. A BODY MASS INDEX (BMI) above 30kg/m^2 is considered to be obesity (and above 40 gross obesity). The desirable range of BMI for optimum life expectancy is 20–25; between 25–30 is considered to be OVER-

WEIGHT rather than obesity. People more than 50% above desirable WEIGHT are twice as likely to die prematurely as those within the desirable weight range. Overweight is often defined as 110–119% of standard, and obesity as 120% or more of standard range.

See also ANORECTIC DRUGS.

ob **gene** See LEPTIN.

obstipation Extreme and persistent CONSTIPATION caused by obstruction of the intestinal tract.

occlusal The biting surface of a premolar or molar tooth.

ochratoxins MYCOTOXINS formed by *Aspergillus* and *Penicillium* spp growing on cereals. They have been associated with nephropathy in both animals and human beings, with evidence that they are carcinogenic and teratogenic. They can accumulate in relatively high concentrations in blood and tissues of monogastric animals but are cleaved by protozoan enzymes in ruminants.

octave A cask for wine containing 1/8 of a PIPE, about 59 L (13 imperial gallons).

octopus Marine creature (*Octopus* spp) with beak-like mouth surrounded by eight tentacles bearing suckers.

odontoblasts Cells in teeth, lining the pulp and forming dentine.

odoratism Disease produced by feeding seeds of the sweet pea, *Lathyrus odoratus*, to rats. The toxin β-aminopropionitrile is present in both *L. odoratus* and the singletary pea (*L. pusillus*), but not the chickling pea, *L. sativa*, which causes LATHYRISM in man. The toxin inhibits lysyl oxidase (EC 1.4.3.13) which oxidises lysine to ALLYSINE for cross-linkage of collagen and elastin, leading to loss of elasticity of elastin and potentially to rupture of the aorta.

oedema Excess fluid in the body; may be caused by cardiac, renal or hepatic failure and by starvation (famine oedema).

oenin An ANTHOCYANIDIN from the skin of purple grapes.

oesophagus The gullet, a muscular tube ~23 cm long, between the pharynx and stomach.

See also GASTROINTESTINAL TRACT.

oestradiol, oestriol, oestrone See OESTROGENS.

oestrogens The female sex hormones; chemically they are STEROIDS, although non-steroidal compounds also have oestrogen activity, including the synthetic compounds stilboestrol and hexoestrol. These have been used for chemical caponisation (see CAPON) of cockerels and to increase the growth rate of cattle. Compounds with oestrogen activity are found in a variety of plants; collectively these are known as phyto-oestrogens.

offal Corruption of 'off-fall'.

(1) With reference to meat, the term includes all parts that are cut away when the carcass is dressed, including liver, kidneys, brain, spleen, pancreas, thymus, tripe and tongue. Known in US as organ meats or variety meat.

(2) With reference to wheat, offal is the bran discarded when milled to white flour. See also WHEATFEED.

ohmic heating Sterilisation by heat generated by passing an electric current through the food or mixture.

oilseed A wide variety of seeds are grown as a source of oils, e.g. cottonseed, sesame, groundnut, sunflower, soya, and nuts such as coconut, groundnut and palm. After extraction of the oil the residue is a valuable source of protein, especially for animal feedingstuffs, oilseed cake.

oils, essential See ESSENTIAL OILS.

oils, fixed The TRIACYLGLYCEROLS (triglycerides), the edible oils, as distinct from the volatile or ESSENTIAL OILS.

okra Also known as gumbo, bamya, bamies and ladies' fingers; the edible seed pods of *Hibiscus esculentus*. Small ridged mucilaginous pods resembling a small cucumber, grown in South America, West Indies and India; used in soups and stews. Two varieties: oblong are gomba, round are bamya.

Composition/100 g: 117 kJ (28 kcal), protein 2.5 g, fat 0.9 g (42.8% saturated, 14.2% mono-, 42.8% polyunsaturated), carbohydrate 2.7 g (2.3 g sugars, 0.5 g starch), dietary fibre 4.1 g, nsp 3.6 g, Na 5 mg, K 310 mg, Ca 120 mg, Mg 57 mg, P 54 mg, Fe 0.6 mg, Cu 0.09 mg, Zn 0.5 mg, Se 1 µg, vitamin A 77 µg (465 µg carotene), B_1 0.13 mg, B_2 0.05 mg, niacin 1.2 mg, B_6 0.19 mg, folate 46 µg, pantothenate 0.2 mg, C 16 mg. A 50 g serving is a source of folate, vitamin C.

olallie berry Cross between LOGANBERRY and YOUNGBERRY.

Olean See OLESTRA.

oleandomycin Antibiotic sometimes used as an additive in chicken feed.

oleic acid Mono-unsaturated FATTY ACID (C18:1 ω9); found to some extent in most fats; olive and rapeseed oils are especially rich sources.

oleomargarine See MARGARINE.

oleo oil See PREMIER JUS; TALLOW, RENDERED.

oleoresins In the preparation of some spices such as pepper, ginger and capsicum, the aromatic material is extracted with solvents which are evaporated off, leaving behind thick oily products known as oleoresins.

oleostearin See PREMIER JUS; TALLOW, RENDERED.

286

oleovitamin Preparation of fish liver oil or vegetable oil containing one or more of the fat-soluble VITAMINS.

Olestra (Olean) Trade name for a sucrose polyester used as a FAT REPLACER since it has the cooking and organoleptic properties of triacylglycerol, but is not hydrolysed by LIPASE, and not absorbed from the intestinal tract.

olfaction The sense or process of smelling. Sensory cells in the mucous membrane lining the nasal cavity communicate with the central nervous system via the olfactory (first cranial) nerve.

oligoallergenic diet Comprising very few foods, or an elemental diet used to diagnose whether particular symptoms are the result of allergic response to food.

oligodipsia Reduced sense of thirst.

oligodynamic Sterilising effect of traces of certain metals. For example, SILVER at a concentration of 1 in 5 million will kill *Escherichia coli* and staphylococci in 3 h.

oligopeptides See PEPTIDES.

oligosaccharides CARBOHYDRATES composed of 3–10 monosaccharide units (with more than 10 units they are termed POLYSACCHARIDES).

See also PREBIOTICS.

olive Fruit of the evergreen tree, *Olea europaea*; picked unripe when green or ripe when they have turned dark blue or purplish, and usually pickled in brine. Olives have been known since ancient times. The tree is extremely slow growing and continues to fruit for many years; there are claims that trees are still fruiting after 1000 years.

Composition /100 g (pickled in brine): 343 kJ (82 kcal), protein 0.7 g, fat 8.8 g (14.4% saturated, 73.4% mono-, 12% polyunsaturated), carbohydrate 0 g, dietary fibre 3.2 g, nsp 2.3 g, Na 1800 mg, K 73 mg, Ca 49 mg, Mg 18 mg, P 14 mg, Fe 0.8 mg, Cu 0.18 mg, vitamin A 24 µg (145 µg carotene), E 1.6 mg, niacin 0.1 mg, B_6 0.02 mg. Serving 25 g (eight olives).

olive oil Pressed from ripe OLIVES, the fruit of *Olea europaea*. Virgin olive oil is not refined and the flavour varies with the locality where it is grown. Other types have been refined to varying extents. Used in cooking, as salad oil, for canning sardines and for margarine manufacture. Apart from the special flavour of olive oil it is valued nutritionally because of its high content, 70%, of mono-unsaturates (mainly oleic acid) and its low content, 15%, of SATURATES; also relatively rich in SQUALENE, which reduces endogenous synthesis of CHOLESTEROL.

omasum See RUMEN.

omega fatty acids Polyunsaturated FATTY ACIDS (PUFA) are described by chain length, number of double bonds and (in biochemistry and nutrition) by the position of their first double bond counting from the terminal methyl group, labelled as omega (ω or n-). In systematic chemical nomenclature the position of a double bond is numbered from the carboxyl end (carbon-1), but what is important nutritionally is that human enzymes can desaturate fatty acids between an existing double bond and the carboxyl group, but not between an existing double bond and the methyl group.

There are three series of PUFA: $\omega3$, $\omega6$ and $\omega9$, derived from linolenic, linoleic and oleic acids, respectively. The first two cannot be synthesised in the body and are the precursors of two families of EICOSANOIDS.

See also FATTY ACIDS, ESSENTIAL; Table 7.

omega-3 ($\omega3$) marine triglycerides A mixture of triacylglycerols (triglycerides) rich in two polyunsaturated FATTY ACIDS, eicosapentaenoic acid (EPA, C20:5 $\omega3$) and docosohexaenoic (DHA, C22:6 $\omega3$).

omentum Double layer of PERITONEUM attached to the STOMACH and linking it to other abdominal organs.

omophagia Eating of raw or uncooked food.

oncogene Any gene associated with the development of cancer. Viral oncogenes are related to, and possibly derived from, normal mammalian genes (proto-oncogenes) that are involved in the regulation of cell proliferation and growth. Mutation to yield an active oncogene involves loss of the normal regulation of the expression of the proto-oncogene.

onglet French; cut of beef corresponding to top of the skirt.

onion Bulb of *Allium cepa*; many varieties with white, brown and red (purple) skins.

Composition /100g: 150kJ (36kcal), protein 1.2g, fat 0.2g, carbohydrate 7.9g (5.6g sugars), dietary fibre 1.5g, nsp 1.4g, Na 3mg, K 160mg, Ca 25mg, Mg 4mg, P 30mg, Fe 0.3mg, Cu 0.05mg, Zn 0.2mg, Se 1μg, I 3μg, vitamin A 1μg (10μg carotene), E 0.3mg, B_1 0.13mg, niacin 1mg, B_6 0.2mg, folate 17μg, pantothenate 0.1mg, biotin 0.9μg, C 5mg. A 160g serving (one medium) is a source of vitamin B_1, B_6, folate, C.

onion, Egyptian (tree onion) *Allium cepa* Proliform group. Type that produces clusters of aerial bulbs which develop shoots to form multitiered plant; the aerial bulbs are cropped.

onion, everlasting *Allium perutile*, similar to Welsh ONION.

onion, green See ONION, SPRING; ONION, WELSH.

onion, Japanese bunching *Allium fistulosum*, similar to Welsh onion, but larger.

onion, perennial See ONION, WELSH.

onion, spring Young plants of *Allium cepa*, generally eaten whole (developing bulb and leaves) as a salad vegetable. Also known as salad onions or scallions.

Composition /100 g: 96 kJ (23 kcal), protein 2 g, fat 0.5 g, carbohydrate 3 g (2.8 g sugars, 0.2 g starch), nsp 1.5 g, Na 7 mg, K 260 mg, Ca 39 mg, Mg 12 mg, P 29 mg, Fe 1.9 mg, Cu 0.06 mg, Zn 0.4 mg, vitamin A 103 µg (620 µg carotene), B_1 0.05 mg, B_2 0.03 mg, niacin 1 mg, B_6 0.13 mg, folate 54 µg, pantothenate 0.1 mg, C 26 mg. Serving 20 g (two onions).

onion, Welsh The perennial onion, *Allium cepa perutile*, leaves are cropped, leaving the plant to grow. Similar to, but smaller, than the Japanese bunching onion, *Allium fistulosum*. Also sometimes used as an alternative name for the LEEK.

opisthorchiasis Infection with the FLUKE *Opisthorchis felineus*; normally a bile duct parasite of fish-eating mammals, but human infection can occur.

opsomania Craving for special food.

optic Dispenser attached to bottles of spirits, etc in bars to ensure delivery of a precise volume.

optical activity (optical rotation) The ability of some compounds to rotate the plane of polarised light because of the asymmetry of the molecule. If the plane of light is rotated to the right, the substance is dextrorotatory and is designated by the prefix (+); if laevorotatory, the prefix is (−). A mixture of the two forms is optically inactive and is termed racemic.

Sucrose is dextrorotatory but is hydrolysed to glucose (dextrorotatory) and fructose, which is more strongly laevorotatory so hydrolysis changes optical activity from (+) to (−); hence, the mixture of glucose and fructose is termed invert sugar.

The obsolete notation for (+) was *d*- and for (−) was *l*-; this is quite separate from D- and L-, which are used to designate stereoisomerism, see D-, L- AND DL-.

opuntia See PRICKLY PEAR.

oral rehydration Administration of an isotonic solution of salt and glucose (or sucrose) to replace fluid and electrolytes lost in DIARRHOEA.

orange CITRUS fruit, from the subtropical tree *Citrus sinensis*.

Composition /100 g: 108 kJ (26 kcal), protein 0.8 g, fat 0.1 g, carbohydrate 5.9 g (5.9 g sugars), dietary fibre 1.3 g, nsp 1.2 g, Na 3 mg, K 110 mg, Ca 33 mg, Mg 7 mg, P 15 mg, Fe 0.1 mg, Cu 0.03 mg, Zn 0.1 mg, Se 1 µg, I 1 µg, vitamin A 3 µg (20 µg carotene), E 0.2 mg, B_1 0.08 mg, B_2 0.03 mg, niacin 0.4 mg, B_6 0.07 mg, folate 22 µg, pantothenate 0.3 mg, biotin 0.7 µg, C 38 mg. A 160 g serving is a source of folate; rich source of vitamin C.

orange, bitter The fruit of the subtropical tree *Citrus aurantium*; known as Seville orange in Spain, bigaradier in France, melangol in Italy and khush-khash in Israel. Used mainly as root stock, because of its resistance to the gummosis disease of citrus. The fruit is too acid to be edible; used in manufacture of MARMALADE; the peel oil is used in the LIQUEUR curaçao; the peel and flower oils (neroli oil) and the oils from the green twigs (petit-grain oils) are used in perfumery.

orange butter   Chopped whole orange, cooked, sweetened and homogenised.

orcanella   See ALKANNET.

oreganum   Or Mexican sage; see MARJORAM.

orekita   See MEZETHAKIA.

orexins   Group of neuropeptides, isolated from the lateral hypothalamic feeding centre, that stimulate appetite and food consumption.

organ meat   See OFFAL (1).

organic   (1) Chemically the term means substances containing carbon in the molecule (with the exception of carbonates and cyanide). Substances of animal and vegetable origin are organic; MINERALS are inorganic.

(2) The term organic foods refers to 'organically grown foods', meaning plants grown without the use of (synthetic) pesticides, fungicides or inorganic fertilisers, without the use of preservatives. Foodstuffs grown on land that has not been treated with chemical fertilisers, herbicides or pesticides for at least three years. Organic meat is from animals fed on organically grown crops without the use of growth promoters, with only a limited number of medicines to treat disease and commonly maintained under traditional, non-intensive, conditions.

organoleptic   Sensory properties, i.e. those that can be detected by the sense organs. For foods used particularly of the combination of TASTE, texture and stringency (perceived in the mouth) and aroma (perceived in the nose).

orlistat   Drug used in the treatment of OBESITY; it inhibits gastric and pancreatic LIPASES (EC 3.1.1.3) and prevents absorption of much of the dietary fat. Trade name Xenical.

ormer   See ABALONE.

ornithine   An AMINO ACID that occurs as a metabolic intermediate (e.g. in the synthesis of UREA), but not involved in protein synthesis, M_r 132.2, pK_a 1.71, 8.69, 10.76. Of no nutritional importance, since it is not found in proteins and can be synthesised in adequate amounts in the body.

orotic acid   An intermediate in the biosynthesis of PYRIMIDINES; a growth factor for some microorganisms and at one time called vitamin B_{13}. There is no evidence that it is a human dietary requirement.

ortanique   A Jamaican CITRUS fruit; cross between orange and tangerine.

Composition /100g: 205 kJ (49 kcal), protein 1 g, fat 0.2 g, carbohydrate 11.7 g (11.7 g sugars), dietary fibre 1.8 g, nsp 1.7 g, Na 5 mg, K 150 mg, Ca 41 mg, Mg 10 mg, P 21 mg, Fe 0.4 mg, Cu 0.05 mg, Zn 0.1 mg, I 2 μg, vitamin A 20 μg (120 μg carotene), E 0.2 mg, B_1 0.1 mg, B_2 0.04 mg, niacin 0.5 mg, B_6 0.1 mg, folate 31 μg, pantothenate 0.4 mg, biotin 1 μg, C 50 mg. A 95 g serving is a source of folate; rich source of vitamin C.

orthophenylphenol (OPP)   A compound used for the treatment of CITRUS fruit and NUTS after harvesting to prevent the growth of moulds (E-231). DIPHENYL (E-230) is also used.

ortolan   Small wild song bird, *Emberisa hortulana*, still caught in the wild and eaten in parts of Europe, where it is prized for its delicate flavour.

oryzenin   The major protein of RICE.

Oslo breakfast   A breakfast requiring no preparation, introduced in Oslo, Norway, in 1929 for school children before classes started. It consisted of rye biscuit, brown bread, butter or vitaminised margarine, whey cheese and cod liver oil paste, 0.3 L milk, raw carrot, apple, half orange.

osmazome   Obsolete name given to an aqueous extract of meat regarded as the 'pure essence of meat'.

osmolality   Concentration of osmotically active particles per kg of solvent.

osmolarity   Concentration of osmotically active particles per litre of solution.

osmole   Unit of OSMOTIC PRESSURE. Equals molecular mass of a solute, in grams, divided by number of ions when it dissociates in solution.

osmophiles   Microorganisms that can flourish under conditions of high OSMOTIC PRESSURE, e.g. in jams, honey, brine pickles; especially yeasts (also called xerophilic yeasts).

osmosis   The passage of water through a semipermeable MEMBRANE, from a region of low concentration of solutes to one of higher concentration. Reverse osmosis (hyperfiltration) is the passage of water from a more concentrated to a less concentrated solution through a semipermeable membrane by the application of pressure. Used for desalination of seawater, concentration of fruit juices and processing of whey. The membranes commonly used are cellulose acetate or polyamide of very small pore size, 10^{-4}–10^{-3} μm.

See also OSMOTIC PRESSURE.

osmotic dehydration   Partial dehydration of fruit by use of a concentrated sugar solution to extract water.

osmotic pressure   The pressure required to prevent the passage of water through a semipermeable MEMBRANE from a region of low concentration of solutes to one of higher concentration, by OSMOSIS.

ossein The organic matrix of the bone left behind when the mineral salts are removed by solution in dilute acid. Mainly collagen, and hydrolysed by boiling water to gelatine.

osteoblasts Cells that are responsible for the formation of bone. Differentiation of osteoblast precursor cells is stimulated by VITAMIN D, after OSTEOCLASTS have been activated.

osteocalcin Calcium-binding protein in bone and cartilage which contains γ-carboxyglutamate (Gla) residues formed by a VITAMIN K-dependent reaction; synthesis regulated by VITAMIN D.

osteoclasts Cells that resorb calcified bone. Activated (*inter alia*) by VITAMIN D to maintain plasma concentration of calcium.

osteomalacia The adult equivalent of RICKETS; bone demineralisation due to deficiency of VITAMIN D and hence inadequate absorption of calcium and loss of calcium from the bones.

osteoporosis Degeneration of the bones with advancing age due to loss of bone mineral and protein; this is largely a result of loss of HORMONES with increasing age (oestrogens in women and testosterone in men). Although there is negative CALCIUM balance (net loss of calcium from the body) this is the result of osteoporosis, not its cause, and there is little evidence that calcium supplements affect the progression of the disease. A high calcium intake in early life may be beneficial, since this may result in greater bone density at maturity, but the most important factor is regular exercise to stimulate bone metabolism. Vitamin D supplements do not improve osteoporosis, and may exacerbate the condition.

Ostermilk Trade name for dried milk for infant feeding. Ostermilk No. 1 is half-cream; No. 2 is full-cream.

ovalbumin The albumin of egg white; comprises 55% of the total solids.

Ovaltine Trade name for a preparation of MALT EXTRACT, milk, eggs, cocoa and soya, for consumption as a beverage when added to milk. Fortified with thiamin, vitamin D and niacin.

oven spring The sudden increases in the volume of a dough during the first 10–12 min of baking, due to increased rate of fermentation and expansion of gases.

overrun In ice-cream manufacture, the percentage increase in the volume of the mix caused by the beating in of air. Optimum overrun, 70–100%. To prevent excessive aeration US regulations state that ice-cream must weigh 4.5 lb/gallon (0.48 kg/L).

overweight Excessive accumulation of body fat, but not so great as to be classified as OBESITY.

ovomucin   A carbohydrate–protein complex in egg white, responsible for the firmness of egg white, 1–3% of the total solids.

ovomucoid   A protein of egg white, 12% of the total solids. It inhibits the digestive enzyme TRYPSIN, but is inactivated by gastric PEPSIN.

oxalic acid   A dicarboxylic acid, chemically COOH—COOH. Poisonous in large amounts; present especially in spinach, chocolate, rhubarb and nuts. The toxicity of rhubarb leaves is due to their high content of oxalic acid.

See also HYPEROXALURIA.

oxidases (oxygenases)   Enzymes that oxidise compounds by removing hydrogen and reacting directly with oxygen to form water (or sometimes hydrogen peroxide). They thus differ from dehydrogenases, which transfer the hydrogen to a COENZYME.

oxidation   The chemical process of removing electrons from an element or compound (e.g. the oxidation of iron compounds from ferrous, Fe^{2+} to ferric, Fe^{3+}); frequently together with the removal of hydrogen ions (H^+). The reverse process, the addition of electrons or hydrogen, is reduction. In biological oxidation and reduction reactions, CYTOCHROMES act to transfer electrons, while COENZYMES derived from the vitamins NIACIN and VITAMIN B_2 are hydrogen carriers, transferring both electrons and H^+ ions.

oxidative phosphorylation   The formation of ATP from ADP and phosphate in the MITOCHONDRIA, linked to the ELECTRON TRANSPORT CHAIN and the oxidation of metabolic fuels.

See also UNCOUPLING PROTEIN.

Oxo   Trade name for a dried preparation of hydrolysed meat, meat extract, salt and cereal in cube form, used as a drink or gravy.

Composition /100 g: 958 kJ (229 kcal), protein 38.3 g, fat 3.4 g, carbohydrate 12 g (12 g starch), Na 10 300 mg, K 730 mg, Ca 180 mg, Mg 59 mg, P 360 mg, Fe 24.5 mg, Cu 0.71 mg, I 44 µg. Serving 5 g.

oxycalorimeter   Instrument for measuring the oxygen consumed and carbon dioxide produced when a food is burned, as distinct from the CALORIMETER, which measures the heat produced.

oxycarotenoids   See XANTHOPHYLLS.

oxygenases   See OXIDASES.

oxyhaemoglobin   HAEMOGLOBIN combined with oxygen; the form in which oxygen is transported in the blood.

oxymyoglobin   MYOGLOBIN is the muscle oxygen-binding protein; it takes up oxygen to form oxymyoglobin, which is bright red, while myoglobin itself is purplish-red. The surface of fresh meat that is exposed to oxygen is bright red from the oxymyoglobin, while the interior of the meat is darker in colour where the myoglobin is not oxygenated.

oxyntic cells See PARIETAL CELLS.

oxytetracycline See TETRACYCLINE.

oxythiamin Antimetabolite of thiamin, used in experimental studies of VITAMIN B₁ deficiency; it inhibits thiamin pyrophosphokinase (EC 2.7.6.2). Unlike PYRITHIAMIN it does not enter the central nervous system.

oxyuriasis Infestation of the large intestine with PINWORM.

oyster Marine bivalve MOLLUSC, *Ostreidae* and *Crassostrea* spp. Composition /100 g: 272 kJ (65 kcal), protein 10.8 g, fat 1.3 g, cholesterol 57 mg, carbohydrate 2.7 g, Na 510 mg, K 260 mg, Ca 140 mg, Mg 42 mg, P 210 mg, Fe 5.7 mg, Cu 7.5 mg, Zn 59.2 mg, Se 23 μg, I 60 μg, vitamin A 75 μg, D 1 μg, E 0.9 mg, B₁ 0.15 mg, B₂ 0.19 mg, niacin 4.1 mg, B₆ 0.16 mg, B₁₂ 17 μg, pantothenate 0.4 mg, biotin 10 μg. A 60 g serving (six oysters weighed without shells) is a source of protein, vitamin D, niacin, Ca; good source of vitamin Fe, I; rich source of vitamin B₁₂, Cu, Se, Zn.

oyster crabs American; small young crabs found inside oysters, cooked and eaten whole, including the soft shell.

oyster mushroom *Pleurotus ostreatus*, see MUSHROOMS.

oyster plant (vegetable oyster) See SALSIFY.

ozone O₃, a powerful germicide, used to sterilise water and in antiseptic ice for preserving fish.

P

P. 4000 A class of synthetic SWEETENERS, chemically nitro-amino alkoxybenzenes. One member of the group, propoxyamino nitrobenzene is 4100 times as sweet as saccharin, but these compounds are not considered harmless and are not permitted in foods.

PA 3679 Designation of a putrefactive anaerobic bacterium widely used in investigations of heat sterilisation.

PABA See *PARA*-AMINO BENZOIC ACID.

pacificarins Compounds present in foods that resist microorganisms; they may be of microbial origin or synthesised by the plant itself. Also known as phytoncides.

packed cell volume (PCV) See HAEMATOCRIT.

paddy RICE in the husk after threshing; also known as rough rice.

pak choy Chinese cabbage or Chinese leaves, *Brassica chinensis*.

PAL See PHYSICAL ACTIVITY LEVEL.

Palatinat Trade name for ISOMALT.

palatinose Isomaltulose, a DISACCHARIDE, α-1,6-glucosyl-fructose.

palatone See MALTOL.

Palestine bee See BEE WINE.

Palestine soup English, nineteenth century, made from Jerusalem

ARTICHOKES and named in the mistaken belief that the artichokes came from Jerusalem.

palmitic acid   A saturated FATTY ACID with 16 carbon atoms (C16:0), common in the triglycerides of many animal and vegetable fats.

palmitoleic acid   A mono-unsaturated fatty acid with 16 carbon atoms (C16:1 ω9), widespread in fats and oils.

palm kernel oil   One of the major oils of commerce, widely used in cooking fats and margarines; oil extracted from the kernel of the nut of the oil palm, *Elaeis guineensis*. Pale in colour in contrast to 'red' PALM OIL from the outer part of the nut; 80% saturated, 15% mono-, 5% polyunsaturated.

palm oil   From outer fibrous pulp of the fruit of the oil palm, *Elaeis guineensis*. Coloured red because of very high content of α-carotene (30 mg per 100 g) and β-carotene (30 mg) together with about 60 mg TOCOPHEROLS but this is usually removed to produce a pale oil; 45% saturated, 40% mono-, 10% polyunsaturated.

palm, wild date   *Phoenix sylvestris*, a relative of the true date palm, *P. dactylifera*, grown in India as a source of sugar, obtained from the sap.

palm wine   Fermented sap from various palm trees, especially date and coconut palms.

pan   See BETEL.

panada   Mixture of fat, flour and liquid (stock or milk) mixed to a thick paste; used to bind mixtures such as chopped meat, and also as the basis of soufflés and choux PASTRY.

panary fermentation   Yeast fermentation of dough in breadmaking.

pancreas   Abdominal gland with two functions: the endocrine pancreas (the islets of Langerhans) secretes the HORMONES INSULIN and GLUCAGON; the exocrine pancreas (acinar cells) secretes the PANCREATIC JUICE. Known by the butcher as sweetbread or gut sweetbread, as distinct from chest sweetbread which is thymus.

pancreatic juice   The alkaline digestive juice produced by the pancreas and secreted into the duodenum. It contains the inactive precursors of a number of PROTEIN digestive enzymes.

Trypsinogen is activated to trypsin (EC 3.4.21.4) by ENTEROPEPTIDASE (EC 3.4.21.9) in the intestinal lumen; in turn, trypsin activates the other enzyme precursors: chymotrypsinogen to chymotrypsin (EC 3.4.21.1), pro-elastase to elastase (EC 3.4.21.36), procarboxypeptidases to carboxypeptidases (EC 3.4.17.1 and 2). Also contains LIPASE (EC 3.1.1.3), AMYLASE (EC 3.2.1.1) and nucleases.

Secretion of alkaline pancreatic juice is stimulated by the hormone secretin; secretion of pancreatic juice rich in enzymes is stimulated by the hormone CHOLECYSTOKININ.

pancreatin Preparation made from the pancreas of animals containing the enzymes of PANCREATIC JUICE. Used to replace pancreatic enzymes in pancreatic insufficiency and CYSTIC FIBROSIS as an aid to digestion.

pancreozymin Obsolete name for CHOLECYSTOKININ.

pan dowdy American; baked apple sponge pudding, served with the apple side up.

pangamic acid N-Di-isopropyl glucuronate, claimed to be an ANTIOXIDANT, and to speed recovery from fatigue. Sometimes called vitamin B_{15}, but no evidence that it is a dietary essential, nor that it has any metabolic function.

panthenol The alcohol of PANTOTHENIC ACID; biologically active.

pantoprazole See PROTON PUMP.

pantothenic acid A vitamin with no numerical designation. Chemically, the β-alanine derivative of pantoic acid. Required for the synthesis of COENZYME A (and hence essential for the metabolism of fats, carbohydrates and amino acids) and of acyl carrier protein (and hence essential for the synthesis of fatty acids).

Dietary deficiency is unknown; it is widely distributed in all living cells. Human requirements are not known with any certainty; average intakes are between 3–7 mg/day, which is therefore considered to be a SAFE AND ADEQUATE level of intake. Experimental deficiency signs in rats include greying of the hair (hence at one time known as the anti-grey hair factor; there is no evidence that it affects greying of human hair with age). Experimental deficiency in human beings leads to fatigue, headache, muscle weakness and gastrointestinal disturbances.

See also BURNING FOOT SYNDROME.

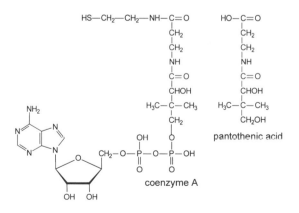

papain   Proteolytic enzyme (see PROTEOLYSIS) (EC 3.4.22.2) from the juice of the PAWPAW (*Carica papaya*) used in tenderising meat; sometimes called vegetable pepsin. The enzyme is obtained as the dried latex on the skin of the fruit by scratching it while still on the tree, and collecting the flow. The rate of reaction is slow at room temperature, increasing to maximum activity at 80°C and rapidly inactivated at higher temperatures; hence, the papain continues to tenderise the meat during the early stages of cooking.

papaw   Purple fruit of *Asiminia triloba*, related to the CUSTARD APPLE; distinct from the PAWPAW or papaya.

papaya   See PAWPAW.

papillote, en   Made or served in a paper case.

Papin's digester   Early version of the pressure cooker. Named after D Papin, French physicist 1647–1712; originally invented for the purpose of softening bones for the preparation of GELATINE. See AUTOCLAVE.

paprika   See PEPPER.

PAR   See PHYSICAL ACTIVITY RATIO.

***para*-amino benzoic acid (PABA)**   Essential growth factor for microorganisms. It forms part of the molecule of FOLIC ACID and is therefore required for the synthesis of this vitamin. Mammals cannot synthesise folic acid, and PABA has no other known function; there is no evidence that it is a human dietary requirement. Sulphanilamides (sulpha drugs) are chemical analogues of PABA, and exert their antibacterial action by antagonising PABA utilisation.

parabens   Methyl, ethyl and propyl esters of *p*-hydroxybenzoic acid used together with their sodium salts as antimicrobials in food (E-214–219). Effective over a wide range of pH; more effective against moulds and yeast than against bacteria.

paracasein   Obsolete name for milk CASEIN after precipitation.

paracrine   Production by a cell of locally acting HORMONE-like substances that act on nearby cells.
See also AUTOCRINE; ENDOCRINE GLANDS.

paraffin, medicinal (liquid)   See MEDICINAL PARAFFIN.

Paraflow   Trade name for a plate heat exchanger used for pasteurising liquids.

parageusia   Abnormality of the sense of taste.
See also DYSGEUSIA; GUSTIN; HYPOGEUSIA.

parakeratosis   Disease of swine characterised by cessation of growth, erythema, seborrhoea and hyperkeratosis of the skin; due to ZINC deficiency and possibly to changes in essential FATTY ACID metabolism.

paralactic acid   See SARCOLACTIC ACID.

paralytic shellfish poisoning   Caused by shellfish that have accumulated toxins from the dinoflagellate plankton, *Gonyaulax* spp.

parasol mushroom   *Macrolepiota procera*, see MUSHROOMS.

paratha   Indian wholewheat unleavened bread.

parathormone   Commonly used as an abbreviation for the parathyroid hormone; correctly a trade name for a pharmaceutical preparation of the hormone.

parathyroid hormone   Hormone secreted by the parathyroid glands; four glands situated in the neck near to the thyroid gland but not connected with its function. The hormone is secreted in response to a fall in plasma calcium, and acts on the kidney to increase the formation of the active metabolite of VITAMIN D (calcitriol), leading to an increase in plasma calcium by increasing intestinal absorption and mobilising the mineral from bones. It also reduces urinary excretion of phosphate.

paratyphoid   See TYPHOID.

parboil   Partially cook. Of special interest in nutrition is the parboiling of brown rice, steaming rice in the husk before milling. The water-soluble vitamins diffuse from the husk into the grain; when the rice is polished, it contains far more of these vitamins than polished raw rice.

parchita   See PASSION FRUIT.

parenteral nutrition   Slow infusion of solution of nutrients into the veins through a catheter. This may be partial, to supplement food and nutrient intake, or total (TPN, total parenteral nutrition), providing the sole source of energy and nutrient intake for patients with major intestinal problems. Parenteral meaning 'not enteral', or through the intestinal tract.

See also ENTERAL NUTRITION; NUTRIENT ENEMATA.

pareve (parve)   Jewish term for dishes containing neither milk nor meat. Orthodox Jewish law prohibits mixing of milk and meat foods or the consumption of milk products for 3 h after a meat meal.

See also MILCHIG; FLEISHIG.

parietal cells   Cells of the gastric mucosa that secrete gastric ACID and INTRINSIC FACTOR. Also known as oxyntic cells.

See also ACHLORHYDRIA; ANAEMIA, PERNICIOUS.

parillin   Highly toxic glycoside from SARSAPARILLA root; consists of glucose, rhamnose and parigenin. Also known as smilacin.

parity   The number of pregnancies that a woman has had that have resulted in the birth of an infant capable of survival.

See also PRIMIPARA.

parmesan cheese   English (and French) name for the hard Italian cheese parmigiana. Made from semi-skimmed cow's milk cooked with RENNET, dried for at least six months. When two years old it is called vecchio, stravecchio is 3 years, stravecchione 4 years old. It is hard and usually served on dishes grated.

PARNUTS   An EU term for foods prepared for particular nutritional purposes (intended for people with disturbed metabolism or in special physiological condition or young children). Also called dietetic foods.

paromomycin   ANTIBIOTIC used to treat intestinal bacterial infections and amoebic DYSENTERY.

parosmia   Any disorder of the sense of smell.

parotid glands   Pair of SALIVARY GLANDS situated in front of the ears, with ducts that open in the cheek, opposite the second molar teeth.

parsley   Leaves of the herb *Petroselinum crispum*, *P. hertense* or *P. sativum*.

Composition/100 g: 142 kJ (34 kcal), protein 3 g, fat 1.3 g, carbohydrate 2.7 g (2.3 g sugars, 0.4 g starch), dietary fibre 8.2 g, nsp 5 g, Na 33 mg, K 760 mg, Ca 200 mg, Mg 23 mg, P 64 mg, Fe 7.7 mg, Cu 0.03 mg, Zn 0.7 mg, Se 1 μg, vitamin A 673 μg (4040 μg carotene), E 1.7 mg, B_1 0.23 mg, B_2 0.06 mg, niacin 1.5 mg, B_6 0.09 mg, folate 170 μg, pantothenate 0.3 mg, biotin 0.4 μg, C 190 mg. A 5 g serving is a source of vitamin C.

parsley, Hamburg   Root of *Petroselinum crispum* var *tuberosum*, grown for its root (also called turnip-rooted parsley); similar in appearance to PARSNIP.

parsnip   Root of *Pastinaca sativa*, eaten as a vegetable.

Composition/100 g: 276 kJ (66 kcal), protein 1.6 g, fat 1.2 g, carbohydrate 12.9 g (5.9 g sugars, 6.4 g starch), dietary fibre 4.4 g, nsp 4.7 g, Na 4 mg, K 350 mg, Ca 50 mg, Mg 23 mg, P 76 mg, Fe 0.6 mg, Cu 0.04 mg, Zn 0.3 mg, vitamin A 5 μg (30 μg carotene), E 1 mg, B_1 0.07 mg, B_2 0.01 mg, niacin 1.1 mg, B_6 0.09 mg, folate 48 μg, pantothenate 0.4 mg, C 10 mg. A 65 g serving is a source of folate, vitamin C.

partial glyceride esters   See ACETOGLYCERIDES.

partridge   GAME bird, *Perdix perdix* and related species.

Composition/100 g: 531 kJ (127 kcal), protein 22 g, fat 4.3 g (26.8% saturated, 48.7% mono-, 24.3% polyunsaturated), carbohydrate 0 g, Na 60 mg, K 240 mg, Ca 28 mg, Mg 22 mg, P 190 mg, Fe 4.6 mg, vitamin niacin 4.1 mg. A 275 g serving ($^1/_2$ bird weighed with bone) is a good source of Mg; rich source of protein, niacin, Fe.

parts per million (ppm)   Method of describing small concentrations and means exactly what the term says; = mg/kg.

pascal (Pa)   SI unit of pressure = 1 Newton/m^2.

passion fruit   Also known as parchita, granadilla and water lemon; fruit of the tropical vine, *Passiflora* spp. Purple or greenish-yellow when ripe, watery pulp containing small seeds.

Composition/100 g: 92 kJ (22 kcal), protein 1.7 g, fat 0.2 g, carbohydrate 3.5 g (3.5 g sugars), nsp 2 g, Na 12 mg, K 120 mg, Ca 7 mg, Mg 18 mg, P 39 mg, Fe 0.8 mg, Zn 0.5 mg, vitamin A 76 µg (460 µg carotene), B_1 0.02 mg, B_2 0.07 mg, niacin 1.1 mg, C 14 mg. Serving 25 g.

pasta (Alimentary paste); dried dough, traditionally made with hard wheat (semolina) but soft wheat may be added, sometimes with egg and milk. Spinach or tomato may be added to the dough to give a green or red colour. The dough is partly dried in hot air, then more slowly. Sold both completely dry, when it can be stored for a long period, or 'fresh', i.e. less dried and keeping for only a week or so.

Made in numerous shapes: spaghetti is a solid rod about 2 mm in diameter; vermicelli is about one-third this thickness, ravioli (envelopes stuffed with meat or cheese), fettucine and linguini (ribbons), and a range of twists, spirals and other shapes. Macaroni is tubular shaped, about 5 mm in diameter; at 10 mm it is known as zitoni, and at 15 mm fovantini or maccaroncelli. Cannelloni are tubes 1.5–2 cm wide and 10 cm long, stuffed with meat; penne are nib-shaped. Lasagne is sheets of pasta. Farfals are ground, granulated or shredded.

Composition/100 g (white pasta, raw): 1431 kJ (342 kcal), protein 12 g, fat 1.8 g (16.6% saturated, 16.6% mono-, 66.6% polyunsaturated), carbohydrate 74.1 g (3.3 g sugars, 70.8 g starch), dietary fibre 5.1 g, nsp 2.9 g, Na 3 mg, K 250 mg, Ca 25 mg, Mg 56 mg, P 190 mg, Fe 2.1 mg, Cu 0.32 mg, Zn 1.5 mg, Se 1 µg, vitamin B_1 0.22 mg, B_2 0.03 mg, niacin 5.6 mg, B_6 0.17 mg, folate 34 µg, pantothenate 0.3 mg, biotin 1 µg. A 30 g serving is a source of Cu.

Composition/100 g (wholemeal pasta, raw): 1356 kJ (324 kcal), protein 13.4 g, fat 2.5 g (22.2% saturated, 16.6% mono-, 61.1% polyunsaturated), carbohydrate 66.2 g (3.7 g sugars, 62.5 g starch), dietary fibre 11.5 g, nsp 8.4 g, Na 130 mg, K 390 mg, Ca 31 mg, Mg 120 mg, P 330 mg, Fe 3.9 mg, Cu 0.51 mg, Zn 3 mg, vitamin B_1 0.99 mg, B_2 0.11 mg, niacin 8.9 mg, B_6 0.39 mg, folate 40 µg, pantothenate 0.8 mg, biotin 1 µg. A 30 g serving is a source of niacin, Mg, Cu; good source of vitamin B_1.

pasteurisation A means of prolonging the storage time of foods for a limited time, by killing the vegetative forms of many pathogenic organisms. These can be killed by mild heat treatment, whereas destruction of all bacteria and spores (sterilisation) requires higher temperatures for longer periods, often spoiling the product in the process.

In flash pasteurisation, the product is held at a higher temperature than for normal pasteurisation, but for a shorter time, so that there is less development of a cooked flavour.

Pasteurisation of milk destroys all pathogens, and although it will sour within a day or two, this is not a source of disease. It is achieved either by heating to 63–66°C for 30 min (holder method), followed by immediate cooling, or (the high-temperature short-time process) heating to 71°C for 15 s. The efficacy of pasteurisation is checked by either the METHYLENE BLUE DYE-REDUCTION TEST or the PHOSPHATASE TEST.

pasteuriser Equipment used to pasteurise liquids such as milk, fruit juices, etc. The material is passed continuously over heated plates, or through pipes, where it is heated to the required temperature, maintained at that temperature for the required time, then immediately cooled.

pastourma Greek and Turkish; black-rinded smoked bacon, highly flavoured with garlic.

pastrami Middle European (especially Rumanian-Jewish); smoked and seasoned beef, also made from turkey. Known in Canada as smoked beef.

pastry Baked dough of flour, fat and water. Six basic types: short-crust in which the fat is rubbed into the flour; suet crust in which chopped suet is mixed with the flour; puff and flaky, in which the fat is rolled into the dough; hotwater crust and choux, in which the fat is melted in hot water before being added to the flour (choux pastry also contains eggs and is whisked to a paste before cooking). PHYLLO PASTRY is made from flour and water only. Suet pastry is raised using baking powder or self-raising flour; puff and flaky and choux pastry are raised by the steam trapped between layers of dough.

pâte French for paste; used for pastry, dough or batter, also for PASTA.

pâté Literally, French for a savoury pie, now used almost exclusively to mean a savoury paste of liver, meat or fish.

patent flour See FLOUR, EXTRACTION RATE.

pathogen Bacterium or other microorganism that causes disease, as opposed to COMMENSAL or SYMBIOTIC organisms.

patty Small savoury pie, normally made with shortcrust pastry; also (in USA) small cakes of minced meat or poultry, like croquettes but not dipped in breadcrumbs before cooking.

patulin Broad-spectrum ANTIBIOTIC, but also a carcinogenic and teratogenic MYCOTOXIN, produced by *Byssochlamys nivea*, *Penicillium* and *Aspergillus* spp; *P. expansum* is the most important because it is a common cause of storage rot in fruit. Inactivated by alcoholic fermentation, pasteurisation or treatment with sulphur dioxide.

patum peperium See GENTLEMAN'S RELISH.

paunching Removing the entrails of rabbit, hare, etc.

paupiette   Small thinly cut piece of meat wrapped round a filling of forcemeat and braised.

pavlova   Australian; meringue cake topped with fruit and whipped cream; created in honour of the Russian ballerina Anna Pavlova on her visit to Australia in the 1920s.

pawpaw (papaya)   Large green or yellow melon-like fruit of the tropical tree *Carica papaya*, widely grown in all tropical regions. The proteolytic enzyme, PAPAIN, is derived from the fruit.

Composition/100 g: 113 kJ (27 kcal), protein 0.4 g, fat 0.1 g, carbohydrate 6.6 g (6.6 g sugars), dietary fibre 1.7 g, nsp 1.7 g, Na 4 mg, K 170 mg, Ca 17 mg, Mg 8 mg, P 10 mg, Fe 0.4 mg, Cu 0.06 mg, Zn 0.1 mg, vitamin A 97 µg (585 µg carotene), B_1 0.02 mg, B_2 0.03 mg, niacin 0.3 mg, B_6 0.02 mg, folate 1 µg, pantothenate 0.2 mg, C 45 mg. A 140 g serving (one slice) is a source of vitamin A, Cu; rich source of vitamin C.

PBI   See PROTEIN-BOUND IODINE.

PCM   Protein–calorie malnutrition; see PROTEIN–ENERGY MAL-NUTRITION.

PCR   See POLYMERASE CHAIN REACTION.

PCV   Packed cell volume, see HAEMATOCRIT.

peach   Fruit of the tree *Prunus persica*.

Composition/100 g: 125 kJ (30 kcal), protein 0.9 g, fat 0.1 g, carbohydrate 6.8 g (6.8 g sugars), dietary fibre 2.1 g, nsp 1.3 g, Na 1 mg, K 140 mg, Ca 6 mg, Mg 8 mg, P 20 mg, Fe 0.4 mg, Cu 0.05 mg, Zn 0.1 mg, Se 1 µg, I 3 µg, vitamin A 8 µg (53 µg carotene), B_1 0.02 mg, B_2 0.04 mg, niacin 0.7 mg, B_6 0.02 mg, folate 3 µg, pantothenate 0.2 mg, biotin 0.2 µg, C 28 mg. A 120 g serving is a rich source of vitamin C.

pea, garden or green   Seed of the LEGUME *Pisum sativum*.

Composition/100 g: 330 kJ (79 kcal), protein 6.7 g, fat 1.6 g, carbohydrate 10 g (1.2 g sugars, 7.6 g starch), dietary fibre 4.7 g, nsp 4.5 g, K 230 mg, Ca 19 mg, Mg 29 mg, P 130 mg, Fe 1.5 mg, Cu 0.03 mg, Zn 1 mg, Se 1 µg, I 2 µg, vitamin A 41 µg (250 µg carotene), E 0.2 mg, B_1 0.7 mg, B_2 0.03 mg, niacin 2.9 mg, B_6 0.09 mg, folate 27 µg, pantothenate 0.2 mg, biotin 0.4 µg, C 16 mg. A 70 g serving is a source of niacin, vitamin C; rich source of vitamin B_1.

pea, mange tout   Immature pods and embryo seeds of the LEGUME *Pisum sativum* var *macrocarpon* or *macrocarpum*, eaten whole. Also known as snap peas or sugar snap peas.

Composition/100 g: 108 kJ (26 kcal), protein 3.2 g, fat 0.1 g, carbohydrate 3.3 g (2.8 g sugars, 0.5 g starch), dietary fibre 4 g, nsp 2.2 g, Na 2 mg, K 170 mg, Ca 35 mg, Mg 22 mg, P 55 mg, Fe 0.8 mg, Cu 0.06 mg, Zn 0.4 mg, vitamin A 110 µg (665 µg carotene), E 0.4 mg, B_1 0.14 mg, B_2 0.16 mg, niacin 0.9 mg, B_6 0.14 mg, folate

6 μg, pantothenate 0.7 mg, biotin 3.7 μg, C 28 mg. A 70 g serving is a rich source of vitamin C.

pea, processed Garden PEAS (*Pisum sativum*) that have matured on the plant and subsequently been canned.

peanut Fruit of *Arachis hypogaea*, also known as earthnut, groundnut, arachis nut, monkey nut; technically a LEGUME, not a nut.

Composition/100 g: 2360 kJ (564 kcal), protein 25.6 g, fat 46.1 g (18.8% saturated, 48.3% mono-, 32.7% polyunsaturated), carbohydrate 12.5 g (6.2 g sugars, 6.3 g starch), dietary fibre 7.3 g, nsp 6.2 g, Na 2 mg, K 670 mg, Ca 60 mg, Mg 210 mg, P 430 mg, Fe 2.5 mg, Cu 1.02 mg, Zn 3.5 mg, Se 3 μg, I 20 μg, vitamin E 10.1 mg, B_1 1.14 mg, B_2 0.1 mg, niacin 19.3 mg, B_6 0.59 mg, folate 110 μg, pantothenate 2.7 mg, biotin 72 μg. A 13 g serving (ten whole nuts) is a source of vitamin E, B_1, niacin, Cu.

peanut butter Ground, roasted peanuts; commonly prepared from a mixture of Spanish and Virginia peanuts, since the first alone is too oily and the second is too dry. Separation of the oil is prevented by partial HYDROGENATION of the oil and the addition of EMULSIFIERS.

Composition/100 g: 2607 kJ (623 kcal), protein 22.6 g, fat 53.7 g (22.7% saturated, 41.4% mono-, 35.7% polyunsaturated), carbohydrate 13.1 g (6.7 g sugars, 6.4 g starch), dietary fibre 6.8 g, nsp 5.4 g, Na 350 mg, K 700 mg, Ca 37 mg, Mg 180 mg, P 330 mg, Fe 2.1 mg, Cu 0.7 mg, Zn 3 mg, Se 3 μg, vitamin E 5 mg, B_1 0.17 mg, B_2 0.09 mg, niacin 17.4 mg, B_6 0.58 mg, folate 53 μg, pantothenate 1.6 mg, biotin 94 μg. A 25 g serving is a source of protein, vitamin E, biotin, Mg; good source of niacin, Cu.

peanut (groundnut, arachis) oil From the peanut or groundnut, *Arachis hypogaea*; 20% saturated, 50% mono-unsaturated, 30% polyunsaturated.

pear Fruit of many species of *Pyrus*; cultivated varieties all descended from *P. communis*. The UK National Fruit Collection has 495 varieties of dessert and cooking pears, and a further 20 varieties of PERRY pears.

Composition/100 g: 150 kJ (36 kcal), protein 0.3 g, fat 0.1 g, carbohydrate 9.1 g (9.1 g sugars), nsp 2 g, Na 3 mg, K 140 mg, Ca 10 mg, Mg 6 mg, P 12 mg, Fe 0.2 mg, Cu 0.05 mg, Zn 0.1 mg, I 1 μg, vitamin A 2 μg (16 μg carotene), E 0.5 mg, B_1 0.02 mg, B_2 0.03 mg, niacin 0.2 mg, B_6 0.02 mg, folate 2 μg, pantothenate 0.1 mg, biotin 0.2 μg, C 5 mg. A 150 g serving is a source of vitamin C.

pear, prickly See PRICKLY PEAR.

pease pudding English; dish prepared from dried peas, soaked, boiled, mashed and sieved, traditionally served with baked ham.

pecan nuts   From the American tree *Carya illinoensis*, species of hickory nut.

Composition/100 g: 2884 kJ (689 kcal), protein 9.2 g, fat 70.1 g (8.5% saturated, 63.5% mono-, 27.9% polyunsaturated), carbohydrate 5.8 g (4.3 g sugars, 1.5 g starch), nsp 4.7 g, Na 1 mg, K 520 mg, Ca 61 mg, Mg 130 mg, P 310 mg, Fe 2.2 mg, Cu 1.07 mg, Zn 5.3 mg, Se 12 μg, vitamin A 8 μg (50 μg carotene), E 4.3 mg, B_1 0.71 mg, B_2 0.15 mg, niacin 5.5 mg, B_6 0.19 mg, folate 39 μg, pantothenate 1.7 mg. An 18 g serving (three nuts) is a good source of Cu.

pectase   An enzyme (EC 3.1.1.11) in the pith (albedo) of CITRUS fruits which removes the methoxyl groups from PECTIN to form water-insoluble pectic acid. The intermediate compounds, with varying numbers of methoxyl groups, are pectinic acids. Also known as pectin esterase, pectin methyl esterase and pectin methoxylase. Unlike PECTINASE, present in ripe and unripe fruit, and not associated with softening and ripening.

pectic acid   Demethylated PECTIN.

pectin   Plant tissues contain hemicelluloses (chemically polymers of galacturonic acid) known as protopectins which cement the cell walls together. As fruit ripens, there is maximum protopectin present; thereafter it breaks down to pectin, pectinic acid and finally pectic acid and the fruit softens as the adhesive between the cells breaks down.

Pectin is the setting agent in JAM; it forms a gel with sugar under acid conditions. Soft fruits, such as strawberry, raspberry and cherry, are low in pectin; plums, apples and oranges are rich. Apple pulp and orange pith are the commercial sources of pectin. Added to jams, confectionery, chocolate, ice-cream as an emulsifier and stabiliser instead of agar; used in making jellies, and as antistaling agent in cakes. Included in NON-STARCH POLYSACCHARIDES.

pectinase   Group of enzymes that hydrolyse PECTIN and pectic acid (demethylated pectin formed by the action of PECTASE). Important in the softening of fruit, by degradation of pectin during ripening, and used commercially to clarify fruit juices. Also known as pectolase, pectozyme.

Two endolyases hydrolyse methylated pectin to yield oligosaccharide fragments: pectin lyase (EC 4.2.2.10) is polymethoxygalacturonide lyase; pectate endolyase (EC 4.2.2.2) is poly α-D-glucuronide lyase. EC 3.2.1.15 is an endopolygalacturonidase, acting on pectic acid to produce oligosaccharides. EC 3.2.1.67 is an exopolygalacturonidase, removing galactonobiose units sequentially from the end of the pectic acid molecule.

See also PECTASE.

pectinesterase See PECTASE.

pectinic acid Partially demethylated PECTIN.

pectins, low-methoxyl Partially demethylated pectins which can form gels with little or no sugar and therefore used in low-calorie jellies.

pectolase, pectozyme See PECTINASE.

pectosase, pectosinase See PROTOPECTINASE.

pedometer Portable device that records number of paces walked, and therefore approximate distance travelled.

Pekar test A comparative test of flour colour.

pekmez Turkish; thick jelly made by evaporating grape juice, the basis of Turkish delight and other sugar confectionery. Also general Balkan name for jam.

Pekoe See TEA.

pelagic fish Fish that swim near the surface, compared with demersal fish, which live on the sea bottom. Pelagic fish are mostly oily, e.g. herring, mackerel and pilchard, containing up to 20% oil.

pellagra The disease due to deficiency of the VITAMIN NIACIN and the AMINO ACID TRYPTOPHAN. Signs include a characteristic symmetrical photosensitive dermatitis (especially on the face and back of hands), resembling severe sunburn; mental disturbances (a depressive psychosis sometimes called dementia); and digestive disorders (most commonly diarrhoea); fatal if untreated. Most commonly associated with a diet based on MAIZE or SORGHUM, which are poor sources of both tryptophan and niacin, with little meat or other vegetables.

PEM See PROTEIN–ENERGY MALNUTRITION.

pemmican Mixture of dried, powdered meat and fat, used as a concentrated food source, e.g. on expeditions.

penicillamine Chelating agent used to enhance the excretion of COPPER in WILSON'S DISEASE.

penicillin The first of the ANTIBIOTICS; found in the culture fluid of the MOULD *Penicillium notatum* in 1929. Active against a wide range of bacteria and of great value clinically. Not used as food preservative because of the danger that repeated small doses will increase the development of penicillin-resistant organisms.

Penicillium A genus of MOULDS; apart from the production of PENICILLIN, several species are valuable in the ripening of CHEESES. *P. roquefortii* is responsible for the blue veining of roquefort, gorgonzola and other blue cheeses. Other species are responsible for spoilage, and may form MYCOTOXINS in foods (e.g. the unidentified nephrotoxin from *P. polonicum*).

pentagastrin Synthetic peptide that has the same effect as the HORMONE GASTRIN on gastric acid secretion.

pentane Hydrocarbon gas (C_5H_{10}) formed in small amounts by breakdown of oxidised linoleic acid, and exhaled on the breath; used as an index of oxygen RADICAL damage to tissue lipids, and indirectly as an index of ANTIOXIDANT status.

See also ETHANE; FATTY ACIDS.

pentosans POLYSACCHARIDES of PENTOSES. Widely distributed in plants, e.g. fruit, wood, corncobs, oat hulls. Not digested in the body, and hence a component of NON-STARCH POLYSACCHARIDES or DIETARY FIBRE.

pentose phosphate pathway Or hexose monophosphate shunt, an alternative pathway of GLUCOSE METABOLISM.

See also FAVISM.

pentoses MONOSACCHARIDE SUGARS with five carbon atoms.

pentosuria The excretion of PENTOSE sugars in the urine. Idiopathic pentosuria is an inherited metabolic disorder almost wholly restricted to Ashkenazi (N European) Jews, which has no adverse effects. Consumption of fruits rich in pentoses (e.g. pears) can also lead to (temporary) pentosuria.

P-enzyme Potato PHOSPHORYLASE (EC 2.4.1.1), an enzyme that cleaves starch to yield glucose-1-phosphate; specific for α-1,4 links.

pepper (1) Bell pepper, bullnose pepper, capsicum, paprika, sweet pepper, Spanish name *pimiento* (not the same as pimento or ALLSPICE); fruits of the annual plant *Capsicum annuum*. Red, yellow, purple or brown fruits, often eaten raw in salads when green and unripe; very variable size and shape; some varieties can be spicy but mostly non-pungent.

Composition/100g (green): 62kJ (15kcal), protein 0.8g, fat 0.3g, carbohydrate 2.6g (2.4g sugars, 0.1g starch), dietary fibre 1.9g, nsp 1.6g, Na 4mg, K 120mg, Ca 8mg, Mg 10mg, P 19mg, Fe 0.4mg, Cu 0.02mg, Zn 0.1mg, I 1μg, vitamin A 44μg (265μg carotene), E 0.8mg, B_1 0.01mg, B_2 0.01mg, niacin 0.2mg, B_6 0.3mg, folate 36μg, pantothenate 0.1mg, C 120mg. An 80g serving (1/2 pepper) is a source of vitamin B_6, folate; rich source of vitamin C.

Composition/100g (red): 133kJ (32kcal), protein 1g, fat 0.4g, carbohydrate 6.4g (6.1g sugars, 0.1g starch), dietary fibre 1.9g, nsp 1.6g, Na 4mg, K 160mg, Ca 8mg, Mg 14mg, P 22mg, Fe 0.3mg, Cu 0.01mg, Zn 0.1mg, I 1μg, vitamin A 640μg (3840μg carotene), E 0.8mg, B_1 0.01mg, B_2 0.03mg, niacin 1.5mg, B_6 0.36mg, folate 21μg, pantothenate 0.1mg, C 140mg. An 80g serving is a source of vitamin B_6; rich source of vitamin A, C.

(2) Red pepper, chilli (or chili), small red fruit of the bushy perennial plant *Capsicum frutescens*. Usually sun-dried and therefore wrinkled. Very pungent, ingredient of CURRY powder,

pickles and TABASCO sauce. Cayenne pepper is made from the powdered dried fruits. Unripe (green) chillis are also very pungent.

(3) Black and white pepper, fruit of the tropical climbing vine, *Piper nigrum*; the fruits are peppercorns. Black pepper is made from sun-dried unripe peppercorns when the red outer skin turns black. White pepper is made by soaking ripe berries and rubbing off outer skin. Usually ground as a condiment. Green peppercorns are dried or pickled unripe fruit. Pungency due to the alkaloids piperine, piperdine and chavicine.

(4) Japan pepper, black seeds of *Zanthoxylum piperitum* with a pungent peppery flavour.

(5) Guinea or melegueta pepper, seeds of the W African tree *Amomum melegueta*, also known as grains of paradise.

peppercorn   See PEPPER.

pepper dulse   Red aromatic seaweed (*Laurencia pinnatifida*), dried and used as a spice in Scotland.

peppergrass   Peppery-tasting cress (*Lepidium sativum*), also known as pepperwort and (in USA) peppermint.

pepper, Jamaican   See ALLSPICE.

peppermint   A hybrid (*Mentha* × *piperita*) between *M. aquatica* and *M. spicata* (SPEARMINT). Not used for flavouring dishes but grown for the essential oil which is used in confectionery (e.g. peppermints) and medicinally.

Pepsi-Cola   Trade name for a COLA beverage. Originally made in 1896 in the USA by Caleb Bradham, druggist.

pepsin   An enzyme (EC 3.4.23.1) in the GASTRIC JUICE; hydrolyses proteins to give smaller polypeptides, known as peptones; an endopeptidase. Active only at acid pH, 1.5–2.5. Secreted as the inactive precursor pepsinogen, which is activated by gastric acid. Vegetable pepsin is PAPAIN.

peptic ulcer   See ULCER.

peptidases   Enzymes that hydrolyse proteins, and therefore important in PROTEIN digestion. Endopeptidases cleave at specific points in the middle of protein molecules (between specific amino acids, depending on the enzyme); exopeptidases remove amino acids sequentially from either the amino terminal (aminopeptidases) or carboxy terminal (carboxypeptidases).

peptide YY   Peptide hormone secreted throughout the gut; decreases pancreatic secretion of fluid, bicarbonate and enzymes.

peptides   Compounds formed when AMINO ACIDS are linked together through the $-CO-NH-$ (peptide) linkage. Two amino acids so linked form a dipeptide, three a tripeptide, etc; medium-length chains of amino acids (4–20) are known as oligopeptides, longer chains are polypeptides or proteins.

peptidoglycans Conjugated proteins with complex chains of carbohydrate, found especially in bacterial cell walls. Especially rich in *N*-acetylglucosamine and *N*-acetylmuramic acid.

peptones Small polypeptides that are intermediate products in the hydrolysis of proteins. The term is often used for any partial hydrolysate of protein, e.g. bacteriological peptone, used as a growth medium for microorganisms.

PER Protein efficiency ratio, a measure of PROTEIN QUALITY.

pericarp The fibrous layers next to the outer husk of cereal grains and outside the testa; of low digestibility and removed from grain during milling. The major constituent of bran.

perigo factor A postulated inhibitory factor produced when bacterial growth medium is autoclaved with nitrite: it is about 10 times more inhibitory to some bacteria than nitrite alone.

perillartine Non-nutritive SWEETENER derived from perillaldehyde, extracted from shiso oil (commercially available in Japan); 2000 times as sweet as sucrose.

perimysium See MUSCLE.

periodontal Relating to the tissues between the teeth; periodontal membrane is the ligament around a tooth, attaching it to the bone.

peristalsis The wavelike rhythmic alternating contraction and relaxation of smooth muscle that forces food through the intestinal tract in peristaltic waves.

peritoneum Serous membrane of the abdominal cavity.

periwinkle See WINKLE.

perleche Dryness of the corners of the mouth; may be infected. See also RIBOFLAVIN deficiency.

Permutit An ION-EXCHANGE RESIN.

pernicious anaemia See ANAEMIA, PERNICIOUS.

peroxidase Enzyme (EC 1.11.1.17) that reduces HYDROGEN PEROXIDE (H_2O_2) to water, while oxidising another substrate. A relatively thermostable enzyme, frequently used as an index of the efficacy of BLANCHING of fruits and vegetables. See also CATALASE.

peroxide Any compound with the peroxy ($-O-O-$) group; atmospheric oxidation of unsaturated FATTY ACIDS produces peroxides. Also used to mean specifically HYDROGEN PEROXIDE (H_2O_2).

peroxide number Or peroxide value; a measure of the oxidative rancidity of fats by determination of the lipid peroxides present.

perry Fermented PEAR juice (in UK may include not more than 25% apple juice) analogous to CIDER from apples. Sparkling perry is sometimes known as champagne perry.

Persian apple See CITRON.

Persian berry   Yellow colour obtained from the berries of the buckthorn, *Rhamnus* spp; legally permitted in food in most countries. Contains the glucosides of rhamnetin and rhamnazin.

persimmon   Fruit of *Diospyros virginiana* (American persimmon or Virginia date) and *D. kaki* (Japanese persimmon, date plum, kaki or sharon fruit). Kaki may be eaten raw or cooked; American persimmon develops a sour flavour if cooked.

Composition/100 g (kaki): 305 kJ (73 kcal), protein 0.8 g, fat 0 g, carbohydrate 18.6 g (18.6 g sugars), nsp 1.6 g, Na 5 mg, K 210 mg, Ca 10 mg, Mg 11 mg, P 19 mg, Fe 0.1 mg, Cu 0.1 mg, Zn 0.1 mg, vitamin A 158 µg (950 µg carotene), B_1 0.03 mg, B_2 0.05 mg, niacin 0.3 mg, folate 7 µg, C 19 mg. A 110 g serving is a source of Cu; good source of vitamin A; rich source of vitamin C.

pervaporation   Evaporation from a colloidal suspension by heating in a bag made from a semipermeable membrane. If there are crystalloids present, they pass through the membrane and are deposited on the outside of the bag.

pescetarian   A partial VEGETARIAN who will eat fish but not meat.

PET   Polyethylene terephthalate; clear plastic used in packaging, especially bottles for drinks.

PET (positron emission tomography) scanning   Radiographic technique that utilises positrons emitted by the decay of ^{15}O after a dose of $H_2{}^{15}O$.

petechiae   Small round, flat, dark red spots caused by bleeding into the skin or under mucous membrane; occur in VITAMIN C deficiency as a result of capillary fragility.

pétillant   French; lightly sparkling wines.

petit-grain oils   Prepared from twigs and leaves of the bitter ORANGE by steam distillation; similar to NEROLI OIL but less fragrant. Petit-grain Portugal prepared from leaves of sweet orange, mandarin petit-grain from TANGERINE leaves, and lemon petit-grain from LEMON leaves.

Peyer's patches   Oval masses of lymphoid tissue in the small intestinal mucous membrane, responsible for the production of lymphocytes (white BLOOD CELLS) and antibodies.

PGA   Pteroylglutamic acid, see FOLIC ACID.

pH   Potential hydrogen, measurement of acidity or alkalinity on a logarithmic scale. Defined as the negative logarithm of the hydrogen ion concentration. The scale runs from 0, which is very strongly ACID, to 14, which is very strongly alkaline. Pure water is pH 7, which is neutral; below 7 is acid, above is alkaline.

See also ACID; BUFFER.

phaeophytin   Brownish-green derivative of CHLOROPHYLL, caused by the loss of MAGNESIUM in acid conditions. The formation of phaeophytin accounts for the colour change when green vegetables are cooked.

phage See BACTERIOPHAGE.

phagomania Morbid obsession with food; also known as sitomania.

phagophobia Fear of food; also known as sitophobia.

phase inversion CREAM is an emulsion of fat in water; BUTTER is an emulsion of water in fat. The change from cream to butter is termed phase inversion.

phase I metabolism The first phase of metabolism of foreign compounds (xenobiotics), involving metabolic activation such as hydroxylation (catalysed by CYTOCHROMES P450), deacylation, etc. Generally regarded as detoxication reactions, but may in fact convert inactive precursors into metabolically active compounds, and involved in activation of precursors to carcinogens.

phase II metabolism The second phase of the metabolism of foreign compounds, in which the activated derivatives formed in PHASE I METABOLISM are conjugated with amino acids (e.g. glycine, alanine), GLUCURONIC ACID or GLUTATHIONE, to yield water-soluble derivatives that can be excreted in the urine or bile.

phaseolin Globulin protein in kidney or haricot BEAN (*Phaseolus vulgaris*).

phaseolunatin Cyanogenic (cyanide-forming) (see CYANOGENIC GLYCOSIDES) GLUCOSIDE found in certain LEGUMES (such as lima bean, chick pea, common vetch), which hydrolyses to glucose, acetone and hydrocyanic acid; not proven harmful when present in the diet.

phasin Originally the LECTIN from the bean *Phaseolus vulgaris*, now used for non-toxic plant lectins in general.

PHB ester See PARABENS.

pheasant GAME bird, *Phasianus colchicus* and related species. Total weight 1.5 kg; traditionally sold as brace, i.e. cock and hen, although now commonly available as single birds; usually hung 3 days (up to 3 weeks in very cold weather) to develop flavour.
    Composition/100 g: 560 kJ (134 kcal), protein 20.3 g, fat 5.9 g (35.7% saturated, 51.7% mono-, 12.4% polyunsaturated), carbohydrate 0 g, Na 66 mg, K 260 mg, Ca 31 mg, Mg 22 mg, P 190 mg, Fe 5.3 mg, Cu 0.05 mg, Zn 0.6 mg, vitamin B_1 0.01 mg, B_2 0.13 mg, niacin 7.9 mg, B_6 0.26 mg, folate 9 µg, B_{12} 1.1 µg. A 200 g serving ($^1/_2$ bird weighed with bone) is a source of vitamin B_2, Mg, Cu; good source of vitamin B_6; rich source of protein, niacin, vitamin B_{12}, Fe.

phenetylurea See DULCIN.

phenol oxidases Group of enzymes that oxidise phenols to quinones, which then undergo non-enzymic polymerisation to red-brown pigments.

Tyrosinase (monophenol oxidase, EC 1.14.18.1) is a copper-dependent enzyme in mammalian tissues, responsible for formation of melanin.

Polyphenol oxidase (catechol oxidase, laccase EC 1.10.3.2) is a calcium-dependent enzyme responsible for browning of cut fruit and vegetables. It acts on catechols and other polyphenols, including FLAVONOIDS. Inhibited by chelating compounds such as EDTA, also by SULPHITES and CYSTEINE.

phenolphthalein See LAXATIVES.

phentermine An anorectic (APPETITE CONTROL, suppressant) drug used in the treatment of obesity, especially in combination with FENFLURAMINE (fen-phen); withdrawn in 1995 in response to reports of heart valve damage.

phenylalanine An essential AMINO ACID; abbr Phe (F), M_r 165.2, pK_a 2.16, 9.18, codons UUPy. In addition to its rôle in protein synthesis, it is the metabolic precursor of the non-essential amino acid TYROSINE (and hence NORADRENALINE, ADRENALINE and the THYROID HORMONES). Tyrosine in the diet spares phenylalanine, so reducing the requirement.

o-**phenylene diamine** Reagent used for determination of total VITAMIN C after oxidation to dehydroascorbic acid with iodine; forms a fluorescent quinoxaline derivative with dehydroascorbic acid.

phenylethylamine The AMINE formed by decarboxylation of the amino acid PHENYLALANINE.

phenylisothiocyanate See EDMAN REAGENT.

phenylketonuria A GENETIC DISEASE affecting the metabolism of PHENYLALANINE. Phenylalanine is normally metabolised to TYROSINE, catalysed by phenylalanine hydroxylase (EC 1.14.16.1). Impairment of this reaction leads to a considerable accumulation of phenylalanine in plasma and tissues (up to 100 times the normal concentration) and metabolism to phenylpyruvate, phenyllactate and phenylacetate, collectively known as phenylketones, which are excreted in the urine. The very high plasma concentration of phenylalanine causes disruption of brain development, and if untreated there is severe mental retardation.

All infants are screened for phenylketonuria shortly after birth (by measurement of plasma phenylalanine); treatment is by very strict limitation of phenylalanine intake, only providing sufficient to meet requirements for protein synthesis. Once brain development is complete (between the ages of 8–12 years) dietary restriction can be relaxed to a considerable extent, since high concentrations of phenylalanine seem to have little adverse effect on the developed brain. There may, however, be benefits from continuing dietary restriction into adult life, and phenylketonuric women require extremely careful dietary control through pregnancy to avoid damage to the foetus' developing brain.

phenylthiohydantoin Reacts with the amino group of AMINO ACIDS; used in separation of amino acids by thin-layer CHROMATOGRAPHY, and for detection in HPLC.

pheophorbide Product of strong acid hydrolysis of CHLOROPHYLL; both the chelated Mg^{2+} ion and the phytol side-chain are lost.
See also CHLOROPHYLLIDE; PHEOPHYTIN.

pheophytin Brown pigment produced from CHLOROPHYLL by removal of the Mg^{2+} ion in dilute acid.
See also CHLOROPHYLLIDE; PHEOPHORBIDE.

phitosite High-calorie food.

phlorizin (phloridzin) A glucoside from the roots and bark of various Rosaceae spp that inhibits the renal tubular reabsorption of glucose. Formerly used as an experimental model of DIABETES mellitus, but it causes glucosuria and hence hypoglycaemia, rather than the hyperglycaemia and subsequent glucosuria seen in uncontrolled diabetes.

phosphatase test A test for the adequacy of PASTEURISATION of milk. The enzyme phosphatase (EC 3.1.3.x), normally present in milk, is denatured at a temperature slightly greater than that required to destroy the tubercle bacillus and other pathogens; therefore the presence of detectable phosphatase activity indicates inadequate pasteurisation. The test can detect 0.2% raw milk in pasteurised milk.

phosphate additives See POLYPHOSPHATES.

phosphates Salts of PHOSPHORIC ACID; the form in which the element PHOSPHORUS is normally present in foods and body tissues.
See also POLYPHOSPHATES.

phosphatides See PHOSPHOLIPIDS.

phosphatidic acid Glycerol esterified to two molecules of fatty acid, with the third hydroxyl group esterified to phosphate; chemically diacylglycerol phosphate; intermediates in the metabolism of PHOSPHOLIPIDS.

phosphatidylcholine A phospholipid containing CHOLINE, see LECITHIN.

phosphatidylethanolamine A PHOSPHOLIPID containing ethanolamine.

phosphatidylinositol A PHOSPHOLIPID containing INOSITOL.

phosphatidylserine A PHOSPHOLIPID containing SERINE.

phospholipids (phosphatides, phospholipins) Glycerol esterified to two molecules of FATTY ACID, one of which is commonly a polyunsaturated fatty acid. The third hydroxyl group is esterified to phosphate and one of a number of water-soluble compounds, including SERINE (phosphatidylserine), ethanolamine (phosphatidylethanolamine), CHOLINE (phosphatidylcholine, also known as LECITHIN) and INOSITOL (phosphatidylinositol).

Cell membranes are a double layer of phospholipids with the fatty acid side-chains on the inside. The water-soluble compound esterified to the phosphate interacts with water. This is why phospholipids can be used to emulsify oils and fats in water and are commonly used in food manufacture as EMULSIFIERS. From the energy point of view they can be regarded as being equivalent to simple fats (TRIACYLGLYCEROLS); they also provide a source of choline and inositol, neither of which is a dietary essential.

phosphoproteins Proteins containing phosphate, other than as NUCLEIC ACIDS (nucleoproteins) or PHOSPHOLIPIDS (lipoproteins), e.g. CASEIN from milk, ovovitellin from egg yolk.

phosphoric acid May be one of three types, orthophosphoric acid (H_3PO_4), metaphosphoric acid (HPO_3) or pyrophosphoric acid ($H_4P_2O_7$). Orthophosphoric acid and its salts are E-338–341, used as ACIDITY REGULATORS and in acid-fruit-flavoured beverages such as lemonade.

phosphorus An essential element, occurring in tissues and foods as phosphate (salts of PHOSPHORIC ACID), PHOSPHOLIPIDS and phosphoproteins. In the body most (80%) is present in the skeleton and teeth as HYDROXYAPATITE; the remainder is in the phospholipids of cell membranes, in NUCLEIC ACIDS and in a variety of metabolic intermediates, including ATP.

The parathyroid glands (see PARATHYROID HORMONE) control the concentration of phosphate in the blood, mainly by modifying its excretion in the urine. Human dietary needs (about 1.3 g per day) are always met; a deficiency never occurs in man. The CALCIUM:phosphate ratio of infant foods is, however, important.

Phosphate deficiency is common in livestock and gives rise to OSTEOMALACIA (also known as sweeny or creeping sickness). Phosphate is also essential for plant growth, hence the use of inorganic phosphate or bone meal as fertiliser. Bone meal (mainly calcium phosphate) is often used as a supplement in human foods but as a source of calcium rather than of phosphate.

phosphorylase Enzyme (EC 2.4.1.1) responsible for the breakdown of glycogen and starch to glucose 1-phosphate. In vegetables associated with formation of sugars during ripening and on storage. Important in potatoes during storage because it remains active at low temperatures whereas enzymes of GLYCOLYSIS are cold labile, so that sugars accumulate rather than being utilised.

photon absorptiometry Technique for determination of BONE density, as an index of CALCIUM and VITAMIN D status.

photosynthesis Sequence of reactions, most commonly in plants, but also in some microorganisms, that leads to synthesis of carbohydrates by reduction of carbon dioxide using light as the primary energy source. Considered in two separate reaction sequences: the light phase, in which light energy is captured by pigments, and eventually transferred to CHLOROPHYLL, leading, via an electron transport chain, to the reduction of NADP$^+$ to NADPH and the synthesis of ATP from ADP and phosphate; the dark phase in which NADPH and ATP are used to reduce carbon dioxide to glucose.

There are two separate pathways for the dark phase reaction: the C3 pathway (Calvin cycle), in which phosphoglyceric acid is the first product of CO_2 fixation, and the C4 pathway (Hatch and Slack pathway), in which four-carbon dicarboxylic acids are the first products of CO_2 fixation. Both pathways may occur together in some plants; the C4 pathway is found especially in maize, sorghum, sugar cane and tropical grasses growing under high light intensity where water is scarce.

phrynoderma Blocked pores or 'toad-skin' (follicular hyperkeratosis of the skin) often encountered in malnourished people. Originally thought to be due to VITAMIN A deficiency but possibly due to other deficiencies, and also occurs mildly in adequately nourished people.

phthisis Obsolete name for any disease resulting in wasting of tissues; see CACHEXIA; MARASMUS.

phulka See CHAPPATI.

phycotoxins Marine biotoxins that accumulate in fish and shellfish from their diet (causing PARALYTIC SHELLFISH POISONING and CIGUATERA poisoning when the fish are eaten), as distinct from toxins naturally present (tetramine poisoning).

phyllo pastry (filo pastry) Plain paper-thin pastry made from flour and water, rolled into small balls then tossed in the air and stretched until it forms an extremely thin sheet. Multiple layers are used as the basis for Greek and Middle-Eastern pastry dishes. Known as mortoban in SE Asia.

phylloquinone See VITAMIN K.

phylloxera An aphid which threatened to destroy the vineyards of Europe in the middle of the nineteenth century. They were saved by grafting susceptible varieties onto resistant American vine rootstock.

physalin A CAROTENOID, zeaxanthin dipalmitate, in the fruits of the CAPE GOOSEBERRY, *Physalis* spp.

physalis See CAPE GOOSEBERRY.

physical activity level (PAL) Total ENERGY cost of physical activity throughout the day, expressed as a ratio of BASAL METABOLIC RATE. Calculated from the PHYSICAL ACTIVITY RATIO for each activity, multiplied by the time spent in that activity. A desirable PAL for health is considered to be 1.7; the average in UK is 1.4.

physical activity ratio (PAR) ENERGY cost of physical activity expressed as a ratio of BASAL METABOLIC RATE.

physin Name given to a growth factor in liver, later identified as vitamin B_{12}.

physiological saline A solution of sodium chloride that is isotonic with blood plasma, 0.15 mol/L (9 g/L).

phytanic acid Tetramethyl hexanoic acid, formed in the body from free (but not combined) phytol; traces in fats. Inability to metabolise phytanic acid leads to Refsum's disease.

phytase Enzyme (inositol hexahydrate phosphohydrolase, EC 3.1.3.26) that hydrolyses PHYTIC ACID to inositol mono- to tetrakis-phosphates (tetraphosphates), which do not chelate minerals, and free phosphate. Occurs in cereal grains, where it is activated by soaking or during germination and malting. Added to poultry feed to increase availability of PHOSPHATE; main commercial source is *Aspergillus* spp, but also expressed in genetically modified rapeseed, tobacco and tomato seeds.

phytate (phytic acid) INOSITOL hexaphosphate, present in cereals, particularly in the bran, dried legumes and some nuts as both water-soluble salts (sodium and potassium) and insoluble salts of calcium and magnesium. Magnesium calcium phytate is phytin. Can bind calcium, iron and zinc to form insoluble complexes; it is not clear how far phytate reduces the availability of these minerals in the diet, especially since there are PHYTASES in yeast and legumes (and possibly in the human gut) which may liberate these minerals.

phytin Magnesium calcium PHYTATE, approximately 12% calcium, 1.5% magnesium and 22% phosphorus.

phytoagglutinins See LECTINS.

phytoalexins Compounds produced by plants under conditions of stress or in response to mechanical or fungal damage which may be toxic, or induce adverse reactions, when the plants are consumed.

phytochromes Also known as florigens. Photosensitive polypeptides with a tetrapyrrole prosthetic group, responsible for day-length sensitivity in plants, and possibly also enhanced germination of seeds that have been vernalised (chilled to 4°C). The protein undergoes a conformational change on exposure to red light (660 nm) and the reverse change on exposure to infrared (735 nm).

phytohaemagglutinins See LECTINS.

phytoncides See PACIFICARINS.

phyto-oestrogens Compounds with OESTROGEN activity found in a variety of plants; see FLAVONOIDS.

phytoplankton See PLANKTON.

phytosterol General name given to sterols occurring in plants, the chief of which is SITOSTEROL.

phytotoxin Any poisonous substance produced by a plant. See also ALKALOIDS.

phytylmenaquinone See VITAMIN K.

pica An unnatural desire for foods; alternative words, cissa, cittosis and allotriophagy. Also a perverted appetite (eating of earth, sand, clay, paper, etc).

piccalilli Mixture of chopped, brine-preserved vegetables in mustard sauce (mustard and vinegar, thickened with tapioca starch, plus turmeric and other spices).

pickling Also called BRINING. Vegetables immersed in 5–10% salt solution (brine) undergo lactic acid fermentation, while the salt prevents the growth of undesirable organisms. The sugars in the vegetables are converted to lactic acid; at 25°C the process takes a few weeks, finishing at 1% acidity.

See also CURING, OF MEAT; HALOPHILIC BACTERIA.

pidan See CHINESE EGGS.

pigeon *Columba livia*; young about four weeks old is squab.

Composition/100 g: 422 kJ (101 kcal), protein 12.2 g, fat 5.8 g, carbohydrate 0 g, Na 46 mg, K 180 mg, Ca 7 mg, Mg 15 mg, P 180 mg, Fe 8.5 mg, Cu 0.15 mg, Zn 0.7 mg, vitamin B_1 0.12 mg, niacin 5.4 mg, B_6 0.36 mg, folate 3 μg. A 240 g serving (weighed with bone) is a source of Mg, Zn; good source of vitamin B_1; rich source of protein, niacin, vitamin B_6; Fe, Cu.

pignoli (pignolias, pinoli) See PINENUTS.

pig nut See EARTH NUT.

pilchard Oily FISH, *Sardina (Clupea) pilchardus*; young is the SARDINE.

Composition/100 g (canned in tomato): 527 kJ (126 kcal), protein 18.8 g, fat 5.4 g (22.4% saturated, 30.6% mono-, 46.9% polyunsaturated), cholesterol 56 mg, carbohydrate 0.7 g (0.6 g sugars, 0.1 g starch), Na 370 mg, K 420 mg, Ca 300 mg, Mg 39 mg, P 350 mg, Fe 2.7 mg, Cu 0.19 mg, Zn 1.6 mg, Se 30 μg, I 64 μg, vitamin A 31 μg (142 μg carotene), D 8 μg, E 0.7 mg, B_1 0.02 mg, B_2 0.29 mg, niacin 11.1 mg, B_6 0.27 mg, B_{12} 12 μg, pantothenate 0.9 mg, biotin 11 μg. A 215 g serving (small tin) is a source of vitamin E, biotin; good source of vitamin B_6, Mg, Zn; rich source of protein, vitamin D, B_2, niacin, B_{12}, pantothenate, Ca, Fe, Cu, I, Se.

piles See HAEMORRHOIDS.

pils Pale type of lager originally made in Czechoslovakia. See BEER.

pimento See ALLSPICE.

pimiento See PEPPER (1).

Pimms Trade name; a ready-mixed cocktail, based on spirits, flavoured with herbs and liqueurs, normally served as a long drink with ice and soda or lemonade, garnished with fruit, cucumber or mint. Originally there were four varieties: No 1 based on gin, No 2 whisky, No 3 brandy, No 4 rum; only No 1, now based on vodka, survives.

pimpernel See BURNET.

pineapple Fruit of the tropical plant *Ananas sativus*, one of the bromeliad family. The fruit contains the proteolytic enzyme bromelain (EC 3.4.22.23), which has been used (like PAPAIN) to tenderise meat.

Composition/100 g: 171 kJ (41 kcal), protein 0.4 g, fat 0.2 g, carbohydrate 10.1 g (10.1 g sugars), dietary fibre 1.3 g, nsp 1.2 g, Na 2 mg, K 160 mg, Ca 18 mg, Mg 16 mg, P 10 mg, Fe 0.2 mg, Cu 0.11 mg, Zn 0.1 mg, vitamin A 3 µg (18 µg carotene), E 0.1 mg, B_1 0.08 mg, B_2 0.03 mg, niacin 0.4 mg, B_6 0.09 mg, folate 5 µg, pantothenate 0.2 mg, biotin 0.3 µg, C 12 mg. An 80 g serving (one slice) is a source of vitamin C, Cu.

pinenuts Or pine kernels, edible seeds of various species of pine cone, especially Mediterranean stone pine, *Pinus pinea*.

Composition/100 g: 2879 kJ (688 kcal), protein 14 g, fat 68.6 g (7% saturated, 30.3% mono-, 62.6% polyunsaturated), carbohydrate 4 g (3.9 g sugars, 0.1 g starch), nsp 1.9 g, Na 1 mg, K 780 mg, Ca 11 mg, Mg 270 mg, P 650 mg, Fe 5.6 mg, Cu 1.32 mg, Zn 6.5 mg, vitamin A 1 µg (10 µg carotene), E 13.7 mg, B_1 0.73 mg, B_2 0.19 mg, niacin 6.9 mg. A 12 g serving is a source of vitamin E, Mg, Cu.

pinnochio See PINENUTS.

pint, reputed $13^1/_3$ fluid oz = 285 mL; half a reputed quart.

pinworm Or threadworm, parasitic nematode worm (*Enterobius* and *Oxyuris* spp) in upper part of large intestine.

pipe Cask for wine; the volume varies with the type of wine, e.g. port, 115 gallons (517 L); Tenerife, 100 gal (450 L); Marsala, 90 gal (418 L).

pipis Edible MOLLUSC, *Plebidonas deltoides*, widely distributed around Australian coastline.

piri-piri Small red chillies (1 cm long), extremely pungent. Also (Portuguese) sauce made from the peppers. See PEPPER (2).

pistachio Fruit of *Pistacchio vera*; yellow-green coloured nut. May be roasted and salted or used as flavouring for ice-cream and (Indian) hot sweet milk beverage.

Composition/100 g (roasted and salted): 2515 kJ (601 kcal), protein 17.9 g, fat 55.4 g (13.9% saturated, 52.1% mono-, 33.8% polyunsaturated), carbohydrate 8.2 g (5.7 g sugars, 2.5 g starch), nsp 6.1 g, Na 530 mg, K 1040 mg, Ca 110 mg, Mg 130 mg, P 420 mg, Fe 3 mg, Cu 0.83 mg, Zn 2.2 mg, Se 6 µg, vitamin A 21 µg (130 µg carotene), E 4.2 mg, B_1 0.7 mg, B_2 0.23 mg, niacin 5.6 mg, folate 58 µg. A 10 g serving (ten nuts) is a source of Cu.

pita (pitta) Middle-Eastern; unleavened flat bread, baked as an oval or circle, which can be opened up as an envelope.

pitanga Surinam cherry, *Eugenia uniflora* or *E. michelii;* small round fruit, deeply ribbed, cherry-like with single stone.

pith See ALBEDO.

pits Stones from cherries, plums, peaches, apricots. Oil extracted from these pits is used in cosmetics and pharmaceuticals, for canning sardines and as table oil. The press cake left behind contains AMYGDALIN.

pitting Removing the stones (pits) from cherries, olives, etc.

pivka Obsolete name for preprothrombin (protein induced by vitamin K absence), the undercarboxylated precursor of PRO-THROMBIN, released into the circulation in VITAMIN K deficiency. May be measured by immunoassay as a sensitive index of vitamin K status.

pizza Originally Italian; savoury tart on a base of yeast dough, traditionally cooked in a wood-burning oven. The topping varies with region and may contain tomatoes, cheese, salami or seafood.

placebo Inactive substance used as a control in trials of drugs, etc, in order to ensure that any response observed is due to the compound under test and not simply the result of an intervention.

plaice Flat FISH, *Pleuronectus platessa.*

Composition/100 g: 330 kJ (79 kcal), protein 16.7 g, fat 1.4 g, cholesterol 42 mg, carbohydrate 0 g, Na 120 mg, K 280 mg, Ca 45 mg, Mg 22 mg, P 180 mg, Fe 0.3 mg, Cu 0.02 mg, Zn 0.5 mg, Se 37 µg, I 33 µg, vitamin B_1 0.2 mg, B_2 0.19 mg, niacin 6.3 mg, B_6 0.22 mg, folate 11 µg, B_{12} 1 µg, pantothenate 0.8 mg, biotin 47 µg. A 130 g serving is a source of vitamin B_1, B_2, B_6, pantothenate; good source of I; rich source of protein, niacin, vitamin B_{12}, biotin, Se.

plankton Minute organisms, both plant (phytoplankton) and animal (zooplankton), drifting in the sea, which serve as the basic foodstuffs of marine life; the basis of the marine food chain.

plansifter A nest of sieves mounted together so that material being sieved is divided into a number of fractions of different size. Widely used in flour milling.

plantago See PSYLLIUM.

plantain   Adam's fig; variety of BANANA (*Musa* spp) with higher starch and lower sugar content than dessert bananas, picked when flesh is too hard to be eaten raw and therefore cooked. Some varieties become sweet if left to ripen, others never develop a high sugar content.

Composition/100 g: 468 kJ (112 kcal), protein 0.8 g, fat 0.2 g, carbohydrate 28.5 g (5.5 g sugars, 23 g starch), dietary fibre 2.2 g, nsp 1.2 g, Na 4 mg, K 400 mg, Ca 5 mg, Mg 33 mg, P 31 mg, Fe 0.5 mg, Cu 0.08 mg, Zn 0.2 mg, Se 2 μg, vitamin A 58 μg (350 μg carotene), E 0.2 mg, B_1 0.03 mg, B_2 0.04 mg, niacin 0.6 mg, B_6 0.24 mg, folate 22 μg, pantothenate 0.3 mg, C 9 mg. A 200 g serving is a source of vitamin A, Cu, Se; good source of vitamin B_6, folate, Mg; rich source of vitamin C.

plaque   (1) Dental plaque is a layer of bacteria in an organic matrix on the surface of teeth, especially around the neck of each tooth. May lead to development of gingivitis, periodontal disease and caries.

(2) Atherosclerotic plaque is the development of fatty streaks in the intima of blood vessels; see also ATHEROSCLEROSIS.

plasma, blood   See BLOOD PLASMA.

plasmid   Small circular region of extrachromosomal bacterial DNA which has an origin of replication and is therefore maintained in a cell line. Especially amenable to the introduction of foreign genes, and widely used in genetic engineering. Between 5–90 kb in size.

plasminogen   Inactive precursor of plasmin in the bloodstream; activation to plasmin is important in the lysis of blood clots.

plate count   To estimate the number of bacteria in a sample, it is poured on to an AGAR plate, when each bacterial cell multiplies to produce a colony of bacteria which is visible to the naked eye. A count of the number of colonies gives the number of bacteria in the portion of the sample that was taken. Pasteurised milk contains about 100 000 bacteria/mL; good quality raw milk contains less than 500 000/mL.

plethysmography   Technique for determination of body volume by immersion in water, for estimation of body fat (see BODY DENSITY).

Pliofilm   Trade name for varieties of rubber hydrochloride, the first transparent wrapping paper (1934) that could be heat sealed.

pluck   Butchers' term for heart, liver and lungs of an animal.

plum   Fruit of numerous species of *Prunus*. Common European plums are *P. domestica*; blackthorn or sloe is *P. spinosa*; bullace is *P. insititia*; damson is *P. damascena*; GREENGAGES are *P. italica*. The UK National Fruit Collection contains 336 varieties.

Composition/100 g: 100–154 kJ (24–37 kcal), protein 0.5 g, fat 0.1 g, carbohydrate 6–9 g (6–9 g sugars), dietary fibre 1.8 g, nsp 1.7 g, Na 2 mg, K 180 mg, Ca 7–10 mg, Mg 5–7 mg, P 15–22 mg, Fe 0.2–0.4 mg, Cu 0.1 mg, vitamin A 20–45 µg (120–275 µg carotene), E 0.6 mg, B_1 0.03 mg, B_2 0.04 mg, niacin 0.6 mg, B_6 0.05 mg, folate 3 µg, pantothenate 0.1 mg, C 6 mg. Serving 55 g (1 plum).

plumcote American; cross between plum and apricot.

pneumatic conveying Transfer of material in powder form by means of air currents. Applied to flour, sugar etc.

pneumatic dryers The material is dried almost instantaneously in a turbulent stream of hot air, which also acts as a conveyor system. Applicable to powdered, granular and flaky materials; used for starch, mashed potato, cereals, flour, powdered soups, etc.

polarimeter, polariscope Instrument used to determine the degree of rotation of POLARISED LIGHT, as a means of measuring concentrations of OPTICALLY ACTIVE compounds.

polarised light Ordinary light vibrates in many planes; after passing through a crystal of quartz or a polarising filter, it vibrates in only one plane, i.e. it is polarised.

Polenske number Measure of the water-soluble fatty acids in a lipid that are not steam volatile.

See also Reichert–Meissl number; steam distillation.

polenta Traditional Italian porridge made from maize meal, often with cheese added. May be further cooked by baking or frying. Also Italian name for coarsely ground maize meal (hominy grits in USA).

pollards See WHEATFEED.

polony Italian smoked pork and veal sausage, ready to slice and eat; also known as bologna.

polydextrose, modified Glucose polymer prepared by heating GLUCOSE and SORBITOL with citric acid. It is more resistant to enzymic digestion than normal POLYSACCHARIDES and 60% is excreted in faeces undigested, so providing only about 4 kJ (1 kcal)/g; hence termed 'non-sweetening sucrose replacement', or BULKING AGENT.

polydipsia Abnormally intense thirst; a typical symptom of DIABETES mellitus and insipidus.

polygalacturonase See PECTINASE.

polyglucose See POLYDEXTROSE.

polymerase chain reaction (PCR) A technique for the rapid amplification of the DNA from a single cell by a repeated cycle of synthesis, denaturation and annealing. Because all new strands act as templates for replication in the next cycle there is exponential amplification of the DNA, 10^6-fold in 20 cycles, each of which takes 4 min.

The basis of DNA fingerprinting techniques, and widely used for rapid identification of potentially pathogenic organisms in foods.

polymorphism (1) The ability to crystallise in two or more different forms. For example, depending on the conditions under which it is solidified, the fat tristearin can form three kinds of crystal, each with a different melting point: 54, 65, 71°C.

(2) Genetic polymorphism is the relatively widespread occurrence in the population of one or more variants of a gene.

polymyxins Antibiotics isolated from *Bacillus polymyxin* (*B. aerosporin*); polymyxin A is aerosporin. They are polypeptides, active against coliform bacteria; apart from clinical use, they are of value in controlling infection in brewing.

polyneuritis Any disease involving inflammation of all of the peripheral nerves.

See also POLYNEUROPATHY.

polyneuropathy Any disease involving all of the peripheral nerves; symptoms first affect the extremities (fingers and toes), then ascend towards the trunk. Occurs in BERIBERI due to VITAMIN B$_1$ deficiency.

See also POLYNEURITIS.

polyols See SUGAR ALCOHOLS.

polyoxyethylene See CRUMB SOFTENERS.

polypeptides See PEPTIDES.

polyphagia Excessive or continuous eating.

polyphenol oxidase See PHENOL OXIDASES.

polyphosphates Complex PHOSPHATES added to foods as EMULSIFIERS, BUFFERS, SEQUESTRANTS, prevent discoloration of sausages, aid mixing of the fat, speed penetration of the brine in curing, hold water in meat and fish products. E-450a, b, c and E-541, 544, 545.

polysaccharides Complex CARBOHYDRATES formed by the condensation of large numbers of MONOSACCHARIDE units, e.g. STARCH, GLYCOGEN, CELLULOSE, DEXTRINS, INULIN. Formerly called polysaccharoses.

See also NON-STARCH POLYSACCHARIDES.

polysome An array of several RIBOSOMES along a molecule of MRNA, engaged in the process of TRANSLATION.

polysorbates See CRUMB SOFTENERS.

polyunsaturated fatty acids (polyunsaturates) Long-chain FATTY ACIDS containing two or more double bonds, separated by methylene bridges: $-CH_2-CH=CH-CH_2-CH=CH-CH_2-$.

polyuria Production of a large volume of dilute urine; may be due simply to high fluid intake, or to kidney disease or DIABETES mellitus or insipidus.

pomace   Residue of fruit pulp after expressing juice: also applied to fish from which oil has been expressed.

pombé   African BEER brewed from millet.

pomegranate   The fruit of the subtropical tree *Punica granatum*. Juice contained in a pulpy sac surrounding each of a mass of seeds, outer skin contains tannin and is therefore bitter. Sweet juice used to prepare grenadine SYRUP for alcoholic and fruit drinks.

Composition/100 g: 138 kJ (33 kcal), protein 0.9 g, fat 0.1 g, carbohydrate 7.7 g (7.7 g sugars), nsp 2.2 g, Na 1 mg, K 160 mg, Ca 8 mg, Mg 7 mg, P 19 mg, Fe 0.5 mg, Cu 0.11 mg, Zn 0.3 mg, vitamin A 3 μg (21 μg carotene), B_1 0.03 mg, B_2 0.03 mg, niacin 0.3 mg, B_6 0.2 mg, pantothenate 0.4 mg, C 8 mg. A 100 g serving is a source of vitamin B_6, C, Cu.

pomelo (pomeloe, pummelo)   Fruit of *Citrus grandis*, from which the GRAPEFRUIT is descended; also called shaddock, after Captain Shaddock, who introduced it into Barbados in the sixteenth century.

Composition/100 g: 75 kJ (18 kcal), protein 0.4 g, fat 0.1 g, carbohydrate 4.1 g (4.1 g sugars), dietary fibre 0.5 g, Na 1 mg, K 140 mg, Ca 16 mg, Mg 4 mg, P 12 mg, Fe 0.2 mg, Cu 0.03 mg, Zn 0.1 mg, vitamin A 2 μg (14 μg carotene), E 0.1 mg, B_1 0.03 mg, B_2 0.02 mg, niacin 0.2 mg, B_6 0.02 mg, folate 16 μg, pantothenate 0.2 mg, biotin 0.6 μg, C 27 mg. A 125 g serving (half fruit) is a source of folate; rich source of vitamin C.

See also CITRUS fruits.

pomes   Botanical name for fruits such as apple or pear, formed by the enlargement of the receptacle which becomes fleshy and surrounds the carpels.

pomfret   See PONTEFRACT CAKES.

ponceau (ponceau 4R)   Strawberry red colour, E-124.

ponderal index   An index of fatness, used as a measure of OBESITY: height divided by cube root of weight. Confusingly, the ponderal index is higher for thin people, and lower for fat people.

See also BODY MASS INDEX.

ponderocrescive   Foods stimulating weight gain.

pondoperditive   Foods stimulating weight loss.

pone bread   Colloquial name for corn bread in the southern states of the USA. (Corn pone are small corn cakes, a speciality of Alabama.)

Pontefract cakes   A round, flat sweetmeat made from LIQUORICE originally in Pontefract in England, also called pomfret.

poonac   The residue of COCONUT after the extraction of the oil.

popcorn   Variety of MAIZE (parch maize, *Zea mays everta*) that expands on heating, also the name of the fluffy white mass so formed.

pope's eye   The small round circle of fat in the centre of a leg of pork or mutton.

poppadom   Indian; thin roasted or fried crisps made from lentil flour; may be spiced.

poppy seed   Seeds of the opium poppy, *Papaver somniferum*, used mixed with honey in cakes, and as a flavouring on the crust of bread and rolls. Also called maw seed.

Population reference intake, PRI   See REFERENCE INTAKES.

pork   Meat from the pig (swine, hog), *Suidae* spp eaten fresh, as opposed to bacon and ham, which are cured.

Composition/100 g: 774 kJ (185 kcal), protein 30.7 g, fat 6.9 g (39.3% saturated, 44.2% mono-, 16.3% polyunsaturated), cholesterol 110 mg, carbohydrate 0 g, Na 79 mg, K 390 mg, Ca 9 mg, Mg 25 mg, P 230 mg, Fe 1.3 mg, Cu 0.29 mg, Zn 3.5 mg, Se 14 µg, I 3 µg, vitamin B_1 0.85 mg, B_2 0.35 mg, niacin 12.3 mg, B_6 0.41 mg, folate 7 µg, B_{12} 2 µg, pantothenate 1.3 mg, biotin 3 µg. A 150 g serving is a source of Mg, Fe; rich source of protein, vitamin B_1, B_2, niacin, B_6, B_{12}, pantothenate, Cu, Se, Zn.

porphyra   Red seaweed used to make LAVERBREAD.

porphyrin   One of a number of pigments consisting of a substituted tetrapyrrole ring and a chelated metal ion, including HAEM and CHLOROPHYLL.

porridge   Oatmeal cooked in water or milk as a breakfast dish; originally Scottish. Also similar thick soups made with other cereals.

Composition/100 g (made with milk): 485 kJ (116 kcal), protein 4.8 g, fat 5.1 g (57.4% saturated, 31.9% mono-, 10.6% polyunsaturated), cholesterol 14 mg, carbohydrate 13.7 g (4.7 g sugars, 9 g starch), dietary fibre 0.8 g, nsp 0.8 g, Na 620 mg, K 190 mg, Ca 120 mg, Mg 29 mg, P 140 mg, Fe 0.6 mg, Cu 0.03 mg, Zn 0.8 mg, vitamin A 56 µg (21 µg carotene), D 0.03 µg, E 0.3 mg, B_1 0.1 mg, B_2 0.17 mg, niacin 1.3 mg, B_6 0.06 mg, folate 7 µg, pantothenate 0.4 mg, biotin 3 µg, C 1 mg. A 110 g serving is a source of protein, vitamin B_2, Ca, Mg.

Composition/100 g (made with water): 205 kJ (49 kcal), protein 1.5 g, fat 1.1 g (20% saturated, 40% mono-, 40% polyunsaturated), carbohydrate 9 g (9 g starch), dietary fibre 0.8 g, nsp 0.8 g, Na 560 mg, K 46 mg, Ca 7 mg, Mg 18 mg, P 47 mg, Fe 0.5 mg, Cu 0.03 mg, Zn 0.4 mg, vitamin E 0.2 mg, B_1 0.06 mg, B_2 0.01 mg, niacin 0.4 mg, B_6 0.01 mg, folate 4 µg, pantothenate 0.1 mg, biotin 2 µg.

See also OATS.

port   Fortified wines from the upper Douro valley of north east Portugal. Mostly aged in wood and bottled when ready for drinking; vintage port is aged in wood for 2 years, then in the bottle for at least 10; late bottled vintage is aged less than 6 years. Crusted port is blended from quality vintages, bottled young and develops a sediment (crust) in the bottle. Ruby port is young, old tawny is aged for 10 or more years; fine old tawny is a blend of young and old wines. Tawny port is aged in wood, vintage in the bottle. White port is made from white grapes; generally served chilled as an aperitif.

Composition/100 g: 657 kJ (157 kcal), protein 0.1 g, fat 0 g, carbohydrate 12 g (12 g sugars), Na 4 mg, K 97 mg, Ca 4 mg, Mg 11 mg, P 12 mg, Fe 0.4 mg, Cu 0.1 mg, vitamin B_2 0.01 mg, niacin 0.1 mg, B_6 0.01 mg.

porter See BEER.

Poskitt index Index of fatness in children; percent of expected weight for age.

posset (1) Drink made from hot milk curdled with ale or wine, sometimes thickened with breadcrumbs and spiced. Formerly used as remedy for colds; popular in late Middle Ages.

(2) Small amount of milk regurgitated by babies after feeding.

post-cibal Occurring after eating.

post-mature Baby born after 42 weeks of gestation.

See also PREMATURE.

post-partum Relating to the first few days after birth.

post-prandial Occurring after eating.

potassium An essential mineral, widespread in nature; the human body contains about 125 g. Mostly present inside the cells. REFERENCE NUTRIENT INTAKE for adults 3.5 g/day; abundant in fruit and vegetables. Important in plant fertilisers.

potassium nitrate See NITRATE; SALTPETRE.

potassium sorbate Potassium salt of SORBIC ACID (E-20(2)).

potato crisps Flavoured thin slices of potato, deep fried and eaten cold, sometimes as an accompaniment to meals, more commonly as a snack. Called chips in USA.

Composition/100 g: 2285 kJ (546 kcal), protein 5.6 g, fat 37.6 g (29.5% saturated, 38.5% mono-, 31.8% polyunsaturated), carbohydrate 49.3 g (0.7 g sugars, 48.6 g starch), dietary fibre 10.7 g, nsp 4.9 g; low fat varieties 2021 kJ (483 kcal), protein 6.6 g, fat 21.5 g (29.8% saturated, 38.4% mono-, 31.7% polyunsaturated), carbohydrate 63 g (1 g sugars, 62 g starch), dietary fibre 13.7 g, nsp 6.3 g; Na 1070 mg, K 1060 mg, Ca 37 mg, Mg 45 mg, P 120 mg, Fe 1.8 mg, Cu 0.13 mg, Zn 0.7 mg, vitamin E 3.1 mg, B_1 0.11 mg, B_2 0.07 mg, niacin 5.9 mg, B_6 0.32 mg, folate 41 µg, C 27 mg. A 30 g serving is a source of vitamin C.

potato, fairy See EARTH NUT.

potato flour Dried potato tuber.

potato, Irish The 'ordinary' potato, tuber of *Solanum tuberosum*.

Composition/100 g: 275–300 kJ (66–72 kcal), protein 1.4–1.8 g, fat 0.1–0.3 g, carbohydrate 15–17 g (1 g sugars, 14–16 g starch), dietary fibre 1.4–1.6 g, nsp 1.2–1.5 g, Na 10 mg, K 280–430 mg, Ca 5–13 mg, Mg 14–18 mg, P 31–54 mg, Fe 0.4–1.6 mg, Cu 0.06 mg, Zn 0.3 mg, Se 1 µg, I 3 µg, vitamin E 0.1 mg, B_1 0.09–0.18 mg, B_2 0.01–0.06 mg, niacin 0.7–0.9 mg, B_6 0.35 mg, folate 10–26 µg, pantothenate 0.4 mg, biotin 0.3 µg, C 6–15 mg. A 175 g serving is a source of pantothenate, Cu; good source of vitamin B_6, C.

potato starch Or farina. Prepared from potato tuber and widely used as a stabilising agent when gelatinised by heat.

potato, sweet Tubers of the herbaceous climbing plant *Ipomoea batatas*, known in Britain before the Irish potato. The flesh may be white, yellow or pink (if carotene is present); the leaves are also edible.

Composition/100 g: 481 kJ (115 kcal), protein 1.6 g, fat 0.4 g, carbohydrate 27.9 g (14.5 g sugars, 13.4 g starch), dietary fibre 3 g, nsp 3.3 g, Na 52 mg, K 480 mg, Ca 31 mg, Mg 23 mg, P 65 mg, Fe 0.9 mg, Cu 0.18 mg, Zn 0.4 mg, Se 1 µg, I 3 µg, vitamin A 856 µg (5140 µg carotene), E 6 mg, B_1 0.09 mg, niacin 0.8 mg, B_6 0.07 mg, folate 9 µg, pantothenate 0.6 mg, C 23 mg. A 130 g serving is a source of pantothenate; good source of Cu; rich source of vitamin A, E, C.

poteen Irish name for illicit home-distilled spirit.

pottle Traditional English wine measure; $^1/_2$ gallon (= 2.25 L).

poularde A neutered hen bird.

poultry General term for farmyard birds (as opposed to wild GAME birds) kept for eggs and/or meat; CHICKEN, DUCK, GOOSE, GUINEA FOWL, PIGEON and TURKEY.

poultry, New York dressed Poultry that have been slaughtered and plucked but not eviscerated.

pound cake American name for Madeira cake; rich cake containing a pound, or equal quantities, of each of the major ingredients, flour, sugar and butter (and eggs).

poussin Young CHICKEN, 4–6 weeks old.

PPAR receptor Peroxisome proliferation activation receptor, a steroid hormone-like nuclear receptor protein that binds long-chain polyunsaturated fatty acids or EICOSANOID derivatives (prostaglandins and leukotrienes). Also activated by FIBRIC ACID derivatives used as hypolipidaemic agents. May act to modulate gene expression alone or as a heterodimer with the RETINOID X receptor.

PP factor or vitamin See NIACIN.

ppm Parts per million (= mg/kg).

prairie chicken American GAME bird, *Tympanuchus cupido* and *T pallidicinctus*.

prairie oyster Traditional cure for a hangover; a raw egg with WORCESTERSHIRE SAUCE and brandy; the egg is swirled with the liquid but the yolk remains intact.

pravastatin See STATINS.

prawns Shellfish of various tribes of suborder *Macrura*. Large fish of species of Palaemonidae, Penaeidae and Pandalidae are prawns; smaller ones are shrimps. The deepwater prawn is *Pandalus borealis*; common pink shrimp is *Pandalus montagui*; brown shrimp is *Crangon* sp.

Composition/100 g (weighed with shells): 171 kJ (41 kcal), protein 8.6 g, fat 0.7 g, cholesterol 31 mg, carbohydrate 0 g, Na 610 mg, K 99 mg, Ca 55 mg, Mg 16 mg, P 130 mg, Fe 0.4 mg, Cu 0.27 mg, Zn 0.6 mg, Se 7 µg, I 11 µg, vitamin B_1 0.01 mg, B_2 0.06 mg, niacin 1.8 mg, B_6 0.03 mg, pantothenate 0.4 mg. A 150 g serving is a source of niacin, Ca, I; good source of protein, Se; rich source of Cu.

See also DUBLIN BAY PRAWN; LOBSTER; SCAMPI.

PRE Protein retention efficiency, a measure of PROTEIN QUALITY.

pre-albumin See TRANSTHYRETIN.

prebiotics Non-digestible OLIGOSACCHARIDES that support the growth of colonies of certain bacteria in the colon. They include derivatives of FRUCTOSE and GALACTOSE, and lead to the growth of bifidobacteria, so changing and possibly improving the colonic flora. PROBIOTICS and prebiotics are sometimes termed synbiotics. They are considered to play a rôle as FUNCTIONAL FOODS.

precision Of an assay; the degree of reproducibility of a result, determined by calculation of the variance between replicate analyses.

See also ACCURACY.

pregnancy, nutritional needs Pregnant women have slightly increased energy and protein requirements compared with their needs before pregnancy, although there are metabolic adaptations in early pregnancy which result in laying down increased reserves for the great stress of the last trimester, and high requirements for iron and calcium. These increased needs are reflected in the increased REFERENCE INTAKES for pregnancy (see Tables 3–5).

premature Usually a PRETERM birth, but also used when the infant weighs less than 2.5 kg, regardless of the length of gestation, as a result of intrauterine undernutrition.

premier jus Best-quality SUET prepared from oxen and sheep kidneys. The fat is chilled, shredded and heated at moderate temperature. When pressed, premier jus separates into a liquid fraction (oleo oil or liquid oleo) and a solid fraction (oleostearin or solid tallow).

preservation Protection of food from deterioration by microorganisms, enzymes and oxidation, by cooling, destroying the microorganisms and enzymes by heat treatment or IRRADIATION, reducing their activity through dehydration or the addition of chemical PRESERVATIVES, and by smoking, SALTING and PICKLING.

preservatives Substances capable of retarding or arresting the deterioration of food; examples are SULPHUR DIOXIDE, BENZOIC ACID, specified ANTIBIOTICS, SALT, acids and essential oils. See Table 6.

pressure cooking See AUTOCLAVE.

preterm Birth before 37 weeks of gestation.
    See also POST-MATURE; PREMATURE.

pretzels German; hard brittle biscuits in the shape of a knot, made from flour, water, shortening, yeast and salt. Also called bretzels.

prevalence rate Measure of morbidity based on current sickness in a population at a particular time (point prevalence) or over a stated period of time (period prevalence).
    See also INCIDENCE RATE.

PRI Population reference intake of nutrients; see REFERENCE INTAKES.

prickly pear Fruit of the cactus *Opuntia* spp, also called Indian fig, barberry fig, tuna or sabra fruit, an important part of the diet in certain areas of Mexico.
    Composition/100g: 205 kJ (49 kcal), protein 0.7 g, fat 0.3 g, carbohydrate 11.5 g (11.5 g sugars), Na 4 mg, K 210 mg, Ca 53 mg, Mg 57 mg, P 27 mg, Fe 0.4 mg, Zn 0.6 mg, vitamin A 7 µg (45 µg carotene), B_1 0.02 mg, B_2 0.04 mg, niacin 0.4 mg, C 22 mg. A 100 g serving is a source of Mg; rich source of vitamin C.

primigravida Woman experiencing her first pregnancy.

primipara Woman who has given birth to one infant capable of survival.
    See also PARITY.

prions Small, glycosylated proteins (M_r 27 000–30 000) in the brain cell membranes; to a considerable extent they are species-specific. A modified prion, designated PrPsc, resistant to digestion, heat and chemical agents, is believed to be the cause of SPONGIFORM ENCEPHALOPATHIES.

probiotics Preparations of microbial culture added to food or animal feed, claimed to be beneficial to health by restoring balance to the intestinal flora. Organisms commonly involved include *Bifidobacterium* spp, *Enterococcus faecium*, *Lactobacillus* spp, *Saccharomyces bulardii*.
    See also ACIDOPHILUS MILK; PREBIOTICS.

probucol Drug used in treatment of primary hypercholesterolaemia; acts by inhibiting synthesis of CHOLESTEROL and increasing catabolism of low-density LIPOPROTEIN.

procarcinogen A compound that is not itself carcinogenic, but undergoes metabolic activation in the body to yield a CARCINOGEN.

See also PHASE I METABOLISM.

processing Any and all processes to which food is subjected after harvesting for the purposes of improving its appearance, texture, palatability, nutritive value, keeping properties and ease of preparation, and for eliminating microorganisms, toxins and other undesirable constituents.

proctitis Inflammation of the rectum.

proctocolitis Inflammation of the colon and rectum.

pro-enzyme See ZYMOGEN.

progoitrins Substances found in plant foods which are precursors of GOITROGENS.

pro-insulin The inactive precursor of INSULIN, in which the A- and B-chains are joined by the C-PEPTIDE; the form in which insulin is stored in pancreatic β-islet cells before release. A small proportion of insulin secretion is pro-insulin.

prolactin Hormone secreted by the anterior pituitary that stimulates milk secretion after childbirth. Also known as lactogenic or luteotrophic hormone, and luteotrophin.

prolamins The major storage proteins of the ENDOSPERM of cereals, including gliadin (wheat), zein (maize), hordein (barley) and avenin (oats). Characterised by solubility in 70% alcohol, but not water or absolute alcohol; especially rich in PROLINE and GLUTAMINE, low in LYSINE.

proline A non-essential AMINO ACID, abbr Pro (P), M_r 115.1, pK_a 1.95, 10.64, CODONS CCNu.

Promega Trade name for mixture of long-chain marine FATTY ACIDS: eicosapentaenoic (EPA, C20:5 ω3) and docosohexaenoic (DHA, C22:6 ω3) acids.

promoter A compound that is not itself carcinogenic, but enhances the activity of a CARCINOGEN if given subsequently.

See also COCARCINOGEN.

Pronutro Protein-rich baby food (22% protein) developed in South Africa; made from maize, skim-milk powder, groundnut flour, soya flour and fish protein concentrate with added vitamins.

proof spirit An old method of describing the ALCOHOL content of SPIRITS; originally defined as a solution of alcohol of such strength that it will ignite when mixed with gunpowder. Proof spirit contains 57.07% alcohol by volume or 49.24% by weight in Great Britain. In the USA it contains 50% alcohol by volume. Pure (absolute) alcohol is 175.25° proof UK or 200° proof USA. Spirits were described as under or over proof; a drink 30° over proof contains as much alcohol as 130 volumes of proof spirit; 30° under proof means that 100 volumes contains as much alcohol as 70 volumes of proof spirit. Nowadays alcohol content is usually measured as percent alcohol by volume.

propanetheline See ATROPINE.

propionates Salts of propionic acid, CH_3CH_2COOH, a normal metabolic intermediate. The free acid and salts are used as mould inhibitors, e.g. on cheese surfaces; to inhibit ROPE in bread and baked goods (E-280–283).

propyl gallate An ANTIOXIDANT, E-310.

Prosparol Trade name for an emulsion containing 50% vegetable fat, 1.7 MJ (405 kcal)/100 g; used as a concentrated source of energy.

prostaglandins Locally acting HORMONES (paracrine agents) synthesised from long-chain polyunsaturated fatty acids; see EICOSANOIDS.

prosthetic group Non-protein part of an enzyme molecule; either a coenzyme or a metal ion. Essential for catalytic activity. The enzyme protein without its prosthetic group is the apo-enzyme and is catalytically inactive. With the prosthetic group, it is known as the holo-enzyme.

See also ENZYME ACTIVATION TESTS.

protamines The simplest natural proteins, containing only a limited number of amino acids, chiefly the basic ones, especially arginine. Soluble in water; not coagulated by heat; so basic that they form salts with strong mineral acids, e.g. salmine from salmon sperm, sturine from sturgeon sperm, clupeine from herring sperm, scombrine from mackerel sperm.

proteans Slightly altered proteins that have become insoluble, probably an early stage of denaturation.

proteases Alternative name for PROTEINASES.

protein All living tissues contain proteins; they are polymers of AMINO ACIDS, joined by PEPTIDE bonds. There are 20 main amino acids in proteins, and any one protein may contain several hundred or thousand amino acids. The sequence of the amino acids in a protein determines its overall structure and function: many proteins are enzymes; others are structural (e.g. COLLAGEN in connective tissue and KERATIN in hair and nails); many HORMONES are polypeptides. Proteins are constituents of all living cells and are dietary essentials. Chemically distinguished from fats and carbohydrates by containing nitrogen.

proteinases Enzymes that hydrolyse proteins, also known as peptidases.

See also CHILLPROOFING; ENDOPEPTIDASES; EXOPEPTIDASES; TENDERISERS.

protein-bound iodine The THYROID HORMONES, tri-iodothyronine and thyroxine are transported in the bloodstream bound to proteins; measurement of protein-bound iodine, as opposed to total plasma iodine, was used as an index of thyroid gland activity before more specific methods of measuring the hormones were developed.

protein calorie malnutrition See PROTEIN ENERGY MALNUTRITION.

protein calories percent See PROTEIN ENERGY RATIO.

protein, conjugated Proteins that include a non-protein prosthetic group, e.g. HAEMOGLOBIN and CYTOCHROMES contain HAEM; many oxidative enzymes contain a prosthetic group derived from VITAMIN B_2; many proteins are conjugated (combined) with carbohydrates (glycoproteins) or fatty acids.

protein conversion factor See NITROGEN CONVERSION FACTOR.

protein, crude Total NITROGEN multiplied by the NITROGEN CONVERSION FACTOR = 6.25.

See also KJELDAHL DETERMINATION; NITROGEN CONVERSION FACTORS.

protein efficiency ratio (PER) A measure of PROTEIN QUALITY.

protein energy malnutrition (PEM) A spectrum of disorders, especially in children, due to inadequate feeding. Marasmus is severe wasting and can occur in adults; the result of a food intake inadequate to meet energy expenditure. Emaciation, similar to that seen in marasmus, occurs in patients with advanced cancer and AIDS; in this case it is known as CACHEXIA.

Kwashiorkor affects only young children and includes severe oedema, fatty infiltration of the liver and a sooty dermatitis; it is likely that deficiency of ANTIOXIDANT nutrients and the stress of infection may be involved. The name kwashiorkor is derived from the Ga language of Ghana to describe the illness of the first child when it is weaned (on to an inadequate diet) on the arrival of the second child.

See also GOMEZ CLASSIFICATION; MARASMIC KWASHIORKOR; WATERLOW CLASSIFICATION; WELLCOME CLASSIFICATION.

protein energy ratio The protein content of a food or diet expressed as the proportion of the total energy provided by protein (17 kJ, 4 kcal, /g). The average requirement for protein is about 7% of total energy intake; average western diets provide about 14%.

protein equivalent A measure of the digestible nitrogen of an animal feedingstuff in terms of protein. It is measured by direct feeding or calculated from the digestible pure protein plus half the digestible non-protein nitrogen.

protein, first class   An obsolete system of classifying proteins into first and second class, to indicate their relative nutritional value or PROTEIN QUALITY. Generally, but not invariably, animal proteins were considered 'first class' and plant proteins 'second class', but this classification has no validity in the diet as a whole.

protein intolerance   An ADVERSE REACTION to one or more specific proteins in foods, commonly the result of an allergy. General protein intolerance may be due to a variety of GENETIC DISEASES affecting amino acid metabolism. Treatment is normally by severe restriction of protein intake.

See also AMINO ACID DISORDERS; HYPERAMMONAEMIA.

protein milk   Partially skimmed lactic acid milk plus milk curd (prepared from whole milk by RENNET precipitation); richer in protein and lower in fat than ordinary milk, supposed to be better tolerated in digestive disorders. Also known as albumin milk and eiweiss milch.

protein quality   A measure of the usefulness of a protein food for maintenance and repair of tissue, growth and formation of new tissues and, in animals, production of meat, eggs, wool and milk. It is only important if the total intake of protein barely meets the requirement. Furthermore, the quality of individual proteins is relatively unimportant in mixed diets, because of COMPLEMENTATION between different proteins. Two types of measurement are used to estimate protein quality: biological assays and chemical analysis.

Biological value (BV) is the proportion of absorbed protein retained in the body (i.e. taking no account of digestibility). A protein that is completely usable (e.g. egg and human milk) has a BV = 0.9–1; meat and fish have BV = 0.75–0.8; wheat protein 0.5; gelatine 0.

Net protein utilisation (NPU) is the proportion of dietary protein that is retained in the body under specified experimental conditions (i.e. it takes account of digestibility; NPU = BV × digestibility). By convention NPU is measured at 10% dietary protein (NPU_{10}) at which level the protein synthetic mechanism of the animal can utilise all of the protein so long as the balance of ESSENTIAL AMINO ACIDS is correct. When fed at 4% dietary protein, the result is NPU standardised. If the food or diet is fed as it is normally eaten, the result is NPU operative (NPU_{op}).

Protein efficiency ratio (PER) is the gain in weight of growing animals per gram of protein eaten.

Net protein retention (NPR) is the weight gain of animals fed the test protein, minus the weight loss of a group fed a protein-free diet, divided by the protein consumed.

Protein retention efficiency (PRE) is the NPR converted into a percentage scale by multiplying by 16; it then becomes numerically the same as net protein utilisation.

Relative protein value (RPV) is the ability of a test protein, fed at various levels of intake, to support NITROGEN BALANCE, relative to a standard protein.

Chemical score is based on chemical analysis of the protein; it is the amount of the limiting AMINO ACID compared with the amount of the same amino acid in egg protein.

Protein score is similar to chemical score, but uses an amino acid mixture as the standard, also known as amino acid score.

Essential amino acid index is the sum of all the essential amino acids compared with those in egg protein or the amino acid target mixture.

protein rating Used in Canadian food regulations to assess the overall protein quality of a food. It is protein efficiency ratio × percent protein content of food × the amount of food that is reasonably consumed. Foods with a rating above 40 may be designated excellent dietary sources; foods with rating below 20 are considered to be insignificant sources; 20–40 may be described as good sources.

protein, reference A theoretical concept of the perfect protein which is used with 100% efficiency at whatever level it is fed in the diet. Used as a means of expressing recommended intakes. The nearest approach to this theoretical protein are egg and human milk proteins, which are used with 90–100% efficiency (BV = 0.9–1.0) when fed at low levels in the diet (4%), but not when fed at high levels (10–15%).

Protein retention efficiency (PRE) A measure of PROTEIN QUALITY.

protein score A measure of PROTEIN QUALITY based on chemical analysis.

protein, second class See PROTEIN, FIRST CLASS.

protein turnover See HALF-LIFE (1).

proteoglycans See GLYCOPROTEINS.

proteolysis The hydrolysis of proteins to their constituent AMINO ACIDS, catalysed by alkali, acid or enzymes.

proteoses Partial degradation products of proteins; soluble in water. The stages of breakdown are protein → proteoses → peptones → polypeptides → oligopeptides → amino acids.

Proteus Genus of flagellate and highly motile rod-like Gram-negative bacteria, common in intestinal flora. Some species are pathogenic.

prothrombin Protein in plasma involved in coagulation of BLOOD. Prothrombin time is an index of the coagulability of blood (and hence of VITAMIN K nutritional status) based on the time taken for a citrated sample of blood to clot when calcium ions and thromboplastin are added.

protogen See LIPOIC ACID.

proton pump Enzyme (H^+/K^+ ATPase, EC 3.6.1.36) in parietal (oxyntic) cells of gastric mucosa that causes secretion of gastric acid; acts by exchanging H^+ and K^+ across the cell membrane. Irreversible inhibitors (lansoprazole, pantoprazole and omeprazole) are used in the treatment of gastric ULCERS.

protopectin See PECTIN.

protoporphyrin The iron-free precursor of HAEM. Normally present in red blood cells in low concentrations, an increased concentration is an early index of IRON deficiency. Also increased by lead toxicity.

See also PORPHYRIN.

proving The stage in bread making when the dough is left to rise.

provitamin A substance that is converted into a vitamin, such as 7-dehydrocholesterol, which is converted into VITAMIN D, or those CAROTENES that can be converted to VITAMIN A.

proximate analysis Analysis of foods and feedingstuffs for NITRO-GEN (for protein), ether extract (for fat), crude FIBRE and ASH (mineral salts) together with soluble carbohydrate calculated by subtracting these values from the total (CARBOHYDRATE by difference). Also known as Weende analysis, after the Weende Experimental Station in Germany, which in 1865 outlined the methods of analysis to be used.

Prozac See FLUOXETINE.

prunin See NARINGIN.

Prunus Genus of plants including PLUMS, PEACHES, NECTARINES, CHERRIES and ALMONDS.

Pruteen Trade name for microbial protein produced by growing bacteria, *Methylophilus methylotrophus*, on methanol (derived from methane or natural gas); 70% protein on dry weight.

pseudoglobulin Water-soluble globulin which is not precipitated from salt solutions by dialysis against distilled water. Pseudo-globulins occur in blood serum, in animal tissues, and in milk.

See also EUGLOBULIN.

pseudokeratins See KERATIN.

pseudoplastic COLLOIDAL SUSPENSION whose observed VISCOSITY decreases with an increase in shear stress.

See also DILATANT; RHEOPEXIC; THIXOTROPIC.

P/S ratio The ratio between polyunsaturated and saturated FATTY ACIDS. In western diets the ratio is about 0.6; it is suggested that increasing to near 1.0 would reduce the risk of atherosclerosis and coronary heart disease.

psychrometry Study of the interrelationships of temperature and humidity relevant to drying with hot air.

psychrophilic organisms Bacteria and fungi that tolerate low temperatures. Their preferred temperature range is 15–20°C, but they will grow in cold stores at or below 0°C; the temperature must be reduced to about –10°C before growth stops, but the organisms are not killed and will regrow when the temperature rises.

Bacteria of the genera *Achromobacter*, *Flavobacterium*, *Pseudomonas* and *Micrococcus*; *Torulopsis* yeasts; and moulds of the genera *Penicillium*, *Cladosporium*, *Mucor* and *Thamnidium* are psychrophiles.

psyllium Also known as plantago or flea seed, *Plantago psyllium*. Small, dark reddish-brown seeds which form a mucilaginous mass with water; used as a bulk-forming LAXATIVE.

pteroylglutamic acid (pteroylglutamate), pteroylpolyglutamic acid (pteroylpolyglutamate) See FOLIC ACID.

ptomaines Loosely used name for amines formed by decarboxylation of amino acids during putrefaction of proteins; putrescine from arginine, cadaverine from lysine, muscarine in mushrooms, neurine formed by dehydration of choline. They have an unpleasant smell and were formerly thought to cause food poisoning, but are in fact harmless, albeit sometimes the products of pathogenic bacteria.

ptyalin Obsolete name for salivary AMYLASE.

ptyalism Or sialorrhoea, excessive flow of SALIVA.

puberty, delayed The normal onset of puberty in boys is between the ages of 12–15; a number of factors may delay this, especially deficiency of ZINC. Severely zinc-deficient boys of 20 are still prepubertal.

PUFA Polyunsaturated FATTY ACIDS.

puffballs Edible wild fungi; mosaic puffball *Calvatia (Lycoperdon) caelata*, giant puffball *C. gigantea* (may grow to 30 cm in diameter), normally eaten while still relatively small and fleshy, much prized for their delicate flavour. See MUSHROOMS.

puffer fish See TETRODONTIN POISONING.

pullulanase See DEBRANCHING ENZYMES.

pulque Sourish beer produced in central and south America by the rapid natural fermentation of aquamiel, the sweet mucilaginous sap of the agave (American aloe or century plant, *Agave americana*). Contains 6% alcohol by volume.

pulses Name given to the dried seeds (matured on the plant) of LEGUMES such as PEAS, BEANS and LENTILS. In the fresh, wet form they contain about 90% water, but the dried form contains about 10% water and can be stored.

pumpernickel Dense sour-flavoured black bread made from rye, originally German; in USA name for any rye bread.

pumpkin A GOURD, fruit of *Cucurbita pepo*.

Composition/100 g: 54 kJ (13 kcal), protein 0.6 g, fat 0.3 g, carbohydrate 2.1 g (1.8 g sugars, 0.1 g starch), dietary fibre 0.5 g, nsp 1.1 g, Na 76 mg, K 84 mg, Ca 23 mg, Mg 7 mg, P 15 mg, Fe 0.1 mg, Cu 0.02 mg, Zn 0.2 mg, vitamin A 159 µg (955 µg carotene), E 1.1 mg, B_1 0.14 mg, niacin 0.2 mg, B_6 0.03 mg, folate 10 µg, pantothenate 0.3 mg, biotin 0.4 µg, C 7 mg. A 65 g serving is a source of vitamin A.

Seeds, composition/100 g: 2381 kJ (569 kcal), protein 24.4 g, fat 45.6 g (19.1% saturated, 30.6% mono-, 50.1% polyunsaturated), carbohydrate 15.2 g (1.1 g sugars, 14.1 g starch), nsp 5.3 g, Na 18 mg, K 820 mg, Ca 39 mg, Mg 270 mg, P 850 mg, Fe 10 mg, Cu 1.57 mg, Zn 6.6 mg, Se 6 µg, vitamin A 38 µg (230 µg carotene), B_1 0.23 mg, B_2 0.32 mg, niacin 8.8 mg. A 15 g serving is a source of Mg, Fe; good source of Cu.

purgative See LAXATIVE.

puri (poori) Indian; unleavened wholewheat bread prepared from a butter-rich dough, shaped into small pancakes and deep fried in hot oil.

purines Nitrogenous bases that occur in NUCLEIC ACIDS (adenine and guanine) and their precursors and metabolites; inosine, caffeine and theobromine are also purines. They are not dietary essentials; both dietary and endogenously formed purines are excreted as URIC ACID.

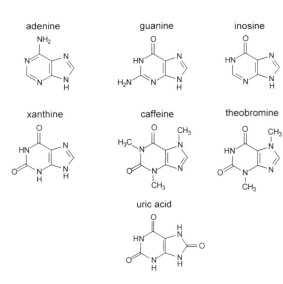

purl Old English winter drink; warmed ale with bitters and brandy or milk, sugar and spirit.

putromaine Any toxin produced by the decay of food within the body.

pylorus Lower end of the stomach, where it enters the duodenum, via the pyloric SPHINCTER. Pyloric stenosis is narrowing of the pylorus, leading to repeated vomiting and sometimes visible distension of the stomach.

pyorrhoea Obsolete name for PERIODONTAL disease.

pyridine nucleotides Obsolete name for the COENZYMES NAD and NADP.

pyridoxal, pyridoxamine, pyridoxine See VITAMIN B$_6$.

4-pyridoxic acid The main urinary metabolite of VITAMIN B$_6$.

pyridoxyllysine A SCHIFF base formed by condensation between pyridoxal and the ε-amino group of lysine in proteins. Renders both the VITAMIN B$_6$ and the LYSINE unavailable, and has antivitamin B$_6$ antimetabolic activity.

pyrimidines Nitrogenous bases that occur in NUCLEIC ACIDS, cytosine, thymidine and uracil.

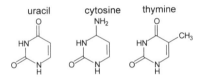

pyrithiamin Antimetabolite of thiamin, used in experimental studies of VITAMIN B$_1$ deficiency; it inhibits thiamin pyrophosphokinase (EC 2.7.6.2) and competes for uptake across the blood–brain barrier, accumulating in the central nervous system. See also OXYTHIAMIN.

pyrocarbonate See DIETHYL PYROCARBONATE.

pyrosis Alternative name for heartburn (USA). See INDIGESTION.

pyruvic acid An intermediate in the metabolism of carbohydrates, formed by the anaerobic GLYCOLYSIS of GLUCOSE. It may then either be converted to acetyl CoA, and oxidised through the CITRIC ACID cycle or be reduced to lactic acid. The oxidation to acetyl CoA is THIAMIN dependent, and blood concentrations of pyruvate and lactate rise in thiamin deficiency.

Q

QUAC stick Quaker arm circumference measuring stick. A stick used to measure height which also shows the 80th and 85th centiles of expected MID-UPPER ARM CIRCUMFERENCE. Developed by a

336

Quaker Service Team in Nigeria in the 1960s as a rapid and simple tool for assessment of nutritional status.

See also ANTHROPOMETRY.

quahog American bivalve mollusc, *Venus mercenaria*.

quail Formerly a GAME bird, now so endangered in the wild that shooting is prohibited, but farmed to some extent. Two main species, *Bonasa umbellus* and *Colinus virginianus*; Californian quail is *Lophortyx californica*. The small eggs are prized as a delicacy.

quamash Or camash; starchy roots of *Camassia quamash*, the staple food of west coast native Americans.

quantitative ingredients declaration (QUID) Will be obligatory on food labels in EU from February 2000; previously legislation only required declaration of ingredients in descending order of quantity, not specific declaration of the amount of each ingredient present.

quark (quarg) When made from skim milk this is a very low fat cheese originating from Germany, containing 80% water.

quart Imperial measure of volume, equal to $^1/_4$ Imperial gallon or 2 pints (i.e. 1.1 L). Reputed quart is the traditional 'bottle' of wine or spirits; approximately $^2/_3$ Imperial quart, or $26^2/_3$ fluid ounces (730 mL). Reputed pint is $13^1/_3$ fluid ounces.

quartern See NOGGIN.

quebracho Or aspidosperma; obtained from the bark of *Aspidosperma quebrachoblanco*; used as source of tannins and alkaloids.

queen substance See ROYAL JELLY.

quercitin A flavone, found in onion skins, tea, hops and horse chestnuts. Not known to be a dietary essential or to have any function in the body, but sometimes called vitamin P. See FLAVONOIDS.

quercitol See ACORN SUGAR.

querns Pair of grinding stones used for pulverising grain (from about 4000–2000 BC). The lower stone was slightly hollowed and the upper stone was rolled by hand on the lower one.

Quetelet's index See BODY MASS INDEX.

quick breads Baked goods such as biscuits, muffins, popovers, griddles, cakes, waffles and dumplings, in which no yeast is used, but the raising carried out quickly with baking powder or other chemical agents.

quick freezing Rapid freezing of food by exposure to a blast of air at a very low temperature. Unlike slow freezing, very small crystals of ice are formed which do not rupture the cells of the food and so the structure is relatively undamaged. A quick-frozen food is commonly defined as one that has been cooled from a temperature of 0°C to –5°C or lower, in a period of not more than 2 h and then cooled to –18°C.

QUID   See QUANTITATIVE INGREDIENTS DECLARATION.

quillaja (quillaia)   Or soapbark; the dried bark of the shrub *Quillaja saponaria*, which contains SAPONINS and TANNINS. Used to produce foam in soft drinks, shampoos and fire extinguishers.

quince   Pear-shaped fruit of *Cydonia oblongata*, with flesh similar to that of the apple; sour but strong aromatic flavour when cooked; rich in pectin and used chiefly in jams and jellies.

Composition/100 g: 108 kJ (26 kcal), protein 0.3 g, fat 0.1 g, carbohydrate 6.3 g (6.3 g sugars), dietary fibre 5.8 g, Na 3 mg, K 200 mg, Ca 14 mg, Mg 6 mg, P 19 mg, Fe 0.3 mg, Cu 0.13 mg, Zn 0.5 mg, vitamin B_1 0.02 mg, B_2 0.02 mg, niacin 0.2 mg, B_6 0.04 mg, pantothenate 0.1 mg, biotin 0.1 µg, C 15 mg. A 150 g serving is a good source of Cu; rich source of vitamin C.

Japanese quince is fruit of the ornamental shrub *Chaenomeles lagenaria*, hard, sour and aromatic, used in preserves and jellies.

quinine   Bitter ALKALOID extracted from bark of the cinchona tree (*Cinchona officinalis*), formerly used to treat or prevent malaria and in apéritif wines, BITTERS and TONIC WATER.

quinoa   Glutinous seeds of the south American plant *Chenopodium album*, used in Chile and Peru to make bread.

Composition/100 g: 1293 kJ (309 kcal), protein 13.8 g, fat 5 g (12.5% saturated, 35% mono-, 52.5% polyunsaturated), carbohydrate 55.7 g (6.1 g sugars, 47.6 g starch), Na 61 mg, K 780 mg, Ca 79 mg, Mg 210 mg P 230 mg, Fe 7.8 mg, Cu 0.82 mg, Zn 3.3 mg, vitamin B_1 0.2 mg, B_2 0.4 mg, niacin 4.8 mg.

quintal   100 kg (220 lb).

Quorn   Trade name for MYCOPROTEIN from the mould *Fusarium graminearum*.

R

***R*- and *S*-**   Systematic chemical nomenclature for assigning conformation of four different groups around an asymmetric carbon atom, in which the two ISOMERS are *R*- (for right) and *S*- (for sinistra, left). It is based on a hierarchy of substituent groups, and does not give the same conformation for all the naturally occurring amino acids, unlike the DL-system. It is little used in biochemistry and nutrition.

See also D-, L- AND DL-; OPTICAL ACTIVITY.

rabbit   (1) *Lepus cuniculus*; both wild and farmed rabbits are eaten.

Composition/100 g: 380 kJ (91 kcal), protein 13.9 g, fat 3.9 g (43.2% saturated, 21.6% mono-, 35.1% polyunsaturated), cholesterol 69 mg, carbohydrate 0 g, Na 16 mg, K 110 mg, Ca 6 mg, Mg 11 mg, P 100 mg, Fe 1 mg, Cu 0.03 mg, Zn 0.9 mg, Se 11 μg, vitamin B_1 0.04 mg, B_2 0.14 mg, niacin 6.9 mg, B_6 0.26 mg, folate 2 μg, B_{12} 6 μg, pantothenate 0.4 mg. A 210 g serving ($^1/_4$ rabbit weighed with bone) is a source of vitamin B_2, pantothenate, Fe, Zn; good source of vitamin B_6; rich source of protein, niacin, vitamin B_{12}, Se.

(2) Original form of rarebit, see WELSH RAREBIT.

racemic The mixture of the D- and L-isomers of a compound, commonly shown as DL-.

rad A non-SI unit of the energy absorbed from ionising radiation; the absorption of 100 ergs per gram of substance. Now superseded by the GRAY.

radappertisation See IRRADIATION.

radiation sterilisation See IRRADIATION.

radical (free radical) A highly reactive molecular species with an unpaired electron.

radicchio Red variety of CHICORY.

radicidation See IRRADIATION.

radioallergosorbent tests (RAST) Tests for food allergy. See ADVERSE REACTIONS TO FOODS.

radio frequency heating See MICROWAVE COOKING.

radioimmunoassay (RIA) Sensitive and specific analytical technique for determination of analytes present at very low concentrations in biological samples. Based on competition between unlabelled and labelled analyte for a limited number of binding sites on an ANTIBODY (or other ligand-binding protein); after calibration, measurement of either the bound or unbound labelled analyte permits determination of the amount present in the sample. Bound and free analyte may be separated by a variety of techniques, including ultrafiltration, solvent extraction, equilibrium dialysis, adsorption onto charcoal, binding of the antiserum to a solid phase, etc.

Also known as saturation analysis or radio-ligand binding assay, especially when a binding protein or plasma transport protein is used rather than an antibody.

See also ELISA; FLUORESCENCE IMMUNOASSAY.

radio-ligand binding assay See RADIOIMMUNOASSAY.

radish The root of *Raphanus* spp.

Composition/100 g: 50 kJ (12 kcal), protein 0.7 g, fat 0.2 g, carbohydrate 1.9 g (1.9 g sugars), dietary fibre 0.9 g, nsp 0.9 g, Na 11 mg, K 240 mg, Ca 19 mg, Mg 5 mg, P 20 mg, Fe 0.6 mg, Cu 0.01 mg, Zn 0.2 mg, Se 2 μg, I 1 μg, vitamin B_1 0.03 mg, niacin 0.5 mg, B_6 0.07 mg, folate 38 μg, pantothenate 0.2 mg, C 17 mg. Serving 30 g (four radishes).

See also MOOLI.

radurisation See IRRADIATION.

raffinade Best-quality refined sugar.

raffinose Trisaccharide, galactosyl-glucosyl-fructose, found in cotton seed, sugar-beet molasses and Australian manna; also known as gossypose, melitose or melitriose. 23% of the sweetness of sucrose. Not digested.

ragi See MILLET.

raisin Dried seedless grapes of several kinds. Valencia raisins from Spanish grapes; Thompson seedless raisins produced mainly in California from the sultanina grape (the skins are coarser than the sultana).

Composition/100 g: 1138 kJ (272 kcal), protein 2.1 g, fat 0.4 g, carbohydrate 69.3 g (69.3 g sugars), dietary fibre 6.1 g, nsp 2 g, Na 60 mg, K 1020 mg, Ca 46 mg, Mg 35 mg, P 76 mg, Fe 3.8 mg, Cu 0.39 mg, Zn 0.7 mg, Se 8 µg, vitamin A 2 µg (12 µg carotene), B_1 0.12 mg, B_2 0.05 mg, niacin 0.8 mg, B_6 0.25 mg, folate 10 µg, pantothenate 0.2 mg, biotin 2 µg, C 1 mg. A 30 g serving (one tablespoon) is a source of Cu.

See also CURRANTS, DRIED; SULTANAS.

Raisin oil is extracted from the seeds of muscat GRAPES, which are removed before drying them to yield raisins. The oil is used primarily to coat the raisins to prevent them sticking together, to render them soft and pliable and less subject to insect infestation.

raising powder See BAKING POWDER.

rambutan Fruit of *Nephelium lappaceum*; covered with yellowish-red soft spines with large seed surrounded by white juicy flesh, similar to LYCHEE, and sometimes called hairy lychee. The name means *hairy man of the jungle* in Bahasa-Malay, reflecting the appearance of the fruit.

Composition/100 g: 288 kJ (69 kcal), protein 1 g, fat 0.4 g, carbohydrate 16.3 g (16.3 g sugars), dietary fibre 1.3 g, Na 1 mg, K 100 mg, Ca 14 mg, Mg 10 mg, P 15 mg, Fe 0.1 mg, Zn 0.6 mg, vitamin B_1 0.02 mg, B_2 0.06 mg, niacin 0.7 mg, C 78 mg. A 95 g serving (four fruits) is a rich source of vitamin C.

ramekin (1) Porcelain or earthenware mould in which mixture is baked and then brought to the table, or the savoury served in a ramekin dish. Paper soufflé cases are called ramekin cases.

(2) Formerly the name given to toasted cheese; now tarts filled with cream cheese.

rancidity The development of unpleasant flavours in oils and fats as a result of LIPASE action or oxidation.

See also ACID NUMBER.

randomisation of fats See INTERESTERIFICATION.

ranitidine See HISTAMINE RECEPTOR ANTAGONISTS.

rape *Brassica napus*, also known as cole, coleseed or colza. Grown for its seed, as source of oil for both industrial and food use. Varieties low in erucic acid are termed '0' or single low; varieties also low in glucosinolates are termed '00' or double low, both these being undesirable constituents of ordinary rapeseed. Oil is very rich in mono-unsaturates (60%), 33% polyunsaturates and only 7% saturates.

rarebit See WELSH RAREBIT.

rasgulla Indian; dessert of small balls of milk curd, ground almond and semolina boiled in syrup.

rasher Slice of BACON or HAM.

raspberry Fruit of *Rubus idaeus*.

Composition/100 g: 104 kJ (25 kcal), protein 1.4 g, fat 0.3 g, carbohydrate 4.6 g (4.6 g sugars), dietary fibre 6.7 g, nsp 2.5 g, Na 3 mg, K 170 mg, Ca 25 mg, Mg 19 mg, P 31 mg, Fe 0.7 mg, Cu 0.1 mg, Zn 0.3 mg, vitamin A 1 μg (6 μg carotene), E 0.5 mg, B_1 0.03 mg, B_2 0.05 mg, niacin 0.8 mg, B_6 0.06 mg, folate 33 μg, pantothenate 0.2 mg, biotin 1.9 μg, C 32 mg. An 80 g serving is a source of folate; rich source of vitamin C.

Black raspberry is *Rubus occidentalis*, native of eastern USA.

RAST Radio-allergosorbent tests for food allergy. See ADVERSE REACTIONS TO FOODS.

rastrello Sharp-edged spoon used to cut out the pulp from halved citrus fruit.

ratafia (1) Flavouring essence made from bitter almonds.
(2) Small macaroon-like biscuits flavoured with almonds.
(3) Almond-flavoured liqueur.

rat line test Biological assay for VITAMIN D. Rats are maintained on a rachitogenic diet, then given the test substance or standard vitamin D for 7–10 days. At post-mortem examination the long bones are stained with silver nitrate; in newly calcified regions silver phosphate is precipitated, and on exposure to light gives a stain that can be quantified.

ravioli Square envelope of PASTA stuffed with minced meat or cheese.

raw sugar Brown unrefined sugar, 96–98% pure, as imported for refining. Contaminated with mould spores, bacteria, cane fibre, and dirt.

ray Cartilaginous FISH, *Raja* spp.

RBP See RETINOL BINDING PROTEIN.

RDA Recommended daily (or dietary) allowance (or amount) of nutrients; see REFERENCE INTAKES.

reactive oxygen species (ROS) A variety of compounds derived from oxygen, including superoxide, hydroxyl and perhydroxy RADICALS, hydrogen peroxide and singlet oxygen.

rebaudioside   Very sweet substance extracted from the leaves of *Stevia rebaudiana* (same source as STEVIOSIDE); 400 times as sweet as sucrose.

recombinant DNA   Product of ligating (joining) two separate pieces of DNA, produced using the same RESTRICTION ENZYME, so as to permit introduction of foreign DNA into a host genome or PLASMID.

recommended daily amount (or allowance), RDA   See REFERENCE INTAKES.

rectal feeding   See NUTRIENT ENEMATA.

red blood cells   See BLOOD CELLS.

red colours   AMARANTH (E-123), CARMOSINE (E-122), COCHINEAL (E-120), ERYTHROSINE (E-127), PONCEAU 4R (E-124), red 2G (E-128).

red cooking   Chinese method of cooking; meat or poultry is first STIR FRIED, then simmered in broth or water.

redcurrants   Fruit of *Ribes sativum* (same species as white currants); the UK National Fruit Collection contains 78 varieties.

Composition/100 g: 87 kJ (21 kcal), protein 1.1 g, fat 0 g, carbohydrate 4.4 g (4.4 g sugars), dietary fibre 7.4 g, nsp 3.4 g, Na 2 mg, K 280 mg, Ca 36 mg, Mg 13 mg, P 30 mg, Fe 1.2 mg, Cu 0.12 mg, Zn 0.2 mg, vitamin A 4 µg (25 µg carotene), E 0.1 mg, B_1 0.04 mg, B_2 0.06 mg, niacin 0.3 mg, B_6 0.05 mg, pantothenate 0.1 mg, biotin 2.6 µg, C 40 mg. An 80 g serving is a source of Cu; rich source of vitamin C.

red herrings   HERRINGS that have been well salted and smoked for about 10 days. Also called Yarmouth bloaters. Bloaters are salted less and smoked for a shorter time; KIPPERS lightly salted and smoked overnight.

red pepper   See PEPPER.

red tide   Sudden, unexplained increase in numbers of toxic dinoflagellate organisms in the sea which cause fish and shellfish feeding on them to become seasonally toxic.

reduced   EU and US legislation state that for a food label or advertising to bear a claim that it contains a reduced amount of fat, saturates, cholesterol, sodium or alcohol it must contain 25% less of the specified nutrient than a reference product for which no claim is made. A food may not claim to have a reduced content of a nutrient if it is already classified as LOW IN or FREE FROM that nutrient.

reducing sugars   SUGARS that are chemically reducing agents, including GLUCOSE, FRUCTOSE, LACTOSE, PENTOSES, but not SUCROSE.

reduction   See OXIDATION.

reduction rolls   See MILLING.

342

reference intakes (of nutrients) Amounts of nutrients greater than the requirements of almost all members of the population, determined on the basis of the average requirement plus twice the standard deviation, to allow for individual variation in requirements, and thus covering the theoretical needs of 97.5% of the population. Reference intakes for energy are based on the average requirement, without the allowance for individual variation. Used for planning institutional catering, assessing the adequacy of diets of groups of people, but not strictly applicable to individuals. Tables of reference intakes published by different national and international authorities differ because of differences in the interpretation of the available data.

Variously called in different countries and by different expert committees: RDA, the recommended daily (or dietary) amount (or allowance); RDI, recommended daily (or dietary) intake; RNI, reference nutrient intake; PRI, population reference intake; safe allowances. See Tables 3–5.

Levels of intake below that at which health and metabolic integrity are likely to be maintained are generally taken as the average requirement minus twice the standard deviation. Variously known as minimum safe intake (MSI), lower reference nutrient intake (LRNI) and lowest threshold intake.

reference man, woman An arbitrary physiological standard; defined as a person aged 25, weighing 65 kg, living in a temperate zone of a mean annual temperature of 10°C. Reference man performs medium work, with an average daily energy requirement of 13.5 MJ (3200 kcal). Reference woman is engaged in general household duties or light industry, with an average daily requirement of 9.7 MJ (2300 kcal).

reference nutrient intake, RNI See REFERENCE INTAKES.

reference protein See PROTEIN, REFERENCE.

refractive index Measure of the bending or refraction of a beam of light on entering a denser medium (the ratio between the sine of the angle of incidence of the ray of light and the sine of the angle of refraction). It is constant for pure substances under standard conditions. Used as a measure of sugar or total solids in solution, purity of oils, etc.

refractometer Instrument to measure the REFRACTIVE INDEX. The Abbé refractometer consists of two prisms between which the substance under examination (jam, fruit juice, sugar syrup, etc) is spread, and light is reflected through the solution. The immersion refractometer dips into the solution.

refried beans See FRIJOLES.

refrigerants Cooling agents in refrigerators and freezers; originally ammonia or carbon dioxide were used, subsequently replaced by chlorofluorocarbons (CFCs), trade names Freons and Arctons. Because of the persistence of CFCs in the upper atmosphere, where they destroy the protective ozone layer, they are considered an environmental hazard, and alternative refrigerants are being developed.

See also HEAT PUMP.

regional enteritis   See CROHN'S DISEASE.

Rehfuss tube   A small diameter tube with a slotted metal tip for removing samples of food from the stomach after a test meal.

See also RYLE TUBE.

Reichert–Meissl number   Measure of the steam-volatile fatty acids in a lipid.

See also POLENSKE NUMBER; STEAM DISTILLATION.

relative dose response test   For vitamin A status. The increase in circulating RETINOL BINDING PROTEIN after an oral dose of vitamin A; greater in vitamin A-deficient subjects because in the absence of vitamin A reserves in the liver there is accumulation of the apo-protein.

relative humidity   See HUMIDITY.

relative protein value   A measure of PROTEIN QUALITY.

release agents   Substances applied to tinned or enamelled surfaces or plastic films to prevent the food adhering, e.g. fatty acid amides, microcrystalline waxes, petrolatums, starch, methyl cellulose.

relish   Culinary term for any spicy or piquant preparation used to enhance flavour of plain food.

See also GENTLEMAN'S RELISH.

remove   Obsolete term for the main course of dinner.

rendering   Liberation of fat from adipose tissue. Dry rendering, heating the fat dry; wet rendering may use steam or hot water, either in open vessels or sealed under a pressure of 280–490 kPa (40–70 psi).

renin   Proteolytic enzyme (angiotensin-forming enzyme, angiotensinogenase, EC 3.4.23.15) secreted by the kidney; specific for the leucine–leucine bond in angiotensinogen, yielding ANGIOTENSIN I. This is then cleaved to yield active angiotensin II by the angiotensin converting enzyme (ACE, EC 3.4.15.1), a peptidase in the blood vessels of the lungs and other tissues.

rennet   Extract of calf stomach; contains the enzyme CHYMOSIN (rennin) which clots milk. Used in cheese-making and for JUNKET. Fungal rennet is a mixture of proteolytic enzymes from *Mucor pusillus*, *M. michei* and *Endothia parasitica*, used as substitutes for RENNET.

Vegetable rennet is the name given to proteolytic enzymes derived from plants, such as BROMELAIN (from the pineapple) and

FICIN (from the fig), as well as biosynthetic CHYMOSIN. Used for the preparation of vegetarian cheeses.

rennin See CHYMOSIN.

rentschlerising Sterilising by treatment with ultraviolet light, named after Dr HC Rentschler, who developed the lamp.

reovirus One of a small group of RNA-containing viruses that infect the intestinal and respiratory tracts without causing specific or serious disease.

See also ECHOVIRUS; ENTEROVIRUS.

repression Inhibition of gene expression leading to a decrease in the rate of synthesis of a protein.

See also INDUCTION.

resazurin test See METHYLENE BLUE DYE-REDUCTION TEST.

resins, ion-exchange See ION-EXCHANGE RESINS.

resistant starch See STARCH, enzyme resistant.

respiratory quotient (RQ) Ratio of the volume of carbon dioxide produced when a substance is oxidised to the volume of oxygen used. The oxidation of carbohydrate results in an RQ of 1.0; of fat, 0.7; and of protein, 0.8.

respirometer See SPIROMETER.

restoration The addition of nutrients to replace those lost in processing, as in milling of cereals.

See also FORTIFICATION.

restriction enzymes (restriction endonucleases) Endonucleases (EC 3.2.21.3–5) that hydrolyse DNA at specific sequences (commonly palindromic sequences of 4–5 nucleotides). Some leave flush ends, others a region of single-stranded DNA (a 'sticky end') that can be annealed with a different fragment of DNA produced using the same enzyme, the basis of genetic engineering and the introduction of DNA from one species into the genome of another. Also used to split genomic DNA into fragments that can be sequenced. More than 160 restriction sites have been identified for different enzymes.

reticulocyte Immature precursor of the red blood cell (normocyte or erythrocyte) in which the remains of the nucleus are visible as a reticulum. Normally ~1% of total red blood cells, but increased on remission of anaemia, when there is a high rate of production.

reticulum See RUMINANT.

retinal (retinaldehyde), retinene, retinoic acid, retinol See VITAMIN A.

retinoid Collective term for compounds chemically related to, or derived from, VITAMIN A. Synthetic retinoids have some of the biological activities of the vitamin, but have lower toxicity, and are used for treatment of serious skin disorders and some cancers.

retinoid receptors Two families of RETINOID BINDING PROTEINS in cell nuclei that bind to retinoid response elements on DNA, and modulate gene expression in response to retinoids. The RAR (retinoic acid receptor) family bind all-*trans* (and 9-*cis*) retinoic acid, the RXR (originally 'unknown retinoid' receptor) family bind 9-*cis* retinoic acid. Retinoid receptors also interact with calcitriol (VITAMIN D) and THYROID HORMONES and other nuclear-acting hormone receptors.

retinol binding protein (1) Plasma protein (RBP) required for transport of retinol; synthesis falls in protein–energy malnutrition and ZINC deficiency, leading to functional VITAMIN A deficiency despite adequate liver reserves. Because apo-retinol binding protein does not occur in plasma, measurement of RBP provides a sensitive index of vitamin A status.

See also RELATIVE DOSE RESPONSE TEST; TRANSTHYRETIN.

(2) Cellular retinol (and retinoic acid) binding proteins (CRBP and CRABP) are essential for uptake of retinol and retinoic acid into cells, before onward metabolism and binding to RETINOID RECEPTORS.

retort In food technology, an AUTOCLAVE.

retrogradation See STALING.

retroretinol Isomer of RETINOL; one of the physiologically active RETINOIDS.

retrovirus RNA-containing virus that can incorporate its genetic material into the DNA of a host cell by making a DNA copy of the RNA using REVERSE TRANSCRIPTASE.

reverse transcriptase Enzyme (EC 2.7.7.49) encoded by RNA viruses that catalyses the synthesis of DNA from an RNA template (the reverse of the process that occurs in TRANSCRIPTION). This permits incorporation of a copy of the virus genome into the host DNA. Reverse transcriptase is widely used in molecular biology and biotechnology to insert novel genes derived from mRNA into PLASMIDS.

Reynolds number (Re) Used to categorise fluid flow = (diameter of pipe × average velocity × fluid density)/ fluid viscosity.

RF heating See MICROWAVE COOKING.

rhamnose A methylated PENTOSE; 33% as sweet as sucrose; widely distributed in plant foods.

rheology The science of the deformation and flow of materials.

rheopexic COLLOIDAL SUSPENSIONS whose VISCOSITY increases over time when subjected to a constant shear stress; there is a reversible change from SOL to GEL under stress.

See also DILATANT; PSEUDOPLASTIC; THIXOTROPIC.

rhizome Botanical term for swollen stem that produces roots and leafy shoots.

rhizopterin Obsolete name for FOLIC ACID.

rhodopsin   The pigment in the cone cells of the retina of the eye, also known as visual purple, consisting of the protein opsin and retinaldehyde, which is responsible for the visual process. In rod cells of the retina the equivalent protein is iodopsin.

See also VITAMIN A; DARK ADAPTATION; VISION.

rhubarb   Leaf-stalks of the perennial plant, *Rheum rhaponticum.* Has a high content of OXALATE (the leaves contain even more, and are toxic).

Composition/100 g: 29 kJ (7 kcal), protein 0.9 g, fat 0.1 g, carbohydrate 0.8 g (0.8 g sugars), dietary fibre 2.3 g, nsp 1.4 g, Na 3 mg, K 290 mg, Ca 93 mg, Mg 13 mg, P 17 mg, Fe 0.3 mg, Cu 0.07 mg, Zn 0.1 mg, vitamin A 10 μg (60 μg carotene), E 0.2 mg, B_1 0.03 mg, B_2 0.03 mg, niacin 0.4 mg, B_6 0.02 mg, folate 7 μg, pantothenate 0.1 mg, C 6 mg. A 140 g serving is a source of vitamin C, Ca, Cu.

RIA   See RADIOIMMUNOASSAY.

Ribena   Trade name for a BLACKCURRANT juice cordial.

riboflavin   See VITAMIN B_2.

ribonucleic acid (RNA)   See NUCLEIC ACIDS.

ribose   A pentose (five-carbon) sugar which occurs as an intermediate in the metabolism of glucose; especially important in the NUCLEIC ACIDS and various COENZYMES: occurs widely in foods.

ribosomes   Intracellular organelles consisting of proteins and RNA that catalyse the synthesis of proteins (TRANSLATION). Ribosomes bind to, and travel along, MRNA, binding aminoacyl TRNA to each CODON in turn, and catalysing the synthesis of peptide bonds. A series of ribosomes translating the same strand of mRNA is known as a polysome. Proteins destined for export from the cell are synthesised by ribosomes attached to the rough endoplasmic reticulum of the cell.

Ribotide   Trade name for a mixture of the PURINE derivatives, disodium inosinate and guanylate, used as a FLAVOUR enhancer for savoury dishes.

ribozyme   An RNA molecule that can catalyse a chemical reaction, an enzyme composed solely of RNA, with no protein.

rice   Grain of *Oryza sativa*; major food in many countries. Rice when threshed is known as paddy, and is covered with a fibrous husk comprising nearly 40% of the grain. When the husk has been removed, brown rice is left.

Composition/100 g (brown rice, raw): 1494 kJ (357 kcal), protein 6.7 g, fat 2.8 g, carbohydrate 81.3 g (1.3 g sugars, 80 g starch), dietary fibre 3.8 g, nsp 1.9 g, Na 3 mg, K 250 mg, Ca 10 mg, Mg 110 mg, P 310 mg, Fe 1.4 mg, Cu 0.85 mg, Zn 1.8 mg, Se 2 μg, vitamin E 0.8 mg, B_1 0.59 mg, B_2 0.07 mg, niacin 6.8 mg, folate 49 μg. A 40 g serving is a source of vitamin B_1, niacin, Mg; rich source of Cu.

When the outer bran layers up to the endosperm and germ are removed, the ordinary white rice of commerce or polished rice is obtained (usually polished with glucose and talc).

Composition/100 g (white rice, raw): 1590 kJ (380 kcal), protein 7.3 g, fat 3.6 g, carbohydrate 85.8 g (85.8 g starch), dietary fibre 2.7 g, nsp 0.4 g, Na 4 mg, K 150 mg, Ca 51 mg, Mg 32 mg, P 150 mg, Fe 0.5 mg, Cu 0.37 mg, Zn 1.8 mg, Se 10 μg, I 14 μg, vitamin E 0.1 mg, B_1 0.41 mg, B_2 0.02 mg, niacin 5.8 mg, B_6 0.31 mg, folate 20 μg, pantothenate 0.6 mg, biotin 3 μg. A 30 g serving is a source of Cu.

rice, American See BULGUR.

rice, glutinous For most dishes, separate rice grains that do not stick together in a glutinous mass are preferred. Glutinous rice is rich in soluble starch, dextrin and maltose and on boiling the grains adhere in a sticky mass; this rice is used for sweetmeats and cakes.

rice grass See INDIAN RICE GRASS.

rice, hungry W African variety of MILLET, *Digitaria exilis*.

rice, maize or mealie See MAIZE RICE.

rice paper Smooth edible white 'paper' made from the pith of the Taiwanese shrub *Tetrapanax papyriferus* and the Indo-Pacific shrub *Scaevola sericea*.

rice, red W African species, *Oryza glaberrima*, with red bran layer.

rice, synthetic See TAPIOCA-MACARONI.

rice, unpolished American term; rice that has been undermilled in that the husk, germ and bran layers have been partially removed.

rice vinegar Japanese; VINEGAR prepared from SAKÉ.

rice, wild Also known as zizanie, Tuscarora rice, Indian rice and American wild rice (American rice is BULGUR); *Zizania aquatica*, native to eastern N America, grows 12 feet high; long, thin, greenish grain; little is grown and difficult to harvest, so is strictly a gourmet food. Higher in protein content than ordinary rice at 14%.

rice wine See SAKÉ.

ricin A LECTIN in the castor oil bean.

ricing Culinary term: cutting into small pieces about the size of rice grains.

rickets Malformation and undermineralisation of the bones in growing children due to deficiency of VITAMIN D, leading to poor absorption of calcium. In adults the equivalent is OSTEOMALACIA. In early (subclinical) rickets there is a marked elevation of plasma ALKALINE PHOSPHATASE.

Refractory or vitamin D-resistant rickets does not respond to normal amounts of vitamin D but requires massive doses.

Usually a result of a congenital defect in the metabolism of vitamin D, may also be due to strontium poisoning.

riffle flumes Washing equipment consisting of stepped channels along which the product being washed is carried in a flow of water; stones and grit are retained on the steps.

rigor mortis Stiffening of muscle that occurs after death. As the flow of blood ceases, anaerobic metabolism leads to the formation of lactic acid and the soft, pliable muscle becomes stiff and rigid. If meat is hung in a cool place for a few days ('conditioned'), the meat softens again. Fish similarly undergo rigor mortis but it is usually of shorter duration than in mammals.
See also DFD MEAT; MEAT CONDITIONING.

rijstaffel Dutch, Indonesian; meal consisting of a variety of different dishes (20 or more) served at the same time.

risk factor A factor that can be measured to indicate the statistical or epidemiological probability of an adverse condition, effect or disease. Does not imply that it is a causative factor, nor that reversing the risk factor will reduce the hazard.

RNA Ribonucleic acid, see NUCLEIC ACIDS.

RNI Reference nutrient intake, see REFERENCE INTAKES.

rocambole Mild variety of GARLIC, *Allium scordoprasum*, also called sand leek.

rock eel, salmon Alternative name for DOGFISH.

rocket Cruciferous plant, *Eruca sativa*, with small spear-shaped leaves and peppery taste, eaten raw in salads or cooked. Also called arugula, rucola, Italian cress.

rock lobster SHELLFISH, family Palinuridae, see LOBSTER.

rocou See ANNATTO.

roe Hard roe is the eggs of the female fish. Soft roe is from the male fish, also known as milt or melt. Hard roe of sturgeon and lumpfish are used to make CAVIARE and mock caviare.

Rohalase Trade name for bacterial and fungal AMYLASES used in brewing.

roller dryer The material to be dried is spread over the surface of internally heated rollers and drying is complete within a few seconds. The rollers rotate against a knife that scrapes off the dried film as soon as it forms. There is little damage to nutrients by this method; for example, roller-dried milk is not scorched, but there is more loss of vitamins B_1 and C than in spray drying.

roller mill Pairs of horizontal cylindrical rollers, separated by only a small gap and revolving at different speeds. The material is thus ground and crushed in one operation. Used in flour milling.

rollmop Filleted uncooked HERRING pickled in spiced vinegar.

roll-on closure (RO) Aluminium or lacquered tinplate cap for sealing on to narrow-necked bottles with a threaded neck. The unthreaded cap is moulded on to the neck of the bottle and forms an airtight seal.

romaine French and American name for COS LETTUCE.

rooibos tea Fermented leaves of the S African bush *Aspalathus linearis*. Contains a unique polyphenol, aspalathin, which becomes red during preparation and produces a reddish herbal tea; free from CAFFEINE and THEAFLAVIN.

root beer American; non-alcoholic carbonated beverage flavoured with extract of SASSAFRAS root and oil of wintergreen.

rope Spore-forming bacteria (*Bacillus mesentericus* and *B. subtilis*) occur on wheat and hence in flour. The spores can survive baking and are present in the bread. Under the right conditions of warmth and moisture the spores germinate and the mass of bacteria convert the bread into sticky, yellowish patches which can be pulled out into rope-like threads, hence the term ropy bread. The bacterial growth is inhibited by acid substances. Can also occur in milk, called long milk in Scandinavia.

roquefort Green-blue marbled French CHEESE made in Roquefort-sur-Soulzon from cow's milk; ripened in limestone caves where the mould, *Penicillium roquefortii* is present and the cheese thus inoculated.

ROS See REACTIVE OXYGEN SPECIES.

Rose-Gottlieb test Gravimetric method for determination of fat in milk, by extraction with diethyl ether and petroleum ether from an ammoniacal alcoholic solution of the sample.

rosella Caribbean plant (*Hibiscus sabdariffa*) grown for its fleshy red sepals, used to make drinks, jams and jelly. Also known as sorrel, flor de Jamaica.

rosemary A bushy shrub, *Rosmarinus officinalis*, cultivated commercially for its essential oil, used in medicine and perfumery. The leaves are used to flavour soups, sauces and meat.

rose water Fragrant water made by distillation or extraction of the ESSENTIAL OILS of rose petals. Used in confectionery (especially TURKISH DELIGHT) and baking.

rotary louvre dryer Hot air passes through a moving bed of the solid inside a rotating drum.

Roth–Benedict spirometer See SPIROMETER.

Rothera's test For KETONES in urine; reaction with ammonium hydroxide, ammonium sulphate and sodium nitroprusside to give a purple colour in the presence of ketones.

roti See CHAPPATI.

rôtisserie Method of cooking which developed from the traditional rotating spit above an open fire; the food is rotated while roasting, so bastes itself.

roughage See DIETARY FIBRE.

round worm See NEMATODE.

roux The foundation of most sauces; prepared by cooking together equal amounts of fat and plain flour, for a short time for white sauces, and longer for blond or brown sauces. The sauce is then prepared by stirring in milk or stock.

Rovimix Trade name for stabilised forms of vitamins as beadlets coated with a gelatine–starch mixture, used to enrich foods.

royal jelly The food on which bee larvae are fed and which causes them to develop into queen bees. Although it is a rich source of PANTOTHENIC ACID and other vitamins, in the amounts consumed it would make a negligible contribution to human intakes. 2% of its dry weight is hydroxydecenoic acid, which is believed to be the active queen substance. Claimed, without foundation, to have rejuvenating properties for human beings.

RPV Relative protein value, a measure of PROTEIN QUALITY.

RQ See RESPIRATORY QUOTIENT.

rubble reel Machine for cleaning materials such as wheat. The material is fed into a long inclined reel made of perforated metal that rotates inside a frame. The perforations become larger nearer the bottom, so that there is a graded sieving of the material as it passes down the reel.

Rubner factors See ENERGY CONVERSION FACTORS.

rum Spirit distilled from fermented sugar cane juice or molasses; may be colourless and light tasting or dark and with a strong flavour. Traditionally rum is darker and more strongly flavoured the further south in the Caribbean it is made. There are three main categories: Cuban, Jamaican and Dutch East Indies; and several types: aguardiente (Spain, Portugal and S America), Bacardi (trade name, originally from Cuba), cachaca (Brazil), cane spirit (S Africa), Demerara rum (Guyana), 35–60% alcohol by volume, 1.0–1.8 MJ (250–420 kcal) per 100 mL.

rumen See RUMINANT.

ruminant Animals such as the cow, sheep and goat, which possess four stomachs, as distinct from monogastric animals, such as man, pig, dog and rat. The four are: the rumen, or first stomach, where bacterial fermentation produces volatile fatty acids, and whence the food is returned to the mouth for further mastication (chewing the cud); the reticulum, where further bacterial fermentation produces volatile fatty acids; the omasum; and the abomasum or true stomach. The bacterial fermentation allows ruminants to obtain nourishment from grass and hay which cannot be digested by monogastric animals.

rumpbone Cut of meat: (USA) = aitchbone, (UK) = loin or haunch.

rush nut   See TIGER NUT.

rusk   (1) Sweetened biscuit or piece of bread or cake crisped in the oven, especially as food for young children when teething. (2) Cereal added to SAUSAGES and HAMBURGERS.

rutabaga   American name for SWEDE.

rutin   The disaccharide derivative of QUERCITIN, containing GLUCOSE and RHAMNOSE. Found in grains, tomato stalk and elderberry blossom. Not known to be a dietary essential or to have any function in the body, but once called VITAMIN P.
See also FLAVONOIDS.

rye   Grain of *Secale cereale*, the predominant cereal in some parts of Europe; very hardy and withstands adverse conditions better than wheat. Rye flour is dark and the dough lacks elasticity; rye bread is usually made with sour dough or leaven rather than yeast.
See also BREAD, rye; CRISPBREADS; PUMPERNICKEL.

Ryle tube   A narrow rubber tube with a blind end containing a lead weight, with holes above this level, for removing samples of the contents from the stomach at intervals after a test meal.
See also REHFUSS TUBE.

Ryvita   Trade name for a rye CRISPBREAD.

S

S- **and** *R-*   See *R-* AND *S-*.

saccharases   Enzymes (including INVERTASE) that HYDROLYSE sugars to their constituent MONOSACCHARIDES.

saccharic acid   The dicarboxylic acid derived from glucose.

saccharimeter   POLARIMETER used to determine the purity of sugar; graduated on the International Sugar Scale, degrees sugar (distinct from SACCHAROMETER).

saccharin   Sulphobenzimide, a synthetic SWEETENER, 550 times as sweet as sucrose. Soluble saccharin is the sodium salt.

saccharometer   Floating device used to determine the specific gravity of sugar solutions (distinct from SACCHARIMETER).

Saccharomyces bulardii   See PROBIOTICS.

saccharose   See SUCROSE.

sachertorte   Austrian; chocolate sponge cake with rich chocolate icing and whipped cream.

sack   Old name for a variety of white wines from Spain and the Canaries, e.g. sherry.

safe allowances, level of intake   See REFERENCE INTAKES.

safe and adequate intake   Where there is inadequate scientific evidence to establish requirements and REFERENCE INTAKES for a nutrient for which deficiency is rarely seen, if ever, the observed levels of intake are assumed to be greater than requirements, and thus provide an estimate of intakes that are safe and (more than) adequate to meet needs.

safflower Oil extracted from the seeds of *Carthamus tinctoria*, 75% polyunsaturated fatty acids. Mexican saffron is a substitute for SAFFRON made from the stigmata.

saffron Deep orange-red powder from the powdered stigmata of the saffron crocus, *Crocus sativus*; 1 g requires stigmata of 1500 flowers and yields about 50 mg of extract. Used as natural dyestuff (permitted food colour, with no E-number) and spice. Very soluble in water. Indian saffron is TURMERIC; Mexican saffron is SAFFLOWER.

sage Leaf of the Dalmatian sage, *Salvia officinalis*, of the mint family; fragrant and spicy and an important herb used in the kitchen for flavouring meat and fish dishes and in poultry stuffing. Other sages (Greek, Spanish, English) differ in flavour from the Dalmatian variety.

sago Starchy grains prepared from the pith of the swamp sago (*Metroxylon sagu*) and the sugar palm (*Arenga pinnuta*); almost pure starch.

Composition/100 g: 1486 kJ (355 kcal), protein 0.2 g, fat 0.2 g (50% saturated, 50% mono-, 0% polyunsaturated), carbohydrate 94 g (94 g starch), nsp 0.5 g, Na 3 mg, K 5 mg, Ca 10 mg, Mg 3 mg, P 29 mg, Fe 1.2 mg, Cu 0.03 mg.

saithe Also known as coley and coal fish, *Polachius virens*.

Composition/100 g: 343 kJ (82 kcal), protein 18.3 g, fat 1 g, cholesterol 40 mg, carbohydrate 0 g, Na 86 mg, K 360 mg, Ca 9 mg, Mg 25 mg, P 250 mg, Fe 0.3 mg, Cu 0.05 mg, Zn 0.5 mg, Se 18 μg, I 36 μg, vitamin A 4 μg, E 0.4 mg, B_1 0.15 mg, B_2 0.2 mg, niacin 5.7 mg, B_6 0.29 mg, B_{12} 3 μg, pantothenate 0.4 mg, biotin 3 μg. A 100 g serving is a source of vitamin B_1, B_2, B_6; good source of I; rich source of protein, niacin, vitamin B_{12}, Se.

saké Japanese wine made from rice. Cooked whole rice grains are fermented with a yeast-like fungus culture for 10–14 days and stored in wooden barrels. Contains about 17% alcohol by volume.

salad dressing Emulsions of oil and vinegar, which may or not contain other flavourings. French dressing (vinaigrette) is a temporary EMULSION of oil and vinegar; heavy French dressing is stabilised with PECTIN or vegetable GUM.

Mayonnaise is a stable emulsion of vinegar in oil, made with egg. Salad cream was originally developed as a commercial substitute for mayonnaise (mid nineteenth century); an emulsion made from vegetable oil, vinegar, salt, spices, emulsified with egg yolk and thickened. Legally, in the UK, must contain not less than 25% by weight of vegetable oil and not less than 1.35% egg yolk solids. Mayonnaise usually contains more oil, less carbohydrate and water.

By US regulations salad dressing contains 30% vegetable oil and 4% egg yolk; mayonnaise contains 65% oil plus egg yolk.

Red mayonnaise is prepared by adding beetroot juice and the coral (eggs) of lobster to mayonnaise; an accompaniment to lobster and other seafood dishes. Russian dressing is in fact American; made from mayonnaise with pimento, chilli sauce, green pepper and celery, or sometimes by mixing mayonnaise with tomato ketchup. Thousand Island dressing is made from equal parts of mayonnaise and Russian dressing, with whipped cream.

salami Type of SAUSAGE speckled with pieces of fat, flavoured with garlic; originally Italian.

Composition/100 g: 2051 kJ (490 kcal), protein 19.3 g, fat 45.2 g, cholesterol 79 mg, carbohydrate 1.9 g (1.9 g starch), Na 1850 mg, K 160 mg, Ca 10 mg, Mg 10 mg, P 160 mg, Fe 1 mg, Cu 0.24 mg, Zn 1.7 mg, Se 7 µg, I 15 µg, vitamin E 0.3 mg, B_1 0.21 mg, B_2 0.23 mg, niacin 8.2 mg, B_6 0.15 mg, folate 3 µg, B_{12} 1 µg, pantothenate 0.8 mg, biotin 3 µg. A 20 g serving (four slices) is a good source of vitamin B_{12}.

salatrim Triacylglycerol whose fatty acid composition has been modified by INTERESTERIFICATION so that it is only partially absorbable.

salep, salepi Turkish, Greek; beverage prepared from orchid tubers. Milky white in appearance, with only a slight flavour.

saline See PHYSIOLOGICAL SALINE.

salinometer (salimeter, salometer) Hydrometer to measure concentration of salt solutions by density.

Salisbury steak American; similar to HAMBURGER, minced beef mixed with bread, eggs, milk and seasoning, shaped into cakes and fried.

saliva Secretion of the salivary glands in the mouth: 1–1.5 L secreted daily. A dilute solution of the protein mucin (which lubricates food) and the enzyme AMYLASE, with small quantities of urea, and mineral salts.

salivary glands Three pairs of glands in the mouth, which secrete SALIVA: parotid, submandibular and submaxillary glands.

Sally Lunn A sweet, spongy, yeast cake, named after a girl who sold her tea cakes in Bath in the eighteenth century. In southern USA a variety of yeast and soda breads.

salmagundi (salamagundi) Old English dish consisting of diced fresh and salt meats mixed with hard-boiled eggs, pickled vegetables and spices, arranged on a bed of salad.

salmine   See PROTAMINES.

salmon   Fish of a number of species including Atlantic salmon (*Salmo salar*), and chinook, chum, coho (or silver), pink (or humpback), sockeye (or red) which are *Oncorhynchus* spp, and in UK must be described as red or pink salmon. Although wild salmon are caught on a large scale, much is farmed in deep inlets of the sea.

Composition/100 g: 753 kJ (180 kcal), protein 20.2 g, fat 11 g (20.2% saturated, 46.8% mono-, 32.9% polyunsaturated), cholesterol 50 mg, carbohydrate 0 g, Na 45 mg, K 360 mg, Ca 21 mg, Mg 27 mg, P 250 mg, Fe 0.4 mg, Cu 0.03 mg, Zn 0.6 mg, Se 26 µg, I 37 µg, vitamin A 13 µg, D 8 µg, E 1.9 mg, B_1 0.23 mg, B_2 0.13 mg, niacin 11 mg, B_6 0.75 mg, folate 16 µg, B_{12} 4 µg, pantothenate 1 mg, biotin 7 µg. A 100 g serving is a source of vitamin E, B_1, pantothenate; good source of I; rich source of protein, vitamin D, niacin, B_6, B_{12}, Se.

***Salmonella* spp**   Bacteria (Enterobacteriaceae) that are a common cause of food poisoning. Found in eggs from infected hens, sausages, etc; can survive in brine and at refrigerator temperatures; destroyed by adequate heating. Most species invade intestinal epithelial cells. Infective dose 10^3–10^6 organisms, onset 6–72 h, duration 2–7 days, TX 4.1.2.2.

S. typhi and *S. paratyphi* cause systemic infection: infective dose 1–10^2 organisms, onset 10–21 days, duration weeks.

There was a large increase in salmonellosis in Britain in the 1980s when *S. enteritidis* became endemic in poultry, levelling off in 1990–1995. Subsequently there was an increase (also in USA) in *S. typhimurium* DT with a relatively high mortality, 3%. Found in cereals, beef, pork and chicken.

salmon, rock   Alternative name for DOGFISH.

salometer   See SALINOMETER.

salsify   (oyster plant, vegetable oyster) Long, white, tapering root of the biennial plant *Tragopogon porrifolius*.

Composition/100 g: 113 kJ (27 kcal), protein 1.3 g, fat 0.3 g, carbohydrate 10.2 g (1.5 g sugars, 3.5 g starch), nsp 3.2 g, Na 5 mg, K 310 mg, Ca 42 mg, Mg 20 mg, P 42 mg, Fe 0.9 mg, Cu 0.01 mg, Zn 0.2 mg, vitamin A 3 µg (20 µg carotene), B_1 0.06 mg, B_2 0.01 mg, niacin 0.4 mg, B_6 0.07 mg, folate 57 µg, C 3 mg. A 50 g serving is a source of folate.

Black salsify is very similar; hardy perennial, *Scorzonera hispanica* (sometimes used roasted as coffee substitute).

salt   Usually refers to sodium chloride, common salt or table salt (chemically any product of reaction between an ACID and an ALKALI is a salt). The main sources are either mining in areas where there are rich deposits of crystalline salt, or evaporation of seawater in shallow pans (known as sea salt).

See also SODIUM; BUFFERS; ESTERS.

salt-free diets Diets low in SODIUM, for the treatment of HYPERTENSION and other conditions. Most of the sodium of the diet is consumed as sodium chloride or SALT, and hence such diets are referred to as salt-restricted or low-salt diets, or sometimes 'salt-free', to emphasise that no salt is added to foods in preparation or at the table. Since foods naturally contain sodium chloride, a truly salt-free diet is not possible. It is the sodium and not the chloride that is important.

See also HYPERTENSION; SODIUM.

salting Method of preserving meat, fish and some vegetables using salt and SALTPETRE.

salt, light (lite) Mixtures of sodium chloride with potassium chloride and/or other substances to reduce the intake of SODIUM.

saltpetre (Bengal saltpetre) Potassium NITRATE.

salts, Indian Ancient Greek and Roman name for sugar.

SAMI Socially acceptable monitoring instrument. A small heart-rate-counting apparatus used to estimate ENERGY EXPENDITURE of human subjects.

samna Clarified butter fat, see BUTTER; GHEE.

samosa Indian; deep-fried stuffed pancakes, rolled into a cone or folded into an envelope.

samp Coarsely cut portions of MAIZE with bran and germ partly removed.

samphire (1) Rock samphire, St Peter's herb, succulent plant of cliffs and salt marshes (*Crithmum maritimum*); grows on coastal rocks, fleshy aromatic leaves may be eaten raw, boiled or pickled.

(2) Marsh samphire (glasswort, sea asparagus), *Salicornia* spp, grows in salt marshes, salty, eaten cooked as a vegetable.

Sanatogen Trade name for a preparation of casein and sodium glycerophosphate for consumption as a beverage when added to milk.

sand leek See ROCAMBOLE.

sandwich Two slices of bread enclosing a filling (meat, cheese, fish, etc). Invention attributed to the fourth Earl of Sandwich (1718–1792), who spent long periods at the gaming table and carried a portable meal of beef sandwiched with bread. Decker sandwiches consist of several layers of bread, each separated by filling; Neapolitan sandwiches are decker sandwiches made with alternating slices of white and brown bread. Open sandwiches (SMØRREBRØD) consist of a single slice of bread, biscuit or small roll.

Sanecta Trade name for ASPARTAME.

Sanka Trade for decaffeinated instant coffee. See CAFFEINE; COFFEE, decaffeinated.

sapodilla Fruit of the sapodilla tree (*Achras sapota*); size of a small apple, rough-grained, yellow to greyish pulp. Chicle, the basis of CHEWING GUM, is made from the latex of the tree. Composition/100 g: 288 kJ (69 kcal), protein 0.6 g, fat 0.9 g, carbohydrate 15.5 g (14.7 g sugars, 0.8 g starch), dietary fibre 8.2 g, Na 7 mg, K 190 mg, Ca 27 mg, Mg 26 mg, P 15 mg, Fe 1.1 mg, Cu 0.36 mg, vitamin A 8 μg (53 μg carotene), B_1 0.01 mg, B_2 0.02 mg, niacin 0.2 mg, B_6 0.04 mg, pantothenate 0.2 mg, C 10 mg. A 100 g serving is a source of vitamin C; rich source of Cu.

saponification Alkaline hydrolysis of FATTY ACID esters (including TRIACYLGLYCEROLS) prior to analysis. The saponification value of a fat or oil is the amount of potassium hydroxide required to hydrolyse (saponify) 1 g of the fat.

saponins Group of substances that occur in plants and can produce a soapy lather with water. Extracted commercially from soapwort (*Saponaria officinalis*) or soapbark (*Quillaja saponaria*) and used as foam producer in beverages and fire extinguishers, as detergents and for emulsifying oils. Bitter in flavour.

See also QUILLAJA.

saracen corn See BUCKWHEAT.

saran Generic name for thermoplastic materials made from polymers of vinylidene chloride and vinyl chloride. They are clear transparent films (cling film) used for wrapping food; resistant to oils and chemicals; can be heat-shrunk on to the product.

sarcolactic acid Obsolete name for (+)lactic acid (which rotates the plane of polarised light to the right), found in muscle, as distinct from the optically inactive LACTIC ACID (a mixture of (+) and (−) isomers) found in sour milk. Also known as paralactic acid.

See also DFD MEAT; MEAT CONDITIONING; RIGOR MORTIS.

sarcolemma See MUSCLE.

sarcomere The basic contractile unit of striated MUSCLE.

sarcosine *N*-Methylglycine, an intermediate in the metabolism of CHOLINE. Found in relatively large amounts in starfish and sea urchins, used as an intermediate in the synthesis of antienzyme agents in toothpaste.

sardell See ANCHOVY.

sardine Young PILCHARD *Sardina (Clupea) pilchardus*; commonly canned in oil, brine or tomato paste. Norwegian canned sardines are salted and smoked before canning; French are salted and steamed.

Composition/100 g (fresh): 690 kJ (165 kcal), protein 20.6 g, fat

9.2 g (34.1% saturated, 31.6% mono-, 34.1% polyunsaturated), carbohydrate 0 g, Na 120 mg, K 360 mg, Ca 84 mg, Mg 31 mg, P 270 mg, Fe 1.4 mg, Cu 0.12 mg, Zn 1 mg, Se 34 μg, I 29 μg, vitamin D 11 μg, E 0.3 mg, B_2 0.22 mg, niacin 10.6 mg, B_6 0.39 mg, folate 4 μg, B_{12} 11 μg, pantothenate 0.8 mg, biotin 6 μg. An 80 g serving (six fish) is a source of vitamin B_2, B_6, pantothenate, Cu, I; rich source of protein, vitamin D, niacin, B_{12}, Se.

Composition/100 g (canned in oil): 908 kJ (217 kcal), protein 23.7 g, fat 13.6 g (22.7% saturated, 38.2% mono-, 39% polyunsaturated), cholesterol 65 mg, carbohydrate 0 g, Na 650 mg, K 430 mg, Ca 550 mg, Mg 52 mg, P 520 mg, Fe 2.9 mg, Cu 0.19 mg, Zn 3 mg, Se 50 μg, I 23 μg, vitamin A 11 μg, D 7.5 μg, E 0.3 mg, B_1 0.04 mg, B_2 0.36 mg, niacin 12.6 mg, B_6 0.48 mg, folate 8 μg, B_{12} 28 μg, pantothenate 0.5 mg, biotin 5 μg. A 100 g serving (four fish) is a source of Mg, I; good source of vitamin B_2, B_6, Fe, Cu, Zn; rich source of protein, vitamin D, niacin, B_{12}, Ca, Se.

Saridele Protein-rich baby food (26–30% protein) developed in Indonesia; extract of soya bean with sugar, calcium carbonate, vitamins B_1, B_{12} and C.

sarsaparilla (1) Flavour prepared from oil of SASSAFRAS and oil of wintergreen or oil of sweet birch,

(2) Roots of a S American plant (*Smilax officinalis*).

Both used to flavour the beverage called sarsaparilla.

sassafras American tree (*Sassafras albidum*) with aromatic bark and leaves. The root is used to make ROOT BEER and the young leaves are powdered to make filé powder, an essential flavouring of GUMBO. Sassafras oil from the rootbark is used medicinally and as a flavour in beverages, but banned in some countries because of its toxicity.

satiety The sensation of fullness after a meal.

satsuma See CITRUS fruit.

saturates Commonly used term for saturated FATTY ACIDS.

saturation analysis See RADIOIMMUNOASSAY.

saturation humidity See HUMIDITY.

sauerkraut German, Dutch, Alsatian; prepared by lactic fermentation of shredded cabbage. In the presence of 2–3% salt, acid-forming bacteria thrive and convert sugars in the cabbage into acetic and lactic acids, which then act as preservatives.

sauerteig See BREAD, sourdough.

sausage Chopped meat, commonly beef or pork, seasoned with salt and spices, mixed with cereal (usually wheat rusk prepared from crumbed unleavened biscuits) and packed into casings made from the connective tissue of animal intestines or cellulose. In UK pork sausages must be 65% meat and beef sausages 50% meat.

Six main types: fresh, smoked, cooked, smoked and cooked, semi-dry and dry. Frankfurters, Bologna, Polish and Berliner sausages are made from cured meat and are smoked and cooked. Thuringer, soft salami, mortadella and soft cervelat are semi-dry sausages. Pepperoni, chorizos, dry salami, dry cervelat are slowly dried to a hard texture.

sausage casings Natural casings are made from hog intestines for fresh frying sausages, and from sheep intestines for chipolatas and frankfurters. Skinless sausages are prepared in cellulose casing, which is then peeled off.

sausage factor See MEAT FACTOR.

savarin See BABA.

saveloy Highly seasoned smoked SAUSAGE; the addition of saltpetre gives rise to the bright red colour. Originally a sausage made from pig brains.

savory Herb with strongly flavoured leaves used as seasoning in sauces, soups, salad dishes. Summer savory is an annual, *Satureja hortensis*; winter savory is a perennial, *Satureja montana*.

savoy Variety of CABBAGE (*Brassica oleracea* var *capitata*) with crimped leaves.

Saxin Trade name for SACCHARIN.

scald (1) Pouring boiling water over a food to clean it, loosen hairs (e.g. on a joint of pork) or remove the skin of fruit and tomatoes.

(2) Heating milk almost to boiling point, to retard souring or to make clotted CREAM.

(3) Defect occurring in stored apples; the formation of brown patches under the skin, with browning and softening of the tissue underneath. Due to accumulation of gases given off during ripening.

scallion Small onion which has not developed a bulb, widely used in Chinese cooking; also used for shallots and spring onion (especially in USA).

See also ONION, SPRING.

scallops Marine bivalve MOLLUSCS, Pectinidae spp; Queen scallop is *Chamys opercularis.*

scampi Shellfish, Norway lobster or Dublin Bay prawn, *Nephrops norvegicus*, see LOBSTER.

scapula The shoulder blade, a triangular BONE.

Scenedesmus See ALGAE.

Schiff base An aldimine linkage formed by condensation between an aldehyde and an amino group.

See also MAILLARD REACTION; PYRIDOXYLLYSINE.

Schilling test For VITAMIN B_{12} absorption; an oral dose of ^{57}Co-labelled vitamin B_{12} is given 1 h after a large (1000 µg) parenteral dose of non-radioactive vitamin, and radioactivity in urine is determined over the next 24–28 h.

See also ANAEMIA, PERNICIOUS; INTRINSIC FACTOR.

schnitzel Austrian, German; cutlet or escalope of veal or pork.

Schoenheimer–Sperry reaction A modification of the LIEBERMANN–BURCHARD reaction for cholesterol.

scifers Cornish name for Welsh ONION.

scintillation counter Instrument for measurement of radioactivity by emission of light from a solid or liquid scintillator that emits a photon after absorbing a β- or γ-particle.

sclerosis Hardening of tissue due to scarring, inflammation or ageing.

See also ARTERIOSCLEROSIS; ATHEROSCLEROSIS.

scolex Head of a TAPEWORM, with hooks or suckers to permit attachment to the intestinal wall.

scombroid poisoning Apparently caused by bacterial spoilage of fish including many of the Scombridae (TUNA, bonito, MACKEREL) but also non-scombroid fish and other foods. Symptoms (including skin rash, nausea, tingling) resemble HISTAMINE poisoning and previously thought to be due to bacterial formation of histamine, now doubted.

scone A variety of tea cake originally made from white flour or barley meal and sour milk or buttermilk in Scone, Scotland; baked on a griddle and cut in quarters. Drop scone is a small pancake made by dropping spoonfuls of batter on to a griddle.

scorbutic See SCURVY.

scorzonera See SALSIFY.

Scotch egg Hard-boiled egg cased in seasoned sausage meat and breadcrumbs, fried and served cold.

scotopic Conditions of poor illumination; hence scotopic VISION is vision in dim light.

See also DARK ADAPTATION.

SCP See SINGLE CELL PROTEIN.

scrapple USA; meat dish prepared from pork carcass trimmings, maize meal, flour, salt and spices, cooked to a thick consistency.

scratchings, pork Small pieces of crisply cooked pork skin.

screening Comparison of measurements made on individuals or population groups using predetermined risk levels or cut-off points of reference ranges.

scrod Young COD.

scrumpy Rough, unsweetened CIDER.

scurvy Deficiency of VITAMIN C, fatal if untreated. Nowadays extremely rare, but in the past a major problem in winter, when there were few sources of the vitamin available. It was especially a problem of long sea voyages during the sixteenth and seventeenth centuries; when fresh supplies of fruit and vegetables were not available the majority of the crew often succumbed to scurvy.

scurvy, Alpine   See pellagra.

scurvy grass   A herb, *Cochlearia officinalis*, recommended as far back as the late sixteenth century as a remedy for scurvy.

scutellum   Area surrounding the embryo of the cereal grain; scutellum plus embryo is the germ; rich in vitamins.

scybalum   Lump or mass of hard FAECES.

SDA   Specific dynamic action, see DIET-INDUCED THERMOGENESIS.

SDS   (1) Sucrose distearate, a SUCROSE ester.

(2) The detergent sodium dodecyl sulphate.

SDS–PAGE   Polyacrylamide gel ELECTROPHORESIS of proteins in the presence of the detergent sodium dodecyl sulphate to cause denaturation and permit estimation of the molecular weight of a protein.

SE   See STARCH EQUIVALENT.

sea kale beet   See SWISS CHARD.

sea slug   See BÊCHE-DE-MER.

seasoning   Normally used to mean salt and pepper, but may include any herbs, spices and condiments added to a savoury dish.

sea truffle   SHELLFISH, a bivalve MOLLUSC, *Venus verrucosa*.

seaweed   Marine algae of interest as food include IRISH MOSS, LAVER bread and KELP, which are eaten as local delicacies and serve as a mineral supplement in animal feed.

second messenger   Small molecule released inside a cell in response to binding of a hormone or neurotransmitter to a receptor on the cell surface, which directly or indirectly activates or inhibits target enzymes.

See also CAMP; DIACYLGLYCEROL; INOSITOL, phosphates.

secretin   Peptide hormone secreted by the S-cells of the duodenum in response to acid food entering from the stomach. Stimulates secretion of alkaline PANCREATIC JUICE containing only low levels of enzyme, and also secretion of bile; decreases gastric secretion and GASTRIN release.

sedoheptulose (sedoheptose)   A seven-carbon sugar, a metabolic intermediate.

Seitz filter   A filter disc with pores so fine that they will not permit passage of bacteria, permitting sterilisation of liquids by filtration.

sekt   German; sparkling WINE, usually dry, made by tank fermentation, not the MÉTHODE CHAMPENOISE.

selenium   A dietary essential mineral, found as SELENOCYSTEINE in the active sites of GLUTATHIONE PEROXIDASE (EC 1.11.1.9) and thyroxine deiodinase EC 3.8.1.4). Through its rôle in glutathione peroxidase it acts as an ANTIOXIDANT, and to some extent can compensate for VITAMIN E deficiency. Similarly, vitamin E can compensate for selenium deficiency to some extent.

Requirements are of the order of 50 µg/day; in parts of New Zealand, Finland and China soils are especially poor in selenium and deficiency occurs. In China selenium deficiency is associated with KESHAN DISEASE and KASHIN–BECK syndrome.

Selenium is toxic in excess; mild selenium intoxication results in production of foul-smelling hydrogen selenide, which is excreted on the breath and through the skin. Intakes above 500 µg (5 µg/kg body weight)/day are considered hazardous.

See also THYROID HORMONES.

selenocysteine   The selenium analogue of the AMINO ACID CYSTEINE. Incorporated during ribosomal protein synthesis, and formed as a result of the action of selenocysteine synthetase (EC 2.9.1.1) on serine bound to tRNA. The codon for selenocysteine is UGA, one of the stop CODONS, read in a context-sensitive manner.

seltzer   Effervescent mineral water, originally from Niederselters, Germany.

See also SODA WATER.

seminose   See MANNOSE.

semipermeable membrane   A membrane with pores that permit the passage of small molecules, but not larger molecules such as proteins.

See also DIALYSIS; ULTRAFILTRATION.

semolina   The inner, granular, starchy endosperm of hard or durum wheat (not yet ground into flour); used to make PASTA and semolina milk pudding.

senna   Dried fruits of *Cassia* spp, used as an irritant LAXATIVE.

sensitivity   Of an assay; the smallest amount that can be determined with acceptable PRECISION.

sensory properties   See ORGANOLEPTIC.

sequestrants, sequestrol   See CHELATING AGENTS.

sequestrene, sequestrol   See EDTA.

sercial   See MADEIRA WINES.

serendipity berry   Or Nigerian berry, fruit of the W African plant *Dioscoreophyllum cumminsii*. It has an extremely sweet taste due to the protein monellin.

serine   A non-essential AMINO ACID; abbr Ser (S), M_r 105.1, pK_a 2.19, 9.21, CODONS UCNu, AGPy.

serotonin   See 5-HYDROXYTRYPTAMINE.

serum   Clear liquid left after protein has been coagulated; the serum from milk, occasionally referred to as lactoserum, is whey. Blood serum is BLOOD PLASMA without the fibrinogen. When blood clots, the fibrinogen is converted to fibrin, which is deposited in strands that trap the red cells and form the clot. The clear liquid that is exuded is the serum.

See also BLOOD CLOTTING.

serving US food labelling legislation (introduced in 1994) requires that nutrients be shown per standard serving of the food. The Food and Drug Administration has defined serving or portion sizes, based on surveys of amounts customarily eaten, so the definition of portions is not left to the manufacturer.

sesame A tropical and subtropical plant, *Sesamum indicum*. Known as sim-sim in East Africa, benniseed in West Africa, gingelly and til in Asia. Seeds are small and, in most varieties, white; used whole in sweetmeats, in stews and to decorate cakes and bread, and for extraction of the oil, which is used as a seasoning.

Composition/100 g: 2503 kJ (598 kcal), protein 18.2 g, fat 58 g (14.9% saturated, 39% mono-, 45.9% polyunsaturated), carbohydrate 0.9 g (0.4 g sugars, 0.5 g starch), nsp 7.9 g, Na 20 mg, K 570 mg, Ca 670 mg, Mg 370 mg, P 720 mg, Fe 10.4 mg, Cu 1.46 mg, Zn 5.3 mg, vitamin A 1 µg (6 µg carotene), E 2.5 mg, B_1 0.93 mg, B_2 0.17 mg, niacin 10.4 mg, B_6 0.75 mg, folate 97 µg, pantothenate 2.1 mg, biotin 11 µg. A 10 g serving (one tablespoon) is a source of Mg, Cu.

See also TAHINI.

sfumatrice Machine for obtaining the oil from the peel of citrus fruit. Based on the principle that the natural turgor of the oil sacs forces out the oil when the peel is folded.

shaddock See POMELO.

shallot Bulb of the plant *Allium escalonium* (*A. cepa aggregatum*) related to the ONION, with similar flavour but less pungent; each plant has a cluster of small bulbs rather than the single large bulb of the onion.

sharon fruit See PERSIMMON.

Sharples centrifuge Continuous high-speed centrifuge (15 000–30 000 rpm), consisting of a vertical cylinder. Used to separate liquids of different densities or to clarify by sedimenting solids.

sharps See WHEATFEED.

shashlik See KEBAB.

shea butter See VEGETABLE BUTTERS.

shearling 15–18 month old sheep. See LAMB.

shellfish A wide range of marine molluscs (ABALONE, CLAMS, COCKLES, MUSSELS, SCALLOPS, OYSTERS, WHELKS, WINKLES) and crustacea (order Decapoda: CRAYFISH, CRABS, LOBSTERS, PRAWNS, SHRIMPS).

sherbet (1) Arabic name for water-ice (sugar, water and flavouring), also known by French name, sorbet, and the Italian name, granita. Used to be served between courses during a meal to refresh the palate.

(2) Originally a middle-eastern drink made from fruit juice, often chilled with snow. Modern version is made with bicarbonate of soda and tartaric acid (to fizz) with sugar and flavours. Sherbet powder is the same mixture in dry form.

sherry Fortified wines (around 15% ALCOHOL by volume) from the south-west of Spain, around Jerez and Cadiz. Matured by the solera process, rather than by discrete vintages; each year 30% of the wine in the oldest barrel is drawn off for bottling and replaced with wine from the next oldest; this in turn is replaced from the next barrel, and so on. In order of increasing sweetness, sherries are: fino (very dry); manzanilla; amontillado; oloroso (may be medium-dry or sweetened and more highly fortified); amoroso or cream.

Dry sherry contains 1–2% sugar and 100 mL supplies 500 kJ (120 kcal); medium sherry 3–4% sugar, 530 kJ (125 kcal); sweet sherry 7% sugar, supplies 590 kJ (140 kcal).

Sherry-type wines are also produced in other countries, including South Africa, Cyprus and Britain (made from imported grape juice) and may legally be described as sherry as long as the country of origin is clearly shown.

***Shigella* spp** Food-poisoning organisms that invade intestinal epithelial cells and cause DYSENTERY. Infective dose 10^2–10^5 organisms; onset 1–7 days; duration weeks; TX 4.1.4.1.

shiitake Or Black Forest mushroom, *Lentinula (Lentinus) edodes*, see MUSHROOMS.

shir To bake food (usually eggs) in a small shallow container or ramekin dish.

shortening Soft fats that produce a crisp, flaky effect in baked products. LARD possesses the correct properties to a greater extent than any other single fat. Shortenings compounded from mixtures of fats or prepared by hydrogenation are still called lard compounds or lard substitutes. Unlike oils, shortenings are plastic and disperse as a film through the batter and prevent the formation of a hard, tough mass.

showarma See KEBAB.

shrimp Small shellfish, Paleamonidea and Pandalidae spp (prawns) and *Crangon crangon* (brown shrimp) and *Pandalus montagui* (pink shrimp).

Composition/100 g: 305 kJ (73 kcal), protein 16.5 g, fat 0.8 g (16.6% saturated, 33.3% mono-, 50% polyunsaturated), cholesterol 200 mg, carbohydrate 0 g, Na 375 mg, K 75 mg, Ca 128 mg, Mg 47 mg, P 150 mg, Fe 2.6 mg, Cu 0.15 mg, Zn 1.1 mg, Se 49 μg, vitamin B_2 0.02 mg, niacin 3.6 mg, folate 14 μg, B_{12} 2.6 μg. A 50 g serving is a source of protein, niacin; rich source of vitamin B_{12}, Se.

sialic acids   *N*-Acetyl-neuraminic acid (amino sugar) derivatives; constituents of gangliosides, glycoproteins and bacterial cell walls.

sialogogue   Substance that stimulates the flow of saliva.

sialorrhoea   Or ptyalism, excessive flow of SALIVA.

sidemeats   See OFFAL.

sideroblast   Red BLOOD CELL precursor in which IRON-containing granules are visible. May be present in normal individuals, absent in iron deficiency ANAEMIA. Sideroblastic anaemia is characterised by the presence of abnormal ringed sideroblasts in the blood.

sideropenia   IRON deficiency.

siderophilin   See iron transport.

siderosis   Accumulation of the iron–protein complex, haemosiderin, in liver, spleen and bone marrow in cases of excessive red cell destruction and in diets exceptionally rich in IRON.
  See also HAEMOCHROMATOSIS.

sigmoidoscope   Instrument that is inserted through the anus to view the interior of the rectum and sigmoid colon.

sign   Indication of a disorder that is observed by a physician but is not apparent to the patient.
  See also SYMPTOM.

sild   Traditional UK name applied to a mixture of young HERRINGS and young SPRATS when canned, since they are caught together and cannot be separated on a commercial scale. When fresh or frozen the mixture is termed WHITEBAIT.

silica gel   A drying agent.

silicones   Organic compounds of silicon; in the food field they are used as antifoaming agents, as semipermanent glazes on baking tins and other metal containers, and on non-stick wrapping paper.

silver beet   See SWISS CHARD.

silver   Not of interest in foods apart from its use in covering 'nonpareils', the silver beads used to decorate confectionery. Present in traces in all plant and animal tissues but not known to be a dietary essential, and has no known function, nor is enough ever absorbed to cause toxicity.
  See also OLIGODYNAMIC.

simethicone   See DIMETHICONE.

simnel cake   Fruit cake with a layer of almond paste on top and sometimes another baked in the middle. Originally baked for Mothering Sunday, now normally eaten at Easter.

Simplesse   Trade name for FAT REPLACER made from milk or egg white. Consists of 0.1–2.0 μm diameter particles which create the feeling of creaminess in the mouth but cannot be used for cooking. Yields 5.2 kJ (1.3 kcal)/g, compared with 37 kJ (9 kcal)/g for fats.

simvastatin See STATINS.

single cell protein Collective term used for biomass of bacteria, algae and yeast, and also (incorrectly) moulds, of potential use as animal or human food.

See also MYCOPROTEIN.

sinharanut See CHESTNUT.

sippy diet For peptic ulcer patients; hourly feeds of small quantities, 150 mL of milk, cream or other milky food.

sitapophasis Refusal to eat as expression of mental disorder.

sitology Science of food (from the Greek *sitos*, food).

sitomania Mania for eating, morbid obsession with food; also known as phagomania.

sitophobia Fear of food; also known as phagophobia.

sitosterol The main STEROL found in vegetable oils, similar in structure to cholesterol; may reduce the absorption of cholesterol from the intestinal tract and has been used in prevention and treatment of HYPERLIPIDAEMIA.

skate Cartilaginous FISH, *Raja undutata*.

Composition/100 g: 267 kJ (64 kcal), protein 15.1 g, fat 0.4 g, carbohydrate 0 g, Na 120 mg, K 260 mg, Ca 40 mg, Mg 30 mg, P 180 mg, Fe 0.5 mg, Cu 0.02 mg, Zn 0.5 mg, I 20 μg, vitamin B_1 0.12 mg, B_2 0.2 mg, niacin 4.8 mg, B_6 0.37 mg, B_{12} 6 μg. A 150 g serving is a source of vitamin B_1, B_2, Mg; good source of vitamin B_6, I; rich source of protein, niacin, vitamin B_{12}.

skinfold thickness Index of subcutaneous fat and hence body fat content. Measured at four sites: biceps (midpoint of front upper arm), triceps (midpoint of back upper arm), subscapular (directly below point of shoulder blade at angle of 45°), supra-iliac (directly above iliac crest in mid-axillary line). Rapid surveys often involve only biceps. Precision calipers for measurement of skinfold thickness exert a pressure of 10 g/mm², with a skin contact (pinch) area of 20–40 mm²; require regular recalibration.

See also ANTHROPOMETRY.

skyr See MILK, FERMENTED.

Slendid See FAT REPLACERS.

sling Drink made from gin and fruit juice.

Slite Trade name for a preparation of 82% SUCROSE with intense SWEETENERS and bulking agents. The mixture has twice the sweetness of sucrose, and is stable to cooking.

slivovitz (sliwowitz) E European (originally Yugoslavia); distilled spirit made from fermented plums; similar to German quetsch and French mirabelle. Some of the stones are included with the fruit and produce a characteristic bitter flavour from the hydrocyanic acid (0.008% cyanide is present in the finished brandy).

sloe Wild PLUM, fruit of the blackthorn (*Prunus spinosa*) with a sour and astringent flavour; almost only use is for the preparation of sloe gin, a liqueur made by steeping wild sloes in gin or neutral spirit. Known in France as prunelle.

sloke See LAVER.

slow virus Obsolete term for infective agents with some properties resembling viruses, but not containing any nucleic acid. Now known as PRIONS.

SMA Trade name (Scientific Milk Adaptation) for a milk preparation for infant feeding modified to resemble the composition of human milk. See MILK, HUMANISED.

smallage Wild celery, *Apium graveolens*.

smell See ORGANOLEPTIC.

smetana Thin soured cream, originally Russian.
Composition/100 g: 544 kJ (130 kcal), protein 4.7 g, fat 10 g (66.3% saturated, 30.5% mono-, 3.1% polyunsaturated), cholesterol 27 mg, carbohydrate 5.6 g (5.6 g sugars), vitamin A 175 µg (65 µg carotene), D 0.07 µg, E 0.2 mg, niacin 1.1 mg, C 1 mg. Serving 45 g (one tablespoon).

smilacin See PARILLIN.

smoke point The temperature at which the decomposition products of frying oils become visible as bluish smoke. The temperature varies with different fats, ranging between 160–260°C.
See also FIRE POINT; FLASH POINT.

smoked beef See PASTRAMI.

smoking The process of flavouring and preserving meat or fish by drying slowly in the smoke from a wood fire; the type of wood used affects the flavour of the final smoked product.

smörgåsbord Scandinavian; buffet table laden with delicacies as a traditional gesture of hospitality, a traditional way of serving meals.

smørrebrød Scandinavian; open SANDWICHES, often on rye bread, with a variety of toppings and garnishes. Literally *smeared bread*.

SMS Sucrose monostearate. See SUCROSE ESTERS.

smut Group of fungi that attack wheat; includes loose or common smut (*Ustilago tritici*) and stinking smut or bunt (*Tilletia tritici*).

snail The small snail eaten in Europe is *Helix pomatia*; giant African snail (which weighs several hundred grams) is *Achatima fulica*.

snap pea, snow pea See PEA, MANGE TOUT.

SNF See solids-not-fat.

snibbing Topping and tailing of GOOSEBERRIES.

SO₂ See SULPHUR DIOXIDE.

soapbark See QUILLAJA.

soapstock In the refining of crude edible oils the free fatty acids are removed by agitation with alkali. The fatty acids settle to the bottom as alkali soaps and are known as soapstock or 'foots'.

SOD See SUPEROXIDE DISMUTASE.

soda bread Irish; made from flour and whey, or buttermilk, using sodium bicarbonate and acid in place of yeast.

soda water Artificially carbonated water, also known as club soda; if sodium bicarbonate is also added, the product is seltzer water.

sodium A dietary essential mineral; requirements are almost invariably satisfied by the normal diet. The body contains about 100 g of sodium and the average diet contains 3–6 g, equivalent to 7.5–15 g of sodium chloride (salt); the requirement is less than 0.5 g sodium/day. The intake varies enormously in different individuals and excretion varies accordingly.

Excessive intake of sodium is associated with high blood pressure, hence often treated with low-salt diets. Sodium controls the retention of fluid in the body, and reduced retention, aided by low-sodium diets, is required in cardiac insufficiency accompanied by OEDEMA, in certain kidney diseases, toxaemias of pregnancy and HYPERTENSION.

Low-sodium diets are usually about 2.3 g and can be as low as 0.6 g. To improve the palatability of such diets, 'salt' mixtures (LIGHT or lite salt) are available, containing potassium and ammonium chlorides together with citrates, formates, phosphates, glutamates, as well as herbs and spices. Such mixtures may be contraindicated in conditions where potassium intake also has to be restricted.

See also 'SALT-FREE' DIETS; SODIUM–POTASSIUM RATIO; WATER BALANCE.

sodium bicarbonate NaHCO₃, also known as baking soda or bicarbonate of soda; liberates carbon dioxide when in contact with acid. Used as a raising agent in baking flour confectionery.

See also BAKING POWDER.

sodium–potassium ratio In the body, the ratio of sodium (in the extracellular fluid) to potassium (in the intracellular fluid) is about 2:3. The ratio in unprocessed food, no salt added, is much lower, and when salt is added during processing it is much higher. Unproven suggestions have been made for the benefits of controlling the sodium–potassium ratio in the diet. Fruits and vegetables are relatively low in sodium and rich in potassium. Animal foods are rich in sodium.

sodom apple Tropical plant, *Calotropis procera*; fruit is inedible, but the leaves are used in W Africa as a source of proteolytic milk-clotting enzymes as an alternative to RENNET in CHEESE production.

soft swell   See SWELLS.

sol   COLLOIDAL SUSPENSION consisting of a solid dispersed in a liquid. In lyophobic sols there is little interaction between the dispersed particles and the dispersing medium; in lyophilic sols there is affinity between the dispersed and dispersant phases.

Solanaceae   Family of plants including AUBERGINE (*Solanum melongena*), CAPE GOOSEBERRY (*Physalis peruviana*), POTATO (*Solanum tuberosum*), TOMATO (*Lycopersicon esculentum*).

solanine   Heat-stable toxic GLYCOSIDE of the ALKALOID solanidine, found in small amounts in potatoes, and larger and sometimes toxic amounts in sprouted potatoes and potato skin when they become green through exposure to light. Causes gastrointestinal disturbances and neurological disorders; 20 mg solanine per 100 g fresh weight of potato tissue is the upper acceptable limit.

sole   Flat FISH, *Solea* spp. Dover sole is S. *solea*.
Composition/100 g: 372 kJ (89 kcal), protein 18.1 g, fat 1.8 g, cholesterol 50 mg, carbohydrate 0 g, Na 100 mg, K 310 mg, Ca 29 mg, Mg 49 mg, P 200 mg, Fe 0.8 mg, Cu 0.02 mg, Zn 0.4 mg, Se 23 µg, vitamin B_1 0.06 mg, B_2 0.1 mg, niacin 6.4 mg. A 250 g serving is a source of vitamin B_1, B_2, Fe; rich source of protein, niacin, Mg, Se.

solera   See SHERRY.

solids-not-fat (SNF)   Refers to the solids of milk excluding the fat, i.e. protein, lactose and salts. Used as an index of milk quality, determined by measuring the specific gravity in the LACTOMETER.

somatomedins   Circulating growth factors, synthesised in the liver, with broad anabolic properties. Their structure resembles that of PRO-INSULIN, and they are sometimes known as insulin-like growth factors. Synthesis is much impaired in children with protein–energy malnutrition, and responds rapidly to nutritional rehabilitation.

somatostatin   Peptide hormone secreted throughout gut; decreases gastric secretion and GASTRIN release, pancreatic secretion of bicarbonate and enzymes, expression and release of gut peptides, gastric emptying, intestinal motility, gall bladder contractility, absorption of glucose, triacylglycerols, amino acids, intestinal ion secretion, splanchnic blood flow.

somatotrophin, bovine (BST)   A peptide hormone produced by cows in the anterior pituitary gland. High-yielding dairy cows have higher circulating levels and injection of BST increases the yield of lower-yielding cows by minimising the rate of yield decline after peak lactation. Such treatment of cows to increase milk yield was started in USA in 1994 and spread to other countries but has been subject to criticism elsewhere.

Differs in structure from human somatotrophin by about 35% and has negligible activity in human beings.

Somogyi–Nelson reagent Cupric tartrate/arsenomolybdate reagent for the detection and semiquantitative determination of glucose and other reducing sugars.

See also BENEDICT'S REAGENT, FEHLING'S REAGENT.

sorbet A water-ice containing sugar, water and flavouring (commonly fruit juice or pulp). Also known as SHERBET or granita.

sorbic acid Hexadienoic acid, $CH_3CH=CH-CH=CH-COOH$, used together with its sodium, potassium and calcium salts to inhibit growth of fungi in wine, cheese, soft drinks, low-sugar jams, flour confectionery, etc (E-200–203).

Sorbistat Trade name for SORBIC ACID and its potassium salt (Sorbistat K).

sorbitol (glycitol, glucitol) A six-carbon SUGAR ALCOHOL found in plums, apricots, cherries and apples; manufactured by reduction of glucose. Although it is metabolised in the body, yielding the same amount of energy as other carbohydrates, 16 kJ (4 kcal)/g, it is only slowly absorbed from the intestine and is tolerated by diabetics. 50–60% as sweet as sucrose. Used in baked products, jam and confectionery suitable for diabetics (E-420).

sorcerer's milk See WITCHES' MILK.

sorghum *Sorghum vulgare, S. bicolor*; cereals that thrive in semi-arid regions, important human food in tropical Africa, central and N India and China. Sorghum produced in the USA and Australia is used for animal feed. Also known as kaffir corn (in S Africa), guinea corn (in W Africa), jowar (in India), Indian millet and millo maize.

The white grain variety is eaten as meal; red grained has a bitter taste and is used for beer; sorghum syrup is obtained from the crushed stems of the sweet sorghum.

See also MILLET.

sorrel A common wild plant (*Rumex acetosa*); the leaves have a strong acid flavour, and are cooked together with spinach or cabbage, used to make soup and used in salads.

See also ROSELLA.

soul food Afro-Caribbean term for food with traditional or cultural links, having emotional significance.

source In this book foods are listed as sources of nutrients. A rich source of a nutrient means that 30% or more, a good source 20–30% and a source 10–20%, of the EU labelling recommended daily amount (see Table 2) of the nutrient is supplied in the stated portion.

soursop See CUSTARD APPLE.

sous vide French-originated term for cooking in special pouches under vacuum, when the food has a shelf life of weeks; claimed also to retain flavour and nutrients. Derived from the French *cuisine en papillote sous vide*, cooking in sealed container (originally a parchment paper case).

Southern blot See BLOTTING.

Soxhlet method For determination of extractable lipids. The sample is extracted by constant perfusion with a stream of freshly distilled solvent.

soya (soy) A BEAN (*Glycine max*) important as a source of both oil and protein. The protein is of high BIOLOGICAL VALUE, higher than that of many other vegetable proteins, and is of great value for animal and human food. When raw it contains a TRYPSIN INHIBITOR, which is destroyed by heat. Native of China, where it has been cultivated for 5000 years; grows 60–100 cm high with 2–3 beans per pod.

Composition/100 g: 590 kJ (141 kcal), protein 14 g, fat 7.3 g (15.5% saturated, 24.1% mono-, 60.3% polyunsaturated), carbohydrate 5.1 g (2.1 g sugars, 1.9 g starch), nsp 6.1 g, Na 1 mg, K 510 mg, Ca 83 mg, Mg 63 mg, P 250 mg, Fe 3 mg, Cu 0.32 mg, Zn 0.9 mg, Se 5 μg, I 2 μg, vitamin A 1 μg (6 μg carotene), E 1.1 mg, B_1 0.12 mg, B_2 0.09 mg, niacin 2.7 mg, B_6 0.23 mg, folate 54 μg, pantothenate 0.2 mg, biotin 25 μg. A 60 g serving is a source of protein, folate, biotin; Mg, Fe; good source of Cu.

soya flour Dehulled, ground SOYA bean. The unheated material is a rich source of AMYLASE and PROTEINASE and is useful as a baking aid.

Composition/100 g (full fat): 1871 kJ (447 kcal), protein 36.8 g, fat 23.5 g (15.4% saturated, 23.9% mono-, 60.6% polyunsaturated), carbohydrate 23.5 g (11.2 g sugars, 12.3 g starch), dietary fibre 10.7 g, nsp 11.2 g, Na 9 mg, K 1660 mg, Ca 210 mg, Mg 240 mg, P 600 mg, Fe 6.9 mg, Cu 2.92 mg, Zn 3.9 mg, Se 9 μg, vitamin E 1.5 mg, B_1 0.75 mg, B_2 0.28 mg, niacin 10.6 mg, B_6 0.46 mg, folate 345 μg, pantothenate 1.6 mg.

Composition/100 g (low fat): 1473 kJ (352 kcal), protein 45.3 g, fat 7.2 g (15.5% saturated, 24.1% mono-, 60.3% polyunsaturated), carbohydrate 28.2 g (13.4 g sugars, 14.8 g starch), dietary fibre 13.3 g, nsp 13.5 g, Na 14 mg, K 2030 mg, Ca 240 mg, Mg 290 mg, P 640 mg, Fe 9.1 mg, Cu 3.12 mg, Zn 3.2 mg, Se 11 μg, vitamin B_1 0.9 mg, B_2 0.29 mg, niacin 13 mg, B_6 0.52 mg, folate 410 μg, pantothenate 1.8 mg.

soybean curd See TOFU.

Soyolk Trade name for full fat SOYA FLOUR.

soy sauce A condiment prepared from fermented SOYA bean, commonly used in China and Japan. Traditionally the bean, often mixed with wheat, is fermented with *Aspergillus oryzae* over a period of 1–3 years. The modern process is carried out at a high temperature or in an autoclave for a short time.

Composition/100 g: 267 KJ (64 kcal), protein 8.7 g, fat 0 g, carbohydrate 8.3 g, Na 5720 mg, K 360 mg, Ca 19 mg, Mg 43 mg, P 210 mg, Fe 2.7 mg, Cu 0.1 mg, Zn 0.2 mg, vitamin B_1 0.05 mg, B_2 0.13 mg, niacin 4.8 mg, folate 11 µg. Serving 5 g.

spaghetti   See PASTA.

spaghetti squash   A GOURD, also called cucuzzi, calabash, Suzza melon; often classed as summer squash but not a true SQUASH. Only after cooking does the flesh resemble spaghetti in appearance.

Spam   Trade name for canned pork luncheon meat; a contraction of 'spiced ham'.

Spanish toxic oil syndrome   Widespread disease in Spain, 1981–1982, with 450 deaths and many people chronically disabled, due to consumption of an oil containing aniline-denatured industrial rape seed oil, sold as olive oil. The disease appears to be unique and the precise cause is unknown.

Spans   Trade name for non-ionic surface agents derived from fatty acids and hexahydric alcohols. Oil soluble, in contrast to TWEENS which are water-soluble or disperse well in water. Used in bread, cakes and biscuits as crumb softeners (antistaling), to improve dough, and as emulsifiers.

spastic colon   See IRRITABLE BOWEL SYNDROME.

spatchcock   Small birds split down the back and flattened before grilling. Spitchcock is eel treated similarly.

SPE   See SUCROSE POLYESTERS.

spearmint   The common garden (culinary) mint; hybrid of *Mentha spicata*, *M. suaveolens* (apple mint) and *M. villosa* (*M. alopecuroides*, Bowles' mint).

specific dynamic action   See DIET-INDUCED THERMOGENESIS.

specificity   (1) Of an assay; the extent to which what is measured is due to the analyte under investigation, rather than other compounds that may also react.

(2) In relation to enzymes, the ability of an enzyme to catalyse only a limited range of reactions, or, in some cases, a single reaction, and to show considerable specificity for the substrates undergoing reaction.

spectrograph   Instrument that produces a photographic record of wavelength and intensity of light or other electromagnetic radiation.

spectrometer   Instrument for measuring wavelength and intensity of light or other electromagnetic radiation.

spectrophotofluorimeter (spectrophotofluorometer) Instrument for measuring wavelength and intensity of light emitted by a solute at right angles to the beam of exciting light of a specific wavelength.

See also FLUORIMETRY.

spectrophotometer Instrument that measures the amount of light absorbed at any particular wavelength, which is directly related to the concentration of the material in the solution. Used extensively to measure substances that have specific absorption in the visible, infrared or ultraviolet range, or can react to form coloured derivatives.

spelt Coarse type of wheat, mainly used as cattle feed.

spent wash Liquor remaining in the whisky still after distilling the spirit. A source of (unidentified) growth factors detected by chick growth. When dried is known as distillers' dried solubles.

spherocyte Abnormal red BLOOD CELL that is spherical rather than disc shaped. Characteristically seen in some types of haemolytic ANAEMIA.

sphincter A ring of concentric muscle that surrounds an orifice and can close it partially or completely on contraction.

sphingolipids Class of phosphatides in which the 18-carbon dihydroxyalcohol sphingosine serves a similar function to GLYCEROL in PHOSPHOLIPIDS. Important in cell membranes, especially in nerve tissue. The major sphingolipid is SPHINGOMYELIN.

sphingomyelin See SPHINGOLIPIDS.

sphygmomanometer Instrument for measuring arterial BLOOD PRESSURE.

spices Distinguished from HERBS in that part, instead of the whole, of the aromatic plant is used: root, stem or seeds. Originally used to mask putrefactive flavours. Some have a preservative effect because of their essential oils, e.g. cloves, cinnamon and mustard.

spina bifida Congenital NEURAL TUBE DEFECT due to developmental anomaly in early embryonic development. Supplements of FOLIC ACID (400 µg/day) begun before conception reduce the risk.

spinach Leaves of *Spinacia oleracea*.

Composition/100 g: 79 kJ (19 kcal), protein 2.2 g, fat 0.8 g, carbohydrate 0.8 g (0.8 g sugars), dietary fibre 3.1 g, nsp 2.1 g, Na 120 mg, K 230 mg, Ca 160 mg, Mg 34 mg, P 28 mg, Fe 1.6 mg, Cu 0.01 mg, Zn 0.5 mg, Se 1 µg, I 2 µg, vitamin A 640 µg (3840 µg carotene), E 1.7 mg, B_1 0.06 mg, B_2 0.05 mg, niacin 1.5 mg, B_6 0.09 mg, folate 90 µg, pantothenate 0.2 mg, biotin 0.1 µg, C 8 mg. A 95 g serving is a source of vitamin E, C, Ca, Mg, Fe; rich source of vitamin A, folate.

spinach beet See SWISS CHARD.

spinach, Chinese   Leaves of *Amaranthus gangeticus*, also known as bhaji and callaloo.

spinach, Philippine   Variety of purslane (*Talinum triangulare*) cultivated in USA and cooked in the same way as SPINACH.

spiny lobster   SHELLFISH, family Palinuridae, see LOBSTER.

spirits   Beverages of high ALCOHOL content made by distillation of fermented liquors, including BRANDY, GIN, RUM, VODKA, WHISKY; usually 40% alcohol by volume (equivalent to 31.7 g per 100 mL). Silent spirit is highly purified alcohol, or neutral spirit, distilled from any fermented material.

spirometer   Or respirometer, apparatus used to measure the amount of oxygen consumed (and in some instances carbon dioxide produced) from which to calculate the energy expended (indirect calorimetry).

spirulina   Blue-green alga which can fix atmospheric nitrogen; eaten for centuries round Lake Chad in Africa and in Mexico. Many health claims are made, but are negated by the small amounts eaten.

splanchnic   Relating to the viscera.

spleen   Abdominal organ whose main function is destruction of aged red blood cells and recycling the iron. As a food it is called melts.

spongiform encephalopathy   Progressive degenerative neurological diseases including scrapie (in sheep), bovine spongiform encephalopathy (in cattle) and Creutzfeldt–Jakob disease (in human beings). Believed to be caused by PRIONS. Bovine spongiform encephalopathy (BSE) is believed to originate from infected meat and bone meal in cattle feed concentrates, and an anomalous form of Creutzfeldt–Jakob disease (new variant or nvCJD) has been linked with consumption of beef from animals affected by BSE.

A ban on the specified bovine offal in food and feedstuffs, and a policy of slaughtering affected animals have resulted in a dramatic fall in the number of confirmed cases of BSE. The important unknown factor is the incubation period in human beings, which could be years.

spores   Bacterial spores are a resting state, resistant to heat, which can germinate to produce bacteria under suitable conditions. Spore formation only occurs in some species, when the organism encounters adverse conditions (e.g. dryness, lack of nutrients, etc). Spore-forming species, especially of *Bacillus* and *Clostridium*, are a health hazard because the spores are resistant to most sterilisation techniques.

sports drinks   Solutions of glucose plus electrolytes to mimic those lost in sweat; generally isotonic with blood plasma to avoid potential problems of water intoxication. Sometimes known as 'bottled sweat'.

sprat Small oily FISH, *Sprattus (Clupea) sprattus,* fresh or frozen; young are canned as brisling.

Composition/100 g: 719 kJ (172 kcal), protein 18.3 g, fat 11 g (22.2% saturated, 47.4% mono-, 30.3% polyunsaturated), cholesterol 93 mg, carbohydrate 0 g, Na 200 mg, K 320 mg, Ca 97 mg, Mg 37 mg, P 240 mg, Fe 1.1 mg, Cu 0.09 mg, Zn 1.7 mg, Se 10 μg, I 64 μg, vitamin A 60 μg, D 13 μg, E 0.5 mg, B_2 0.2 mg, niacin 6.4 mg, B_6 0.27 mg, B_{12} 7 μg, pantothenate 0.7 mg, biotin 4 μg. An 80 g serving is a source of vitamin B_6; good source of protein, niacin, Se; rich source of vitamin D, B_{12}, I.

See also HERRING; WHITEBAIT.

spray dryer Equipment in which the material to be dried is sprayed as a fine mist into a hot-air chamber and falls to the bottom as dry powder. Period of heating is very brief and so nutritional and functional damage are avoided. Dried powder consists of hollow particles of low density.

springers See SWELLS.

spring greens Young leafy CABBAGE eaten before the heart has formed, or leaf sprouts formed after cutting off the head.

Composition/100 g: 83 kJ (20 kcal), protein 1.9 g, fat 0.7 g, carbohydrate 1.6 g (1.4 g sugars, 0.2 g starch), dietary fibre 3.4 g, nsp 2.6 g, Na 10 mg, K 160 mg, Ca 75 mg, Mg 8 mg, P 29 mg, Fe 1.4 mg, Cu 0.02 mg, Zn 0.3 mg, vitamin A 378 μg (2270 μg carotene), B_1 0.05 mg, B_2 0.06 mg, niacin 1.5 mg, B_6 0.18 mg, folate 66 μg, pantothenate 0.3 mg, biotin 0.4 μg, C 77 mg. A 95 g serving is a rich source of vitamin A, folate, C.

See also COLLARD.

spring rolls Chinese (and general SE Asian); pancakes filled with quick fried vegetables and meat; may be served as soft pancakes prepared at the table or rolled and deep fried. Also known as pancake rolls and Imperial rolls; loempia in Indonesian and nem in Vietnamese cuisine.

sprouts (1) See BRUSSELS SPROUTS (2) See BEANSPROUTS.

spruce beer Western Canada; branches, bark and cones of black spruce (*Picea mariana*) boiled for several hours, then put in a cask with molasses, hops and yeast, and allowed to ferment.

sprue, tropical Name given (by Dutch in Java) to a tropical disease characterised by atrophy of the intestinal VILLI, with fatty diarrhoea and sore mouth, and signs of undernutrition due to poor absorption of nutrients. Both an unidentified infectious agent and folic acid deficiency have been suggested as causes.

spurtle Scottish; wooden stick traditionally used to stir porridge. Also known as theevil.

squab   Young PIGEON; squab pie is W of England dish made from meat, apples and onions.

squalene   Acyclic intermediate (triterpene hydrocarbon) in the synthesis of CHOLESTEROL. Acts as a feedback inhibitor and repressor of the rate-limiting enzyme of cholesterol synthesis (HMG COA reductase, EC 1.1.1.34), so has a useful hypocholesterolaemic effect. Found in small amounts in fish liver oils and in relatively large amounts in OLIVE OIL, but only small amounts in most other plant oils.

squash   (1) Varieties of the GOURD *Cucurbita pepo*. Grouped with courgettes, squashes and pumpkins.

Composition/100 g (acorn squash): 234 kJ (56 kcal), protein 1.1 g, fat 0.1 g, carbohydrate 12.6 g (1.6 g sugars, 10.8 g starch), nsp 3.2 g, Na 4 mg, K 440 mg, Ca 44 mg, Mg 43 mg, P 45 mg, Fe 0.9 mg, Cu 0.09 mg, Zn 0.2 mg, vitamin A 43 μg (260 μg carotene), B_1 0.17 mg, B_2 0.01 mg, niacin 1.2 mg, B_6 0.19 mg, folate 19 μg, pantothenate 0.5 mg, biotin 0.6 μg, C 11 mg. A 65 g serving is a source of vitamin C.

Composition/100 g (spaghetti squash): 96 kJ (23 kcal), protein 0.7 g, fat 0.3 g, carbohydrate 4.3 g (3.4 g sugars, 0.6 g starch), nsp 2.1 g, Na 18 mg, K 120 mg, Ca 21 mg, Mg 11 mg, P 14 mg, Fe 0.3 mg, Cu 0.03 mg, Zn 0.2 mg, vitamin A 11 μg (66 μg carotene), B_1 0.04 mg, B_2 0.02 mg, niacin 1 mg, B_6 0.1 mg, folate 8 μg, pantothenate 0.4 mg, biotin 0.4 μg, C 3 mg. Serving 65 g. Courgettes and zucchini are varieties that have been developed for cutting when small.

(2) Fruit squash is a concentrated sweetened fruit juice preparation which is diluted before drinking.

squid (calamar)   Marine creature with elongated body and eight arms, *Loligo* and *Illex* species.

Composition/100 g: 339 kJ (81 kcal), protein 15.4 g, fat 1.7 g, cholesterol 225 mg, carbohydrate 1.2 g, Na 110 mg, K 280 mg, Ca 13 mg, Mg 28 mg, P 190 mg, Fe 0.5 mg, Cu 0.98 mg, Zn 1.1 mg, Se 66 μg, I 20 μg, vitamin A 15 μg, E 1.2 mg, B_1 0.1 mg, B_2 0.12 mg, niacin 6.7 mg, B_6 0.69 mg, folate 13 μg, B_{12} 3 μg, pantothenate 0.7 mg. A 65 g serving is a good source of protein, niacin, vitamin B_6; rich source of vitamin B_{12}, Cu, Se.

SRD   State registered dietitian; legal qualification to practise as a dietitian in UK.

stabilisers   Substances that stabilise emulsions of fat and water, e.g. GUMS, AGAR, egg albumin, CELLULOSE ethers; used to produce the texture of meringues and marshmallow, LECITHIN (E-322) for crumb softening in bread and confectionery, glyceryl monostearate (E-471) and polyoxyethylene stearate (E-430–436) for crumb softening. The legally permitted list includes also SUPER-

GLYCERINATED FATS, propylene glycol alginate and stearate (E-570), methyl-, methylethyl-, and sodium carboxymethyl-celluloses (E-466), stearyl tartrate (E-483), sorbitan esters of fatty acids (E-491–495). Bread may contain only superglyceri-nated fats and stearyl tartrate.

See also EMULSIFYING AGENTS.

stachyose Tetrasaccharide, galactosyl-galactosyl-glucosyl-fructose not hydrolysed in the human digestive tract, passing to the large intestine, where it is fermented by bacteria. Present in SOYA beans and some other LEGUMES; gives rise to the flatulence commonly associated with eating beans. Also known as man-notetrose or lupeose.

stachys See ARTICHOKE, CHINESE.

stackburn The deterioration in colour and quality of canned foods which have not been sufficiently cooled after canning, then stored in stacks which cool slowly.

stadiometer Portable device for measuring height, with a vertical measuring board and a horizontal headboard.

stagnant loop syndrome See BLIND LOOP SYNDROME.

staling Starch has a crystalline structure which is lost during baking. Subsequently the starch recrystallises, i.e. it retrogrades and, in the instance of bread, the crumb loses its softness and the bread goes stale. Staling can be delayed by emulsifiers (CRUMB SOFTENERS) such as polyoxyethylene and monoglyceride deriva-tives of fatty acids. Retrogradation of starch also takes place in dehydrated potatoes.

St Anthony's Fire See ERGOT.

Staphylococcus aureus Food poisoning organism that produces ENTEROTOXINS (TX 1.2.3.1–7) in the food. Onset of symptoms 1–6 h, duration 8–24 h.

starch POLYSACCHARIDE, a polymer of GLUCOSE units; the form in which carbohydrate is stored in the plant, and does not occur in animal tissue. (GLYCOGEN is sometimes referred to as animal starch.) Starch is broken down by acid or enzymic hydrolysis (AMYLASE), ultimately yielding glucose; it is the principal carbo-

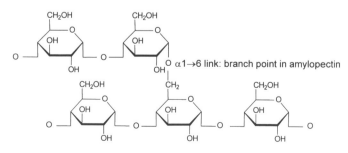

hydrate of the diet and, hence, the major source of energy for man and animals.

Starches from different sources (e.g. potato, maize, cereal, arrowroot, sago, etc) have different structures, and contain different proportions of two major forms: AMYLOSE, which is a linear polymer and AMYLOPECTIN, which has a branched structure. The mixture of dietary starches consists of about one-quarter amylose and three-quarters amylopectin.

starch, A and B   Refers to larger granules of wheat starch, A 25–35 μm, and smaller particles, B 2–8 μm.

starch, animal   See GLYCOGEN.

starch, arum   From root of the arum lily (*Arum maculatum* and other spp); similar to SAGO and ARROWROOT.

starch, derivatised   See STARCH, MODIFIED.

starch, enzyme-resistant   Starch that escapes digestion in the small intestine but can be fermented in the large intestine. According to the method of analysis used, enzyme-resistant starch may be included with DIETARY FIBRE. Chemically it is a glucan formed when starch is heated (apparently formed after gelatinisation by spontaneous self-association of hydrated amylose).

starch equivalent   A measure of the energy value of animal feed-ingstuffs; the number of parts of pure starch that would be equivalent to 100 parts of the ration as a source of energy.

starch, inhibited   See STARCH, MODIFIED.

starch, modified   Starch altered by physical or chemical treatment to give special properties of value in food processing, e.g. change in gel strength, flow properties, colour, clarity, stability of the paste.

Acid-modified starch: acid treatment reduces the viscosity of the paste (used in sugar confectionery, e.g. gum drops, jelly beans).

Oxidised starch: peroxide, permanganate, chlorine, etc, alter viscosity, clarity and stability of the paste (major use is outside the food industry).

Derivatised starch: chemical derivatives such as ethers and esters show properties such as reduced gelatinisation in hot water and greater stability to acids and alkalis (inhibited starch); useful where food has to withstand heat treatment, as in canning or in acid foods. Further degrees of treatment can result in starch being unaffected by boiling water and losing its gel-forming properties.

See also STARCH, PREGELATINISED.

starch, oxidised   See STARCH, MODIFIED.

starch, pregelatinised   Raw starch does not form a paste with cold water and therefore requires cooking if it is to be used as a food thickening agent. Pregelatinised starch, mostly maize starch, has been cooked and dried. Used in instant puddings, pie fillings, soup mixes, salad dressings, sugar confectionery, as binder in meat products. Nutritional value the same as that of the original starch.

See also STARCH, MODIFIED.

starch, resistant See STARCH, ENZYME-RESISTANT.

starch, waxy Starches containing a high percentage of AMYLOPECTIN; they form soft pastes rather than rigid gels when gelatinised (see GELATINISATION).

See also MAIZE STARCH, WAXY.

starter Culture of bacteria used to inoculate or start growth in a fermentation, e.g. milk for cheese production, or butter to develop the flavour.

statins A family of related compounds (lovastatin, pravastatin, simvastatin) used to treat hypercholesterolaemia. They act by inhibiting hydroxymethylglutaryl CoA reductase (HMG CoA reductase, EC 1.1.1.34), the first and rate-limiting enzyme of CHO-LESTEROL synthesis.

steam baking In baking an even temperature is maintained in the oven by means of closed pipes through which steam circulates. This is sometimes erroneously taken to mean that the bread is baked in live steam.

steam distillation Process for removal of volatile components by passing steam through the heated mixture, followed by condensation of the steam and volatiles. May be used either to purify a volatile compound such as an ESSENTIAL OIL or to remove undesirable flavours from oils and fats.

steapsin Obsolete name for LIPASE.

stearic acid Saturated FATTY ACID with 18 carbon atoms (C18:0); present in most animal and vegetable fats.

steatopygia Accumulation of large amounts of fat in the buttocks.

steatorrhoea Excretion of faeces containing a large amount of fat (>5 g/day), and generally foul smelling. May be due to lack of BILE, lack of LIPASE in the digestive juices, or defective absorption of fat. Treatment by feeding low-fat diet.

See also COELIAC DISEASE.

steatosis Fatty infiltration of the liver; occurs in PROTEIN–ENERGY MALNUTRITION and alcoholism.

steep The process of leaving a food to stand in water, either to soften it or to extract its flavour and colour. Also the preparation of fruit liqueurs by steeping fruit in SPIRIT.

stenosis Abnormal narrowing of blood vessels or heart valves.

stercobilin One of the brown pigments of the faeces; formed from the BILE pigments, which, in turn, are formed as breakdown products of HAEMOGLOBIN.

stercolith   Stone formed of dried compressed FAECES.

sterculia   A bulk-forming LAXATIVE. See KARAYA GUM.

stereoisomerism   See ISOMERS.

sterigmatocystin   A MYCOTOXIN.

sterile   Free from all microorganisms, bacteria, moulds and yeasts. When foods are sterilised, as in canning, they are preserved indefinitely, since they are protected from recontamination in the can, and also from chemical and enzymic deterioration.

sterilisation, cold   Applied to preservation with SULPHUR DIOXIDE or by IRRADIATION, high pressure, ULTRASONICATION or ELECTRO-PORATION.

sterilisation, radiation   See IRRADIATION.

sterility, commercial   Canned foods that are not STERILE but which will not spoil during storage, because of the high acid content of the food, or the presence of pickling salts, or a high concentration of sugar.

steroids   Chemically, compounds that contain the cyclopenteno-phenanthrene ring system. All the biologically important steroids are derived metabolically from CHOLESTEROL; they include VITAMIN D (chemically a secosteroid rather than a steroid), and hormones including the sex hormones (androgens, oestrogens and progesterone) and the hormones of the adrenal cortex.

   See also PHYTOSTEROLS; SITOSTEROL.

stevia leaves   Leaves of the Paraguayan shrub, *Stevia rebaudiana*, the source of STEVIOSIDE and REBAUDIOSIDE, also known as yerba dulce.

stevioside   Naturally occurring GLUCOSIDE of steviol, a STEROID derivative, which is 300 times as sweet as sucrose. Isolated from leaves of the Paraguayan shrub, yerba dulce (*Stevia rebaudiana*), the same source as REBAUDIOSIDE.

Stevix   Trade name for mixture of the sweet GLYCOSIDES extracted from STEVIA LEAVES.

stickwater   The aqueous fraction from pressing cooked fish in the manufacture of FISH MEAL. Contains amino acids, vitamins and minerals, and is either added to animal feed or mixed back with the fish meal and dried. Also known as fish solubles.

stilboestrol   Dihydroxystilbene, synthetic substance with potent activity as female sex hormone; the first non-steroid compound developed to have oestrogen activity (1938). Formerly widely used both clinically and for chemical caponisation of cockerels and to stimulate the growth of cattle.

   See also CAPON.

Stilton   Semi-hard, creamy white or blue-veined English CHEESE made only in a very restricted area of the Vale of Belvoir in Leicestershire UK, but named after the village of Stilton,

Huntingdonshire. Matured 3–4 months; for production of blue Stilton the cheese is pricked with stainless steel wires during ripening to encourage growth of the mould *Penicillium roquefortii*.

stiparogenic   Foods that tend to cause constipation.

stiparolytic   Foods that tend to prevent or relieve constipation.

stirabout   Irish name for PORRIDGE.

stir fry   Chinese method of cooking; sliced vegetables and meat fried for a short time in a small amount of oil, normally in a WOK, over high heat with constant stirring.

St John's bread   See CAROB.

stobb   Strawberry stalk.

stockfish   Unsalted fish that has been dried naturally in air and sunshine; mostly prepared in Norway. Contains 12–15% water; 4.5 kg of fresh fish yield 1 kg stockfish.

See also KLIPFISH.

stomatitis   Inflammation of the mucous lining of the mouth.

stork process   The process of ultra-high temperature sterilisation of milk followed by sterilisation again inside the bottle.

stout   See BEER.

strawberry   Fruit of *Fragaria* spp, a perennial herb of American origin, introduced into UK around 1600.

Composition/100 g: 113 kJ (27 kcal), protein 0.8 g, fat 0.1 g, carbohydrate 6 g (6 g sugars), dietary fibre 2 g, nsp 1.1 g, Na 6 mg, K 160 mg, Ca 16 mg, Mg 10 mg, P 24 mg, Fe 0.4 mg, Cu 0.07 mg, Zn 0.1 mg, I 9 µg, vitamin A 1 µg (8 µg carotene), E 0.2 mg, B_1 0.03 mg, B_2 0.03 mg, niacin 0.7 mg, B_6 0.06 mg, folate 20 µg, pantothenate 0.3 mg, biotin 1.1 µg, C 77 mg. A 100 g serving is a source of folate; rich source of vitamin C.

Alpine strawberry is *Fragaria vesca semperflorens*, a variety of the European wild strawberry.

straw mushroom   *Volvariella volvacea*, see MUSHROOMS.

straw potatoes   Very thin strips of potato, deep fried. Also known as pommes allumettes.

Strecker degradation   A non-enzymic BROWNING REACTION between free amino acids and di- or tri-carbonyl compounds to form pyrazine derivatives. Will lead to loss of amino acids, and may be aesthetically damaging to food, but also exploited to yield desirable flavours in chocolate, honey and a variety of cooked and baked products.

See also MAILLARD REACTION.

streptavidin   Protein from *Streptomyces* spp that is similar to AVIDIN, and binds BIOTIN with high affinity.

streptozotocin   ANTIBIOTIC isolated from *Streptomyces achromo-*

genes culture broth; specifically cytotoxic to the β-cells of the pancreatic islets, and used to induce experimental insulin-dependent DIABETES mellitus.

See also ALLOXAN.

stroke Also known as cerebrovascular accident (CVA); damage to brain tissue by hypoxia due to blockage of a blood vessel as a result of thrombosis, atherosclerosis or haemorrhage. The severity and nature of the effects of the stroke depend on the region of the brain affected and the extent of damage. HYPERTENSION and HYPERCHOLESTEROLAEMIA are major risk factors.

Strongyloides Genus of small nematode worms that infest the small intestine.

struvite Small crystals of magnesium ammonium phosphate that occasionally form in canned fish, resembling broken glass.

Stubbs and More factor For calculating the amount of fat-free meat in a product from total NITROGEN content.

See also KJELDAHL DETERMINATION; NITROGEN CONVERSION FACTOR.

stunting Reduction in the linear growth of children, leading to lower height for age than would be expected, and generally resulting in life-long short stature. A common effect of PROTEIN–ENERGY MALNUTRITION, and associated especially with inadequate protein intake.

See also ANTHROPOMETRY; HARVARD STANDARD; NCHS STANDARDS; NUTRITIONAL STATUS ASSESSMENT; TANNER STANDARD; WATERLOW CLASSIFICATION.

sturgeon White FISH, *Acipenser* spp. See CAVIAR.

submaxillary gland One of the SALIVARY GLANDS.

submucosa Layer of loose (areolar) connective tissue underlying a mucous membrane.

substantial equivalence Term used to denote oil, starch, etc, from genetically modified crop, that does not contain protein or DNA, and cannot be distinguished from the same product from the unmodified crop. Hence not subject to regulations concerning novel foods.

substrate (1) The substance on which an enzyme acts.

(2) The medium on which MICROORGANISMS grow.

subtilin Antibiotic isolated from a strain of *Bacillus subtilis* grown on a medium containing asparagine. Used as a food preservative (not permitted in UK), as it reduces the thermal resistance of bacterial SPORES and so permits a reduction in the processing time.

Sucaryl Trade name for sodium or calcium salt of cyclohexyl sulphamate (CYCLAMATE).

succory See CHICORY.

succotash American; sweetcorn (MAIZE) kernels cooked with green or lima (butter) beans.

succus Any juice or secretion of animal or plant origin. Succus entericus is the INTESTINAL JUICE.

suchar Activated charcoal, used to decolorise solutions.
See also CHARCOAL.

sucking pig Piglet aged 4–5 weeks, usually stuffed and roasted whole.

sucralfate Complex of aluminium hydroxide and sulphated sucrose used to form a protective coat over the gastric or duodenal mucosa in treatment of peptic ULCERS.

Sucralose Trade name for chlorinated sucrose (trichlorogalacto-sucrose); 2000 times as sweet as sucrose, stable to heat and acid.

sucrase (sucrase-isomaltase) See INVERTASE.

sucrol See DULCIN.

Sucron Trade name for mixture of SACCHARIN and SUCROSE, four times as sweet as sucrose alone.

sucrose Cane or beet SUGAR. A DISACCHARIDE, glucosyl-fructose.

sucrose distearate See SUCROSE ESTERS.

sucrose esters Di- and trilaurates and mono- and distearates of sucrose. Used as emulsifiers, wetting agents and surface active agents, e.g. for washing fruits and vegetables, as antispattering agents, antifoam agents and antistaling or crumb-softening agents (E-473).

sucrose intolerance See DISACCHARIDE INTOLERANCE.

sucrose monostearate See SUCROSE ESTERS.

sucrose polyesters (SPE) Mixtures of hexa- hepta- and octa-esters of sucrose and common FATTY ACIDS (C-12 to C-20 and above). Can replace fats and oils in foods and food preparation but pass through the gastrointestinal tract without being absorbed, hence known as fat substitutes or FAT REPLACERS.
See also OLESTRA.

Sudan gum See GUM ARABIC.

suet Solid white fat around the kidneys of oxen and sheep, used in baking and frying.
Composition/100 g: 3457 kJ (826 kcal), protein 0 g, fat 86.7 g (58.3% saturated, 39% mono-, 2.5% polyunsaturated), cholesterol 82 mg, carbohydrate 12.1 g (0.2 g sugars, 11.9 g starch), dietary fibre 0.6 g, nsp 0.5 g, I 5 µg, vitamin A 64 µg (73 µg carotene), E 1.5 mg. A 100 g serving is a source of vitamin E.

suet crust See PASTRY.

sufu Fermented product made by inoculating soybean curd (TOFU) with the mould, *Actinomucor elegans*; stored after adding salt and alcohol.

sugar (1) Commonly table sugar or SUCROSE, which is extracted from the SUGAR BEET or SUGAR CANE, concentrated and refined. MOLASSES is the residue left after the first stage of crystallisation and is bitter and black. The residue from the second stage is TREACLE, less bitter and viscous than molasses. The first crude crystals are Muscovado or Barbados sugar, brown and sticky. The next stage is light brown, Demerara sugar. Refined white sugar is essentially 100% pure sucrose; technically described as semi-white, white and extra-white (EU definitions). Yields 16 kJ (3.9 kcal)/g. Soft sugars are fine grained and moister, white or brown (excluding large-grained Demerara sugar).

(2) Chemically a group of compounds of carbon, hydrogen and oxygen (carbohydrates). The simplest sugars are monosaccharides. They may contain three (triose), four (tetrose), five (pentose), six (hexose) or seven (heptose) carbon atoms, with hydrogen and oxygen in the ratio $C_nH_{2n}O_n$.

The nutritionally important monosaccharides are hexoses: glucose (grape sugar), fructose (fruit sugar) and galactose. Two pentoses are also important: ribose and deoxyribose. Disaccharides consist of two monosaccharide units, linked by condensation (elimination of water). The nutritionally important disaccharides are SUCROSE (cane or beet sugar, a disaccharide of glucose + fructose), lactose (milk sugar, a disaccharide of glucose + galactose) and maltose (malt sugar, a disaccharide of glucose).

Trisaccharides consist of three monosaccharide units and tetrasaccharides of four monosaccharide units. Larger numbers of monosaccharide units make up oligosaccharides. Most tri-, tetra- and oligosaccharides are not digested by human enzymes, but are substrates for bacterial fermentation in the large intestine.

See also CARBOHYDRATES.

sugar alcohols Also called polyols, chemical derivatives of SUGARS that differ from the parent compounds in having an alcohol group (CH_2OH) instead of the aldehyde group (CHO); thus MANNITOL from MANNOSE, XYLITOL from XYLOSE, LACTICOL from LACTULOSE (also SORBITOL, ISOMALT and hydrogenated glucose SYRUP). Several occur naturally in fruits, vegetables and cereals. They range in sweetness from equal to sucrose to less than half. They provide bulk in foods such as confectionery (in contrast to INTENSE SWEETENERS), and so are called bulk sweeteners.

They are slowly and incompletely metabolised so that they are tolerated by diabetics and provide less energy than sucrose: they are less CARIOGENIC than sucrose, especially hydrogenated glucose syrup, isomalt, sorbitol and xylitol. The energy yields differ, but the EU has adopted a value of 10 kJ (2.4 kcal)/g for all polyols (compared with 16 for carbohydrates).

Considered safe and have no specified ADI, meaning that they can be used in foods in any required amount; however a fairly large amount, more than 20–50 g per day, varying with the rest of the diet and the individual, can cause gastrointestinal discomfort and osmotic DIARRHOEA. For labelling purposes they are included with carbohydrates not sugars; they do not ferment and so do not damage teeth.

See also TOOTH-FRIENDLY SWEETS.

sugar beet *Beta vulgaris* subsp *cicla*, biennial plant related to the garden BEETROOT but with white, conical roots; the most important source of SUGAR (SUCROSE) in temperate countries; contains 15–20% sucrose.

sugar cane The tropical grass, *Saccharum officinarum*; the juice of the stems contains about 15% SUCROSE and provides about 70% of the world's sugar production.

sugar, canners' Sugar with a higher standard of microbiological quality control than highly refined table sugar because some bacterial spores can survive the high temperatures of canning and even small numbers can damage canned food. Similarly bottlers' sugar must be virtually free from yeasts, moulds and certain bacteria.

sugar, caster Ordinary SUGAR (sucrose) crystallised in small crystals.

sugar confectionery A range of sugar-based products, including boiled sweets (hard glasses), fatty emulsions (toffees and caramels), soft crystalline products (fudges), fully crystalline products (fondants) and gels (gums, pastilles and jellies).

sugar doctor To prevent the crystallisation or 'graining' of SUGAR in sugar confectionery, a substance called the sugar doctor or candy doctor is added. This may be a weak acid, such as cream of tartar, which 'inverts' (HYDROLYSES) part of the sugar during the boiling, or invert sugar or starch syrup.

sugar esters See SUCROSE ESTERS.

sugar, icing Powdered SUGAR.

sugaring A type of deterioration of dried fruit on storage, most frequently on prunes and figs. A sugary substance appears on the surface or under the skin, consisting of glucose and fructose, with traces of citric and malic acids, lysine, asparagine and aspartic acid. When occurring under the skin of prunes, it is called 'red sugar'.

sugar, London Demerara White sugar coloured with molasses to resemble partly refined sugar.

sugar maple N American tree; *Acer saccharum*. See MAPLE SYRUP.

sugar palm *Arenga saccharifera*; grows wild in Malaysia and Indonesia; sugar (sucrose) is obtained from the sap.

sugar pea See PEA, MANGE-TOUT.

sugar tolerance See GLUCOSE TOLERANCE.

sugarware Edible seaweed, *Laminaria saccharina*.

sulforaphane Isothiocyanate derivative in *Brassica* spp that induces PHASE II METABOLISM of XENOBIOTICS, and hence has a potentially anticarcinogenic action.

sulphaguanidine (sulfaguanidine) Poorly absorbed antibacterial agent (a sulphonamide) used in treatment of persistent bacterial DIARRHOEA and gastrointestinal infection.

sulphasalazine (sulfasalazine) A sulphonamide drug (salicyl-azosulphapyridine) used in treatment of inflammatory bowel disease. Inhibits absorption of folic acid.

See also AMINOSALICYLATES.

sulphites Salts of sulphurous acid (H_2SO_3) used as sources of SULPHUR DIOXIDE (E-221–227).

sulphonamides (sulfonamides) Family of drugs derived from sulphanilamide that prevent the growth of bacteria (i.e.bacteriostatic, not bactericidal).

sulphonylureas See HYPOGLYCAEMIC AGENTS.

sulphur An element that is part of the amino acids cysteine and methionine and therefore present in all proteins. It is also part of the molecules of vitamin B_1 and biotin and occurs in foods and in the body as sulphates. Apart from these amino acids and vitamins, there appears to be no requirement for sulphur in any other form and no deficiency has ever been observed, although it is essential for plants. Not only was the old-fashioned remedy of sulphur and molasses (brimstone and treacle) quite unnecessary, but elemental sulphur is not used by the body.

sulphur dioxide (SO_2) Preservative used in gaseous form or as salts (SULPHITES) for fruit drinks, wine, comminuted meat, as a processing aid to control physical properties of flour; also prevents enzymic and non-enzymic browning (see BROWNING REACTIONS) by inhibition of PHENOL OXIDASES. Protects vitamin C but destroys vitamin B_1. Prepared by ancient Egyptians and Romans by burning sulphur and used to disinfect wine (E-220).

sulphuring Preservation by SULPHUR DIOXIDE.

sultanas Made by drying the golden sultana grapes grown in Turkey, Greece, Australia, and S Africa; the bunches are dipped in alkali, washed, sulphured and dried. Sultanas of the European type produced in the USA are termed seedless raisins.

Composition/100 g: 1151 kJ (275 kcal), protein 2.7 g, fat 0.4 g, carbohydrate 69.4 g (69.4 g sugars), dietary fibre 6.3 g, nsp 2 g, Na

19 mg, K 1060 mg, Ca 64 mg, Mg 31 mg, P 86 mg, Fe 2.2 mg, Cu 0.4 mg, Zn 0.3 mg, vitamin A 2 μg (12 μg carotene), E 0.7 mg, B_1 0.09 mg, B_2 0.05 mg, niacin 1 mg, B_6 0.25 mg, folate 27 μg, pantothenate 0.1 mg, biotin 4.8 μg. A 30 g serving (one tablespoon) is a source of Cu.

See also CURRANTS, DRIED; RAISIN.

summer pudding   Cold sweet of stewed fruit cased in bread or sponge cake.

sum-sum   See SESAME.

Sunett   Trade name for ACESULPHAME K.

sunflower   Annual plant, *Helianthus annuus*. Seeds.

Composition/100 g: 2432 kJ (581 kcal), protein 19.8 g, fat 47.5 g (9.9% saturated, 21.6% mono-, 68.4% polyunsaturated), carbohydrate 18.6 g (1.7 g sugars, 16.3 g starch), nsp 6 g, Na 3 mg, K 710 mg, Ca 110 mg, Mg 390 mg, P 640 mg, Fe 6.4 mg, Cu 2.27 mg, Zn 5.1 mg, Se 49 μg, vitamin A 2 μg (15 μg carotene), E 37.8 mg, B_1 1.6 mg, B_2 0.19 mg, niacin 9.1 mg. A 15 g serving (one tablespoon) is a source of vitamin B_1; Mg, Se; rich source of vitamin E, Cu.

sunlight flavour   Name given to unpleasant flavours developing in foods after exposure to sunlight. In milk it is said to be due to the oxidation of METHIONINE in the presence of vitamin B_2. At the same time riboflavin undergoes photolysis to metabolically inactive lumichrome, a significant loss of the vitamin can occur when milk is exposed to sunlight. In beer due to a change in the bitter principles from the hops.

superchill   Cool to temperature −1 to −4°C (chill temperature is usually +2°C).

supercritical fluid extraction   Technique for extraction especially of non-polar compounds, e.g. decaffeination of coffee. A gas (commonly carbon dioxide) is compressed to above its critical pressure, but above its critical temperature, to yield a supercritical fluid with physical properties intermediate between those of a dense gas and a liquid with low viscosity and surface tension, high solvating properties and a high diffusion constant of solutes.

superglycerinated fats   Neutral fats are triacylglycerols, i.e. with three molecules of fatty acid to each molecule of glycerol. Mono- and diacylglycerols (sometimes called mono- and diglycerides) are known as superglycerinated high ratio fats or fat extenders (E-471).

Glyceryl monostearate (GMS) is solid at room temperature, flexible and non-greasy; used as a protective coating for foods, as plasticiser for softening the crumb of bread, to reduce spattering in frying fats, as emulsifier and stabiliser. Glyceryl mono-oleate (GMO) is semiliquid at room temperature.

superoxide dismutase (SOD) COPPER- and ZINC-containing enzyme (EC 1.15.1.1), important as a scavenger of the superoxide radical. Activity in red BLOOD CELLS may be an index of copper status.

supplementation See FORTIFICATION.

suprarenal glands See ADRENAL GLANDS.

surface area See BODY SURFACE AREA.

surfactants Surface active agents; compounds that are both hydrophobic and hydrophilic, so act to emulsify lipids and water, e.g. soaps and detergents. Used as wetting agents to assist the reconstitution of powders, including dried foods, to clean and peel fruits and vegetables, also in baked goods and comminuted meat products.

surimi Water extract of minced flesh of low-oil FISH (mostly myofibrillar protein) with gelling properties, used to prepare a range of foods. It is white, relatively tasteless and odourless. Introduced from Japan into the United States in 1979, as the basis for SEAFOOD analogues but with broad potentialities.

surveillance Continuous monitoring of (the nutritional status of) selected population groups. Differs from surveys in that data are collected and analysed over a prolonged period of time, hence longitudinal rather than cross-sectional data.

susceptor plates Special metallic films (usually powdered ALUMINIUM) deposited inside the packets of foods intended for microwave cooking; they concentrate the energy on the outside of the food and brown and crisp it.

sushi Japanese; thinly sliced raw fish.

suspensoids See COLLOID, lyophobic.

süssreserve Unfermented grape juice added to wines after fermentation to increase sweetness, especially in Germany, England and New Zealand.

Sustagen Trade name for a food concentrate in powder form; mixture of whole and skim milk, casein, maltose, dextrins and glucose.

Svedberg Unit of the rate of sedimentation of biological particles and proteins in centrifugation = 10^{-13} s.

swainsonine See LOCOWEED.

swede Root of *Brassica rutabaga* or Swedish turnip; called rutabaga in the USA.

Composition/100 g: 46 kJ (11 kcal), protein 0.3 g, fat 0.1 g, carbohydrate 2.3 g (2.2 g sugars, 0.1 g starch), dietary fibre 1.2 g, nsp 0.7 g, Na 14 mg, K 86 mg, Ca 26 mg, Mg 4 mg, P 11 mg, Fe 0.1 mg, Zn 0.1 mg, Se 1 µg, vitamin A 27 µg (165 µg carotene), B_1 0.13 mg, B_2 0.01 mg, niacin 1.1 mg, B_6 0.04 mg, folate 18 µg, pantothenate 0.1 mg, C 15 mg. A 60 g serving is a source of vitamin C.

sweeney OSTEOMALACIA in livestock due to PHOSPHATE deficiency.

sweetbread Butchers' term for PANCREAS (gut sweetbread) or thymus (chest sweetbread).

sweet cecily See CHERVIL (3).

sweetcorn See MAIZE.

sweeteners Four groups of compounds are used to sweeten foods:
(1) The SUGARS, of which the commonest is SUCROSE. FRUCTOSE has 173% of the sweetness of sucrose; GLUCOSE, 74%; MALTOSE, 33% and LACTOSE, 16%. HONEY is a mixture of glucose and fructose.

(2) Bulk sweeteners, including SUGAR ALCOHOLS.

(3) Synthetic non-nutritive sweeteners (intense sweeteners), which are many times sweeter than sucrose, such as ACESUL-PHAME-K, ASPARTAME, CYCLAMATE, DULCIN, P4000, SACCHARIN, SUCARYL.

(4) Various other chemicals such as GLYCEROL and GLYCINE (70% as sweet as sucrose), and certain PEPTIDES.

sweeteners, artificial See SWEETENERS, INTENSE.

sweeteners, bulk Used to replace sucrose and glucose syrups. One example is hydrogenated glucose syrup, in which the free aldehyde groups of glucose have been reduced to sorbitol by catalytic hydrogenation; effectively a mixture of glucose and sorbitol. Used in soft drinks and sugar confectionery, and in some diabetic foods as a partial substitute for sorbitol; 70–80% as sweet as sucrose.

See also SUGAR ALCOHOLS.

sweeteners, intense (non-nutritive) Chemical substances that have no calorific value but are intensely sweet and so are useful as a replacement for sucrose in foods intended for diabetics and those on slimming regimes, but unlike bulk sweeteners (SUGAR ALCOHOLS) do not replace the bulk of sucrose.

See also ACESULPHAME, ASPARTAME, CYCLAMATE, MIRACLE BERRY, MONELLIN, NEOHESPERIDIN, SACCHARIN, STEVIOSIDE, THAUMATIN.

Sweetex Trade name for SACCHARIN.

sweetness One of the five basic senses of TASTE.

sweet sop See CUSTARD APPLE.

swells Infected cans of food swollen at the ends by gases produced by fermentation. A 'hard swell' has permanently extended ends. If the ends can be moved under pressure, but not forced back to the original position, they are 'soft swells'. 'Springers' can be forced back, but the opposite end bulges. A 'flipper' is a can of normal appearance in which the end flips out when the can is struck. Hydrogen swells are harmless, and due to acid fruits attacking the can.

Swift stability test See ACTIVE OXYGEN METHOD.

Swiss chard The spinach-like leaves and broad mid-rib of *Beta* *vulgaris* var. *cicla*, also known as leaf beet, leaf chard, sea kale beet, silver beet, white leaf beet, spinach beet.

Composition/100 g: 83 kJ (20 kcal), protein 1.9 g, fat 0.1 g, carbohydrate 3.2 g (0.4 g sugars, 2.8 g starch), Na 180 mg, K 550 mg, Ca 58 mg, Mg 86 mg, P 33 mg, Fe 2.3 mg, vitamin A 727 µg (4365 µg carotene), B_1 0.03 mg, B_2 0.09 mg, niacin 0.7 mg, folate 100 µg, pantothenate 0.2 mg, C 18 mg. A 90 g serving is a source of Fe; good source of vitamin C, Mg; rich source of vitamin A, folate.

Also blanched summer shoots of globe ARTICHOKE and inner leaves of CARDOON, *Cynara cardunculus*.

swordfish   Oily FISH, *Xiphias gladius*.

Composition/100 g: 456 kJ (109 kcal), protein 18 g, fat 4.1 g (25% saturated, 44.4% mono-, 30.5% polyunsaturated), cholesterol 41 mg, carbohydrate 0 g, Na 130 mg, K 350 mg, Ca 4 mg, Mg 27 mg, P 260 mg, Fe 0.5 mg, Se 45 µg, vitamin B_1 0.16 mg, B_2 0.17 mg, niacin 11.7 mg, B_6 0.51 mg, B_{12} 4 µg, pantothenate 0.4 mg. A 140 g serving is a source of vitamin B_1, $B_{2;}$ Mg; rich source of protein, niacin, vitamin B_6, B_{12}, Se.

syllabub (sillabub)   Elizabethan dish made of cream curdled with white wine or cider; thickened version as a dessert and a thinner version as a drink.

symbiotic   Organisms (commonly microorganisms) that have a close and obligatory relationship of mutual benefit with another organism.

See also COMMENSAL; PATHOGEN.

symptom   Indication of a disease or condition noticed by the patient.

See also SIGN.

synbiotic   A food or ingredient that contains both a PREBIOTIC and a PROBIOTIC.

syndrome   Combination of SIGNS and/or SYMPTOMS that form a distinct clinical picture.

syneresis   Oozing of liquid from gel when cut and allowed to stand (e.g. jelly or baked custard or clotted blood).

synsepalum   See MIRACLE BERRY.

synthetic rice   See TAPIOCA-MACARONI.

syrup   A solution of sugar which may be from a variety of sources, such as maple or sorghum, or stages in refining cane and beet sugar such as top syrup, refiner's syrup, sugar syrup, golden syrup or by hydrolysis of STARCH (glucose or corn syrup).

Glucose syrup is the concentrated solution of sugars from the acid or enzymic hydrolysis of starch (usually maize or potato starch); a mixture of varying amounts of glucose, maltose and glucose complexes. The CODEX ALIMENTARIUS definition is: purified, concentrated, aqueous solutions of nutritive saccharides from starch. Usually 70% total solids by weight, containing glucose, maltose and oligomers of glucose of three, four or more units. May be in dried form. Used as a sweetening agent in sugar confectionery; also termed corn syrup, corn starch hydrolysate, starch syrup, confectioners' glucose and uncrystallisable syrup.

See also DEXTROSE EQUIVALENT VALUE; FRUCTOSE SYRUPS.

T

T3, T4 Tri-iodothyronine and thyroxine (tetra-iodothyronine), the THYROID HORMONES.

tabasco A thin piquant sauce prepared by fermentation of powdered dried fruits of chilli PEPPER, mixed with spirit vinegar and salt.

tachycardia Rapid heartbeat, as occurs after exercise; may also occur, without undue exertion, as a result of anxiety and in ANAEMIA and VITAMIN B_1 deficiency.

tachyphagia Rapid eating.

taeniasis Infection with TAPEWORMS of the genus *Taenia*.

taette See MILK, FERMENTED.

tagliatelle See PASTA.

tahini (tahina) Middle East; paste made from SESAME seeds, usually eaten as a dip; also used in preparation of HUMMUS.

takadiastase Or koji, an enzyme preparation produced by growing the fungus *Aspergillus oryzae* on bran, leaching the culture mass with water and precipitating with alcohol. Contains a mixture of enzymes, largely diastatic (i.e. AMYLASES), used for the preparation of starch hydrolysates.

Talin Trade name for thaumatin, an extract of the berry *Thaumatococcus danielli*, about 3000 times as sweet as sucrose. See KATEMFE.

tallow, rendered Beef or mutton fat prepared from parts other than the kidney, by heating with water in an autoclave. When pressed, separates to a liquid fraction, oleo oil, used in margarine, and a solid fraction, oleostearin, used for soap and candles.

See also PREMIER JUS.

tamal (tamales) Mexican; maize meal pancake, similar to TORTILLA, but made with fat. Traditionally cooked inside the soft husks of maize.

tamarillo Reddish yellow or purple fruit of *Cyphomandra betacea*, also called tree or English tomato.

Composition/100g: 117 kJ (28 kcal), protein 2 g, fat 0.3 g, carbohydrate 4.7 g (4.7 g sugars), Na 1 mg, K 300 mg, Ca 10 mg, Mg 19 mg, P 43 mg, Fe 0.8 mg, Cu 0.05 mg, Zn 0.1 mg, vitamin A 153 µg (920 µg carotene), E 1.9 mg, B_1 0.06 mg, B_2 0.03 mg, niacin

0.6 mg, B_6 0.19 mg, C 23 mg. A 100 g serving is a source of vitamin A, E; rich source of vitamin C.

tamarind Leguminous tree, *Tamarindus indica*, with pods containing seeds embedded in brown pulp, eaten fresh, and used to prepare beverages and seasonings in oriental cuisine (e.g. the Indian sauce, imli).

Composition/100 g: 996 kJ (238 kcal), protein 2.3 g, fat 0.3 g, carbohydrate 56.5 g, Na 15 mg, K 600 mg, Ca 77 mg, Mg 92 mg, P 94 mg, Fe 1.8 mg, vitamin A 2 µg (14 µg carotene), B_1 0.29 mg, B_2 0.1 mg, niacin 1.4 mg, B_6 0.08 mg, pantothenate 0.2 mg, C 3 mg. A 100 g serving is a source of Fe; good source of vitamin B_1; rich source of Mg.

tammy To squeeze a sauce through a fine woollen cloth (a tammy cloth) to strain it.

tandoori (tanduri) Indian term for food cooked in a clay oven (tandoor). The meat is marinated with aromatic herbs and spices before cooking.

tangelo CITRUS fruit, cross between TANGERINE and POMELO.

tangerine A CITRUS fruit, *Citrus reticulata*, also called mandarin; satsuma is a variety of tangerine.

Composition/100 g: 104 kJ (25 kcal), protein 0.7 g, fat 0.1 g, carbohydrate 5.8 g (5.8 g sugars), dietary fibre 1.2 g, nsp 0.9 g, Na 1 mg, K 120 mg, Ca 31 mg, Mg 8 mg, P 12 mg, Fe 0.2 mg, Cu 0.01 mg, Zn 0.1 mg, vitamin A 11 µg (71 µg carotene), B_1 0.05 mg, B_2 0.01 mg, niacin 0.2 mg, B_6 0.05 mg, folate 15 µg, pantothenate 0.2 mg, C 22 mg. A 95 g serving is a rich source of vitamin C.

tangors See CITRUS.

tanier See TANNIA.

tankage Residue from slaughterhouse excluding all the useful tissues; fertiliser or animal feed.

Tanner standard Tables of height and weight for age used as reference values for the assessment of growth and nutritional status in children, based on data collected in England. Now largely replaced by the NCHS (US National Center for Health Statistics) standards.

See also ANTHROPOMETRY.

tannia (tanier) The corm of *Xanthosoma sagittifolium*; known as new cocoyam or yautia in West Africa; same family as TARO.

Composition/100 g: 447 kJ (107 kcal), protein 1.3 g, fat 0.4 g, carbohydrate 24.5 g (0.2 g sugars, 24.3 g starch), nsp 2.3 g, Na 4 mg, K 480 mg, Ca 14 mg, Mg 22 mg, P 55 mg, Fe 0.6 mg, Cu 0.18 mg, Zn 0.6 mg, vitamin A 4 µg (29 µg carotene), B_1 0.02 mg, B_2 0.05 mg, niacin 0.6 mg, C 16 mg. A 130 g serving is a good source of Cu; rich source of vitamin C.

tannic acid See TANNINS.

tannins Compounds present in dark-coloured sorghum, carob bean, unripe fruits, tea, etc; they give an astringent effect in the mouth, precipitate proteins and are used to clarify beer and wines. Also called tannic acid and gallotannin.

tanrogan Manx name for SCALLOPS.

tansy A herb, *Tanacetum vulgare*. Leaves and young shoots used for flavouring puddings and omelettes. Tansy cakes made with eggs and young leaves used to be eaten at Easter. Tansy tea made by infusing the herb, formerly used as tonic and for intestinal worms. Root, preserved in honey or sugar, was used to treat gout.

tapas Spanish; small savoury dishes served with wine in bars.

tapeworm Parasitic intestinal worms; infection is acquired by eating raw or undercooked infected pork (*Taenia solium*), beef (*T. saginata*) or fish (*Diphyllobothrium latum*). Eggs are shed in the faeces and infect the animal host. Cysticercosis is infection of human beings with the larval stage by ingestion of eggs from faecal contamination of food and water.

tapioca Starch prepared from the root of the CASSAVA plant (*Manihot utilissima*), only traces of nutrients. The starch paste is heated to burst the granules, then dried either in globules resembling SAGO or in flakes. The name is also used of starch in general, as in manioc tapioca and potato flour tapioca.

Composition/100 g: 1502 kJ (359 kcal), protein 0.4 g, fat 0.1 g, carbohydrate 95 g (95 g starch), nsp 0.4 g, Na 4 mg, K 20 mg, Ca 8 mg, Mg 2 mg, P 30 mg, Fe 0.3 mg, Cu 0.07 mg, vitamin niacin 0.1 mg.

tapioca-macaroni A mixture of either 80–90 parts TAPIOCA flour, with 10–20 parts of peanut flour, or tapioca, peanut, and semolina, 60:15:25, baked into shapes resembling rice grains or macaroni shapes; developed in India. Also referred to as synthetic rice.

taramasalata Greek; fish roe (commonly smoked cod roe), whipped with oil, garlic and lemon juice, then thickened with bread, to make a dip.

tares Traditional English name for the vetches, which are PULSES.

taro Corm of *Colocasia esculenta* and *C. antiquorum*; called eddo or dasheen in Caribbean, old cocoyam in W Africa.

Composition/100 g: 380 kJ (91 kcal), protein 1.2 g, fat 0.2 g, carbohydrate 22.4 g (0.9 g sugars, 21.5 g starch), dietary fibre 3 g, nsp 2.1 g, Na 3 mg, K 200 mg, Ca 27 mg, Mg 31 mg, P 56 mg, Fe 0.8 mg, Cu 0.18 mg, Zn 1.3 mg, vitamin A 5 µg (32 µg carotene), B_1 0.05 mg, B_2 0.02 mg, niacin 0.8 mg, B_6 0.05 mg, C 7 mg. A 130 g serving is a source of vitamin C; Mg, Zn; good source of Cu.

Leaves, composition/100 g: 79 kJ (19 kcal), protein 2.4 g, fat 0.5 g, carbohydrate 1.4 g (1.2 g sugars, 0.2 g starch), dietary fibre

2.2 g, Na 2 mg, K 360 mg, Ca 86 mg, Mg 20 mg, P 27 mg, Fe 1.2 mg, Cu 0.18 mg, Zn 0.5 mg, vitamin A 638 µg (3830 µg carotene), B_1 0.14 mg, B_2 0.38 mg, niacin 1.7 mg, folate 27 µg, C 35 mg. A 95 g serving is a source of folate, Ca; good source of vitamin B_2, Cu; rich source of vitamin A, C.

tarragon Leaves and flowering tops of the bushy perennial plant *Artemisia dracunculus*.

tartar Hard gritty deposit of PLAQUE and minerals that accum lates on and between teeth, also known as calculus. Originally the name given by alchemists to animal and vegetable concretions, such as wine lees, stone, gravel and deposits on teeth, since they were all attributed to the same cause.

tartar emetic Potassium antimonyl tartrate, produces inflammation of the gastrointestinal MUCOSA; formerly used as an emetic.

tartaric acid Dihydroxysuccinic acid, a dibasic acid. Occurs in fruits, the chief source is grapes; used in preparing lemonade, added to jams when the fruit is not sufficiently acidic (citric acid is also used) and in baking powder (E-334). Wine lees is a mixture of tartrates. Rochelle salt is potassium sodium tartrate (E-337).

See also CREAM OF TARTAR; TARTAR EMETIC.

tartrazine A yellow colour (E-102), called Yellow No. 5 in the USA.

taste The tongue can distinguish five separate tastes: sweet, salt, sour (or acid), bitter and savoury (sometimes called UMAMI, from the Japanese word for a savoury flavour), due to stimulation of the TASTE BUDS. The overall taste or flavour of foods is due to these tastes, together with astringency in the mouth, texture and AROMA.

taste buds Situated mostly on the tongue; about 9000 elongated cells ending in minute hairlike processes, the gustatory hairs.

tatare (steak tatare) Dish prepared from minced beef or other meat, eaten uncooked.

taurine Aminoethane sulphonic acid, derived from CYSTEINE by oxidation of the sulphydryl group and decarboxylation. Known to be a dietary essential for cats (deficient kittens are blind) and possibly essential for human beings, since the capacity for synthesis is limited, although deficiency has never been observed.

taurochenodeoxycholic acid The TAURINE conjugate of CHENODEOXYCHOLIC ACID, see BILE.

taurocholic acid The TAURINE conjugate of CHOLIC ACID, see BILE.

TBARS (thiobarbituric acid reactive substances) Colorimetric method of determination of dialdehydes formed by breakdown of lipid peroxides, by reaction with thiobarbituric acid; used as an index of RADICAL attack on unsaturated fatty acids, and hence as an inverse index of antioxidant status.

tea A beverage prepared by infusion of the young leaves, leaf buds and internodes of varieties of *Camellia sinensis* and *C. assamica*, originating from China. Green tea is dried without further treatment. Black tea is fermented (actually an oxidation) ' before drying; Oolong tea is lightly fermented. Among the black teas, flowering Pekoe is made from the top leaf buds, orange Pekoe from first opened leaf, Pekoe from third leaves, and Souchong from next leaves.

See also CAFFEINE; TISANE; XANTHINES.

tea, Brazilian (Paraguayan) See MATÉ.

teaseed oil Oil from the seed of *Thea sasangua*, cultivated in China; used as salad oil and for frying.

TEF Thermic effect of food, see DIET-INDUCED THERMOGENESIS.

teff A tropical MILLET, *Eragrostis abyssinica*, the dietary staple in Ethiopia; little grown elsewhere.

teg Two year old sheep. See LAMB.

tempeh SOYA bean cake fermented by *Rhizopus* spp mould.

Composition/100g: 694kJ (166kcal), protein 20.7g, fat 6.4g (16% saturated, 24% mono-, 60% polyunsaturated), carbohydrate 6.4g (0.9g sugars, 4.6g starch), dietary fibre 4.1g, nsp 4.3g, Na 6mg, K 370mg, Ca 120mg, Mg 70mg, P 200mg, Fe 3.6mg, Cu 0.67mg, Zn 1.8mg, vitamin A 5µg (30µg carotene), B_1 0.19mg, B_2 0.48mg, niacin 7.9mg, B_6 1.86mg, folate 76µg, B_{12} 0.1µg, pantothenate 1.1mg, biotin 53µg. A 100g serving is a source of vitamin B_1, B_{12}, pantothenate, Ca, Zn; good source of Mg, Fe; rich source of protein, vitamin B_2, niacin, B_6, folate, biotin, Cu.

tempering As applied to CHOCOLATE manufacture this is the process of converting unstable forms of fats (polymorphs) into the stable β-forms (mp 34.5°C). It involves controlled cooling and reheating. If not properly carried out crystals of fat can separate out on the surface of the chocolate causing the harmless but unsightly effect of 'fat bloom'.

Templein Trade name for textured vegetable protein.

tenderiser PROTEINASES (endopeptidases) used to hydrolyse COLLAGEN and ELASTIN in the SARCOLEMMA, and so tenderise meat. Enzymes used include: actinidain (EC 3.4.22.14) from KIWI fruit, bromelain (EC 3.4.22.33) from PINEAPPLE, ficin (EC 3.4.22.3) from FIGS, papain (EC 3.4.22.2) from PAWPAW, and proteases from *Aspergillus oryzae* and *Bacillus subtilis*.

See also MUSCLE.

tenderometer Instrument to measure the stage of maturity of peas to determine whether they are ready for cropping. Measures the force required to effect a shearing action.

tenesmus Persistent ineffective spasms of bladder or rectum;

intestinal tenesmus commonly occurs in IRRITABLE BOWEL SYNDROME.

tensiometer   Instrument for measuring the surface tension of a liquid.

tenuate   Anorectic (appetite suppressing, see APPETITE CONTROL) drug, used in the treatment of OBESITY.

tepary bean   *Phaseolus acutifolius*, also known as frijole, Mexican haricot bean or pinto. Able to grow during drought.

tequila   Mexican; SPIRIT (40–50% alcohol by volume) prepared by double distillation of fermented sap of the cultivated agave or maguey, *Agave tequilana*. Mescal and pulque are similar, made from various species of wild agave, and have a stronger flavour.

teratogen   A compound that is capable of causing developmental defects in the foetus *in utero*, and hence non-genetic congenital defects.

terpeneless oil   See TERPENES.

terpenes   Chemically consist of multiple isoprenoid (five-carbon) units. Monoterpenes consist of two isoprenoids; sesquiterpenes of three, diterpenes of four, triterpenes of six, and tetraterpenes of eight. Phytol and RETINOL are diterpenes; CAROTENES are tetraterpenes.

Major components of the ESSENTIAL OILS of citrus fruits, but not responsible for the characteristic flavour, and since they readily oxidise and polymerise to produce unpleasant flavours, removed from citrus oils by distillation or solvent extraction, leaving the so-called terpeneless oils for flavouring foods and drinks.

terramycin   One of the TETRACYCLINE antibiotics, also known as oxytetracycline.

testa   The fibrous layer between the pericarp and the inner aleurone layer of a cereal grain.

test meal   See FRACTIONAL TEST MEAL.

tetany   Spasm of twitching of muscles, caused by oversensitivity of motor nerves to stimuli; particularly affects face, hands and feet. Caused by reduction in the level of ionised CALCIUM in the bloodstream and may occur in RICKETS.

tetracyclines   A group of closely related ANTIBIOTICS including tetracycline, oxytetracycline (terramycin) and aureomycin. The last two are used in some countries for preserving food and as growth improvers, added to animal feed at the rate of a few milligrams per tonne.

tetraenoic acid   FATTY ACID with four double bonds, e.g. ARACHIDONIC ACID.

tetramine poisoning   Paralysis similar to that caused by curare, caused by a toxin in the salivary glands of the red whelk,

Neptunea antiqua (distinct from the edible whelk *Buccinum undatum*).

tetrodontin poisoning Caused by a toxin, tetrodotoxin, in fish of the Tetrodontidae family (puffer fish) and amphibia of the Salamandridae family. Occurs in Japan from Japanese puffer fish or fugu (*Fuga rubripes*), eaten for its gustatory and tactile pleasure since traces of the poison cause a tingling sensation in the extremities (larger doses cause respiratory failure). The toxin is acquired via the food chain from bacteria in the coral reef, rather than synthesised by the fish. Lethal dose 10 μg/kg body weight.

tetrodotoxin See TETRODONTIN POISONING.

tewfikose Name given to a sugar isolated from a sample of buffalo milk obtained from Egypt in 1892, later found to be an artefact; named after Tewfik Bey Pasha, Governor of Egypt.

Texatrein, Texgran Trade names for textured vegetable proteins.

texture Combination of physical properties perceived by senses of kinaesthesis (muscle–nerve endings), touch (including mouth-feel), sight and hearing. Physical properties may include shape, size, number and conformation of constituent structural elements.

The texture profile is an ORGANOLEPTIC analysis of the complex of food in terms of mechanical and geometrical characteristics, fat and moisture content, including the order in which they appear from the first bite to complete mastication.

textured vegetable protein Spun or extruded vegetable protein, usually made to simulate meat.

TGS Trichlorogalactosucrose, see SUCRALOSE.

thaumatin The intensely sweet protein of the African fruit, *Thaumatococus danielli*, 1600 times as sweet as sucrose. Called katemfe in Sierra Leone and miracle fruit in the Sudan (not the same as MIRACLE BERRY).

theaflavins Reddish-orange pigments formed in TEA during fermentation; responsible for the colour of tea extracts and part of the astringent flavour.

theanine γ-*N*-Ethylglutamine, the major free amino acid in tea, 1–2% dry weight of leaf.

theine Alternative name for CAFFEINE.

theobromine 3,7-Dimethylxanthine, an ALKALOID found in cocoa, chemically related to CAFFEINE, and with similar effects.

theophylline 1,3-Dimethylxanthine, an ALKALOID found in tea, chemically related to CAFFEINE, and with similar effects.

therapeutic diets Those formulated to treat disease or metabolic disorders.

therapeutic index Ratio of the dose of a drug that causes tissue or cell damage to that required to have a therapeutic effect.

therm   Obsolete unit of heat = 1.055×10^8 J.

thermal death time (TDT)   Measure of heat resistance of an organism, enzyme or chemical component at a particular temperature, usually 121°C.

Thermamyl   Trade name for heat-stable α-AMYLASE from *Bacillus licheniformis*, active up to 100°C; used in manufacture of glucose SYRUP from STARCH.

thermic effect of food   See DIET-INDUCED THERMOGENESIS.

thermisation   Heat treatment, less severe than PASTEURISATION, e.g. heat treatment of milk for cheese-making whereby the number of organisms is diminished.

thermoduric   Bacteria that are heat resistant but not THERMOPHILIC (see THERMOPHILES) i.e. they survive, but do not develop, at PASTEURISATION temperatures. Usually not pathogens but indicative of insanitary conditions.

thermogenesis   Increased heat production by the body, either to maintain body temperature (by either shivering or non-shivering thermogenesis) or in response to food intake (DIET-INDUCED THERMOGENESIS).

   See also BROWN ADIPOSE TISSUE; UNCOUPLING PROTEINS.

thermogenic drugs   Substances that stimulate body heat output, and thus of interest in 'slimming'.

thermogenin   See UNCOUPLING PROTEINS.

thermography   Technique for measuring and recording heat output by regions of the body, using a film sensitive to infrared radiation.

thermopeeling   A method of peeling tough-skinned fruits in which the fruit is rapidly passed through an electric furnace at about 900°C then sprayed with water.

thermophiles   Bacteria that prefer temperatures above 55°C and can tolerate temperatures up to 75–80°C. Extreme thermophiles can live in boiling water, and have been isolated from hot springs.

thiamin   See VITAMIN B₁.

thiaminases   Enzymes that cleave thiamin (VITAMIN B₁). Thiaminase I (EC 2.5.1.2) is found in freshwater fish, ferns and some bacteria; it catalyses an exchange reaction between the thiazole ring and a variety of bases. Thiaminase II (EC 3.5.99.2) occurs in a small number of microorganisms; it catalyses hydrolysis of the methylene–thiazole bond, releasing TOXOPYRIMIDINE.

thiobendazole   Drug used to treat intestinal infestation with *STRONGYLOIDES* spp, and antifungal agent used for surface treatment of bananas.

thiochrome   Fluorescent product of the oxidation of thiamin (VITAMIN B₁) in alkaline solution; the basis of an assay of the vitamin.

thioctic acid See LIPOIC ACID.

thirst See WATER BALANCE.

thixotropic COLLOIDAL SUSPENSIONS whose VISCOSITY decreases over time when subjected to a constant shear stress; there is a reversible change from GEL to SOL under stress.
See also DILATANT; PSEUDOPLASTIC; RHEOPEXIC.

thoracic duct One of two main trunks of the lymphatic system, receives lymph from the legs and lower abdomen, and drains into the left innominate vein. The main point of entry of CHYLO-MICRONS into the bloodstream.

threonine An essential AMINO ACID, chemically amino-hydroxybutyric acid, abbr Thr (T), M_r 119.1, pK_a 2.09, 9.10, CODONS ACNu.

thrombin Plasma protein involved in the COAGULATION of blood formed in the circulation by partial proteolysis of PROTHROMBIN.
See also VITAMIN K.

thromboembolism Condition in which a blood clot formed in the circulation becomes detached and lodges elsewhere.

thrombokinase (thromboplastin) An enzyme (clotting factor Xa, EC 3.4.21.6) liberated from damaged tissue and blood platelets; converts prothrombin to THROMBIN in the coagulation of blood.

thrombolysis Dissolution of blood clots.

thromboplastin See THROMBOKINASE.

thrombosis Inappropriate formation of blood clots in blood vessels. Antagonists of VITAMIN K, including WARFARIN, are comonly used to reduce clotting in people at risk of thrombosis.

thrombus Blood clot that remains stationary in a blood vessel.
See also EMBOLUS.

thuricide Name given to a living culture of *Bacillus thuringiensis* which is harmless to man but kills insect pests. Known as a micro-bial insecticide. Used to treat certain foods and fodder crops to destroy pests such as corn earworm, flour moth, tomato fruit worm, cabbage looper, etc.

thyme The aromatic leaves and flowering tops of *Thymus vulgaris* used as flavouring.

thymidine, thymine A PYRIMIDINE; see NUCLEIC ACIDS.

thymonucleic acid Obsolete name for DEOXYRIBONUCLEIC ACID.

thymus Chest (neck) sweetbread; a ductless gland in the chest, as distinct from gut sweetbread or PANCREAS.

thyrocalcitonin See CALCITONIN.

thyroglobulin The protein in the thyroid gland (M_r 660000) which is the precursor for the synthesis of the THYROID HORMONES as a result of iodination of tyrosine residues. The thyroid-stimulating hormone (THYROTROPIN) stimulates hydrolysis of thyroglobulin and secretion of the HORMONES into the bloodstream.

thyroid hormones The thyroid is an endocrine gland situated in the neck, which takes up IODINE from the bloodstream and synthesises two HORMONES, tri-iodothyronine (T3) and thyroxine (T4, tetra-iodothyronine). The active hormone is T3; thyroxine is converted to T3 in tissues by the action of a SELENIUM-dependent de-iodinase (EC 3.8.1.4). T3 controls the BASAL METABOLIC RATE.

Enlargement of the thyroid gland is GOITRE; it may be associated with under- or overproduction of the thyroid hormones. Severe iodine deficiency in children leads to goitrous CRETINISM.

See also HYPOTHYROIDISM; IODINE, PROTEIN-BOUND; THYROTOXI-COSIS; TRANSTHYRETIN.

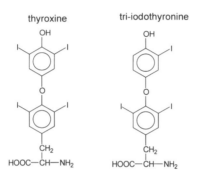

thyroxine   tri-iodothyronine

thyroid-releasing hormone (TRH) Hormone secreted by the hypothalamus which stimulates secretion of THYROID HORMONES.

thyrotoxicosis Overactivity of the thyroid gland, leading to excessive secretion of THYROID HORMONES and resulting in increased BASAL METABOLIC RATE. Hyperthyroid subjects are lean and have tense nervous activity. May be due to overstimulation of the thyroid gland. Iodine-induced thyrotoxicosis affects mostly elderly people who have lived for a long time in iodine-deficient areas, have a long-standing goitre, and have then been given extra iodine. Also known as Jodbasedow, Basedow's disease and Graves' disease.

thyrotropin Thyroid-stimulating hormone (see THYROID HOR-MONES) secreted by the anterior pituitary; regulates the activity of the thyroid gland.

thyroxine One of the THYROID HORMONES.

thyroxine binding pre-albumin See TRANSTHYRETIN.

TIA See TRANSIENT ISCHAEMIC ATTACK.

TIBC Total iron binding capacity. See TRANSFERRIN.

tierce   Obsolete measure of wine cask; one-third of a PIPE, i.e. about 160 L (35 Imperial gallons).

tiffin   Anglo-Indian name for a light mid-day meal.

tiger nut   Tuber of grass-like sedge, *Cyperus esculentus*, also earth or ground almond, chufa nut, rush nut, nut sedge, 5–20 mm long, usually available in partly dried condition.

Composition/100 g: 1686 kJ (403 kcal), protein 4.3 g, fat 23.8 g (17.6% saturated, 72.5% mono-, 9.7% polyunsaturated), carbohydrate 45.7 g (16.1 g sugars, 29.6 g starch), dietary fibre 17.4 g, nsp 11.7 g, Na 1 mg, K 14 mg, Ca 48 mg, P 210 mg, Fe 3.2 mg, vitamin B_1 0.23 mg, B_2 0.1 mg, niacin 1.8 mg, C 6 mg.

tikka   Indian; marinated chicken (or other meat) threaded on skewers and grilled.

til   See SESAME.

timbale   Round fireproof china or tinned copper mould, used for moulding meat or fish mixtures; also the dishes cooked in the mould. For hot timbales the mould is lined with potato, pastry or pasta; for cold the lining is aspic.

tin   A metal; a dietary essential for experimental animals, but so widely distributed in foods that no deficiency has been reported in man, and its function, if any, is not known. In the absence of oxygen tin is resistant to corrosion; hence widely used in tinned cans for food containers.

tipsy cake   Sponge cake soaked in wine and fruit juice, made into a trifle and reassembled into the original tall shape. The wine and fruit juice may cause the cake to topple sideways in drunken (tipsy) fashion.

tiramisu   Italian; dessert made of coffee-flavoured sponge or biscuit filled with sweetened cream cheese (MASCARPONE) and cream, doused with syrup.

tisane   French term for an infusion made from herbs, fruits or flowers (camomile, lime blossoms, fennel seeds, etc), believed to have medicinal properties. Also known as herb or herbal tea. Medicinal or health claims are sometimes made, largely on traditional rather than scientific grounds.

titre   A measure of the amount of antibody in an antiserum, the extent to which the antiserum can be diluted and still retain the ability to cause agglutination of the antigen.

TK$_{ac}$ Transketolase activation coefficient, the result of the TRANSKETOLASE test for VITAMIN B_1 nutritional status, an enzyme activation assay.

TNF   See TUMOUR NECROSIS FACTOR.

toad skin   See PHRYNODERMA.

TOBEC   See TOTAL BODY ELECTRICAL CONDUCTIVITY.

tocol, tocopherol   See VITAMIN E.

tocopheronic acid   Water-soluble metabolite isolated from the urine of animals fed tocopherol (VITAMIN E); has vitamin E activity.

tocotrienol   See VITAMIN E.

toenail analysis   Measurement of various minerals (including ZINC) in toenails has been proposed as an index of status. Adsorption of minerals from sweat confounds the results.

toffee   A sweet made from butter or other fat, milk and sugar boiled at a higher temperature than caramels. Called candy or taffy USA (originally the UK name). Variants include butterscotch and glessie (Scots). Toffee apples are apples coated with hardened syrup (caramel apples, USA).

tofu   Japanese; soybean curd precipitated from the aqueous extract of the SOYA bean.

   Composition/100 g: 305 kJ (73 kcal), protein 8.1 g, fat 4.2 g (15.1% saturated, 24.2% mono-, 60.6% polyunsaturated), carbohydrate 0.7 g (0.3 g sugars, 0.3 g starch), dietary fibre 0.3 g, Na 4 mg, K 63 mg, Ca 510 mg, Mg 23 mg, P 95 mg, Fe 1.2 mg, Cu 0.2 mg, Zn 0.7 mg, vitamin E 1 mg, B_1 0.06 mg, B_2 0.02 mg, niacin 1.4 mg, B_6 0.07 mg, folate 15 µg, pantothenate 0.1 mg. A 60 g serving is a source of Cu; rich source of Ca.

tolazamide, tolbutamide   See HYPOGLYCAEMIC AGENTS.

tomatillo   Or ground tomato, husk-covered fruit of *Physalis ixocarpa*, resembles a small, green tomato.

tomato   The fruit of *Lycopersicon esculentum*.

   Composition/100 g: 71 kJ (17 kcal), protein 0.7 g, fat 0.3 g, carbohydrate 3.1 g (3.1 g sugars), dietary fibre 1.3 g, nsp 1 g, Na 9 mg, K 250 mg, Ca 7 mg, Mg 7 mg, P 24 mg, Fe 0.5 mg, Cu 0.01 mg, Zn 0.1 mg, I 2 µg, vitamin A 106 µg (640 µg carotene), E 1.2 mg, B_1 0.09 mg, B_2 0.01 mg, niacin 1.1 mg, B_6 0.14 mg, folate 17 µg, pantothenate 0.3 mg, biotin 1.5 µg, C 17 mg. An 85 g serving (one medium) is a source of vitamin A, E; good source of vitamin C.

tomato, English or tree   See TAMARILLO.

tomography   Technique for visualisation of organs and generation of a three-dimensional image, by analysis of successive images produced using X-rays or ultrasound sharply focused at a given depth within the body.

   See also CAT SCANNING; PET SCANNING.

tonic water   A sweetened carbonated beverage flavoured with quinine, commonly used as a mixer with GIN or VODKA. Originally invented by the British in India as a pleasant way of taking a daily dose of quinine to prevent malaria; sometimes known as Indian tonic water.

tonka bean   Seed of the S American tree *Dipteryx odorata* with a sweet pungent smell, used like VANILLA for flavouring.

toothfriendly sweets   Name given to sugar confectionery made with SUGAR ALCOHOLS and/or BULK SWEETENERS which are not fermented in the mouth and so do not damage teeth.

topepo   Hybrid between tomato and sweet pepper.

tophus (plural tophi)   Hard deposit of URIC ACID under skin, in cartilage or joints, as occurs in GOUT.

toppings   See WHEATFEED.

topside   Boneless cut of BEEF from the top of the hind leg.

torte   Open tart or rich cake mixture baked in a pastry case, filled with fruit, nuts, chocolate, cream, etc.

tortilla   (1) Mexican; thin maize pancake. Traditionally prepared by soaking the grain in alkali and pressing it to form a dough, which is then baked on a griddle. Tortillas filled with meat, beans and spicy sauce are TACOS.

See also TAMALES.

(2) In Spain, an omelette made by frying potatoes and onions with eggs; may be served hot or cold; also used for a variety of filled omelettes.

torulitine   See VITAMIN T.

total body electrical conductivity (TOBEC)   A method of measuring the proportion of fat in the body by the difference in the electrical conductivity of fat and lean tissue. Depends on the induction of a magnetic field by a high frequency (5 MHz) alternating current in a solenoid above the body, and detection of the evoked field by a secondary coil.

See also BIOELECTRICAL IMPEDANCE.

total iron binding capacity   See TRANSFERRIN.

total parenteral nutrition (TPN)   See PARENTERAL NUTRITION.

toxic oil syndrome   See SPANISH TOXIC OIL SYNDROME.

Toxocara   Genus of intestinal parasitic nematode worms, especially in domestic cats and dogs; human beings can become infected by larvae from eggs in the faeces of pets (toxocariasis).

toxoid   Chemically inactivated derivative of the toxin produced by a pathogenic organism; harmless, but stimulates the synthesis of antibodies; used in vaccines.

toxopyrimidine   Antimetabolite of vitamin B_6 released by the action of THIAMINASE II on thiamin.

TPN   Total PARENTERAL NUTRITION.

trabecular bone   Thin bars of bony tissue in spongy bone.

trace elements   See MINERALS, TRACE; MINERALS, ULTRATRACE.

tracers   See ISOTOPES.

traife   Foods that do not conform to Jewish dietary laws; the opposite of KOSHER.

trans-   See ISOMERS (3).

transaminase   Enzymes (EC 2.6.1.x, also known as aminotransferases) that catalyse the reaction of transamination; the transfer of the amino group from an amino acid donor onto a keto-acid acceptor, yielding the keto-acid carbon skeleton of the donor and the amino acid corresponding to the acceptor. The enzymes are pyridoxal phosphate (VITAMIN B_6)-dependent, and the activation of either alanine (EC 2.6.1.2) or aspartate (EC 2.6.1.1) aminotransferase apo-enzyme in red blood cells by pyridoxal phosphate added *in vitro* provides an index of vitamin B_6 status. An activation coefficient above 1.25 (alanine aminotransferase) or 1.8 (aspartate aminotransferase) is indicative of deficiency.

transcription The process whereby one strand of the region of DNA containing the information for one or more proteins is copied to yield RNA. Transcription factors are the various proteins that are required for transcription of DNA to form mRNA, in addition to RNA polymerase (EC 2.7.7.6) itself.

See also TRANSLATION.

transferrin The main IRON transport protein in plasma. Fractional saturation of transferrin with iron provides a sensitive index of iron status, but transferrin synthesis is impaired in some chronic diseases, so fractional saturation may be inappropriately high. This also limits the usefulness of transferrin measurement as an index of protein–energy nutrition. Total iron binding capacity of plasma is the sum of free plus iron-containing transferrin.

transferrin receptor A transmembrane protein for uptake of TRANSFERRIN (and hence IRON) into cells. The extracellular region is cleaved and enters the circulation, where it can be measured by immunoassay. In early iron deficiency there is induction of the transferrin receptor, and an elevated plasma concentration of the extracellular fragment thus provides a sensitive index of iron status.

transient ischaemic attack (TIA) Temporary disruption of the blood supply to part of the brain, due to EMBOLISM, THROMBOSIS or a spasm of the arterial wall.

transit time The time taken between ingestion of a food and elimination in faeces, commonly measured by including radio-opaque plastic markers in the test food, followed by X-ray examination of faeces.

transketolase Enzyme (EC 2.2.1.1) in the pentose phosphate pathway of GLUCOSE METABOLISM; requires thiamin diphosphate as cofactor, so activation of apo-transketolase in red blood cells by thiamin diphosphate added *in vitro* provides an index of vitamin B_1 status. An activation coefficient above 1.25 indicates deficiency.

translation The process of synthesising protein on the RIBOSOME, by translating the information in mRNA into the amino acid sequence.

See also TRANSCRIPTION.

transthyretin THYROID HORMONE binding protein in plasma, formerly known as pre-albumin. Also forms a complex with the small plasma RETINOL BINDING PROTEIN to prevent loss of bound VITAMIN A by renal filtration. It has a half-life of 2–3 days, and may provide an index of nutritional status because synthesis decreases rapidly in protein–energy malnutrition; however, synthesis is also affected by trauma and sepsis.

treacle First product of refining of MOLASSES from beet or sugar cane extract is black treacle, slightly less bitter; will not crystallise.

Composition/100 g: 1075 kJ (257 kcal), protein 1.2 g, fat 0 g, carbohydrate 67.2 g (67.2 g sugars), Na 96 mg, K 1470 mg, Ca 500 mg, Mg 140 mg, P 31 mg, Fe 9.2 mg, Cu 0.43 mg, Zn 0.9 mg. Serving 15 g.

trehalose Mushroom sugar, or mycose, a DISACCHARIDE of glucose. Found in some fungi (*Amanita* spp), MANNA and some insects.

trematode See FLUKE.

tremorgens A group of neurotoxins produced by various moulds (*Penicillium* spp, *Aspergillus* spp, *Claviceps* spp) which cause sustained whole body tremors leading to convulsive seizures which may be fatal. Possible cause of endemic afflictions in human beings in Nigeria and India (alfatrem from *A. flavus*, penitrem from *Penicillium* spp).

trepang See BÊCHE-DE-MER.

tretinoin Synthetic RETINOID used in treatment of acne.

TRH See THYROID-RELEASING HORMONE.

triacylglycerols Sometimes called triglycerides, simple fats or LIPIDS consisting of glycerol esterified to three FATTY ACIDS (chemically acyl groups). The major component of dietary and tissue fat. Also known as saponifiable fats, since on reaction with sodium hydroxide they yield glycerol and the sodium salts (or soaps) of the fatty acids.

trichinosis (trichinellosis, trichiniasis) Disease that can arise from eating undercooked pork or pork sausage meat; due to *Trichinella spiralis*, a worm that is a parasite in pork muscle; destroyed by heat and by freezing. Adult worms live in the small intestine; larvae bore through the intestinal wall and migrate around the body, causing fever, delirium and limb pain.

trichlorogalactosucrose See SUCRALOSE.

trichobezoar Or hairball, a mass of swallowed hair in the stomach. See also BEZOAR.

trichology Study of hair. See HAIR ANALYSIS.

Trichomonas Genus of parasitic flagellate protozoans. *T. hominis* infests the large intestine, *T. tenax* the mouth.

trichuriasis Infestation of the large intestine by the whipworm, *Trichuris trichiura*.

trientine Chelating agent used to enhance the excretion of COPPER in WILSON'S DISEASE.

trifluoracetyl chloride Used to prepare volatile trifluoracetyl derivatives of AMINO ACIDS for gas–liquid CHROMATOGRAPHY.

Trifyba Trade name for processed wheat bran from husk of *Testa triticum tricum* containing 80 g dietary fibre/100 g with reduced content of PHYTATE.

triglycerides See TRIACYLGLYCEROLS.

trigonelline *N*-Methyl nicotinic acid, a urinary metabolite of NICOTINIC ACID. There is a relatively large amount in green COFFEE beans, much of which is demethylated during roasting, so coffee is a significant source of NIACIN.

tri-iodothyronine One of the THYROID HORMONES.

tripe Lining of the first three stomachs of ruminants, usually calf or ox. Sold 'dressed', i.e. cleaned and treated with lime. According to the part of the stomach there are various kinds such as blanket, honeycomb, book, monk's hood and reed tripe. Contains a large amount of CONNECTIVE TISSUE which is changed to GELATINE on boiling.

Composition/100 g: 418 kJ (100 kcal), protein 14.8 g, fat 4.5 g (63.1% saturated, 34.2% mono-, 2.6% polyunsaturated), cholesterol 160 mg, carbohydrate 0 g, Na 73 mg, K 100 mg, Ca 150 mg, Mg 15 mg, P 90 mg, Fe 0.7 mg, Cu 0.14 mg, Zn 2.3 mg, vitamin E 0.1 mg, B_2 0.08 mg, niacin 3.2 mg, B_6 0.02 mg, folate 1 µg, pantothenate 0.2 mg, biotin 2 µg, C 3 mg. A 150 g serving is a good source of niacin, Ca, Cu, Zn; rich source of protein.

triticale Cross between WHEAT (*Triticum* spp) and RYE (*Secale* spp) which combines the winter hardiness of the rye with the special baking properties of wheat.

tRNA (transfer RNA) The family of small RNA species that have both an anticodon region which binds to the CODON on mRNA on the RIBOSOME and also a specific amino acid binding site, so that the appropriate amino acid is brought to the ribosome for protein synthesis.

Trolox Trade name for a water-soluble VITAMIN E analogue, 6-hydroxy-2,5,7,8-tetramethyl-chroman-2-carboxylic acid.

tropical oils Suggested term (USA) for vegetable oils that contain little polyunsaturated fatty acids, such as coconut and palm oils.

trout Freshwater oily FISH, brown trout is *Salmo trutta*, rainbow trout is *S. gairdneri*.

Composition/100 g: 523 kJ (125 kcal), protein 19.6 g, fat 5.2 g (23.9% saturated, 39.1% mono-, 36.9% polyunsaturated), cholesterol 67 mg, carbohydrate 0 g, Na 45 mg, K 420 mg, Ca 18 mg, Mg 27 mg, P 240 mg, Fe 0.3 mg, Cu 0.04 mg, Zn 0.5 mg, Se 18 µg, I

13 µg, vitamin A 49 µg, D 10.6 µg, E 0.7 mg, B_1 0.2 mg, B_2 0.11 mg, niacin 8.2 mg, B_6 0.34 mg, folate 9 µg, B_{12} 5 µg, pantothenate 1.5 mg, biotin 3 µg. A 230 g serving (whole fish) is a source of vitamin A, E, B_2, folate, Cu, I; good source of Mg; rich source of protein, vitamin D, B_1, niacin, B_6, B_{12}, pantothenate, Se.

trub   See HOT BREAK.

truffles   (1) Edible fungi growing underground, associated with roots of oak trees; very highly prized for their aroma and flavour. Most highly prized is French, black or Perigord truffle, *Tuber melanosporum*, added to pâté de foie gras. Others include: white Piedmontese truffle, *T. magnatum*; summer truffle *T. aestivum* and violet truffle *T. brumale*;
See also MUSHROOMS.

(2) Chocolate truffles, mixture of chocolate, sugar, cream and often rum covered with chocolate strands or cocoa powder.

Trusoy   Trade name for heat-treated full-fat soya flour.

trypsin   A proteolytic enzyme (EC 3.4.21.4) in pancreatic juice, an ENDOPEPTIDASE. Active at pH 8–11. Secreted as the inactive precursor, trypsinogen, which is activated by ENTEROPEPTIDASE.

trypsin inhibitors   Low molecular weight proteins in raw soya beans and other legumes that inhibit trypsin and thus impair the digestion of proteins. Inactivated by heat, but the nutritional quality of some animal feeds containing trypsin inhibitors is not improved by heating.

trypsinogen   See TRYPSIN.

tryptophan   An essential AMINO ACID, abbr Trp (W), M_r 204.2, pK_a 2.43, 9.44, codon UGG. In addition to its rôle in protein synthesis, it is the precursor of the neurotransmitter 5-HYDROXYTRYPTAMINE (serotonin) and of NIACIN. Average intakes of tryptophan are more than adequate to meet niacin requirements without the need for any preformed niacin in the diet.

Destroyed by acid, and therefore not measured when proteins are hydrolysed by acid before analysis; determination of tryptophan requires alkaline or enzymic hydrolysis of the protein.

tryptophan load test   For assessment of VITAMIN B_6 status; measurement of urinary excretion of xanthurenic and kynurenic acids after a test dose of 2 or 5 g of tryptophan. The enzyme kynureninase (EC 3.7.1.3) is pyridoxal phosphate-dependent, and especially sensitive to deficiency.

Tshugaeff reaction   Colorimetric reaction for CHOLESTEROL; the development of a cherry red colour on reaction with zinc chloride and acetyl chloride.

TSP   Trade name for textured SOYA protein, prepared by extrusion through fine pores to give a fibrous, meat-like, texture to the final product.

tube feeding See ENTERAL NUTRITION.

tuber Botanical term for underground storage organ of some plants, e.g. POTATO (Irish), Jerusalem ARTICHOKE, sweet POTATO, YAM.

tuberin The major protein of POTATO, a globulin.

tumour necrosis factor Two CYTOKINES produced by monocytes and macrophages (cachectin, TNF-α) or lymphocytes (lymphotoxin, TNF-β); cytotoxic to a variety of cancer cells, but also act on other cells. TNF action is responsible for much of the hypermetabolism seen in CACHEXIA.

tun Obsolete measure; large cask holding 216 Imperial gallons (972 L) of ale; 252 gallons (1134 L) of wine.

tuna See PRICKLY PEAR.

tuna fish (tunny) Species of *Thunnus* and *Neothunnus*, oily FISH. Albacore tuna is specifically *Thunnus alalunga*; bonita tuna and skipjack tuna are different species.

Composition/100 g: 569 kJ (136 kcal), protein 23.7 g, fat 4.6 g (30% saturated, 30% mono-, 40% polyunsaturated), cholesterol 28 mg, carbohydrate 0 g, Na 47 mg, K 400 mg, Ca 16 mg, Mg 33 mg, P 230 mg, Fe 1.3 mg, Cu 0.15 mg, Zn 0.7 mg, Se 57 µg, I 30 µg, vitamin A 26 µg, D 7.2 µg, B_1 0.1 mg, B_2 0.13 mg, niacin 17.2 mg, B_6 0.38 mg, folate 15 µg, B_{12} 4 µg, pantothenate 0.7 mg. A 120 g serving is a source of pantothenate, Mg, Fe; good source of vitamin B_6, Cu, I; rich source of protein, vitamin D, niacin, B_{12}, Se.

turanose A DISACCHARIDE, α-1,3-glucosyl-fructose.

turbidimetry Measurement of the turbidity (or optical density) of a culture as an index of growth in microbiological assays.

turbidity See TYNDALL EFFECT.

turkey A poultry bird, *Meleagris gallopavo*.

Composition/100 g roast meat and skin: 715 kJ (171 kcal), protein 28 g, fat 6.5 g (34.4% saturated, 44.2% mono-, 21.3% polyunsaturated), cholesterol 191 mg, carbohydrate 0 g, Na 52 mg, K 280 mg, Ca 9 mg, Mg 24 mg, P 200 mg, Fe 0.9 mg, Cu 0.14 mg, Zn 2.1 mg, vitamin niacin 5.2 mg. A 90 g serving is a source of Cu, Zn; good source of niacin; rich source of protein.

turkey X disease See AFLATOXINS.

Turkish delight Sweet made from gelatine and concentrated grape juice, flavoured with rose water. Also sometimes made with marshmallow (Turkish *rahat lokum*).

Composition/100 g: 1234 kJ (295 kcal), protein 0.6 g, fat 0 g, carbohydrate 77.9 g (68.6 g sugars, 9.3 g starch), Na 31 mg, K 4 mg, Ca 10 mg, Mg 2 mg, P 7 mg, Fe 0.2 mg, Cu 0.12 mg, Zn 0.7 mg, vitamin B_1 0.13 mg. Serving 15 g (one square).

See also PEKMEZ.

turmeric Dried rhizome of *Curcuma longa* (ginger family), grown in India and S Asia. Deep yellow and used both as condiment and food colour; used in curry powder and in prepared mustard. Its pigment is used as a dye under the name curcumin or Indian saffron (E-100).

turnip Root of *Brassica campestris* eaten as a cooked vegetable. Composition/100 g: 50 kJ (12 kcal), protein 0.6 g, fat 0.2 g, carbohydrate 2 g (1.9 g sugars, 0.1 g starch), dietary fibre 2 g, nsp 1.9 g, Na 28 mg, K 200 mg, Ca 45 mg, Mg 6 mg, P 31 mg, Fe 0.2 mg, Cu 0.01 mg, Zn 0.1 mg, Se 1 µg, vitamin A 3 µg (20 µg carotene), B_1 0.05 mg, B_2 0.02 mg, niacin 0.3 mg, B_6 0.04 mg, folate 8 µg, pantothenate 0.1 mg, C 10 mg. A 60 g serving is a source of vitamin C.
See also HAMBURG PARSLEY; SWEDE.

turtle Marine reptile; the main species for food is the green turtle, *Chelonia mydas*, so-called because of the greenish tinge of its fat. Farmed to a small extent, but mainly caught in the wild.
See also MOCK TURTLE.

Tuscorora rice See RICE, WILD.

Tuxford's index Formula for assessing height relative to weight in children. The index is >1 for heavier than average children and <1 for lighter than average. For boys, TI = (weight (lb)/height (in)) × (336 – age (m)/270); for girls, TI = (weight (lb)/height (in)) × (308 – age (m)/235).

TVP See TEXTURED VEGETABLE PROTEIN.

Twaddell Scale for measurement of density of solutions; only for density greater than 1. Density = 1 + (°Twaddell/200):
1% salt = 1.4° Twaddell, density = 1.007
2% salt = 2.8° Twaddell, density = 1.014
4% salt = 5.6° Twaddell, density = 1.028
10% salt = 14.6° Twaddell, density = 1.073
20% salt = 30.2° Twaddell, density = 1.151.

Tweens Trade name for nonionic surface agents derived from SPANS by adding polyoxyethylene chains to the non-esterified hydroxyl groups, so making them water-soluble. Polysorbate 40 is a mixture of polyoxyethylene esters of oleic esters of sorbitol anhydrides used in medicinal products as an emulsifying agent.

TX numbers Systematic classification of toxins produced by food poisoning bacteria according to: type of infection: 1 = intoxication, 2 = toxin produced in host without adherence, 3 = toxin produced in host with adherence to cells, 4 = toxin produced by invasive bacteria, 5 = toxin produced by bacteria causing systemic infection; type of toxin: 1 = enterotoxin, 2 = neurotoxin, 3 = non-protein toxin; target or mechanism of action; individual toxin number. Shown as TX x. x. x. x.

Tyndall effect Dispersion of light by a COLLOIDAL SUSPENSION, commonly determined as turbidity by measuring the light emitted at 90° to the direction of incident light.

typhoid Gastrointestinal infection caused by *Salmonella typhi*, transmitted by food or water contaminated by faeces of patients or asymptomatic carriers. Paratyphoid is due to *S. paratyphi*.

tyramine The AMINE formed by decarboxylation of the amino acid TYROSINE; chemically *p*-hydroxyphenylethylamine.

tyrosinase See PHENOL OXIDASES.

tyrosine A non-essential AMINO ACID, abbr Tyr (Y), M_r 181.2, pK_a 2.43, 9.11, 10.13 (−OH), CODONS UAPy, that can be formed from the essential amino acid PHENYLALANINE, hence it has some sparing action on phenylalanine. In addition to its rôle in proteins, tyrosine is the precursor for the synthesis of melanin (the black and brown pigment of skin and hair), and for ADRENALINE and NORADRENALINE.

tyrosinosis GENETIC DISEASE due to lack of *p*-hydroxyphenylpyruvate oxidase (EC 1.13.11.27), affecting the metabolism of TYROSINE and leading to excretion of *p*-hydroxyphenylpyruvic acid in the urine. Treatment is by restriction of dietary intake of PHENYLALANINE and tyrosine.

tzatziki Greek; grated cucumber in yoghurt, flavoured with garlic, olive oil and vinegar.

U

ubichromenol Cyclised derivatives of UBIQUINONES.

ubiquinones Coenzymes in the respiratory (electron transport) chain in mitochondria, also known as coenzyme Q or mitoquinones; widely distributed in nature. Chemically derivatives of benzoquinone with isoprene side-chains. There is no evidence that they are dietary essentials; they may have ANTIOXIDANT activity.

UFA Unesterified FATTY ACIDS, see FATTY ACIDS, NON-ESTERIFIED.

ugli CITRUS fruit, cross between grapefruit and tangerine, also called tangelo (USA); first produced in Jamaica in 1930.

UHT See ULTRA HIGH TEMPERATURE STERILISATION.

UL Tolerable upper intake level of a nutrient; maximum intake (from supplements and enriched foods) that is unlikely to pose a risk of adverse effects on health.

ulcer A crater-like lesion of the skin or a mucous membrane resulting from tissue death associated with inflammatory disease, infection or cancer. Peptic ulcers affect regions of the GASTROINTESTINAL TRACT exposed to gastric juices containing acid and PEPSIN: gastric ulcer in the stomach and duodenal ulcer in the duodenum. Treatment was formerly conservative, with a bland

diet, followed if necessary by surgery; specific antagonists of HISTAMINE receptors have improved treatment enormously. May be caused or exacerbated by infection with *Helicobacter pylori*.
See also HISTAMINE RECEPTOR ANTAGONISTS; PROTON PUMP.

ulcerative colitis   See COLITIS.

ullage   Liquid left in cask or bottle after some has been removed.

ultracentrifuge   See CENTRIFUGE.

ultrafiltration   Procedure for removal of low molecular weight compounds from plasma, protein solutions, etc, using a SEMIPERMEABLE MEMBRANE and either hydrostatic pressure or centrifugation.

ultra high temperature sterilisation (UHT)   Sterilisation at higher temperatures and for shorter times, than HIGH TEMPERATURE-SHORT TIME sterilisation.

ultrasonic homogeniser   Used to form emulsions of immiscible liquids. High-frequency sound waves (18–20 kHz) giving a cavitation force of 10 tonnes/cm^2 cause alternate cycles of compression and tension, forming emulsions of droplet size 1–2 μm. The mixture is pumped through the homogeniser at a pressure of 340–1400 kPa.

ultrasound   Sound above the normal range of human hearing, commonly above 20 kHz.

ultraviolet (UV) irradiation   Light of wavelength below the visible range. Wavelength for maximal germicidal action is 260 nm; poor penetrating power and only of value for surface sterilisation or sterilising air and water. Also used for tenderising and ageing of meat, curing cheese, and prevention of mould growth on the surface of bakery products. Ultraviolet from sunlight is responsible for skin tanning, and the formation of VITAMIN D from 7-dehydrocholesterol in the skin.

umami   Name given to the special taste of MONOSODIUM GLUTAMATE, protein, certain amino acids and the RIBONUCLEOTIDES (inosinate and guanylate). The Japanese name for a savoury flavour, now considered one of the five basic senses of TASTE.

umbles   Edible entrails of any animal (especially deer) which used to be made into pie, umble pie or humble pie.

uncoupling proteins   Proteins in MITOCHONDRIA that act to uncouple the processes of electron transport and oxidative phosphorylation, so permitting more or less uncontrolled oxidation of metabolic fuels, with production of heat. An important part of maintenance of body temperature by non-shivering thermogenesis.

UCP-1 (thermogenin) is the best studied. It occurs only in BROWN ADIPOSE TISSUE, and is activated by free fatty acids produced in response to β-adrenergic stimulation. UCP-2 occurs in a variety of tissues, including skeletal muscle and lung; UCP-3 occurs only in skeletal muscle.

uncrystallisable syrup   See SYRUP.

unesterified fatty acids (UFA)   See FATTY ACIDS, NON-ESTERIFIED.

universal product codes (UPC)   Standard multidigit numbers that represent product, size, manufacturer and nature of contents, on food and other labels as machine-readable bar codes.

unsaturated fatty acids   See FATTY ACIDS.

UPC   See UNIVERSAL PRODUCT CODES.

uperisation   A method of sterilising milk by injecting steam under pressure to raise the temperature to 150°C. The added water is evaporated off.

uracil   A PYRIMIDINE; see NUCLEIC ACIDS.

urataemia   High blood concentration of URIC ACID and its salts, as in GOUT.

uraturia   Urinary excretion of high concentrations of URIC ACID and its salts.

urea $CO(NH_2)_2$, the end-product of nitrogen metabolism in most mammals, excreted in the urine. Synthesised in the liver from ammonia (arising from the deamination of amino acids) and the amino acid ASPARTIC ACID. It is the major nitrogenous compound in urine, and the major component of the non-protein nitrogen in blood plasma.

urease   Intestinal bacterial enzyme (EC 3.5.1.5) that hydrolyses urea to ammonia and carbon dioxide. Important in the entero-hepatic cycling of urea. Also found in some beans.

urethane   Ethyl carbamate, used as intermediate in organic syn-theses, as a solubiliser and as the precursor for polyurethane foam. Found in small amounts in liqueurs made from stone fruits, wines and some distilled spirits where it is formed by reaction between alcohol and nitrogenous compounds; cause for concern since it is genotoxic.

uric acid   The end-product of PURINE metabolism in man and other apes; other mammals have the enzyme uricase (EC 1.7.3.3), which oxidises uric acid to allantoin, which is more soluble in water. Gout is the result of excessive formation of uric acid, and/or impaired excretion; it is only slightly soluble in water, and in excess it crystallises in joints, as gouty nodules under the skin and sometimes in the kidney.

urobilinogen   Pigment in urine derived from the bile pigments, which, in turn, are formed from haemoglobin. When urine is left to stand, the urobilinogen is oxidised in air to urobilin.

urogastrone   Hormone similar to GASTRIN, found in urine; little known of its function.

UV   See ULTRAVIOLET.

V

vacherin (1) Circular cakes of meringue and cream.

(2) French mild cheeses made from cow's milk; traditionally moulded in flat circles and wrapped in a border of bark.

vac-ice process Alternative name for FREEZE DRYING.

vacreation DEODORISATION of cream by steam distillation under reduced pressure; developed in New Zealand.

vacuum contact drying Or vacuum contact plate process, a method of drying food in a vacuum oven in which the material is heated by hot plates both above and below. As the material shrinks due to water loss, continuous contact is maintained by closing the plates; supplies heat to the food more effectively than a simple vacuum oven.

vagotomy Surgical cutting of part of the vagus (10th cranial) nerve, usually to reduce secretion of acid and PEPSIN by the gastric mucosa.

valgus Any deformity that displaces the hand or foot away from the mid-line of the body; e.g. genu valgus is knock knees, as seen in RICKETS.

See also VARUS.

validity Of an assay, the extent to which a method measures what it purports to measure.

See also ACCURACY; PRECISION; SENSITIVITY; SPECIFICITY.

valine An essential AMINO ACID, abbr Val (V), M_r 117.1, pK_a 2.29, 9.74, CODONS GUNu; rarely, if ever, limiting in foods. Chemically, aminoisovaleric acid.

valzin, valzol See DULCIN.

vanadium A MINERAL known to be essential to experimental animals, although sufficiently widespread for human dietary deficiency to be unknown. Its precise function is unknown, although it acts as an activator of a number of enzymes.

vanaspati Indian; purified hydrogenated vegetable oil; similar to MARGARINE and usually fortified with vitamins A and D. Also used to prepare GHEE (vanaspati ghee).

vanilla Extract of the vanilla bean, fruit of the tropical orchid *Aracus* (or *Vanilla*) *aromaticus* and related species. Discovered in Mexico in 1571 and could not be grown elsewhere, because pollination could be effected only by a small Mexican bee, until artificial pollination was introduced in 1820. Main growing regions now Madagascar and Tahiti.

The major flavouring principle is vanillin (chemically methyl protocatechuic aldehyde), but other substances present aid the flavour. Ethyl vanillin is a synthetic substance which does not occur in the vanilla bean; $3^1/_2$ times as strong in flavour, and more stable to storage than vanillin, but does not have the true flavour.

vanillin   See VANILLA.

variety meat   American name for OFFAL.

varus   Any deformity that displaces the hand or foot towards the mid-line of the body; e.g. genu varus is bow legs, as seen in RICKETS. See also VALGUS.

vasoactive intestinal peptide (VIP)   Protein secreted by the PAN-CREAS; oversecretion can cause severe DIARRHOEA.

vasoconstriction   Constriction of the blood vessels; the reverse of VASODILATATION.

vasodilatation (vasodilation)   Dilation of the blood vessels; the reverse is VASOCONSTRICTION. Caused by a rise in body temperature; serves to lose heat from the body.

vasopressin   Antidiuretic hormone secreted by the pituitary, acts to increase resorption of water in the kidneys and to constrict blood vessels.

VCD   See VACUUM CONTACT DRYING.

veal   Meat of young calf (*Bos taurus*) $2^{1}/_{2}$–3 months old.
Composition/100 g: 962 kJ (230 kcal), protein 31.6 g, fat 11.5 g (35.5% saturated, 47.1% mono-, 17.3% polyunsaturated), cholesterol 155 mg, carbohydrate 0 g, Na 97 mg, K 430 mg, Ca 14 mg, Mg 28 mg, P 360 mg, Fe 1.6 mg, Cu 0.05 mg, Zn 2.1 mg, Se 8 μg, vitamin B_1 0.06 mg, B_2 0.27 mg, niacin 13.7 mg, B_6 0.32 mg, folate 4 μg, B_{12} 1 μg, pantothenate 0.5 mg. A 150 g serving is a source of pantothenate.

Vegans   Those who consume no foods of animal origin. See VEGETARIANS.

Vegemite   Australian; trade name for YEAST EXTRACT.

vegetable butters   Naturally occurring fats that melt rather sharply because they contain a preponderance of a single TRIACYLGLYCEROL. Cocoa butter from the COCOA bean, used in CHOCOLATE; Borneo tallow or green butter from Malaysian and Indonesian plant, *Shorea stenopiera*, resembles cocoa butter; shea butter from African plant, *Butyrospermum parkii*, softer than cocoa butter. Mowrah fat or illipé butter from Indian plant, *Bassia longifolia*.

vegetable oyster   See SALSIFY.

vegetable pepsin   See PAPAIN.

vegetable protein products   General term to include textured SOYA and other bean products often made to simulate meat. Basic material is termed flour when the protein content is not less than 50%; concentrate, not less than 65%; isolate, not less than 90% protein.
See also TEXTURED VEGETABLE PROTEIN.

vegetable spaghetti See SPAGHETTI SQUASH.

vegetarians Those who do not eat meat or fish, either for ethical/religious reasons or because they believe that a meat-free diet confers health benefits. Apart from a risk of VITAMIN B$_{12}$ deficiency (vitamin B$_{12}$ is found only in meat and meat products), there are no adverse effects of a wholly meat-free diet, although vegetarian women are more at risk of IRON deficiency than those who eat meat. Vitamin B$_{12}$ supplements prepared by bacterial fermentation (and hence ethically acceptable to the strictest of vegetarians) are available.

The strictest vegetarians are vegans, who consume no products of animal origin at all. Those who consume milk and milk products are termed lacto-vegetarians; those who also eat eggs, ovo-lacto-vegetarians. Some vegetarians (pescetarians) will eat fish, but not meat; demi-vegetarians eat little or no meat, or eat poultry but not red meat.

veltol See MALTOL.

venison Meat of deer (*Odocoileus* spp); traditionally GAME, but now mainly farmed.

Composition/100 g: 828 kJ (198 kcal), protein 35 g, fat 6.4 g, carbohydrate 0 g, Na 86 mg, K 360 mg, Ca 29 mg, Mg 33 mg, P 290 mg, Fe 7.8 mg, Cu 0.36 mg, Zn 3.9 mg, vitamin B$_1$ 0.22 mg, B$_2$ 0.69 mg, niacin 12 mg, B$_6$ 0.65 mg, folate 6 µg, B$_{12}$ 0.8 µg. A 120 g serving is a source of vitamin B$_1$, Mg; rich source of protein, vitamin B$_2$, niacin, B$_6$, B$_{12}$, Fe, Cu, Zn.

verbascose A non-digestible tetrasaccharide, galactosyl-galactosyl-glucosyl-fructose, found in LEGUMES; fermented by intestinal bacteria and causes flatulence.

verdoflavin Name given to a substance isolated from grass, later shown to be riboflavin (VITAMIN B$_2$).

verjuice Literally green juice; sour juice of crab apples (and sometimes unripe grapes) formerly used in cooking meat, fish and game dishes. Now normally replaced by lemon juice.

vermicelli See PASTA.

vermicide Any drug used to kill or expel intestinal parasitic worms.

vermouth Fortified wine (about 16% alcohol by volume) flavoured with herbs and QUININE. French vermouth is dry and colourless; Italian may be red or white and is sweet. Drunk as an apéritif, either with soda or with gin or vodka (when called a martini). Name originally derived from German *Wermut* for wormwood, a toxic ingredient that was included in early vermouths (as in ABSINTHE).

Sweet or Italian vermouth, 15–17% alcohol (by volume), 12–20% sugar (by weight). Dry or French type 18–20% alcohol, 3–5% sugar.

Versene   Trade name for ethylenediamine tetra-acetic acid, see EDTA.

Verv   Trade name for calcium stearyl-2-lactate, used to reduce baking variations in flour. It produces a more extensible dough, more easily machined, and gives a loaf with better keeping properties and more uniform structure.

very low-density lipoproteins (VLDL)   See LIPIDS, PLASMA.

vetch   Old term applied generally to LEGUMES; originally *Vicia* spp, also called tares.

Vibrio cholerae   The causative agent of cholera, bacterium transmitted especially through water; forms an ENTEROTOXIN after adhering to epithelial cells in gut. Infective dose 10^8 organisms, onset 2–5 days, duration 4–6 days, TX 3.1.2.2.

vichyssoise   Cold leek and potato cream soup.

vicilin   Globulin protein in pea and lentil.

vicine   One of the toxins in broad beans, responsible for acute haemolytic anaemia or FAVISM.

Vienna flour   Specially fine flour used to make strudel PASTRY, Vienna bread and cakes.

Viennese coffee   Ground coffee containing dried figs.

villi, intestinal   Small, finger-like processes covering the surface of the small intestine in large numbers ($20–40/mm^2$), projecting some 0.5–1 mm into the lumen. They provide a surface area of about $300 m^2$ for the absorption of nutrients from the small intestine.

vinasses   The residual liquors from sugar beet MOLASSES; contain appreciable quantities of BETAINE.

vinegar   Not less than 4% solution of acetic acid; the product of two fermentations, first with yeast to convert sugars into alcohol; this liquor, called gyle (6–9% alcohol), is then fermented with *Acetobacter* spp to form acetic acid.

In most countries vinegar is made from grape juice (wine vinegar, may be from red, white or rosé wine).

Malt vinegar is made from malted barley and may be distilled to a colourless liquid with the same acetic acid content but a more mellow flavour.

Cider vinegar (simply known as vinegar in USA) is made from apple juice; vinegars may be flavoured with a variety of herbs.

Non-brewed condiment (once called non-brewed vinegar) is a solution of acetic acid, 4–8%, coloured with caramel.

Balsamic vinegar is made from grape juice that has been concentrated over a low flame and fermented slowly in a series of wooden barrels; made only around Modena, Italy.

Rice vinegar is made from SAKE.

viosterol   Irradiated ergosterol; VITAMIN D_2.

VIP   See VASOACTIVE INTESTINAL PEPTIDE.

Virginia date   See PERSIMMON.

Virol   Trade name for a vitamin preparation based on malt extract.

viscera   The organs within a body cavity, used especially for the abdominal viscera, LIVER, SPLEEN, GASTROINTESTINAL TRACT, kidneys, etc.

viscogen   Thickening agent for whipping CREAM. Two parts of lime (calcium oxide) in six parts of water, added to five parts of sugar in ten parts of water; used at the rate of 3–6 g/L of cream.

viscometer   Instrument for measuring the VISCOSITY of liquids.

viscosity   The resistance to flow of a liquid, due to cohesion and adhesion.

vision   The process of vision is mediated by photosensitive pigments formed by reaction between retinaldehyde (VITAMIN A aldehyde) and the protein opsin. The pigments are known variously as visual purple (because of the colour), rhodopsin (in the rod cells of the retina) and iodopsin (in the cone cells, with sensitivity to different wavelengths of light in different cells). Exposure to light results in bleaching of the pigment, with loss of the retinaldehyde and a conformational change in the protein, which leads to closure of a sodium channel in the retinal cell, and initiation of a nerve impulse.

visual pigments, visual purple   See VISION.

vitamers   Chemical compounds structurally related to a VITAMIN, and converted to the same overall active metabolites in the body. They thus possess the same kind of biological activity, although sometimes with lower potency.

When there are several vitamers, the group of compounds exhibiting the biological activity of the vitamin is given a GENERIC DESCRIPTOR (e.g. VITAMIN A is the generic descriptor for retinol and its derivatives as well as several CAROTENOIDS).

vitamin   There are 13 organic substances (thus excluding trace minerals) essential to human life in very small amounts. Eleven of these must be supplied in the diet (vitamins A, B_1, B_2, B_6, B_{12}, C, E, K, folate, biotin and pantothenate); two (niacin and vitamin D) can be made in the body if there is sufficient of the AMINO ACID, TRYPTOPHAN, and sunlight, respectively. The word may be pronounced either *veitamin* or *vittamin*.

Vitamins A, D, E and K are grouped together as fat-soluble vitamins, because they are soluble in lipids, but not in water. Vitamin C and the B vitamins (including pantothenic acid, biotin and folate) are grouped together as the water-soluble vitamins since they are all soluble in water, but not lipids.

According to the UK Code of Practice, no claims for the presence of a vitamin (or mineral) in a food should be made unless the amount ordinarily consumed in a day contains one-sixth of the daily requirements. No claim should be made that the food is a rich or excellent source unless half of the daily requirement is present; no reference to the prevention of disease unless the full day's requirement is present. EU labelling regulations only permit claims to be made if a food provides more than 15% of the labelling reference value (see Table 2)/100 g or 100 mL.

vitamin A   Fat soluble vitamin, occurring either as the preformed vitamin (retinol) found in animal foods or as a precursor, CAROTENES found in plant foods. Required for control of growth, cell turnover and foetal development, maintenance of fertility and maintenance of the normal moist condition of epithelial tissues lining the mouth and respiratory and urinary tracts; is essential in VISION.

Deficiency leads to slow adaptation to see in dim light (poor DARK ADAPTATION), later to night blindness; then drying of the tear ducts (xerophthalmia) and ulceration of the cornea (keratomalacia) resulting in blindness.

The vitamin A content of foods is expressed as retinol equivalents, i.e. retinol plus carotene; 1 μg retinol = 6 μg β-carotene = 12 μg other active carotenoids = 3.33 INTERNATIONAL UNITS.

See also CONJUNCTIVAL IMPRESSION CYTOLOGY; RELATIVE DOSE RESPONSE TEST; RETINOL BINDING PROTEIN; VISION.

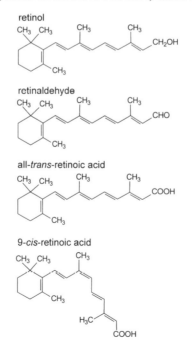

418

vitamin A toxicity   Retinol in excess of requirements is stored in the liver, bound to proteins, and is a cumulative poison. When the storage capacity is exceeded, free retinol causes damage to cell membranes. CAROTENE is not toxic in excess, since there is only a limited capacity to form retinol from carotene.

The recommended upper limits of habitual daily intake of retinol are about $12.5 \times$ REFERENCE INTAKE for adults, but only $2.5 \times$ reference intake for infants. Retinol is also TERATOGENIC in excess, and for pregnant women the recommended upper limit of daily intake is $3300\,\mu g$.

vitamin A_2   Old name for dehydroretinol, the form found in livers of freshwater fish; has 40% of the biological activity of retinol.

vitamin B complex   Old-fashioned term for the various B vitamins: VITAMIN B_1 (thiamin), VITAMIN B_2 (riboflavin), NIACIN, VITAMIN B_6, VITAMIN B_{12}, FOLATE, BIOTIN and PANTOTHENIC ACID. These vitamins occur together in cereal germ, liver and yeast; function as coenzymes; and historically were discovered by separation from what was known originally as 'vitamin B'; hence, they are grouped together as the B complex.

vitamin B_1   Thiamin. Thiamin diphosphate is a coenzyme in metabolism of glucose, and in the citric acid cycle. Thiamin triphosphate has a rôle in nerve conduction. Deficiency, especially when associated with a carbohydrate-rich diet, results in the disease BERIBERI, degeneration of the sensory nerves in the hands and feet fast spreading through the limbs, with fluid retention and heart failure. Relatively acute deficiency, especially associated with alcohol abuse, results in central nervous system damage, the WERNICKE–KORSAKOFF SYNDROME.

See also THIOCHROME; TRANSKETOLASE.

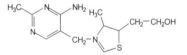

vitamin B_1 dependency syndromes   A very small number of children have been reported with a variant form of MAPLE SYRUP URINE DISEASE in which the defect is in the binding of thiamin diphosphate to the branched chain keto acid dehydrogenase (EC 1.2.4.4). These children respond well to supplements of large amounts of vitamin B_1, without the need for strict control of their intake of the amino acids.

vitamin B_2   Riboflavin. Coenzyme in a wide range of oxidation reactions of fats, carbohydrates and amino acids, as riboflavin phosphate (flavin mononucleotide), flavin adenine dinucleotide or covalently bound riboflavin at the active site of the enzyme. Riboflavin-dependent enzymes are collectively known as flavoproteins.

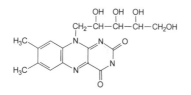

Deficiency impairs energy-yielding metabolism and results in a group of symptoms known as ariboflavinosis, including cracking of the skin at the corners of the mouth (angular stomatitis), fissuring of the lips (cheilosis) and tongue changes (glossitis); seborrhoeic accumulations appear around the nose and eyes. Not fatal because there is very efficient recycling of riboflavin in deficiency.

See also GLUTATHIONE REDUCTASE; LUMICHROME; LUMIFLAVIN.

vitamin B₃ Non-existent; term once used for PANTOTHENIC ACID and sometimes, incorrectly, used for NIACIN.

vitamin B₄ Name given to what was later identified as a mixture of the amino acids arginine, glycine and cystine.

vitamin B₅ Name given to a substance later presumed to be identical with vitamin B₆ or possibly nicotinic acid: also sometimes used for PANTOTHENIC ACID.

vitamin B₆ Generic descriptor for three compounds (chemically derivatives of 2-methylpyridine):

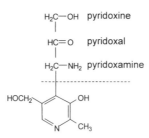

(1) the hydroxyl (alcohol) compound, pyridoxine (previously known as adermin and pyridoxol);

(2) the aldehyde, pyridoxal; and

(3) the amine, pyridoxamine; and their phosphates.

All are equally active biologically. The active metabolite is pyridoxal 5′-phosphate, which acts as a coenzyme in decarboxylation and transamination of amino acids, and in glycogen phos-

420

phorylase (EC 2.4.1.1), also a rôle in terminating the actions of STEROID hormones.

Deficiency causes abnormalities in the metabolism of the amino acids TRYPTOPHAN and METHIONINE; in rats convulsions and skin lesions (acrodynia) and in dairy cows and dogs, anaemia with abnormal red blood cells. Dietary deficiency leading to clinical signs is not known in human beings, apart from a single outbreak in babies fed a severely overheated preparation of formula milk in the 1950s; they showed abnormalities of amino acid metabolism and convulsions resembling epileptic seizures, which responded to supplements of the vitamin.

See also METHIONINE LOAD TEST; TRANSAMINASE; TRYPTOPHAN LOAD TEST.

vitamin B_6 dependency syndromes   A very small number of children suffer from GENETIC DISEASES affecting the binding of pyridoxal phosphate to an enzyme. The abnormality is corrected by the administration of large supplements of vitamin B_6.

vitamin B_6 toxicity   High intakes of supplements of vitamin B_6, in excess of 200–1000 mg/day (far in excess of what could be obtained from foods) cause peripheral sensory neuropathy.

vitamin B_7, B_8 and B_9   In the early days of nutrition research, when a new factor was discovered which was claimed to be essential for chick growth and feathering, the claimant stated that since nine factors were known the new factors should be called vitamins B_{10} and B_{11}. In fact, the B vitamins had been numbered only up to B_6, hence B_7, B_8 and B_9 have never existed. B_9 is sometimes (incorrectly) used for FOLATE.

vitamin B_{10} and B_{11}   The names given to two factors claimed to be essential for chick growth and feathering; they were later shown to be a mixture of vitamin B_1 and folic acid.

vitamin B_{12}   Cobalamin; coenzyme for methionine synthetase (EC 2.1.1.13, important in metabolism of FOLIC ACID) and methylmalonyl CoA mutase (EC 5.4.99.2).

Deficiency leads to pernicious ANAEMIA when immature red blood cells are released into the bloodstream, and there is degeneration of the spinal cord. The anaemia is the same as seen in folate deficiency, and is due to impairment of folate metabolism. There is also urinary excretion of METHYLMALONIC ACID.

Absorption of vitamin B_{12} requires INTRINSIC FACTOR, a protein secreted in the gastric juice. Failure of absorption, rather than dietary deficiency, is the main cause of pernicious anaemia. However, B_{12} is found only in animal foods so strict VEGETARIANS are at risk.

See also DUMP SUPPRESSION TEST; METHYL FOLATE TRAP; SCHILLING TEST.

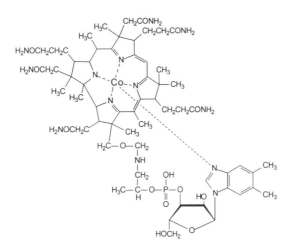

vitamin B$_{13}$ Orotic acid, an intermediate in PYRIMIDINE synthesis; no evidence that it is a dietary essential; not a vitamin.

vitamin B$_{14}$ Not an established vitamin; name originally given to a substance found in human urine that increases the rate of cell proliferation in bone marrow culture.

vitamin B$_{15}$ PANGAMIC ACID; no evidence that it has any physiological function in the body; not a vitamin.

vitamin B$_{16}$ This term has never been used.

vitamin B$_{17}$ AMYGDALIN (laetrile); no evidence that it has any physiological function in the body; not a vitamin.

vitamin B$_c$ Obsolete name for FOLIC ACID.

vitamin B$_p$ Called the antiperosis factor for chicks, but can be replaced by MANGANESE and CHOLINE (not a dietary essential for human beings).

vitamin B$_T$ CARNITINE; an essential dietary factor for the mealworm *Tenebrio molitor*, and certain related species, but not a dietary essential for human beings.

vitamin B$_w$ Or factor W; probably identical to BIOTIN.

vitamin B$_x$ Non-existent; has been used in the past for both PANTOTHENIC ACID and *p*-amino benzoic acid.

vitamin C   ASCORBIC ACID. Historically an inadequate intake of vitamin C led to SCURVY, especially common among sailors unable to obtain fruits and vegetables.

Three main areas of function:

(1) as a general (non-enzymic) antioxidant, including the reduction of oxidised VITAMIN E in cell membranes;

(2) as a coenzyme in the hydroxylation of LYSINE and PROLINE

in the synthesis of COLLAGEN, hence essential for the normal formation of CONNECTIVE TISSUE;

(3) as a coenzyme in the formation of NORADRENALINE.

Deficiency results in scurvy: seepage of blood from capillaries, subcutaneous bleeding, weakness of muscles, soft, spongy gums and loss of dental cement, leading to loss of teeth and in advanced cases deep bone pain. A lesser degree of deficiency results in impaired healing of wounds.

The requirement to prevent scurvy is less than 10 mg/day; reference intakes are 30 mg/day (FAO); 40 mg/day (UK); 45 mg/day (EU); 60 mg/day (USA and Codex Alimentarius); 85 mg/day (Netherlands). All of these differing figures can be justified, depending on the criteria of adequacy adopted and the assumptions made in the interpretation of experimental data. At intakes above 100 mg/d the vitamin is excreted in the urine; there is no evidence of any adverse effects at intakes up to 4000 mg/day.

Fruits and vegetables are rich sources; also used in curing ham, and as an antioxidant and bread improver.

See also DICHLOROPHENOL INDOPHENOL; ERYTHORBIC ACID; IRON; O-PHENYLENE DIAMINE.

vitamin D   Vitamin D_3 is calciol or cholecalciferol; formed in the skin by the action of ultraviolet light on 7 DEHYDROCHOLESTEROL, hence not strictly a vitamin. However, in northern latitudes sunlight exposure may not be adequate to meet requirements, and a dietary source becomes essential.

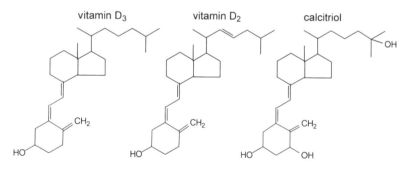

Vitamin D_2 (ercalciol or ergocalciferol) is a synthetic VITAMER produced by irradiation of ergosterol. The name vitamin D_1 was given originally to an impure mixture and is not used now.

The main storage form of the vitamin is the 25-hydroxy derivative, calcidiol, in plasma; the active metabolite is the 1,25-dihydroxy derivative, calcitriol. Formation of calcitriol is regulated by the state of CALCIUM balance.

The function of calcitriol is in regulation of calcium metabolism; it acts via nuclear receptors, like a STEROID hormone, and also via cell–surface receptors. Stimulates absorption of dietary calcium from the small intestine and calcium turnover in bone, by activating osteoblasts to mobilise calcium, then later recruiting and stimulating differentiation of osteoblast precursors for bone formation.

Deficiency causes RICKETS in young children, OSTEOMALACIA in adults.

Not widely distributed in foods, egg yolk, butter, oily fish and enriched margarine are the only significant sources. There are no REFERENCE INTAKES for adults, since it is assumed that normal sunlight exposure will meet requirements; for the housebound elderly the REFERENCE INTAKE is 10 µg. The obsolete international unit of vitamin D = 25 ng calciol; 1 mg calciol = 40 iu.

vitamin D resistant rickets   See RICKETS, vitamin D resistant.

vitamin D toxicity   Excessive intake of vitamin D results in disturbance of calcium metabolism, resulting in hypercalcaemia, dangerously raised blood calcium concentrations, leading to raised blood pressure, and calcinosis, inappropriate deposition of calcium in soft tissues, leading to brain and kidney damage. Excessive exposure to sunlight does not lead to excessive formation of vitamin D because previtamin D undergoes further light-catalysed reactions to inactive compounds, and there is only limited availability of 7-DEHYDROCHOLESTEROL in the skin.

vitamin E   Two main groups of compounds have vitamin E activity: the tocopherols and the tocotrienols; there are four isomers of each: α-, β-, γ- and δ-tocopherols and α-, β-, γ- and δ-tocotrienols, with differing potencies.

Deficiency symptoms vary considerably in different animal species, sterility in mouse, rat, rabbit, sheep and turkey; muscular dystrophy in several species; capillary permeability in chick and turkey; anaemia in monkey. Human dietary deficiency is unknown, but hereditary lack of β-lipoprotein leads to functional deficiency, with severe neurological damage. Premature infants may show haemolytic ANAEMIA as a result of vitamin E deficiency.

Functions as an ANTIOXIDANT in cell membranes, protecting unsaturated fatty acids from oxidative damage.

The vitamin E content of foods is expressed as milligrams α-tocopherol equivalent (based on the different potency of the different vitamers). The obsolete INTERNATIONAL UNIT of vitamin E activity was equal to 1 mg of synthetic α-tocopherol; on this basis natural source α-tocopherol is 1.49 iu/mg.

424

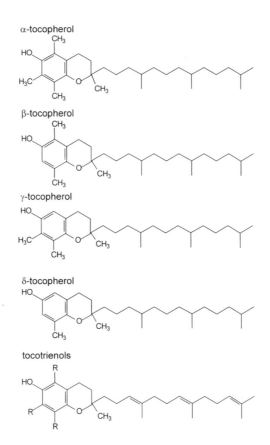

α-tocopherol

β-tocopherol

γ-tocopherol

δ-tocopherol

tocotrienols

vitamin F   Sometimes used for the essential FATTY ACIDS.

vitamin G   Obsolete name for VITAMIN B₂.

vitamin H   See BIOTIN.

vitamin K   Two groups of compounds have vitamin K activity: phylloquinones (vitamin K_1), found in all green plants, and a variety of menaquinone (vitamin K_2) synthesised by intestinal bacteria. Vitamin K_3 is a synthetic analogue, MENADIONE.

Functions as coenzyme in carboxylation of glutamate to γ-CARBOXYGLUTAMATE in a number of calcium binding proteins, including PROTHROMBIN and other proteins involved in the BLOOD CLOTTING system, and the bone protein OSTEOCALCIN.

Dietary deficiency is unknown, except associated with general malabsorption diseases. However, some newborn infants are at risk of developing haemorrhagic disease as a result of low vitamin K status, and it is general practice to give a single relatively large dose of the vitamin by injection.

See also ANTICOAGULANTS; DICOUMAROL; WARFARIN.

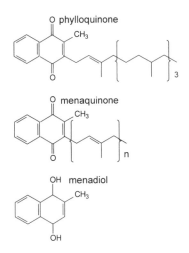

vitamin L Factors extracted from yeast and thought at the time to be essential for lactation; they have not become established vitamins.

vitamin M Obsolete name for FOLIC ACID.

vitamin P Name given to a group of plant FLAVONOIDS (sometimes called bioflavonoids) which affect the strength of blood capillaries: rutin (in buckwheat), hesperidin, eriodictin and citrin (a mixture of hesperidin and eriodictin in the pith of citrus fruits). Now considered that the effect is pharmacological and that they are not dietary essentials, although they may have ANTIOXIDANT activity; however, there is little evidence that they can be absorbed from the gut. Called vitamin P from the German *permeabilitäts vitamin*, because of the effect on capillary permeability and fragility.

vitamin PP The PELLAGRA-preventing vitamin, an old name for NIACIN before it was identified.

vitamin T Factor found in insect cuticle, mould mycelia and yeast fermentation liquor, claimed to accelerate maturation and promote protein synthesis. Also known as torulitine. Said to be a mixture of folic acid, vitamin B_{12} and deoxyribosides (DNA); hence not a particular vitamin.

vitaminoids Name given to compounds with 'vitamin-like' activity; considered by some to be vitamins or partially to replace vitamins. Include FLAVONOIDS (VITAMIN P), INOSITOL, CARNITINE, CHOLINE, LIPOIC ACID and the essential FATTY ACIDS. With the exception of the essential fatty acids, there is no evidence that any of them is a dietary essential.

vitellin The major protein of egg yolk; approximately 80% of the total; a phosphoprotein accounting for 30% of the phosphorus of egg yolk.

VLDL Very low-density lipoprotein, see LIPOPROTEINS, PLASMA.

vodka Made from neutral spirit, i.e. alcohol distillate mainly from potatoes, with little or no acid, so that there is no ester formation and hence no flavour. Polish vodka is flavoured with a variety of herbs and fruits.

Vol Trade name for commercial ammonium carbonate, a mixture of ammonium bicarbonate and carbamate. Used as aerating agent in baking, as it breaks down to carbon dioxide, ammonia and steam on heating, without leaving any residue.

volvulus Twisting of part of the gastrointestinal tract, leading to partial or complete obstruction.

votator Machine used for the continuous manufacture of margarine; the fat and water are emulsified, and the subsequent conditioning process carried out in the same machine.

W

waist:hip circumference ratio Simple method for describing the distribution of subcutaneous and intra-abdominal ADIPOSE TISSUE.

walnuts The rough shelled English walnut, black walnut, hickory nut and butternut are all botanically walnuts. Common English walnut (so-called because carried round the world for centuries in English ships) is *Juglans regia*.

Composition /100 g (shelled): 2879 kJ (688 kcal), protein 14.7 g, fat 68.5 g (8.5% saturated, 18.9% mono-, 72.5% polyunsaturated), carbohydrate 3.3 g (2.6 g sugars, 0.7 g starch), dietary fibre 5.9 g, nsp 3.5 g, Na 7 mg, K 450 mg, Ca 94 mg, Mg 160 mg, P 380 mg, Fe 2.9 mg, Cu 1.34 mg, Zn 2.7 mg, Se 19 μg, I 9 μg, vitamin E 3.9 mg, B_1 0.4 mg, B_2 0.14 mg, niacin 4 mg, B_6 0.67 mg, folate 66 μg, pantothenate 1.6 mg, biotin 19 μg. A 20 g serving (three nuts) is a source of Mg; rich source of Cu.

Warfarin Synthetic compound that acts as a VITAMIN K antagonist, by inhibiting vitamin K epoxide reductase (EC 1.1.4.1). Used clinically to impair blood clotting in patients at risk of THROMBOSIS, and as a rodenticide. Named for the Wisconsin Alumnus Research Fund, which sponsored the research that led to its discovery (1951).

wasabe Japanese; pungent condiment prepared from dried HORSERADISH and MUSTARD.

wash, spent See SPENT WASH.

wassail (1) Spiced ale.

(2) Salutation or toast drunk to a person's health.

water activity (a_w)   Ratio between vapour pressure of water in the food and that of pure water at the same temperature. Most bacteria cannot grow at a_w below 0.9, yeasts below 0.85 and moulds below 0.7. So-called dehydrated foods have a_w lower than 0.6.

water balance   The balance between intake and excretion of fluids. Average daily intakes are: as drinks 1–1.5 L; as aqueous part of food, 0.5 L; and formed in the body by oxidation of foodstuffs (METABOLIC WATER), 300–500 mL; total 2–3 L. Losses from the lungs, 400–500 mL; through the skin 400–500 mL; in faeces 80–100 mL; in urine 1–1.8 L.

Total body water 40–44 L as: blood plasma (2–3 L), extracellular fluid (between cells) 10 L and intracellular fluid (within cells) 27–30 L.

The kidney controls the volume of extracellular water by excreting water. Ingestion of sodium chloride (SALT) raises the OSMOTIC PRESSURE of the extracellular water, causing thirst.

water biscuit   See CRACKERS.

waterbrash   Sudden filling of the mouth with dilute SALIVA.

water chestnut   Seeds of *Trapa natans* and *T. bicornis*; see CHESTNUT.

watercress   Leaves of *Nasturtium officinale* (green watercress, remains green in autumn and is susceptible to frost) and *N. microphyllum × officinale* (brown or winter watercress); eaten raw in salads.

Composition /100 g: 92 kJ (22 kcal), protein 3 g, fat 1 g (37.5% saturated, 12.5% mono-, 50% polyunsaturated), carbohydrate 0.4 g (0.4 g sugars), dietary fibre 3 g, nsp 1.5 g, Na 49 mg, K 230 mg, Ca 170 mg, Mg 15 mg, P 52 mg, Fe 2.2 mg, Cu 0.01 mg, Zn 0.7 mg, vitamin A 420 µg (2520 µg carotene), E 1.5 mg, B_1 0.16 mg, B_2 0.06 mg, niacin 0.8 mg, B_6 0.23 mg, pantothenate 0.1 mg, biotin 0.4 µg, C 62 mg. A 20 g serving ($^1/_4$ bunch) is a source of vitamin A; good source of vitamin C.

water, demineralised   Water that has been purified by passage through a bed of ION-EXCHANGE RESIN which removes mineral salts. Demineralised or deionised water is at least as pure as distilled water, and may be purer.

water, extracellular, intracellular   See WATER BALANCE.

water-glass   Sodium silicate; used at one time to preserve eggs, by forming a layer of insoluble calcium silicate around the shell, and so sealing the pores.

water hardness   Soap-precipitating power of water due to the formation of insoluble calcium and magnesium salts of the soap. Temporary hardness (carbonates) is removed by boiling, permanent hardness (sulphates) is not. May be measured in degrees Clarke; one degree = 10 ppm calcium carbonate.

water ice See SORBET.

water lemon See PASSION FRUIT.

waterless cooking Cooking in a heavy pan with tightly fitting lid, with a steam vent; only a minimal amount of cooking liquid is needed, but the food is not cooked under pressure.

Waterlow classification A system for classifying PROTEIN–ENERGY MALNUTRITION in children based on wasting (the percentage of expected weight for height) and the degree of stunting (the percentage of expected height for age).

See also GOMEZ CLASSIFICATION; WELLCOME CLASSIFICATION.

watermelon Fruit of *Citrullus vulgaris*.

Composition /100 g: 129 kJ (31 kcal), protein 0.5 g, fat 0.3 g, carbohydrate 7.1 g (7.1 g sugars), dietary fibre 0.3 g, nsp 0.1 g, Na 2 mg, K 100 mg, Ca 7 mg, Mg 8 mg, P 9 mg, Fe 0.3 mg, Cu 0.03 mg, Zn 0.2 mg, vitamin A 38 µg (230 µg carotene), E 0.1 mg, B_1 0.05 mg, B_2 0.01 mg, niacin 0.1 mg, B_6 0.14 mg, folate 2 µg, pantothenate 0.2 mg, biotin 1 µg, C 8 mg. A 200 g serving is a source of vitamin B_6; good source of vitamin C.

water, metabolic See METABOLIC WATER; WATER BALANCE.

water, mineral (natural) See MINERAL WATER.

waxes ESTERS of FATTY ACIDS with long-chain monohydric alcohols (fats are esters of fatty acids with the trihydric alcohol glycerol). For example, beeswax, myricyl palmitate; spermaceti, cetyl palmitate. Animal waxes are often esters of the steroid alcohol CHOLESTEROL.

waxing Coating fruits and vegetables with a thin layer of edible wax. In the case of apples and oranges this replaces the natural wax that is removed when the crop is washed; in the case of vegetables it is an addition; in both instances the waxing prevents loss of moisture, prolongs storage life and improves the appearance.

weaning foods Foods specially formulated for infants aged between 3–9 months for the transition between breast or bottle feeding and normal intake of solid foods.

Weende analysis See PROXIMATE ANALYSIS.

weenie American name for small sausages, abbreviation of wienerwurst.

weight, desirable (ideal) Standardised tables of desirable (or ideal) weight for height for adults are based on life expectancy; both undernutrition and obesity are associated with increased risk of premature death.

See also BODY MASS INDEX.

weight-for-age An index of the adequacy of the child's nutrition to support growth. Standard weight-for-age is the 50th centile of the weight-for-age curves of well-fed children.

See also ANTHROPOMETRY.

weight-for-height   For children, can be used as an alternative to WEIGHT-FOR-AGE as an index of nutritional adequacy; for adults it is the only acceptable way of expressing weight relative to ideal or desirable weight.

See also ANTHROPOMETRY; BODY MASS INDEX; WEIGHT, DESIRABLE.

weighting oils   See BROMINATED OILS.

Wellcome classification   A system for classifying PROTEIN–ENERGY MALNUTRITION in children based on percentage of expected weight for age and the presence or absence of OEDEMA. Between 60–80% of expected weight is underweight in the absence of oedema, and is kwashiorkor if oedema is present; under 60% of expected weight is marasmus in the absence of oedema, and is marasmic kwashiorkor if oedema is present.

See also GOMEZ CLASSIFICATION; WATERLOW CLASSIFICATION.

Welsh rarebit   (Originally rabbit), melted cheese, mixed with mustard powder, pepper and brown ale, served on toast. Buck rarebit is Welsh rarebit topped with a poached egg.

Wernicke–Korsakoff syndrome   The result of damage to the brain as a result of VITAMIN B$_1$ deficiency, commonly associated with alcohol abuse. Affected subjects show clear signs of neurological damage, including NYSTAGMUS (Wernicke's encephalopathy) with psychiatric changes (Korsakoff's psychosis) characterised by loss of recent memory and confabulation, the invention of fabulous stories.

See also ALCOHOLISM; BERIBERI.

western blot   See BLOTTING.

Wetzel Grid   Children are grouped by physique into five groups, ranging from tall and thin to short and thick-set. A healthy child will grow, as measured by height and weight, along one of these channels at a standard rate, if s/he deviates from the channel, malnutrition is suspected.

See also ANTHROPOMETRY; WEIGHT-FOR-AGE; WEIGHT-FOR-HEIGHT.

wey   Obsolete measure; 48 bushels of oats or 40 bushels of salt or corn.

wheat   The most important of the cereals and one of the most widely grown crops. Many thousand varieties are known but there are three main types: *Triticum vulgare*, used mainly for BREAD; TRITICUM DURUM (Durum wheat), largely used for PASTA; and *Triticum compactum* (club wheat), too soft for ordinary bread. The berry is composed of the outer branny husk, 13% of the grain, the germ or embryo (rich in nutrients) 2%, and the central endosperm (mainly starch) 85%.

See also FLOUR, EXTRACTION RATE; GERM, WHEAT.

wheatfeed   Also called millers' offal and wheat offals; by-product from milling of WHEAT, other than the GERM; bran of various particle sizes and varying amounts of attached endosperm.

wheatmeal, national   Name given to the 85% extraction flour (see FLOUR, EXTRACTION RATE) when introduced in UK in February 1941; later called national flour. The term is now obsolete and replaced by 'brown'.

whelks   SHELLFISH; several types of spiral-shelled marine MOLLUSCS, *Buccinum undatum, Fusus antiquus.*

Composition /100 g: 58 kJ (14 kcal), protein 2.8 g, fat 0.3 g, cholesterol 19 mg, carbohydrate 0 g, Na 40 mg, K 47 mg, Ca 8 mg, Mg 24 mg, P 34 mg, Fe 0.9 mg, Cu 1.1 mg, Zn 1.1 mg, vitamin E 0.1 mg, B_1 0.01 mg, B_2 0.03 mg, niacin 0.8 mg, B_6 0.01 mg, B_{12} 3.1 µg. A 200 g serving (weighed with shells) is a source of protein, Mg, Fe, Zn; rich source of vitamin B_{12}, Cu.

whey   The residue from milk after removal of the casein and most of the fat (as in cheese-making); also known as lactoserum. Contains about 1% protein (lactalbumin and lactoglobulin) together with all the lactose, water-soluble vitamins and minerals, and therefore has some food value, although it is 92% water.

Whey cheese can be made by heat coagulation of the protein and whey butter from the small amount of fat (0.25%). Dried whey is added to processed cheese; most whey is fed in liquid form to pigs.

Whipple's disease   Rare GENETIC DISEASE occurring only in males, in which intestinal absorption is impaired, accompanied by skin pigmentation and arthritis.

whipworm   Whip-like nematode worm (*Trichuris trichiura* or *Trichocephalus dispar*) parasitic in the large intestine.

whiskey, whisky   A grain SPIRIT distilled from BARLEY, RYE, MAIZE or other cereal which has first been malted (see MALT) and then fermented. Most brands of whisky are a blend of malt whisky with spirit distilled from grain. The distilled spirit is diluted to about 62% alcohol and matured in wooden casks; Irish and Scotch whisky, made from malted barley, are matured for at least three years. Bourbon, made from malted maize, for at least one year. Sour mash bourbon is made from mash that has yeast left in it from a previous fermentation. Other American and Canadian whiskies are made from rye.

Diluted after maturation and generally around 40% ALCOHOL by volume, 920 kJ (220 kcal) /100 mL.

Both spellings permitted but generally whisky is the Scotch variety and whiskey the Irish and American varieties. Name derived from the Gaelic *uisge beatha*, water of life.

whitebait   Traditionally a mixture of young HERRINGS and SPRATS (fresh or frozen); they are caught together and are impossible to separate on a commercial scale.

Composition /100 g floured and fried: 2197 kJ (525 kcal), protein 19.5 g, fat 47.5 g, carbohydrate 5.3 g (0.1 g sugars, 5.2 g starch), dietary fibre 0.2 g, nsp 0.2 g, Na 230 mg, K 110 mg, Ca 860 mg, Mg 50 mg, P 860 mg, Fe 5.1 mg. An 80 g serving is a source of Mg, a good source of Fe; rich source of protein, Ca.

white blood cells See LEUCOCYTES.

white foots Fine white precipitate of calcium and other salts deposited in jars of meat cured with rock salt.

white pudding Sausage made from white meat (chicken, rabbit, pork), cereal and spices. The French version, *boudin blanc*, includes eggs and onions. Irish white pudding is made from flake or leaf lard and oatmeal, spiced; served sliced and fried.

white spirits Distilled SPIRITS from fermented fruit; *eau de vie* or *alcool blanc* in French, *schnapps* in German.

whiting White FISH, *Merlangius merlangus*.

Composition /100 g: 339 kJ (81 kcal), protein 18.7 g, fat 0.7 g, cholesterol 46 mg, carbohydrate 0 g, Na 90 mg, K 330 mg, Ca 18 mg, Mg 22 mg, P 170 mg, Fe 0.1 mg, Cu 0.01 mg, Zn 0.4 mg, Se 21 µg, I 67 µg, vitamin B_1 0.05 mg, B_2 0.26 mg, niacin 5.2 mg, B_6 0.17 mg, pantothenate 0.3 mg, biotin 1 µg. A 150 g serving is a source of vitamin B_6, Mg; good source of vitamin B_2; rich source of protein, niacin, I, Se.

wholefoods Foods that have been minimally refined or processed, and are eaten in their natural state. In general nothing is removed from, or added to, the foodstuffs in preparation. Wholegrain cereal products are made by milling the complete grain.

wholesome Description applied to food that is hygienically fit for human consumption.

wholewheat meal Flour or meal prepared by milling the whole wheat grain, i.e. 100% extraction rate. See FLOUR, EXTRACTION RATE.

whortleberry See BILBERRY.

Wilson's disease Inborn error of metabolism (deficiency of caeruloplasmin) affecting COPPER metabolism, leading to accumulation of copper in liver and brain. Also known as hepatolenticular degeneration.

windberry See BILBERRY.

wine Fermented juice from grapes (varieties of *Vitis vinifera*), also made with other fruits and even vegetables with the addition of sugar. Red wines are made by fermenting the juice together with the skins at 21–29°C; white wines normally from white grapes by fermenting the juice alone at 15–17°C; rosé by removing the skins after 12–36 h, or by mixing red and white wines.

Beverages made by fermenting other fruit juices and sugar in the presence of vegetables or leaves or roots are also called wines (elderberry, elder flower, parsnip, peapod, rhubarb etc), although the legal definition may be restricted to the fermented grape. See also ALCOHOLIC BEVERAGES.

Wines generally contain 9–14% alcohol, dry wines 290 kJ (70 kcal), sweet wines 500 kJ (120 kcal), and about 1 mg iron /100 mL; only traces of vitamins.

wine, apéritif Slightly bitter-tasting fortified wines drunk before meals, VERMOUTH, including (trade names) Amer Picon, Bonal, Byrrh, Campari, Dubonnet, Fernet-Branca, Martini, Saint Raphaël. Made from red or white wine fortified with spirit and flavoured with herbs and quinine. 15–25% alcohol by volume, 5–10% sugars, 75–130 kcal (320–550 kJ) per 100 mL.

wineberry Orange coloured fruit of the Japanese and Chinese wild raspberry, *Rubus phoenicolasius*, and now also hybrids with European cultivated raspberries.

wine, British Made in Great Britain from imported grape juice or concentrated grape juice, as distinct from English wine, which is made from grapes grown in England.

wine classification Many of the major wine producing countries have legally enforced systems of classification of wines based on grape varieties used and regions of production. Other countries have a system of denomination of origin for wines grown in defined regions which may or may not reflect quality. The national classifications are as follows (in increasing order of quality for each country).

Austria: As for Germany, with an additional classification of QmP wines, ausbruch, intermediate in sweetness between beerenauslese and trockenbeerenauslese.

Bulgaria: Three grades: wines of declared variety of brand; wine of declared geographical origin (DGO); controliran, which are specific varieties grown in specific areas. The best of DGO and controliran wines can be offered as reserve, and in exceptional years as special reserve.

France: Vin de table (or vin ordinaire); vin de pays (subdivided into vin de pays de zone for wines from a single area; départementaux for wines from one département; régionaux for wines from more than one département); vin délimité de qualité supérieure (VDQS); appellation contrôlée (AC) or appellation d'origine contrôlée (AOC) for wines from a specified area, from specified grape varieties grown under controlled conditions.

Germany: Tafelwein (Deutscher Tafelwein is of German origin; wine labelled simply as Tafelwein may be of mixed origin); Landwein (dry or half-dry wines from one of 15 designated areas); Qualitätswein bestimmer Anbaugebeite, QbA (from 11 designated areas and approved grape varieties, sugar may be added to increase sweetness, each bottle carries a batch number (*Amtliche Prüfungsnummer*, AP), as proof that it complies with QbA status); Qualitätswein mit Prädikat, QmP (with six quality gradings based on the level of natural sugar at harvest and extra sugar may not be added: kabinett, light, fruity and delicate, usually dry; spätlese, late picked grapes, dry to sweet; auslese, selected late picked grapes, rich and sweet; beerenauslese, late picked grapes affected by 'NOBLE ROT', always sweet; trockenbeerenauslese, late picked grapes that have dried to raisins on the vine, strong and sweet; eiswein, rare, made from grapes that have frozen on the vine, very sweet.

Italy: Vini de tavola (Vdt); vini di tavola con indicazione geografica (from a particular area); vini tipici (equivalent to French vin de pays); denominazione di origine controllata (DOC, from specified areas and grape varieties); denominazione di origine controllata e garantita (DOCG, as DOC but with more stringent regulations and control).

Luxembourg: Appellation Contrôlée wines must carry a vintage; bottles carry a neck label awarded by the state controlled Marque Nationale after tasting, according to the strength of the wine; in order of increasing alcohol content the grades are: non admis, marque nationale, vin classé, premier cru, grand premier cru.

Portugal: Indicação de proveniencia regulamentada (IPR); região demarcada (RD, the same as appellation contrôlée). Table wines are vinho de mesa, wines aged more than 1 year are vinho maduro.

South Africa: Classification by variety of grape and area of production; coloured seals used as: blue band indicates that origin is certified; red band guarantees vintage year; green band certifies grape varieties; 'estate' certifies that it is from one estate; 'superior' on gold seal indicates superior quality. Wines also carry identification numbers to testify that controls have been adhered to during production.

Spain: Vinos de la tierra (two thirds of the grapes must come from the region named on the label); denominacion de origen (DO).

USA: Each state has its own appellation of origin; in addition *American wine* or *vin de table* is blended wine from one or more areas; multistate appellation is wine from two or three neighbouring states (the percentage from each must be shown on the label); for State and County appellation at least 75% must come from the designated area. *Approved viticultural areas* must have defined boundaries, specific characteristics and a proven reputation for quality; 85% of the grapes used must come from the defined area; when an individual vineyard is named, 95% of the grapes must have been grown there. For tax purposes a table wine must be between 10–14% alcohol, stronger wines are classified as dessert wines, even if dry; dessert wines between 17–21% alcohol are classified by alcoholic strength, not sweetness. US Wines may be sold by a generic classification (e.g. Chablis or Loire); such names are prohibited from export to the EU.

wine, fortified   Made by adding BRANDY or SPIRITS to increase the ALCOHOL content of the wine to 15–18% and so prevent further fermentation (to acids) in warm climates, e.g. MADEIRA, marsala, PORT, SHERRY.

wine, sparkling   Wine containing bubbles of carbon dioxide, bottled under pressure. Three methods of production:

(1) The méthode champenoise in which the wine undergoes a second fermentation in the bottle. Wine produced outside the Champagne region of France may not be called champagne, even if made by this method.

(2) The tank or bulk method, in which the wine is bottled while still fermenting slightly.

(3) The addition of carbon dioxide gas while bottling. Lightly sparkling wines are known as pétillante or frizzante; they are often young wines, bottled while still fermenting.

wine, sweetness   The UK Wine Promotion Board classifies white and rosé wines from 1 for very dry wines (0.6% sugars) to 9 (very sweet, 6% sugars).

For red wines the classification is from A (light and dry) to E (full-bodied heavy wines).

German and Austrian labelling is: trocken (dry), halbtrocken (half dry), halbsüss or lieben (medium sweet) and süss (very sweet).

winkle (periwinkle)   Small snail-like, marine MOLLUSCS, *Littorina littorea*.

Composition /100 g: 58 kJ (14 kcal), protein 2.9 g, fat 0.3 g, cholesterol 20 mg, carbohydrate 0 g, Na 220 mg, K 29 mg, Ca 26 mg, Mg 68 mg, P 42 mg, Fe 2.9 mg, Cu 0.25 mg, Zn 1.1 mg, vitamin B_1 0.05 mg, B_2 0.07 mg, niacin 0.9 mg, B_6 0.02 mg, B_{12} 6.9 µg, pantothenate 0.1 mg, biotin 1 µg. A 100 g serving (weighed with shells) is a good source of Mg, Fe; rich source of vitamin B_{12}, Cu.

winter berry   Fruit of the American evergreen shrub *Gaultheria* *procumbens*, red, with a spicy flavour; used mainly for pies and sauces.

winterisation Process involving slow cooling of oils and removal of the precipitated fats which have a relatively high melting point, so that the final product remains clear when refrigerated.

wisdom teeth Third molar tooth on each side of both jaws; usually erupt around age 20.

witches' milk Secretion of the mammary gland of the newborn of both sexes, due to the presence of the hormone prolactin which travels from the blood of the mother into the fetus. Also known as sorcerers' milk.

witchetty grubs Australian edible grubs, species of longicorn beetle (*Xylentes* spp).

witloof See CHICORY.

wok Chinese vessel for STIR FRYING; a shallow bowl-shaped pan in which food can be fried rapidly in a small amount of oil over a high heat.

wood alcohol See METHANOL.

wood sugar See XYLOSE.

wool green S A green COLOUR, Green S (E-142).

Worcestershire sauce Characterised by spicy flavour, sediment and thin supernatant liquid. Recipes usually secret but basically soya, tamarinds, anchovies, garlic and spices, plus sugar, salt and vinegar, matured 6 months in oak casks.

work See ENERGY.

wort Aqueous extract of MALT in brewing. See BEER.

wraplings See WUNTUN.

wuntun (wonton) Chinese; small dough parcels containing meat, boiled or deep fried. Also known as chiao-tzu or wraplings.

X

xanthaemia See CAROTINAEMIA.

xanthan gum Complex polymer made by bacterial fermentation; stable to wide range of pH and temperatures; used as thickening agent to form gels, increase viscosity in foods.

xanthelasma Yellow plaques around the eyelids. Common in elderly people; in younger people may be a sign of HYPERLIPIDAEMIA.

xanthine A PURINE, intermediate in the metabolism of adenine and guanine to URIC ACID. CAFFEINE (in coffee and tea) is 1,3,7-trimethylxanthine; THEOPHYLLINE (in tea) is 1,3-dimethylxanthine; THEOBROMINE (in cocoa) is 3,7-dimethylxanthine.

xanthoma Yellow skin lesion associated with disorders of lipid metabolism, and especially HYPERLIPIDAEMIA.

xanthophylls Hydroxylated CAROTENOIDS. Occur in all green leaves together with CHLOROPHYLL and CAROTENE, also present in egg yolk, CAPE GOOSEBERRY, etc. Most have no VITAMIN A activity. Include flavoxanthin (E-161a), lutein (161b), cryptoxanthin (E-161c, is vitamin A precursor), rubixanthin (161e), rhodoxanthin (161f), canthaxanthin (161g).

xanthoproteic reaction Test for proteins (actually for the aromatic rings of PHENYLALANINE, TYROSINE and TRYPTOPHAN). Yellow colour on boiling with nitric acid, turns orange on adding ammonia.

Xenical See ORLISTAT.

xenobiotic Substances foreign to the body, including drugs and some food additives.

xerophilic See OSMOPHILES.

xerophthalmia Advanced VITAMIN A deficiency in which the epithelium of the cornea and conjunctiva of the eye deteriorates because of impairment of the tear glands, resulting in dryness then ulceration, leading to blindness.

xerosis Abnormal dryness of conjunctiva, skin or mucous membranes.

xerostomia Dry mouth, a common side effect of a variety of drugs.

See also PTYALISM.

X-ray diffraction Technique for determination of crystal structures (e.g. of proteins) by analysis of the diffraction pattern of a beam of X-rays shone through the crystal.

xylanase Mixture of enzymes of fungal or bacterial origin that hydrolyse XYLANS: β-1,4-endoxylanase (EC 3.2.1.8) and β-D-xylosidase (EC 3.2.1.32). Sometimes added to poultry and pig feed to increase the digestibility of cereal NON-STARCH POLYSACCHARIDES.

xylans Polysaccharides of XYLOSE, not digested, part of NON-STARCH POLYSACCHARIDE.

xylitol A five-carbon SUGAR ALCOHOL found in raspberries, endive, lettuce; 80–100% of the sweetness of sucrose; used in sugar-free hard sweets and gelatine gums. Apart from being of low cariogenicity, xylitol is said to have an effect in suppressing the growth of some of the bacteria associated with dental CARIES. See TOOTH-FRIENDLY SWEETS.

xyloascorbic acid Term used to distinguish VITAMIN C (ASCORBIC ACID) from isoascorbic acid (ERYTHORBIC ACID), which is araboascorbic acid and has only slight vitamin C activity.

xyloglucan One of the hemicelluloses in plant cell walls, linking CELLULOSE fibres.

See also NON-STARCH POLYSACCHARIDE.

xylose   Pentose (five-carbon) sugar found in plant tissues mainly as polysaccharides (XYLANS); 40% as sweet as sucrose. Also known as wood sugar. Mainly excreted unmetabolised, and used to test carbohydrate absorption.

Y

YAC   Yeast artificial chromosome, a specialised cloning vector that can carry large DNA inserts.

yam   Tubers of perennial climbing plants of a number of species of *Dioscorea, D. rotundala* white yam, and *D. cayenensis*, yellow or Guinea yam, water, trifoliate or Chinese yam. A major food in parts of Africa and also the Far East. In USA sweet POTATOES (see POTATO, SWEET) are sometimes called yam.

Composition/100 g: 556 kJ (133 kcal), protein 1.7 g, fat 0.3 g, carbohydrate 33 g (0.7 g sugars, 32.3 g starch), dietary fibre 3.5 g, nsp 1.4 g, Na 17 mg, K 260 mg, Ca 12 mg, Mg 12 mg, P 21 mg, Fe 0.4 mg, Cu 0.03 mg, Zn 0.4 mg, vitamin B_1 0.14 mg, B_2 0.01 mg, niacin 0.6 mg, B_6 0.12 mg, folate 6 µg, pantothenate 0.3 mg, C 4 mg. A 130 g serving is a source of vitamin B_1.

yang   See MACROBIOTIC DIET.

Yarmouth bloater   See RED HERRINGS.

yautia   See TANNIA.

yeast   Unicellular organisms, grouped with the fungi; eukaryotic organisms with more complex subcellular organisation than BACTERIA. Some types are of major importance in the food industry. *Saccharomyces cerevisiae* and *S. carlsbergensis* are used in brewing, wine-making and baking.

Yeasts such as *Candida utilis* (formerly *Torula utilis*) are grown on carbohydrate or hydrocarbon media as animal feed and potential human food, since they contain about 50% protein (dry weight) and are very rich in B vitamins.

Some yeasts are pathogenic (especially *Candida* spp, which cause thrush); many are used in biotechnology for production of human hormones (see HORMONES, HUMAN) and other proteins.

yeast extract   A preparation of the water-soluble fraction of autolysed brewers' YEAST, valuable both as a source of B vitamins and for its strong savoury flavour. Commercial preparations include Marmite, Yeastrel, Yeatrex, Vegemite, used as a drink or a breadspread.

Composition/100 g: 719 kJ (172 kcal), protein 39.7 g, fat 0.7 g, carbohydrate 1.8 g (1.8 g starch), Na 4500 mg, K 2600 mg, Ca 95 mg, Mg 180 mg, P 1700 mg, Fe 3.7 mg, Cu 0.3 mg, Zn 2.1 mg, I 49 µg, vitamin B_1 3.1 mg, B_2 11 mg, niacin 67 mg, B_6 1.3 mg, folate

$1010\,\mu g$, B_{12} $0.5\,\mu g$. A $4\,g$ serving is a source of niacin; good source of vitamin B_2, folate.

yeast fermentation, bottom Or deep fermentation; fermentation during the manufacture of BEER with a yeast that sinks to the bottom of the tank. Most beers are produced this way; ale, porter and stout being the principal beers produced by top fermentation.

Yeastrel, Yeatex Trade names for YEAST EXTRACT.

yellow fats See FAT SPREAD.

yerba dulce The leaves of the Paraguayan shrub, *Stevia rebaudiana*, the source of STEVIOSIDE and REBAUDIOSIDE.

yerba maté See MATÉ.

Yersinia enterocolitica Food poisoning organism that invades intestinal epithelial cells. Infective dose 10^6–10^7 organisms; onset 3–5 days; duration weeks; TX 4.1.3.1.

Yestamin Trade name for a variety of preparations of dried *Saccharomyces* YEAST (debittered brewers' yeast) used to enrich foods.

yin See MACROBIOTIC DIET.

yogurt Milk (from a variety of animals but usually cows) coagulated and fermented with two types of bacteria, *Streptococcus thermophilus* and *Lactobacillus bulgaricus*; may be stirred or set. The two organisms are symbiotic; each produces compounds that promote the growth of the other. Both act to precipitate and gel proteins; main flavour development is from the slower formation of D-lactic acid by *L. bulgaricus*, although *S. thermophilus* has a greater capacity to metabolise LACTOSE to L-lactate.

May be pasteurised, when most of the bacteria are destroyed, otherwise termed live yogurt. Bioyogurts also contain *Lactobacillus acidophilus* (see ACIDOPHILUS MILK) and *Bifidobacterium bifidum*, which are claimed to enhance the growth of beneficial bacteria in the intestine.

See also MILK, FERMENTED.

Composition/100 g full cream plain: 330 kJ (79 kcal), protein 5.7 g, fat 3 g (60.7% saturated, 32.1% mono-, 7.1% polyunsaturated), cholesterol 11 mg, carbohydrate 7.8 g (7.8 g sugars); full cream fruit: 439 kJ (105 kcal), protein 5.1 g, fat 2.8 g (60% saturated, 32% mono-, 8% polyunsaturated), cholesterol 10 mg, carbohydrate 15.7 g (15.7 g sugars); low fat plain: 234 kJ (56 kcal), protein 5.1 g, fat 0.8, cholesterol 4 mg, carbohydrate 7.5 g (7.5 g sugars); low fat flavoured: 376 kJ (90 kcal), protein 3.8 g, fat 0.9, cholesterol 4 mg, carbohydrate 17.9 g (17.9 g sugars).

Composition/100 g Greek cow's milk: 481 kJ (115 kcal), protein 6.4 g, fat 9.1 g (61.9% saturated, 32.1% mono-, 5.9% polyunsaturated), carbohydrate 2 g (2 g sugars); Greek sheep milk: 443 kJ

(106 kcal), protein 4.4 g, fat 7.5 g (67.6% saturated, 26.7% mono-, 5.6% polyunsaturated), cholesterol 14 mg, carbohydrate 5.6 g (5.6 g sugars); Na 80–150 mg, K 190–280 mg, Ca 150–200 mg, Mg 16–19 mg, P 130–170 mg, Fe 0.1–0.3 mg, Zn 0.5–0.7 mg, Se 2 μg, I 63 μg, vitamin A 31 μg (21 μg carotene), D 0.04 μg, E 0.1 mg, B_1 0.06 mg, B_2 0.27 mg, niacin 1.5 mg, B_6 0.1 mg, folate 10–18 μg, B_{12} 0.2 μg, pantothenate 0.5 mg, biotin 2.6 μg, C 1 mg. A 60 g serving (small pot) a source of vitamin B_2, Ca; good source of I.

yolk index Index of freshness of an egg; ratio between height and diameter of yolk under defined conditions. As the egg deteriorates, the yolk index decreases.

youngberry Cross between BLACKBERRY and DEWBERRY.

Yusho disease Caused by leakage of polychlorinated biphenyls which contaminated edible oil on the Japanese island of Kyushu in 1968.

Z

zabaglione (zabaione) Italian; frothy dessert made from egg yolks, sugar and wine (usually marsala) whisked over gentle heat until thick. French sabayon is similar.

zearalenone See MYCOTOXINS.

zeaxanthin One of the carotenoid pigments in maize, egg yolk and *Physalis* (CAPE GOOSEBERRY); has no vitamin A activity; used as a colouring.

zébrine Variety of AUBERGINE with purple and white stripes.

zedoary root Root of the Indian plant *Curcuma zedoaria*, a member of the ginger family. Used in the manufacture of flavours and BITTERS.

zein A PROLAMIN, the major protein of MAIZE (*Zea mays*), very poor in lysine and tryptophan.

Z-enzyme enzyme (β-1,3-glucosidase, EC 3.2.1.58) found associated with AMYLASES, that hydrolyses the few β-1,3-links present in AMYLOSE. Pure, crystalline β-amylase will convert only 70% of amylose to maltose; it requires the presence of the Z-enzyme for complete conversion.

Zeocarb An ION-EXCHANGE RESIN.

zest Outer skin of citrus fruits. See FLAVEDO.

zinc An essential mineral which forms the PROSTHETIC GROUP of a large number of enzymes, and the receptor proteins for STEROID and THYROID HORMONES and VITAMINS A and D. Deficiency results in hypogonadism and delayed puberty, small stature and mild anaemia; it occurs mainly in subtropical regions where a great deal of zinc is lost in sweat, and the diet is largely based on unleavened wholemeal bread, in which much of the zinc is unavailable because of the high content of PHYTATE. Intestinal absorption of zinc requires an (as yet unidentified) organic zinc binding ligand secreted in pancreatic juice. Deficiency may also lead to functional vitamin A deficiency because of impaired synthesis of RETINOL BINDING PROTEIN.

zitoni   See PASTA.

zizanie   See RICE, WILD.

Zollinger–Ellison syndrome   Excessive secretion of gastric acid due to high levels of circulating GASTRIN secreted by a pancreatic tumour.

zomotherapy   Treatment of convalescents with raw meat or meat juice, long since discontinued.

zoopherin   Obsolete name for VITAMIN B_{12}.

zooplankton   See PLANKTON.

zucchini   Italian variety of MARROW developed to be harvested when small. American and Australian name for COURGETTE.

Zucker rat   A genetically obese strain of rat used in research.

z-value   See DECIMAL REDUCTION TIME.

zwieback   German; twice-baked bread or rusk.

zwitterion   An ionised molecule with both positive and negative charges, e.g. the AMINO ACIDS.

zymase   The mixture of enzymes in YEAST which is responsible for FERMENTATION.

zymogens   The inactive form in which some enzymes, especially the PROTEIN digestive enzymes, are secreted, being activated after secretion. Also called proenzymes, or enzyme precursors.

zymotachygraph   An instrument that measures the gas produced in a fermenting dough and the amount escaping from the dough, as an index of breadmaking properties.

Appendix

Table 1 Units of physical quantities and multiples and submultiples of units

Physical quantity	Unit	Symbol	Definition
Amount of substance	mole	mol	SI base unit
Electric charge	coulomb	C	sA
Electric conductance	siemens	S	AV^{-1}
Electric current	ampere	A	SI base unit
Electric potential difference	volt	V	$JA^{-1}s^{-1}$
Electric resistance	ohm	Ω	VA^{-1}
Electrical capacitance	farad	F	AsV^{-1}
Energy	joule	J	$m^2 kg s^{-1}$
	calorie	cal	$4.186J$
Force	newton	N	Jm^{-1}
Frequency	hertz	Hz	s^{-1}
Illuminance	lux	lx	$cd\,sr\,m^{-2}$
Length	metre	m	SI base unit
Length	ångstrom	Å	$10^{-10}m$
Luminous flux	lumen	lm	$cd\,sr$
Luminous intensity	candela	cd	SI base unit
Magnetic flux	weber	Wb	Vs
Magnetic flux density	tesla	T	$Vs\,m^{-2}$
Mass	kilogram	kg	SI base unit
Plane angle	radian	rad	SI base unit
Power	watt	W	Js^{-1}
Pressure	pascal	Pa	Nm^{-2}
	bar	bar	$10^5 Pa$
Radiation dose absorbed	gray	Gy	Jkg^{-1}
Radioactivity	becquerel	Bq	s^{-1}
Solid angle	steradian	sr	SI base unit
Temperature	degree Celsius	°C	thermodynamic temperature $-273.15K$
Temperature (thermodynamic)	kelvin	K	SI base unit
Time	second	s	SI base unit
Volume	litre (cubic decimetre)	L (dm³)	$10^{-3}m^3$

	Name	Symbol		Name	Symbol
$\times10^{21}$	zetta	Z	$\times10^{-1}$	deci	d
$\times10^{18}$	exa	E	$\times10^{-2}$	centi	c
$\times10^{15}$	peta	P	$\times10^{-3}$	milli	m
$\times10^{12}$	tera	T	$\times10^{-6}$	micro	μ (or mc)
$\times10^{9}$	giga	G	$\times10^{-9}$	nano	n
$\times10^{6}$	mega	M	$\times10^{-12}$	pico	p
$\times10^{3}$	kilo	k	$\times10^{-15}$	femto	f
$\times10^{2}$	centa	ca	$\times10^{-18}$	atto	a
$\times10$	deca	da	$\times10^{-21}$	zepto	z

Table 2 Labelling reference values for foods

	USA	European Union	
	Reference daily intake	Proposed by Scientific Committee for Food, 1993	Required by EU Directive
Vitamin A, µg	1500	500	800
Vitamin D, µg	10	5	5
Vitamin E, mg	30	–	10
Vitamin C, mg	60	30	60
Thiamin, mg	1.5	0.8	1.4
Riboflavin, mg	1.7	1.3	1.6
Niacin, mg	20	15	18
Vitamin B_6, mg	2.0	1.3	2.0
Folate, µg	400	140	200
Vitamin B_{12}, µg	6.0	1.0	1.0
Biotin, µg	300	–	150
Pantothenic acid, mg	10	–	6
Calcium, mg	1000	550	800
Copper, mg	2.0	0.8	–
Iodine, µg	150	100	150
Iron, mg[a]	18	7, 14	14
Magnesium, mg	400	–	300
Phosphorus, mg	1000	–	800
Selenium, µg	–	40	–
Zinc, mg	15	7.5	15

[a] The Scientific Committee for Food proposed separate figures for iron for women (14 mg) and men (7 mg).

Table 3 US recommended daily amounts of nutrients, 1989, updated 1997, 1998

Age (months, m years, y)	Protein (g)	Vit A (μg)	Vit D (μg)	Vit E (mg)	Vit K (mg)	Vit C (mg)	Vit B₁ (mg)	Vit B₂ (mg)	Niacin (mg)	Vit B₆ (mg)
0–6 m	13	375	5*	3	5	30				
6–12 m	14	375	5*	4	10	35				
0–5 m							0.2*	0.3*	2*	0.1*
6–11 m							0.3*	0.4*	3*	0.3*
1–3 y	16	400	5*	6	15	40	0.5	0.5	6	0.5
4–8 y			5*				0.6	0.6	8	0.6
4–6 y	24	500		7	20	45				
7–10 y	28	700		7	30	45				
Males										
9–13 y			5*				0.9	0.9	12	1.0
14–18 y			5*				1.2	1.3	16	1.3
19–30 y			5*				1.2	1.3	16	1.3
31–50 y			5*				1.2	1.3	16	1.3
51–70 y			10*				1.2	1.3	16	1.7
>70 y			15*				1.2	1.3	16	1.7
11–14 y	45	1000		10	45	50				
15–18 y	59	1000		10	65	60				
19–24 y	58	1000		10	70	60				
25–50 y	63	1000		10	80	60				
51+ y	63	1000		10	80	60				

Females										
9–13y			5*				0.9	0.9	12	1.0
14–18y			5*				1.0	1.0	14	1.2
19–30y			5*				1.1	1.1	14	1.3
31–50y			5*				1.1	1.1	14	1.3
51–70y			10*				1.1	1.1	14	1.5
>70y			15*				1.1	1.1	14	1.5
11–14y	46	800		8	45	50				
15–18y	44	800		8	55	60				
19–24y	46	800		8	60	60				
25–50y	50	800		8	65	60				
51+y	50	800		8	65	60				
Pregnant	60	800	5*	10	65	70	1.4	1.4	18	1.9
Lactating	65	1300	5*	10	65	95	1.5	1.6	17	2.0

Table 3 (*continued*)

Age (months, m years, y)	Folate (µg)	Vit B_{12} (µg)	Pantothenate (mg)	Biotin (µg)	Choline (mg)	Ca (mg)	P (mg)	Mg (mg)	Fe (mg)	Zn (mg)	I (µg)	Se (µg)
0–6m						210*	100*	30*	6	5	40	10
6–12m						270*	275*	75*	10	5	50	15
0–5m	65*	0.4*	1.7*	5*	125*							
6–11m	80*	0.5*	1.8*	6*	150*							
1–3y	150	0.9	2*	8*	200*	500*	460	80	10	10	70	20
4–8y	200	1.2	3*	12*	250*	800*	500	130				
4–6y									10	10	90	20
7–10y									10	10	120	30
Males												
9–13y	300	1.8	4*	20*	375*	1300*	1250	240				
14–18y	400	2.4	5*	25*	550*	1300*	1250	410				
19–30y	400	2.4	5*	30*	550*	1000*	700	400				
31–50y	400	2.4	5*	30*	550*	1000*	700	420				
51–70y	400	2.4	5*	30*	550*	1200*	700	420				
>70y	400	2.4	5*	30*	550*	1200*	700	420				
11–14y									12	15	150	40
15–18y									12	15	150	50
19–24y									10	15	150	70
25–50y									10	15	150	70
51+y									10	15	150	70

	C1	C2	C3	C4	C5	C6	C7	C8	C9	C10	C11	C12
Females												
9–13y	300	1.8	4*	20*	375*	1300*	1250	240				
14–18y	400	2.4	5*	25*	400*	1300*	1250	360				
19–30y	400	2.4	5*	30*	435*	1000*	700	310				
31–50y	400	2.4	5*	30*	425*	1000*	700	320				
51–70y	400	2.4	5*	30*	425*	1200*	700	320				
>70y	400	2.4	5*	30*	425*	1200*	700	320				
11–14y									15	12	150	45
15–18y									15	12	150	50
19–24y									15	12	150	55
25–50y									15	12	150	55
50+y									10	12	150	55
Pregnant	600	2.6	6*	30*	450*	a1000*	a700	a360	30	15	175	65
Lactating	500	2.8	7*	35	550*	a1000*	a700	a310	15	19	200	75

* Starred values are adequate intakes, where there is insufficient evidence to establish RDAs.

a For pregnancy and lactation in women aged up to 18 the adequate intake for calcium is 1300 mg, RDA for phosphorus 1250 mg, RDA for magnesium 400 mg (pregnancy) and 360 mg (lactation).

Source: National Research Council / National Academy of Sciences 1989, Food and Nutrition Board, 1997, 1998.

Table 4 UK reference nutrient intakes, 1991

Age (months, m years, y)	Vit B₁ (mg)	Vit B₂ (mg)	Niacin (mg)	Vit B₆ (mg)	Vit B₁₂ (µg)	Folate (µg)	Vit C (mg)	Vit A (µg)	Vit D (µg)	Ca (mg)	P (mg)	Mg (mg)	Na (mg)	Fe (mg)	Zn (mg)	Cu (mg)	Se (µg)	I (µg)
0–3 m	0.2	0.4	3	0.2	0.3	50	25	350	8.5	525	400	55	210	1.7	4.0	0.2	10	50
4–6 m	0.2	0.4	3	0.2	0.3	50	25	350	8.5	525	400	60	280	4.3	4.0	0.3	13	60
7–9 m	0.2	0.4	4	0.3	0.4	50	25	350	7	525	400	75	320	7.8	5.0	0.3	10	60
10–12 m	0.3	0.4	5	0.4	0.4	50	25	350	7	525	400	80	350	7.8	5.0	0.3	10	60
1–3 y	0.5	0.6	8	0.7	0.5	70	30	400	7	350	270	85	500	6.9	5.0	0.4	15	70
4–6 y	0.7	0.8	11	0.9	0.8	100	30	500	–	450	350	120	700	6.1	6.5	0.6	20	100
7–10 y	0.7	1.0	12	1.0	1.0	150	30	500	–	550	450	200	1200	8.7	7.0	0.7	30	110
Males																		
11–14 y	0.9	1.2	15	1.2	1.2	200	35	600	–	1000	775	280	1600	11.3	9.0	0.8	45	130
15–18 y	1.1	1.3	18	1.5	1.5	200	40	700	–	1000	775	300	1600	11.3	9.5	1.0	70	140
19–50	1.0	1.3	17	1.4	1.5	200	40	700	–	700	550	300	1600	8.7	9.5	1.2	75	140
50+ y	0.9	1.3	16	1.4	1.5	200	40	700	10	700	550	300	1600	8.7	9.5	1.2	75	140
Females																		
11–14 y	0.7	1.1	12	1.0	1.2	200	35	600	–	800	625	280	1600	14.8	9.0	0.8	45	130
15–18 y	0.8	1.1	14	1.2	1.5	200	40	600	–	800	625	300	1600	14.8	7.0	1.0	60	140
19–50 y	0.8	1.1	13	1.2	1.5	200	40	600	–	700	550	270	1600	14.8	7.0	1.2	60	140
50+ y	0.8	1.1	12	1.2	1.5	200	40	600	10	700	550	270	1600	8.7	7.0	1.2	60	140
Pregnant	+0.1	+0.3	–	–	–	+100	+10	+100	10	–	–	–	–					
Lactating	+0.1	+0.5	+2	–	+0.5	+60	+30	+350	10	+550	+440	+50	–		+6.0	+0.3	+15	

Source: Department of Health 1991.

Table 5 EU population reference intakes of nutrients

Age (months, m years, y)	Protein (g)	Vit A (µg)	Vit B_1 (mg)	Vit B_2 (mg)	Niacin (mg)	Vit B_6 (mg)	Folate (µg)	Vit B_{12} (µg)	Vit C (mg)	Ca (mg)	P (mg)	Fe (mg)	Zn (mg)	Cu (mg)	Se (µg)	I (µg)
6–12 m	15	350	0.3	0.4	5	0.4	50	0.5	20	400	300	6	4	0.3	8	50
1–3 y	15	400	0.5	0.8	9	0.7	100	0.7	25	400	300	4	4	0.4	10	70
4–6 y	20	400	0.7	1.0	11	0.9	130	0.9	25	450	350	4	6	0.6	15	90
7–10 y	29	500	0.8	1.2	13	1.1	150	1.0	30	550	450	6	7	0.7	25	100
Males																
11–14 y	44	600	1.0	1.4	15	1.3	180	1.3	35	1000	775	10	9	0.8	35	120
15–17 y	55	700	1.2	1.6	18	1.5	200	1.4	40	1000	775	13	9	1.0	45	130
18+ y	56	700	1.1	1.6	18	1.5	200	1.4	45	700	550	9	9.5	1.1	55	130
Females																
11–14 y	42	600	0.9	1.2	14	1.1	180	1.3	35	800	625	18	9	0.8	35	120
15–17 y	46	600	0.9	1.3	14	1.1	200	1.4	40	800	625	17	7	1.0	45	130
18+ y	47	600	0.9	1.3	14	1.1	200	1.4	45	700	550	16[a]	7	1.1	55	130
Pregnant	57	700	1.0	1.6	14	1.3	400	1.6	55	700	550	[a]	7	1.1	55	130
Lactating	63	950	1.1	1.7	16	1.4	350	1.9	70	1200	950	16	12	1.4	70	160

[a] 8 mg iron postmenopausally; supplements required in latter half of pregnancy.

Table 6 Permitted food additives in the European Union (Those without the prefix E- are permitted in UK but not throughout the EU)

Colouring materials	*Used to make food more colourful and attractive, or to replace colour lost in processing*

Yellow and orange colours

E-100	Curcumin
E-101	Riboflavin, riboflavin phosphate (vitamin B_2)
E-102	Tartrazine (= FD&C Yellow no 6)
E-104	Quinoline yellow
107	Yellow 2G
E-110	Sunset yellow FCF or orange yellow S (= FD&C Yellow no 6)

Red colours

E-120	Cochineal or carminic acid
E-122	Carmoisine or azorubine
E-123	Amaranth
E-124	Ponceau 4R or cochineal red A
E-127	Erythrosine BS (= FD&C Red no 3)
E-128	Red 2G
E-129	Allura red (= FD&C Red no 40)

Blue colours

E-131	Patent blue V
E-132	Indigo carmine or indigotine (= FD&C Blue no 2)
E-133	Brilliant blue FCF (= FD&C Blue no 1)

Green colours

E-140	(i) Chlorophylls, the natural green colour of leaves (ii) chlorophyllins
E-141	Copper complexes of (i) chlorophylls, (ii) chlorophyllins
E-142	Green S or acid brilliant green BS

Brown and black colours

E-150a	Plain caramel (made from sugar in the kitchen)
E-150b	Caustic sulphite caramel
E-150c	Ammonia caramel
E150d	Sulphite ammonia caramel
E-151	Black PN or brilliant black BN
E-153	Carbon black or vegetable carbon (charcoal)
E-154	Brown FK
E-155	Brown HT (Chocolate brown HT)

Derivatives of carotene

E-160(a)	(i) Mixed carotenes, (ii) β-carotene
E-160(b)	Annatto, bixin, norbixin
E-160(c)	Paprika extract, capsanthin or capsorubin
E-160(d)	Lycopene
E-160(e)	β-Apo-8′-carotenal (vitamin A active)
E-160(f)	Ethyl ester of β-apo-8′-carotenoic acid

Other plant colours

E-161(a)	Flavoxanthin
E-161(b)	Lutein
E-161(c)	Cryptoxanthin

Table 6 (*continued*)

Colouring materials	Used to make food more colourful and attractive, or to replace colour lost in processing

E-161(d)	Rubixanthin
E-161(e)	Violaxanthin
E-161(f)	Rhodoxanthin
E-161(g)	Canthaxanthin
E-162	Beetroot red or betanin
E-163	Anthocyanins (the pigments of many plants)

Inorganic compounds used as colours

E-170	(i) Calcium carbonate (chalk), (ii) calcium hydrogen carbonate
E-171	Titanium dioxide
E-172	Iron oxides and hydroxides
E-173	Aluminium
E-174	Silver
E-175	Gold
E-180	Pigment rubine or lithol rubine BK

Preservatives	Compounds that protect foods against microbes that cause spoilage and food poisoning. They increase the safe storage life of foods

Sorbic acid and its salts

E-200	Sorbic acid
E-201	Sodium sorbate
E-202	Potassium sorbate
E-203	Calcium sorbate

Benzoic acid and its salts

E-210	Benzoic acid (occurs naturally in many fruits)
E-211	Sodium benzoate
E-212	Potassium benzoate
E-213	Calcium benzoate
E-214	Ethyl *p*-hydroxybenzoate
E-215	Ethyl *p*-hydroxybenzoate sodium salt
E-216	Propyl *p*-hydroxybenzoate
E-217	Propyl *p*-hydroxybenzoate sodium salt
E-218	Methyl *p*-hydroxybenzoate
E-219	Methyl *p*-hydroxybenzoate sodium salt

Sulphur dioxide and its salts

E-220	Sulphur dioxide (also used to prevent browning of raw peeled potatoes)
E-221	Sodium sulphite
E-222	Sodium hydrogen sulphite
E-223	Sodium metabisulphite
E-224	Potassium metabisulphite
E-226	Calcium sulphite
E-227	Calcium hydrogen sulphite
E-228	Potassium hydrogen sulphite

454

Table 6 (*continued*)

Preservatives	*Compounds that protect foods against microbes that cause spoilage and food poisoning. They increase the safe storage life of foods*

Biphenyl and its derivatives

E-230	Biphenyl or diphenyl (for surface treatment of citrus fruits)
E-231	Orthophenylphenol (2-Hydroxybiphenyl) (for surface treatment of citrus fruits)
E-232	Sodium orthophenylphenol (sodium biphenyl-2-yl oxide)

Other preservatives

E-233	2-(Thiazol-4-yl) benzimidazole (thiobendazole) (for surface treatment of citrus fruits and bananas)
E-234	Nisin
E-235	Natamycin (NATA) (for surface treatment of cheeses and dried cured sausages)
E-239	Hexamethylene tetramine (hexamine)
E-242	Dimethyl dicarbonate
E-912	Montan acid esters (for surface treatment of citrus fruits)
E-914	Oxidized polyethylene wax (for surface treatment of citrus fruits)

Pickling salts

E-249	Potassium nitrite
E-250	Sodium nitrite
E-251	Sodium nitrate
E-252	Potassium nitrate (saltpetre)

Acids and their salts	*Used as flavourings and as buffers to control the acidity of foods, in addition to their antimicrobial properties*

E-260	Acetic acid
E-261	Potassium acetate
E-262	(i) Sodium acetate, (ii) sodium hydrogen acetate (sodium diacetate)
E-263	Calcium acetate
E-270	Lactic acid
E-280	Propionic acid
E-281	Sodium propionate
E-282	Calcium propionate
E-283	Potassium propionate
E-284	Boric acid (as preservative in caviare)
E-285	Sodium tetraborate (borax) (as preservative in caviare)
E-290	Carbon dioxide
E-296	Malic acid
E-297	Fumaric acid

Table 6 (*continued*)

Antioxidants	*Compounds used to prevent fatty foods going rancid, and to protect fat-soluble vitamins (A, D, E and K) against the damaging effects of oxidation*

Vitamin C and derivatives
E-300	L-Ascorbic acid (vitamin C)
E-301	Sodium-L-ascorbate
E-302	Calcium-L-ascorbate
E-304	(i) Ascorbyl palmitate, (ii) ascorbyl stearate
E-315	Erythorbic acid (*iso*-ascorbic acid)
E-316	Sodium erythorbate (sodium *iso*-ascorbate)

Vitamin E
E-306	Natural extracts rich in tocopherols
E-307	Synthetic α-tocopherol
E-308	Synthetic γ-tocopherol
E-309	Synthetic δ-tocopherol

Other antioxidants
E-310	Propyl gallate
E-311	Octyl gallate
E-312	Dodecyl gallate
E-320	Butylated hydroxyanisole (BHA)
E-321	Butylated hydroxytoluene (BHT)
E-322	Lecithins

More acids and their salts	*Used as flavourings and as buffers to control the acidity of foods, in addition to other special uses*

Salts of lactic acid (E270)
E-325	Sodium lactate
E-326	Potassium lactate
E-327	Calcium lactate
E-585	Ferrous lactate

Citric acid, its salts and esters
E-330	Citric acid (formed in the body, and present in many fruits)
E-331	(i) Monosodium citrate, (ii) disodium citrate, (iii) trisodium citrate
E-332	(i) Monopotassium citrate, (ii) dipotassium citrate, (iii) tripotassium citrate
E-333	(i) Monocalcium citrate, (ii) dicalcium citrate, (iii) tricalcium citrate
E-1505	Triethyl citrate

Tartaric acid and its salts
| E-334 | L(+)Tartaric acid (tartaric acid occurs naturally; as well as their properties as acids, tartrates are often used as sequestrants and emulsifying agents) |

Table 6 (*continued*)

More acids and their salts	*Used as flavourings and as buffers to control the acidity of foods, in addition to other special uses*
E-335	(i) Monosodium tartrate, (ii) disodium tartrate
E-336	(i) Monopotassium tartrate (cream of tartar), (ii) dipotassium tartrate
E-337	Sodium potassium tartrate

Phosphoric acid and its salts

E-338	Phosphoric acid
E-339	(i) Monosodium phosphate, (ii) disodium phosphate, (iii) trisodium phosphate
E-340	(i) Monopotassium phosphate, (ii) dipotassium phosphate, (iii) tripotassium phosphate
E-341	(i) Monocalcium phosphate, (ii) dicalcium phosphate, (iii) tricalcium phosphate
E-450	Diphosphates: (i) disodium diphosphate, (ii) trisodium diphosphate, (iii) tetrasodium diphosphate, (iv) dipotassium diphosphate, (v) tetrapotassium diphosphate, (vi) dicalcium diphosphate, (vii) calcium dihydrogen diphosphate
E-451	Triphosphates: (i) pentasodium triphosphate, (ii) pentapotassium triphosphate
E-452	Polyphosphates: (i) sodium polyphosphate, (ii) potassium polyphosphate, (iii) sodium calcium polyphosphate, (iv) calcium polyphosphate
E-540	Dicalcium diphosphate
E-541	Sodium aluminium phosphate, acidic
E-542	Edible bone phosphates (bone meal, used as anticaking agent)
E-544	Calcium polyphosphates (used as anticaking agent)
E-545	Ammonium polyphosphates (used as anticaking agent)

Salts of malic acid (E-296)

E-350	Sodium malate
E-351	Potassium malate
E-352	Calcium malate

Other acids and their salts

E-353	Metatartaric acid
E-354	Calcium tartrate
E-355	Adipic acid
E-356	Sodium adipate
E-357	Potassium adipate
E-363	Succinic acid
E-370	1,4-Heptonolactone
E-375	Nicotinic acid
E-380	Triammonium citrate
E-381	Ammonium ferric citrate
E-385	Calcium disodium EDTA

Table 6 (*continued*)

Emulsifiers and stabilisers	*Used to enable oils and fats to mix with water, to give a smooth and creamy texture to food, and slow the staling of baked goods. Many of these compounds are also used to make jellies.*

Alginates
E-400	Alginic acid (derived from seaweed)
E-401	Sodium alginate
E-402	Potassium alginate
E-403	Ammonium alginate
E-404	Calcium alginate
E-405	Propane-1,2-diol alginate

Other plant gums
E-406	Agar (derived from seaweed)
E-407	Carrageenan (derived from the seaweed Irish moss)
E-410	Locust bean gum (carob gum)
E-412	Guar gum
E-413	Tragacanth
E-414	Gum acacia (gum Arabic)
E-415	Xanthan gum
E-416	Karaya gum
E-417	Tara gums
E-418	Gellan gums

Fatty acid derivatives
E-430	Polyoxyethylene (8) stearate
E-431	Polyoxyethylene (40) stearate
E-432	Polyoxyethylene (20) sorbitan monolaurate (Polysorbate 20)
E-433	Polyoxyethylene (20) sorbitan mono-oleate (Polysorbate 80)
E-434	Polyoxyethylene (20) sorbitan monopalmitate (Polysorbate 40)
E-435	Polyoxyethylene (20) sorbitan monostearate (Polysorbate 60)
E-436	Polyoxyethylene (20) sorbitan tristearate (Polysorbate 65)

Pectin and derivatives
E-440	(i) Pectin, (ii) Amidated pectin (pectin occurs in many fruits, and is often added to jam to help it set)

Other compounds
E-322	Lecithins
E-442	Ammonium phosphatides
E-444	Sucrose acetate isobutyrate
E-445	Glycerol esters of wood rosins

Cellulose and derivatives
E-460	(i) Microcrystalline cellulose, (ii) powdered cellulose
E-461	Methyl cellulose
E-463	Hydroxypropyl cellulose
E-464	Hydroxypropylmethyl cellulose
E-465	Ethylmethyl cellulose
E-466	Carboxymethylcellulose, sodium carboxymethylcellulose

Table 6 (*continued*)

Emulsifiers and stabilisers	*Used to enable oils and fats to mix with water, to give a smooth and creamy texture to food, and slow the staling of baked goods. Many of these compounds are also used to make jellies.*

Salts or esters of fatty acids

E-470a	Sodium, potassium and calcium salts of fatty acids
E-470b	Magnesium salts of fatty acids
E-471	Mono- and diglycerides of fatty acids
E-472a	Acetic acid esters of mono- and diglycerides of fatty acids
E-472b	Lactic acid esters of mono- and diglycerides of fatty acids
E-472c	Citric acid esters of mono- and diglycerides of fatty acids
E-472d	Tartaric acid esters of mono- and diglycerides of fatty acids
E-472e	Mono- and diacetyl tartaric esters of mono- and diglycerides of fatty acids
E-472f	Mixed acetic and tartaric acid esters of mono- and diglycerides of fatty acids
E-473	Sucrose esters of fatty acids
E-474	Sucroglycerides
E-475	Polyglycerol esters of fatty acids
E-476	Polyglycerol esters of polycondensed esters of castor oil (polyglycerol polyricinoleate)
E-477	Propane-1,2-diol esters of fatty acids
E-478	Lactylated fatty acid esters of glycerol and propane-1,2-diol
E-479b	Thermally oxidized soya bean oil interacted with mono- and diglycerides of fatty acids
E-481	Sodium stearoyl-2-lactylate
E-482	Calcium stearoyl-2-lactylate
E-483	Stearyl tartrate
E-491	Sorbitan monostearate
E-492	Sorbitan tristearate
E-493	Sorbitan monolaurate
E-494	Sorbitan mono-oleate
E-495	Sorbitan monopalmitate
E-1518	Glyceryl triacetate (triacetin)

Acids and salts used for special purposes	*Buffers, emulsifying salts, sequestrants, stabilisers, raising agents, anti-caking agents*

Carbonates

E-500	(i) Sodium carbonate, (ii) sodium bicarbonate (sodium hydrogen carbonate), (iii) sodium sesquicarbonate
E-501	(i) Potassium carbonate, (ii) potassium bicarbonate (potassium hydrogen carbonate)
E-503	(i) Ammonium carbonate, (ii) ammonium hydrogen carbonate

Table 6 (*continued*)

Acids and salts used for special purposes	Buffers, emulsifying salts, sequestrants, stabilisers, raising agents, anti-caking agents
E-504	(i) Magnesium carbonate, (ii) magnesium hydrogen carbonate (magnesium hydroxide carbonate)

Hydrochloric acid and its salts
E-507	Hydrochloric acid (ordinary salt is sodium chloride)
E-508	Potassium chloride (sometimes used as a replacement for ordinary salt)
E-509	Calcium chloride
E-510	Ammonium chloride
E-511	Magnesium chloride
E-512	Stannous chloride

Sulphuric acid and its salts
E-513	Sulphuric acid
E-514	(i) Sodium sulphate, (ii) sodium hydrogen sulphate
E-515	(i) Potassium sulphate, (ii) potassium hydrogen sulphate
E-516	Calcium sulphate
E-517	Ammonium sulphate
E-518	Magnesium sulphate
E-520	Aluminium sulphate
E-521	Aluminium sodium sulphate
E-522	Aluminium potassium sulphate
E-523	Aluminium ammonium sulphate

Alkalis	Used as bases to neutralise acids in foods
E-524	Sodium hydroxide
E-525	Potassium hydroxide
E-526	Calcium hydroxide
E-527	Ammonium hydroxide
E-528	Magnesium hydroxide
E-529	Calcium oxide
E-530	Magnesium oxide

Other salts
E-535	Sodium ferrocyanide
E-536	Potassium ferrocyanide
E-538	Calcium ferrocyanide
E-540	Dicalcium diphosphate
E-541	Sodium aluminium phosphate, acidic

Compounds used as anticaking agents, and other uses

E-542	Edible bone phosphate (bone meal)
E-544	Calcium polyphosphates
E-545	Ammonium polyphosphates

460

Table 6 (*continued*)

Compounds used as anticaking agents, and other uses

Silicon salts
E-551	Silicon dioxide (silica, sand)
E-552	Calcium silicate
E-553a	(i) Magnesium silicate, (ii) magnesium trisilicate
E-553b	talc
E-554	Sodium aluminium silicate
E-555	Potassium aluminium silicate
E-556	Calcium aluminium silicate

Other compounds
E-558	Bentonite
E-559	Kaolin (aluminium silicate)
E-570	Fatty acids
E-572	Magnesium stearate
E-574	Gluconic acid
E-575	Glucono-δ-lactone
E-576	Sodium gluconate
E-577	Potassium gluconate
E-578	Calcium gluconate
E-579	Ferrous gluconate
E-585	Ferrous lactate

Compounds used as flavour enhancers

E-620	L-Glutamic acid (a natural amino acid)
E-621	Monosodium glutamate (MSG)
E-622	Monopotassium glutamate
E-623	Calcium diglutamate
E-624	Monoammonium glutamate
E-625	Magnesium diglutamate
E-626	Guanylic acid
E-627	Disodium guanylate
E-628	Dipotassium guanylate
E-629	Calcium guanylate
E-630	Inosinic acid
E-631	Disodium inosinate
E-632	Dipotassium inosinate
E-633	Calcium inosinate
E-634	Calcium 5'-ribonucleotides
E-635	Disodium 5-ribonucleotides
E-636	Maltol
E-637	Ethyl maltol
E-640	Glycine and its sodium salt (a natural amino acid)
E-900	Dimethylpolysiloxane

Table 6 (*continued*)

Compounds used as glazing agents

E-901	Beeswax
E-902	Candelilla wax
E-903	Carnauba wax
E-904	Shellac
E-912	Montan acid esters
E-914	Oxidized polyethylene wax

Compounds used to treat flour

E-920	L-Cysteine hydrochloride (a natural amino acid)
924	Potassium bromate
925	Chlorine
926	Chlorine dioxide
927	Azodicarbamide

Propellant gases

E-938	Argon
E-939	Helium
E-941	Nitrogen
E-942	Nitrous oxide
E-948	Oxygen

Sweeteners and sugar alcohols

E-420	(i) Sorbitol, (ii) sorbitol syrup
E-421	Mannitol
E-422	Glycerol
E-927a	Azodicarbonamide
E-927b	Carbamide
E-950	Acesulfame K
E-951	Aspartame
E-952	Cyclamic acid and its sodium and calcium salts
E-953	Isomalt
E-954	Saccharine and its sodium, potassium and calcium salts
E-957	Thaumatin
E-959	Neohesperidin didihydrochalcone
E-965	(i) Maltitol, (ii) maltitol syrup
E-966	Lactitol
E-967	Xylitol

Table 6 (*continued*)

Miscellaneous compounds

E-999	Quillaia extract
E-1105	Lysozyme
E-1200	Polydextrose
E-1201	Polyvinyl pyrrolidone
E-1202	Polyvinyl polypyrrolidone
E-1505	Triethyl citrate
E-1518	Glyceryl triacetate (triacetin)

Modified starches

E-1404	Oxidised starch
E-1410	Monostarch phosphate
E-1412	Distarch phosphate
E-1413	Phosphated distarch phosphate
E-1414	Acetylated distarch phosphate
E-1420	Acetylated starch
E-1422	Acetylated starch adipate
E-1440	Hydroxypropyl starch
E-1442	Hydroxypropyl distarch phosphate
E-1450	Starch sodium octanoyl succinate

Table 7 Nomenclature of fatty acids

Trivial name	Systematic name	Shorthand code
Acetic	ethanoic	C2:0
Propionic	propanoic	C3:0
Butyric	butanoic	C4:0
Caproic	hexanoic	C6:0
Caprylic	octanoic	C8:0
Capric	decanoic	C10:0
Lauric	dodecanoic	C12:0
Myristic	tetradecanoic	C14:0
Palmitic	hexadecanoic	C16:0
Stearic	octadecanoic	C18:0
Arachidic	eicosanoic	C20:0
Behenic	docosanoic	C22:0
Lignoceric	tetracosanoic	C24:0
Palmitoleic	9-hexadecenoic	C16:1 ω6
Oleic	9-octadecenoic	C18:1 ω9
Elaidic	trans-9-octadecenoic	trans-C18:1 ω9
Vaccenic	11-octadecenoic	C18:1 ω9
Petroselinic	6-octadecenoic	C18:1 ω6
Gadoleic	9-eicosaenoic	C20:1 ω9
Erucic	13-docosenoic	C22:1 ω9
Brassidic	trans-13-docosenoic	trans-C22:1 ω9
Cetoleic	11-docosenoic	C22:1 ω11
Nervonic	15-tetracosenoic	C24:1 ω9
α-Linolenic	9,12,15-octadecatrienoic	C18:3 ω3
Parinaric	9,11,13,15-octadecatetraenoic	C18:4 ω3
Eicosapentaenoic (timnodonic)	5,8,11,14,17-eicosapentaenoic	C20:5 ω3
Docosapentaenoic (clupanodonic)	7,10,13,16,19-docosapentaenoic	C22:5 ω3
Docosahexaenoic (cervonic)	4,7,10,13,16,19-docosahexaenoic	C22:6 ω3
Linoleic	9,12-octadecadienoic	C18:2 ω6
γ-Linolenic	6,9,12-octadecatrienoic	C18:3 ω6
α-Eleostearic	9,11 trans,13, trans-octadecatrienoic	trans-C18:3 ω6
Dihomo-γ-linolenic	8,11,14-eicosatrienoic	C20:3 ω6
Arachidonic	5,8,11,14-eicosatetraenoic	C20:4 ω6
Docosatetraenoic (adrenic)	7,10,13,16-docosatetraenoic	C22:4 ω6
Docosapentaenoic	4,7,10,13,16-docosapentaenoic	C22:5 ω6
Mead	5,8,11-eicosatricnoic	C20:3 ω9